NURSES and
FAMILY HEALTH
PROMOTION
Concepts, Assessment, and Interventions

D0817416

NURSES and FAMILY HEALTH PROMOTION
Concepts, Assessment, and Interventions

2nd Edition

Perri J. Bomar, PhD, RN

Professor, Parent-Child Nursing Department
School of Nursing
East Carolina University
Greenville, North Carolina

W.B. SAUNDERS COMPANY
A Division of Harcourt Brace & Company
Philadelphia London Toronto Montreal Sydney Tokyo

W. B. SAUNDERS COMPANY

A Division of Harcourt Brace & Company

The Curtis Center
Independence Square West
Philadelphia, Pennsylvania 19106

Library of Congress Cataloging in Publication Data

Nurses and family health promotion / [edited by] Perri J. Bomar. —
    2nd ed.
        p. cm.
    Includes bibliographical references.
    ISBN 0-7216-3795-7
    1. Family nursing. 2. Health promotion. 3. Family—Health and
hygiene. I. Bomar, Perri J.
    [DNLM: 1. Nursing Process. 2. Family. 3. Family Health.
4. Health Promotion—nurses' instruction. WY 100 N97416 1996]
RT120.F34N874 1996
613—dc20
DNLM/DLC
                                                                95-19486

NURSES AND FAMILY HEALTH PROMOTION   ISBN 0-7216-3795-7

Printed in United States of America.

Last digit is the print number: 9   8   7   6   5   4   3   2   1

This second edition is lovingly dedicated to my husband, Guy,
who helped in many ways,
sacrificed countless hours of our couple time,
and who, with God, was the wind under my wings
during the writing and editing of this second edition
and my entire career.

FOREWORD

The immense popularity of Perri Bomar's first edition of *Nurses and Family Health Promotion: Concepts, Assessment, and Interventions* spoke to the need for a comprehensive text dealing with the many aspects of family health nursing from the perspective of health promotion. In this second edition, her contributors have updated their chapters with the most recent research in their respective areas. Dr. Bomar has added two new chapters, "Family Spirituality," and "Social Political Environment and Family Health Promotion," both topics which are currently on the front burner in the debate regarding how values drive our national agenda.

The current national focus on health care reform reflects the need for a book of this scope and quality. Nurses long have been promoting and providing high quality, comprehensive, cost effective *health* care for all of our many publics. After years of sporadic concern, there now is widespread agreement that stabilization of the American family is of crucial importance to the survival of this country and the values for which it stands. This is an exciting time for nurses. Nurses have been concerned with promoting healthy life styles with the goal of preventing illness for a long time. The public finally has had enough rampant individualism—coming to realize that this nation can no longer afford a costly, mismanaged, and ineffective health care system that is illness-oriented and also leaves the health needs of a very large proportion of the population covered inadequately.

Just as the first edition of *Nurses and Family Health Promotion* met the needs for both clinicians and students in nursing, the second edition makes a very timely and vital contribution to the understanding and solution of our current crisis in health care. It dovetails nicely with *Nursing's Agenda for Health Care Reform,* which emphasizes increased access and higher quality health care for broad segments of the population through primary health care delivery that emphasizes disease prevention and health promotion. The book is also an excellent fit with the position statement of the American Association of Colleges of Nursing, Nursing Education's Agenda for the 21st Century, which delineates a new role for nursing education and strategies for preparing nurses to carry out this role. Dr. Bomar and her colleagues are to be complimented for their contribution to the understanding of the importance of the family unit in the promotion of health.

Janet A. Rodgers, PhD, RN, FAAN
Dean and Professor
Philip Y. Hahn School of Nursing
University of San Diego
San Diego, California

PREFACE

The first edition of *Nurses and Family Health Promotion: Concepts, Assessment, and Interventions* was written for two reasons. First, it was a response to my frustration with teaching family nursing (with an emphasis on family health promotion) without adequate sources and assessment instruments. Second, it was generated in answer to my graduate students' questions, "Why isn't there a book on family health promotion?" and "Are there any instruments to assess family health promotion?" The second edition of this book (1) continues to respond to the void that my students and teaching colleagues noted, (2) provides selected assessment tools relevant to family health promotion and protection, and (3) supplies a resource for undergraduate and graduate students as well as clinicians practicing in the area of family health promotion.

As consumers recognize the need for self-management beliefs and behaviors that will improve the quality of their health, health professionals will need a greater understanding of how the family unit influences the level of health promotion and protection for individuals. The family experience of health occurs in an ever-changing social, economic, cultural, and political climate. Subsequently, individuals and families are encouraged to be more knowledgeable about their health, assume more self-responsibility that will promote health, maintain wellness, and prevent disease.

Although the current health care economy supports disease-related care more than wellness care, there is a national, state, and regional trend toward creating health policies that support health promotion. The beginning of federal support for health promotion began with the historic federal document *Healthy People: The Surgeon General's Report on Health Promotion and Disease Prevention* (1979). This report emphasized the need for family and individual health promotion and protection. The follow-up report, *Health of the Nation 2000* (1990), sets forth 22 objectives for national health promotion and disease prevention. The report reflects a concern for the promotion of health within individuals, families, and communities. The objectives are to be attained in the 21st century. Most of them cannot be attained without the participation of health professionals in collaboration with families. Health promotion for individuals, families, and communities will be a major component of the health care agenda in the next decade; therefore, it is crucial that nurses have texts that provide information on understanding family processes and family assessment and intervention to help them enhance the well-being of their clients.

Although families will be more diverse in the 21st century, the major roles of family health clinicians will be: (1) *competence* in providing holistic care to families and individuals in a family context; (2) *commitment* to efforts to strengthen families in adapting to life transitions and situations; (3) *collaboration/empowerment* of family units by providing families with the knowledge, skills, and resources necessary for health promotion and protection; and (4) *communication* with families through interviewing, assessment, and interaction to provide culturally sensitive care (Durand, 1993).

Currently there are not sufficient resources that address family health from the perspective of health promotion and protection. The purpose of this book, then, is to (1) describe the development of family health nursing; (2) provide nurses with selected theories, frameworks, and concepts that will assist in understanding family dynamics and their relationship to family health promotion; (3) supply a text on health promotion and health protection that will aid nurses in helping families promote, attain, and regain health; and (4) provide guidelines and family measurement tools for assessing, contracting, and collaborating with families in their efforts to attain higher levels of health.

The first edition of this text was an initial effort to compile the writings of family nurse scholars on the topic of family health promotion in one text. The current thrust on health promotion and disease prevention for the remainder of this decade and the 21st century creates a need for family nurses to focus on all the realms of the family health experience. A crucial aspect of family health that has not received attention from nurses is health promotion of the family unit. This text is written in an effort to provide a resource for nurses to empower families toward higher levels of wellness in a changing health care climate.

The author recognizes that the area of family health promotion is broad, fuzzy, and inconsistent in definition. This book is written to provide an overview of selected topics, and highlight classic and/or recent references.

Unit I (Chapters 1-3) provides a foundation for understanding the emerging specialty of family nursing with a focus on family health promotion. Chapter 1 introduces family health nursing, traces its origins, discusses contemporary influences, and projects the future of the specialty. Family health nursing shares many of the characteristics of other nursing specialties; however, it is distinctly different because of the theoretical basis of family and its focus on the family unit's health promotion and protection, separate from individual health. In Chapter 2, Carol Loveland-Cherry presents a revised theoretical framework of family health promotion. Chapter 3 presents a historical overview of the contemporary American family.

Unit II (Chapters 3-11) provides an overview of both theories and concepts, thus enhancing the understanding of family processes. Theories and concepts reviewed include system, culture and ethnicity, communication, family roles, family self-care, family stress, and social support. A new chapter in the second edition is Chapter 11, Family Spirituality. In order to facilitate data collection about family health in each of these areas, an assessment tool or literature review of family measures is included in each chapter.

Each chapter in Unit III (Chapters 12-21) uses the nursing process to discuss family health promotion and protection in such areas as nutrition, stress management, sleep, recreation, sexuality, protective health behaviors, and environmental health. Each chapter includes an assessment instrument specific to that topic. Chapter 12 discusses the nursing process and family health assessment based on Neuman's Systems Model. Berkey and Hanson's Family Strengths and Stressors Inventories are revised in Chapter 12. An overview of the impact of family transitions on family health is discussed in Chapter 20, Family

Health Promotion During Transitions. Specific transitions reviewed include addition of family members, remarriage, loss of family members, unemployment of providers, single parenthood, effects of retirement, and the stress of grief and loss. The final chapter, Chapter 21, Social Political Environment and Family Health Promotion, is new to this edition. It addresses current issues in family policy, the impact of these policies on family health, and the role of the family nurse in health and family policy.

The concept of family health nursing emerged in the late 1970s. Family health nurses are those with graduate education in the specialty of family health nursing. The primary focus of their practice has been the well and worried-well families. The goal was to improve the quality of family health in an ever-changing and complex society. However, more recently, family nurse scholars agree that family nurses provide nursing care to families experiencing illness, transitions, and crises. Throughout the book, the terms *family nurse, nurse,* and *family health nurse* are used interchangeably. In addition, *client* and *family* are used interchangeably by different authors to express the same meaning.

Because the emphasis on family health promotion is a recent development, there is lack of consensus in defining it. Each contributing author was asked to address his or her topic using family and family health promotion as a framework. The following definitions were incorporated throughout the book. A **family** is a group of individuals closely related by blood, marriage, or friendship ties with a common goal or purpose. **Family health** is the family's quality of life from a holistic perspective as it is affected by such variables as spirituality, nutrition, stress, environment, recreation and exercise, sleep, and sexuality. **Family health promotion** is the family behaviors that are undertaken to increase the family's well-being or quality of life.

Because family health promotion is a relatively recent area of study, some contributors experienced difficulty in locating references on their topic. Inevitably, the text will stimulate new ideas for research and, as a result, will further the knowledge-base for family health nursing.

The intended readers of this book are undergraduate nursing students working with well families, graduate students in family health nursing, and clinicians whose goals include empowerment of families in any setting to attain, regain, or maintain a health promotion and health protection family lifestyle.

Perri J. Bomar

REFERENCES

Durand, B.A. (1993). Preface. In Feetham, S.L., Meister, S.B., Bell, J.M., Gillis, C.L. (Eds.) *The nursing of families; Theories, research, education, and practice.* Newbury Park, CA: Sage.

ACKNOWLEDGMENTS

The revision of this second edition is the result of two years of fruitful labor and struggle. Many people—individuals, colleagues, friends, families, students, and organizations—contributed both knowingly and unknowingly to the completion of this second edition.

As with any major project that requires considerable energy, time, and concentration, the writing and editing of this book permeated all aspects of my personal and professional life. The many hours at the computer and reading and editing three drafts were made possible by the cooperation, patience, and sacrifice of my friend and husband, Guy. He was there to read proofs, pray with me, and share exhilarating moments and disappointments. I am deeply indebted to my extended family (particularly my grandsons, Derek and Dustin) who continued their support despite the infrequency of my visits, calls, and letters during this project. A sincere thanks to my dear friends who sustained our friendships during this endeavor, although our times together were briefer than usual.

New friendships developed during this project and others were strengthened. I remain deeply indebted to Rev. Carmen Warner, friend, Christian sister, and colleague who has an incredible ability to inspire others. Carmen was instrumental in encouraging me to create the first edition and contributed the new chapter on Family Spirituality for this edition. I am deeply indebted to friends and colleagues such as Shirley Hanson and Kathryn Anderson who encouraged me to revise and continue the second edition of this text.

I am extremely appreciative for the contributing authors who remained committed to this project. A special thank you to new contributors Evelyn Anderson, Sherry Cooper, Rosemary Goodyear, Kathleen Groves, Kathleen Heinrich, and Carmen Warner. My indebtedness continues to Lillian DeYoung, former dean and professor of the University of Akron School of Nursing, and to former colleagues and family health nursing faculty, Ella Kick, Patricia Putnam Godfrey, JoAnne Marchione, and Delores Vandervort. Together we defined family health nursing and family health promotion as we developed one of the early graduate curriculums in family health nursing in the United States.

I appreciate students and faculty both around the country and internationally who read the first edition, believed in the importance of family health promotion, and inquired about the second edition. Special thanks to graduates who have taken the concept of family health promotion, developed innovative family nursing practices, and have shared information on their implementation with me. Also, special thanks to former graduate assistants Gloria Reed and Ana-Marie Gallo for their valuable assistance in literature review and other details.

A special thank you to my friend and colleague, Janet Rodgers, dean and professor of the University of San Diego School of Nursing for her support. I am also indebted to the faculty of the University of San Diego School of Nursing for being supportive listeners and remaining supportive through both the first and second editions. Also, the contributions of the University of San Diego (a grant for literature review and provision of graduate assistants) are acknowledged and appreciated.

I am indebted to the fine editorial staff at W.B. Saunders for fostering the quality production for this book. Special thanks to Ilze Rader, Senior Editor of Nursing Books, for belief in the continuing value of this book, and the encouragement to begin a second edition. The prompt response to my questions and requests by Marie Thomas, editorial assistant, is greatly appreciated. Lastly, a special thank you is expressed to Marty Tenney of Textbook Writers Associates and her staff for their invaluable editorial talents that contributed to making this book more readable and visually appealing.

Although I am new to the East Carolina University (ECU) School of Nursing, I want to express appreciation to Dr. Phyllis Horns, Dean; Dr. Jo Ann Neff, Chair of Parent-Child Nursing; and Dr. Dixie Koldjeski, Associate Dean for Research and Evaluation for their support of my scholarly endeavors as I simultaneously completed the last stages of this edition. Special thanks to the faculty and students at East Carolina Nursing who believe that families are important to the care of the individual and encourage my continued interest in family health promotion.

Perri J. Bomar

CONTRIBUTORS

Evelyn Anderson, PhD, RN
CoCoordinator of Menopause Clinic
Assistant Clinical Professor
Department of Reproductive Medicine
University of California
San Diego, California
Lecturer, University of San Diego
University of Phoenix at San Diego
Philip Y. Hahn School of Nursing
San Diego, California

Chapter 6: Family Roles

Perri J. Bomar, PhD, RN
Professor
Parent-Child Nursing Department
School of Nursing
East Carolina University
Greenville, North Carolina

*Chapter 1: Family Health Nursing Role: Past,
Present, and Future*
Chapter 10: Family Stress

Barbara A. Casey, MSN, RN
Clinical Specialist, Adult Psych-Mental Health
Nursing
Program Coordinator, Mood Disorders Clinic
VA Medical Center
San Diego, California

Chapter 4: The Family as a System

Sherry Cooper, MSN, RN, FNP
Family Nurse Practitioner
Child/Adolescent Psychiatry
University of California at San Diego Medical
Center
San Diego, California

Chapter 10: Family Stress

Gretchen Dimico, PhD, RN, IBCLC
Associate Professor
Lewis-Clark State College
Coeur d'Alene, Idaho

Chapter 14: Family Stress Management

V. Ruth Gray, EdD, RN
Professor and Dean
The University of Akron
College of Nursing
Akron, Ohio

Chapter 7: Family Self-Care

Rosemary Goodyear, EdD, RN
Professor of Nursing
Coordinator MS Program
Director, C.A.R.E.S.
Texas Woman's University
Denton, Texas

*Chapter 21: Social Political Environment and
Family Health Promotion*

Kathleen A. Grove, PhD
Department of Sociology
University of San Diego,
San Diego, California

*Chapter 3: The American Family: History and
Development*

**Shirley M. H. Hanson, PMHNP, PhD, RN,
FAAN, LMFT, CFLE**
Licensed Marriage and Family Therapist
Professor, School of Nursing
Oregon Health Science University
Portland, Oregon

*Chapter 12: Family Health Assessment and
Intervention*

Kathleen Heinrich, PhD, RN
Adjunct Professor
University of Hartford
West Hartford, Connecticut

Chapter 17: Family Sexuality

Jeanne Hoffer, EdD, RN
Graduate Nursing Education Consultant and
Professor
St. Francis College
Fort Wayne, Indiana

Chapter 8: Family Communication

Kathy Shadle James, DNSC, RN
Lecturer, School of Nursing
University of San Diego
San Diego, California
Statewide Nursing Program
Carson, California

Chapter 13: Family Nutrition and Weight Control

Ella Kick, PhD, RN
Professor and Dean
Ashland University School of Nursing
Ashland, Ohio

Chapter 15: Sleep and the Family

John M. Lantz, PhD, RN
Interim Associate Dean for Academic Programs
University of San Francisco
San Francisco, California

Chapter 5: Family Culture and Ethnicity

Carol J. Loveland-Cherry, PhD, RN
Associate Professor and Director
Division of Health Promotion and Risk
  Reduction Programs
The University of Michigan
School of Nursing
Ann Arbor, Michigan

*Chapter 2: Family Health Promotion and
  Health Protection*

Darlene E. McCown, PhD, RN, FNPC, PNP
Family Nurse Practitioner
Associate Professor
St. John Fisher College
Rochester, New York

Chapter 16: Family Recreation and Exercise

A. Gretchen McNeely, DNSc, RNC
Assistant Professor and Assistant Dean
Montana State University
College of Nursing
Bozeman, Montana

*Chapter 1: Family Health Nursing Role: Past,
  Present, and Future*

Anne Roe Mealey, PhD, ARNP
Professor
Intercollegiate Center for Nursing Education
Spokane, Washington

Chapter 14: Family Stress Management

Karen B. Mischke, WHCNI, PhD, RN, CFLE
Independent Practitioner
Beaverton, Oregon

*Chapter 12: Family Health Assessment and
  Intervention*

Haroldyne Scott Richardson, MN, ARNP, CS
Faculty (Retired)
Intercollegiate Center for Nursing Education
Spokane, Washington
Advance Registered Nurse Practitioner
Clinical Nurse Specialist in Psychiatric and
  Mental Health Nursing
Psychotherapist and Consultant
Spokane, Washington

Chapter 14: Family Stress Management

Patricia Roth, EdD, RN
Professor of Nursing
University of San Diego
Phillip Y. Hahn School of Nursing
San Diego, California

Chapter 9: Family Social Support
*Chapter 20: Family Health Promotion During
  Transitions*

Karen K. Szafran, MSN, RN
Assistant Professor
Catholic University of America
School of Nursing
Washington, DC

Chapter 18: Family Health Protective Behaviors

Rev. Carmen Germaine Warner, MSN, RN, FAAN
Chaplain, Vista Jail
Chaplain, Donovan State Prison
San Diego California
Minister, Milagro Ministry
Tijuana, Mexico
Publishing Consultant
Mercy Hospital and Medical Center
VA Medical Center
Leucadia, California

Chapter 11: Family Spirituality

Dorothy J. D. Wiley, PhD, RN
Epidemiologist
Los Angeles County Department of Health
  Services
Los Angeles, California

Chapter 19: Family Environmental Health

CONTENTS

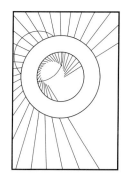

UNIT I

Introduction to Family Health Nursing and Family Health Promotion

FAMILY HEALTH NURSING ROLE: PAST, PRESENT, AND FUTURE

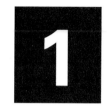

PERRI J. BOMAR and GRETCHEN MCNEELY

Nursing's goal is to facilitate the health of the family . . . facilitating the development of an increased range of responses of family members to each other and to the world outside the family.

MARGARET A. NEWMAN

OBJECTIVES

On completion of this chapter, the reader will be able to:

1. Describe the specialty of family health nursing.
2. Trace the historical development of family health nursing as a specialty.
3. Discuss factors that have influenced the evolution of family health nursing.
4. List a variety of settings for family health nursing practice that focuses on health promotion and health protection.
5. Identify characteristics of family health nursing practice.
6. Examine trends that will affect the future practice of family health nursing.

This book focuses on family health nursing and strategies to promote family health. Although families have been the concern of nursing care for centuries, family health nursing as we know it today emerged in the 1970s when nurses began to consider health promotion, in addition to illness care, as a legitimate concern for the nursing profession. Therefore, since the family is the environment where health promotion is taught, provided, carried out, supported, or undermined, it is crucial for nurses to understand their role in empowering families, both individual members and as a unit, to reach their highest potential in health promotion. This chapter will acquaint the reader with definitions of family health nursing, the historical evolution of family health nursing, factors influencing its evolution, characteristics of family health nursing practice and the potential impact of future societal trends on this specialty.

DEFINING FAMILY HEALTH NURSING

Until recently, nurses who focused on families as the unit of care used a variety of titles that included "family" or "health," but only since the 1970s has the title "Family Health Nurse" emerged. Initially, nursing care involving families was called family-centered care (Cunningham, 1978);

The authors want to express appreciation to Irene S. Palmer, RN, PhD, FAAN for her contributions in writing this chapter for the first edition. Dr. Palmer is former Dean and Professor Emeritus at the University of San Diego School of Nursing, a nurse historian, and a Florence Nightingale scholar.

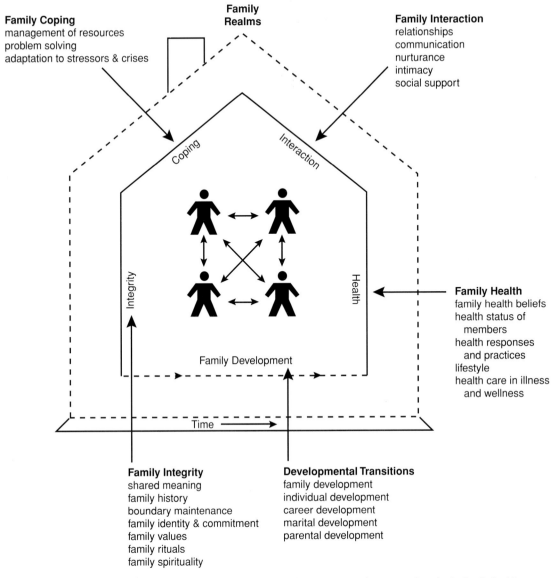

Family Coping
management of resources
problem solving
adaptation to stressors & crises

Family Realms

Family Interaction
relationships
communication
nurturance
intimacy
social support

Coping

Interaction

Integrity

Health

Family Development

Time

Family Health
family health beliefs
health status of
    members
health responses
    and practices
lifestyle
health care in illness
    and wellness

Family Integrity
shared meaning
family history
boundary maintenance
family identity & commitment
family values
family rituals
family spirituality

Developmental Transitions
family development
individual development
career development
marital development
parental development

FIGURE 1–1. Realms of Family Health Nursing Practice. (Data from Anderson K.K., Tomlinson P.S., (1992). The family health system: An emerging paradigmatic view for nursing. *Image,* 24(1), 57–63.)

family-focused care (Janosik & Miller, 1980); or family nursing (Friedman, 1992). The specialty has its roots in the specialties of maternal child nursing, community nursing, and psychiatric mental health nursing, and in the family nurse practitioner. There is controversy and ambiguity regarding the focus, education, and clients of the family health nurse. Questions often asked include "Is family health nursing synonymous with community health nursing or psychiatric nursing?" "Is it a distinct specialty?" Although it overlaps with other specialties, family health nursing is a distinct specialty that still is in its infancy. In other words, the specialty of family health nursing is both old and new and incorporates theories, concepts, and

interventions from past nursing specialties while building on the new areas such as family science and health promotion.

This new (revived) specialty has a cadre of nursing scholars who have authored textbooks, organized national and international family nursing conferences, conducted research on issues of families in sickness and wellness across the life span, and published numerous articles on family nursing and research. And in February 1995 the inaugural issue of the *Journal of Family Nursing* was published (Bell, 1995).

Based on Schlotfeldt's (1987) definition of nursing, family health nursing is defined here as the assessment and enhancement of family health

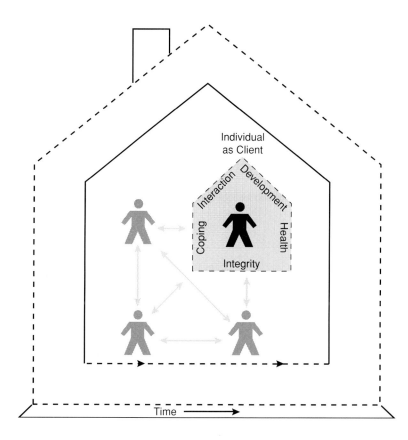

FIGURE 1–2. Individual as Client in the Family Context.

status, family health assets, and family potentials. Assessment of families includes systematic appraisal of the family processes of development, interaction, coping, integrity, and family health (Anderson & Tomlinson, 1992; see Fig. 1–1). The literature suggests that the client of the family nurse may be the individual as client in the family context; the family interactional system of dyads, triads, or other groupings; the entire family unit as a system; or family aggregates (groups) (Friedemann, 1989; Wright, & Leahey, 1994; Swanson & Albrecht, 1993).

INDIVIDUAL AS CLIENT. In the past, health care was provided to the individual, with limited focus on the family unit. In this type of nursing, the individual is the primary focus (Fig. 1–2), and the family system is the background or context (Friedemann, 1989; Wright & Leahey, 1990). The primary focus is on the health status of each member of the family (e.g., recovery from illness, change in diet or exercise, or preventative health practices). In the past, family was of interest primarily because of its role in caregiving. However, in order to provide competent care to an individual, the nurse needs to assess family variables that may affect the individual's health status and the outcome of interventions. For example, if the goal is to lower dietary fat in one family member, attaining and maintaining this change will be difficult unless family environment, nutrition, re-

sources, and internal social support are considered. Family members continually interact with each other and self-care decisions are subtly influenced by the family. There will be a need to coordinate family grocery shopping and meal preparation and obtain social support if the individual is to succeed in making this change in lifestyle permanent.

INTERPERSONAL FAMILY NURSING. As depicted in Figure 1–3, the focus of family nursing assessment and enhancement is on family interactions (e.g., parenting, communication, decision making, limit setting, and negotiation of family roles) between family dyads, triads, and larger groupings (Anderson, & Tomlinson, 1992; Wright & Leahey, 1994). This type of family nursing is also called *family systems nursing* by Wright and Leahey (1990, 1994). To illustrate, when a family system experiences continuing spousal conflict other aspects of family life are affected. Nursing intervention would focus on resolution of the conflict with the dyad while recognizing the import of family data and processes that will influence the outcome. If the issue is lack of couple time and sexual intimacy, contributing factors from the family system may be household upkeep and child care responsibilities that cause fatigue and take up time. In this example, although the problem is dyadic and interactive in nature, a healthy resolution will involve changes in the family system. The

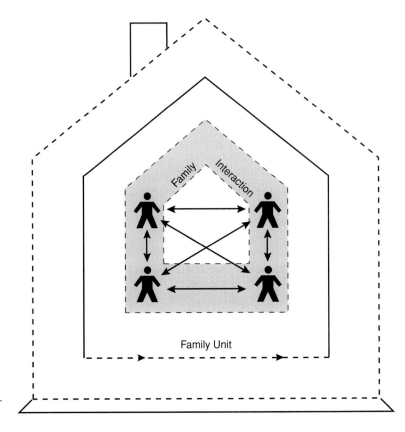

FIGURE 1-3. Family Systems Nursing (Interpersonal Family Nursing).

nurse's role in this type of family nursing is to facilitate functional family interaction or to serve as the moderator as family members explore issues and problem solve as a unit.

FAMILY UNIT AS CLIENT. When the problem is a family systems issue, the entire family unit is the focus of holistic assessment and intervention (Fig. 1–4). The nurse assesses each of the five family processes and assumes a partnership with the family in decision making about interventions. For example, a change in the family system (e.g., chronic disease, a new family member, death of a family member) creates a need for family solutions through minor adjustments or adaptations in family patterns. In a family whose problem is lack of time together because they are a dual earner family, the nurse would assist the family in negotiating and implementing a plan to have routine family time.

FAMILY AGGREGATES. Some families share similar issues, and therefore issues can be dealt with at the group (aggregate) level. At the aggregate level, the family nurse provides assessment and intervention to groups of families. Examples of family nursing to family aggregates include leading support groups for mothers, helping single parent teenagers to continue their education, teaching parenting to couples, and providing health teaching to families who have members with chronic diseases such as Alzheimer's Disease, AIDS, dia-

betes, or cancer. Most family and community health nursing graduate programs focus on family aggregates.

Conceptualization of family nursing as previously discussed helps the family nurse to understand who the client is, and thus focus assessment and intervention appropriately. The skills and knowledge needed differ with each type of family nursing practice.

HISTORICAL FACTORS INFLUENCING THE DEVELOPMENT OF FAMILY HEALTH NURSING

It is crucial for family nurses to understand the historical legacy of this evolving specialty. Family health nursing has its roots in prehistoric times. The role of women has always been inextricably interwoven with the family, for it was the responsibility of women to care for family members who fell ill and to seek herbs or remedies. Also, in their housekeeping, women made an effort to provide an environment for the maintenance of health and wellness. Ham and Chamings (1983) have noted that "in the preindustrial era, the home and family were basic units of society, and . . . informal nursing was the work of women in general and encompassed the care of whole families" (p. 34). According to Ford (1979), "The concept of family

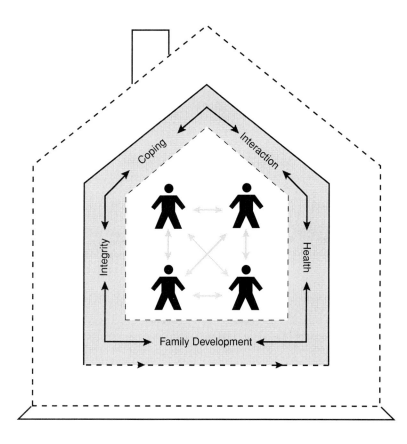

FIGURE 1–4. Family Unit as Client.

nursing has always been with us" (p. 88). Historical events that have affected the development of current family nursing practice are traced in the following discussion and depicted in Table 1–1.

The Nightingale Era

Florence Nightingale influenced both district nursing of the sick and poor and the work of "health missioners" through "health-at-home" teaching. The exorbitant mortality and morbidity of British troops during the Crimean War convinced Nightingale that British soldiers were subject more "to death in the barracks" than to death by bullets and bayonets. This confirmed for Nightingale the vital importance of improving the health of the British citizenry, the source of the British army. She realized that the health of the citizen was a paramount obligation of the mother of the family. Nightingale wrote: "Upon womanhood the national health, as far as the household goes, depends. . . . I know of no systematic teaching for the ordinary mother, how to keep the baby in health, certainly the most important function to make a healthy nation" (1893, p. 24). From this philosophical and practical perspective, she also promoted the concept that people should to be taught the laws of health and how to use them in order to improve their own condition.

In her book *Notes on Nursing: What It Is, and What It Is Not,* Nightingale (1859) admonished mothers not to say, "I am not a doctor. I must leave this to doctors" (p. 6). She referred to the fact that girls in her society were being taught such things as astronomy but not "those laws which God has assigned to the relations of our bodies with the world in which He has put them" (p. 7). She went on to say that those "laws of life" are not considered by mothers to be worthwhile to study in order "to give their children healthy existences. . . . They call it medical . . . knowledge, fit only for doctors" (p. 7). Nightingale realized that the high infant mortality rate in London was related to mothers' lack of knowledge regarding sanitation. She believed that the cleanliness or hygiene of the home could contribute greatly to eradication of the problem. The use of district nurses and health missioners was part of the plan to teach women how to keep their homes healthy and care for those who were ill (Ham & Chamings, 1983).

Nurses in Colonial America

Colonial women in America continued the century-old tradition of the female householder in nurturing and sustaining the wellness of the family and caring for those who became ill. "Nursing care" during the Revolutionary War was provided

TABLE 1–1. FACTORS CONTRIBUTING TO THE DEVELOPMENT OF FAMILY HEALTH AS A FOCUS IN NURSING

Pre-Nightingale era	Revolutionary War "camp followers"—example of family health focus prior to Nightingale
Mid-1800s	Nightingale influences district nurses and health missioners to maintain clean environment for patients' home and family
	Family members provide for soldiers' needs during Civil War through Ladies Aid Societies and Women's Central Association for Relief
Late 1800s	Industrial Revolution and immigration influence focus of public health nursing on prevention of illness, health education, and care of the sick for both families and communities
	Lillian Wald establishes Henry Street Visiting Nurse Service (1893)
	Focus on family during childbearing by maternal-child nurses and midwives
Early 1900s	School nursing established in New York City (1903)
	First White House Conference on Children (1909)
	Red Cross Town and Country Nursing Service (1912)
	Margaret Sanger opens first birth control clinic (1916)
	Family planning and quality care available for families
	Mary Breckinridge forms Frontier Nursing Service (1925)
	Nurses assigned to families
	Red Cross Public Health Nursing Service meets rural health needs following stock market crash (1929)
	Federal Emergency Relief Act passed (1933)
	Social Security Act passed (1935)
	Psychiatric/Mental Health begins family therapy focus (late 1930s)
1960s	Concept of family as a unit of care introduced into basic nursing curriculum
	NLN requires emphasis on families and communities in nursing curriculum
	Family-centered approach in maternal-child nursing and midwifery programs
	Nurse practitioner movement—programs to provide primary care to children (1965)
	Shift from public health nursing to community health nursing
	Family studies and research produce family theories
1970s	Changing health care system with focus on maintaining health and returning emphasis on family health
	Development and refinement of nursing conceptual models that consider the family as a unit of analysis or care (i.e., King, Newman, Orem, Rogers, and Roy)
	Many specialties focus on the family (e.g., hospice, oncology, geriatrics, school health, psychiatric/mental health, occupational health, and home health)
	Master's and doctoral programs focus on the family (e.g., Family Health Nursing, Community Health Nursing, Psychiatric/Mental Health and Family Counseling and Therapy)
	ANA Standards of Nursing Practice (1973)
	Surgeon General's Report (1979)
1980s	ANA Social Policy Statement (1980)
	White House Conference on Families
	Greater emphasis on health from very young to very old
	Increasing emphasis on obesity, stress, chemical dependency, and parenting skills
	Graduate level specialization with emphasis on primary care outside of acute care settings, health teaching, and client self-care
	Increased use of wellness and nursing models in providing care
	Promoting Health/Preventing Disease: Objectives for The Nation (1980) by U.S. Department of Health and Human Services
	Development of family science as a discipline
	Increased family nursing research
	National Center for Nursing Research founded with a Health Promotion and Prevention Research section
	First International Family Nursing Conference (1988)
1990s	*Healthy People 2000: National Health Promotion and Disease Prevention Objectives* (1990) by U.S. Department of Health and Human Services.
	Nursing's Agenda for Health Care Reform (ANA, 1991)
	Family Leave legislation (1991)
	Journal of Family Nursing (1995)

by women called "camp followers." These untrained "nurses" were often the wives of soldiers and performed a number of functions, such as providing comfort, cheer, encouragement, mending uniforms, darning socks, preparing meals, cleaning, and doing the laundry. Caring for the sick and wounded was done with the other duties. One camp follower who gained national recognition was Mary Ludwig Hays McCauley, who became known as "Molly Pitcher" because she carried water to thirsty soldiers in her husband's, John Hays, regiment (Selavan, 1975).

The Civil War (1861–1865)

With rumors of an imminent Civil War, American women prepared to care for ill and wounded soldiers. They organized Ladies' Aid Societies, known by various names and led by various women. The ladies met regularly to sew, prepare food, gather clothing, collect books, prepare medicines, and provide other items that might be needed by the soldiers (Kalisch & Kalisch, 1986; Matejski, 1986).

Among the leaders were Dr. Elizabeth Blackwell, who contributed to the New York Women's Central Association for Relief, and Dorothea Dix, who was named the Superintendent of Women Nurses of the Army. According to Matejski (1986), "Thousands of women whose husbands, sons, and brothers had volunteered for the Army reported for nursing duty" (p. 45). One hundred women received a month's training either at Bellevue Hospital or at New York Hospital to prepare them for nursing work. They were then assigned actual hospital and nursing duties in the Army. Others served without formal training. All of the women fed and bathed injured men and dressed their wounds. Other hospital duties entailed housekeeping, cleaning, and cooking.

The Industrial Revolution and Immigration

During the industrial revolution of the late 18th century, family members began to work outside the home instead of working on the family farm or in the family business. Men especially began to work in factories, leaving the running of the home and the care of children to women. During the late 19th century in the United States, the increase in immigration produced a population of families who needed the income of children for economic survival. This resulted in an increase in child labor and difficulty in keeping children in school and contributed to the increase in the spread of contagious diseases.

The beginning of public health nursing in the United States and the contributions of Lillian Wald, Lina Rogers, and others in the establishment of the Henry Street Visiting Nurse Service (1893) and school nursing (1903) were the result of the postindustrial environment. This was coupled with the influx of immigrants, particularly in New York City's Lower East Side. Wald established the Henry Street Settlement House in the immigrant slums in 1893 (Christy, 1970). "The public health nurses of the 19th century were involved in the beginning of the labor movement, concerned with the health of industrial workers, immigrants and their families, and the exploitation of women and children" (Heinrich, 1983, p. 318). Although the family and the community were the intended focus of public health nursing practice, the individual continued to receive primary attention. Maternal child nursing courses and the concepts of family care with specialized clinical experiences were incorporated into the basic nursing curriculum of training schools as an outgrowth of public health nursing and school nursing (Ford, 1979; Whaley & Wong, 1995).

Maternity Nursing and Midwifery

Maternity nursing, nurse midwifery, and community nursing also focused on the quality of family health. For example, Margaret Higgins Sanger Slee fought for family planning information to be made available to American women, particularly in the state of New York. She became aware of the contraceptive needs of poor women during her training at White Plains Hospital. Many women who could not afford to have more children asked the young nurse for contraceptive advice, which she felt inadequate to provide. Later, in the immigrant tenements in the Lower East Side of Manhattan, Margaret Sanger dealt with the horrors of botched illegal abortions that women had resorted to. Desperate families received limited practical family planning information from their physicians or clergy. To correct a social injustice, Sanger opened the first birth control clinic in the United States in 1916 (Forster, 1984; Ham & Chamings, 1983; Kalisch & Kalisch, 1986) and was pilloried for her efforts. Undaunted, she continued a lifelong fight for the rights of women.

Mary Breckinridge, another nurse, made her contribution to family health nursing by forming the Frontier Nursing Service to provide trained nurses to meet the health needs of the mountain families of Leslie County, Kentucky. Breckinridge's interest in the care of sick children developed when she worked as a volunteer in France, after World War I. In 1925, following her midwifery training in London, she returned to Wendover, Kentucky to serve the families of the community. Along with two other nurses, she practiced midwifery in Leslie County until her death in 1965 (Ham & Chamings, 1983; Kalisch & Kalisch, 1986; Pletsch, 1981). Her focus on maternity care contributed to the family-centered approach to nursing care.

Expansion of Public Health Nursing Services during the Depression

After the stock market crash of 1929, the health care needs of families in rural America were met primarily by the Red Cross Public Health Nursing Service. This was begun by Lillian Wald in 1912 as the Red Cross Town and Country Nursing Service. More nurses were needed in rural areas for public health work during the depression; however, those who had lost their jobs in the urban areas were not educationally prepared to be employed as rural nurses. This situation forced the nursing profession to reevaluate nursing education and to assist those who were willing to be reeducated for this new area of practice (Fitzpatrick, 1975).

Many federal programs that provided help for families, women, and children were established during the 1930s as a result of the depression. The Federal Emergency Relief Act (FERA), passed in 1933, provided for reimbursement of voluntary nursing agencies. In 1935, the Social Security Act provided for adequate public health services. Aid to crippled children and child health services was provided through Title V. Fitzpatrick (1975) summarized the period by stating that the "precedents set by government during the Great Depression and through the programs of the 'New Deal' changed the complexion of all that was to follow in health care and nursing services" (p. 2190).

The Nurse Practitioner Movement

Expansion of the nurse's role in well-child care and maternal-child nursing during the 1960s paved the way for the establishment of pediatric and family nurse practitioner programs later in the decade. Initially, nurse practitioners focused on primary care for families as a unit. Today, there are two types of nurse practitioners. The first type practice as physician extenders in a medical model practice. The second type use a nursing model practice focusing on individuals in the family context rather than solely on pathology. Education for nurse practitioners has progressed from continuing education programs to graduate preparation, with a heavy concentration on family theory and family nursing. Today, the practice of many practitioners is oriented toward health promotion, and they maintain an independent nursing role while collaborating interdependently with physicians in ambulatory settings. The definition of family nurse often is considered to be synonymous with the definition of nurse practitioner, but in fact they are different.

Psychiatric/Mental Health Nursing

Although family therapy had its roots in the work of Ackerman in the late 1930s, it was not until the 1970s that the family mental health nursing role with families began to emerge (Ham & Chamings, 1983). Ford (1979) notes that "early hospital discharge of the mentally ill forced public health nurses to examine their abilities to cope with family problems in this relocation effort and seek consultation from psychiatric nurse clinicians and others in the mental health field" (p. 91). The evolution of concepts such as family systems and family stress influenced the incorporation of the family as a unit of care into psychiatric nursing. As a result, educational programs in the 1960s and 1970s began to integrate psychiatric mental health nursing concepts into all aspects of the baccalaureate curriculum and to include the family as a major concept in graduate psychiatric mental health nursing curricula.

The Shift from Public Health Nursing to Community Health Nursing

In the 1960s there was a subtle shift from the term "public" health nursing to "community" health nursing, and to some authorities it was more than just a matter of semantics (Logan & Dawkins, 1986; Clements & Roberts, 1983). The shift increased the focus on community and family health. In fact, by the mid-1960s, a number of factors had emerged that would contribute to the creation of community health nursing as a specialty. These factors included recognition of the importance of community health nursing in nursing education, confusion about the role and responsibilities of the community health nurse, and changes in society and health care delivery (Spradley, 1985). "In 1966, the American Public Health Association and the National League for Nursing jointly launched a program for the accreditation of community health nursing services" (Tinkham et al., 1984, p. 86). By the 1970s, other factors such as the consumer movement, the women's movement, educational changes, and advanced technology contributed to the growth of this specialty (Spradley, 1985).

Archer (1982) described community health nursing as a "synthesis of public health science and nursing science" (p. 442). According to Spradley (1985), "The purpose of this synthesis is to improve the health of the entire community" (p. 59). Other characteristics of community health nursing seen as salient to the development of family health nursing are its focus on the family and community as the unit of concern, emphasis on health promotion and disease prevention, interdisciplinary collaboration, and client participation.

Impact of Family Studies and Family Research

Since the 1950s, over 20 disciplines have studied the family and through research have produced family assessment inventories and theoretical frameworks. These disciplines include sociology, psychology, family ecology, home economics, educational psychology, health education, behavioral health, preventive medicine, theology, and law. Nursing not only has used theories from these related fields but has developed some of its own theories and carried out its own research on the family as a unit of measurement. In the 1980s and 1990s, the interdisciplinary work has become known as "family science" and it is considered by some to be a distinct discipline with its own body of knowledge (Burr & Leigh, 1983). Building on the developments in family studies and family research, many graduate programs have been established in family science, family and community health nursing, and family health nursing (Hanson & Heims, 1992; Murphy, 1986).

THE 1990S

With the escalating costs of health care in the United States, a decreasing percentage of the population are able to obtain appropriate care at a price they can afford. Many proposals have been presented for reforming the health care system. Among them is *Nursing's Agenda for Health Care Reform* (ANA, 1991), endorsed by 62 nursing organizations as well as a number of non-nursing organizations. The plan proposes to assure "access, quality, and service at affordable costs." Nursing's plan calls for a restructured health care system that focuses on the health of consumers and offers services to consumers in familiar and convenient sites such as schools, workplaces, and the home. The goal is to facilitate consumer access to competently provided health care. The plan also calls for a shift from a focus on illness care and cure to wellness care. Vulnerable populations such as women and children are given priority in the plan as an investment in the future health and prosperity of the United States.

CONTEMPORARY FACTORS INFLUENCING THE DEVELOPMENT OF FAMILY HEALTH NURSING

Multiple changes continue to shape family health nursing. As shown in Figure 1–5, numerous factors affect this dynamic and revived specialty. An in-depth discussion of each of these factors is beyond the scope of this chapter; therefore only selected contributions from the nursing profession, related disciplines, service and professional organizations, and policy-making organizations are highlighted. Factors that have most significantly affected family health nursing are the following:

- Professionalization of nursing practice and nursing education
- Development of nursing theories, family nursing frameworks, and family nursing research
- Evolution of the concept of health promotion, family health, and related family theories and concepts
- Evolution of the disciplines of family social science and behavioral health
- Emphasis of professional organizations on families and health
- Health objectives of national and international organizations
- Dynamic nature of society and public policy
- Family research and family assessment measures
- National and international family health promotion and prevention agenda

Contemporary Nursing

NURSING PROFESSION. The nursing profession has mandated family health care in a number of documents. For example, many of the American Nurses' Association (ANA) *Standards of Nursing Practice* (1973a) for clinical specialties such as community health nursing (ANA, 1973b), maternal-child health nursing (ANA, 1973c), and pediatric oncology nursing (ANA, 1978) emphasize family as focal phenomenon for nursing practice (Whall & Fawcett, 1991). Other examples of the linkage of family and nursing practice are noted in the ANA's *Social Policy Statement* (1980) and *Nursing's Agenda for Health Care Reform* (ANA, 1991). Standards have not been developed for family health nursing, suggesting that this area of nursing practice is still in its formative stages.

In the past decade, as the attention of health professionals turned to promoting health and the preventing of dysfunction in families, nursing began to incorporate such concepts as wellness, health promotion, self-care, and family health into family nursing.

Within many nursing organizations (e.g., the ANA's Council of Nurse Researchers and the Western Nursing Research Society), there are interest groups on family nursing research and health promotion. The First International Family Nursing Conference was held in 1987 in Calgary, Alberta, while the third conference (1994), held in Montreal, Canada, coincided with the International Year of the Family. Families will continue to be a focus of nursing's attention as family nursing research and theory advances.

NURSING THEORIES. The evolution of nursing science and theories of nursing by theorists such as King (1981), Neuman (1982), Newman (1994), Orem (1985), Rogers (1990), and Roy (1984) have contributed to the development of family health nursing. The nursing paradigm includes the concepts of person, nursing, health, and environment.

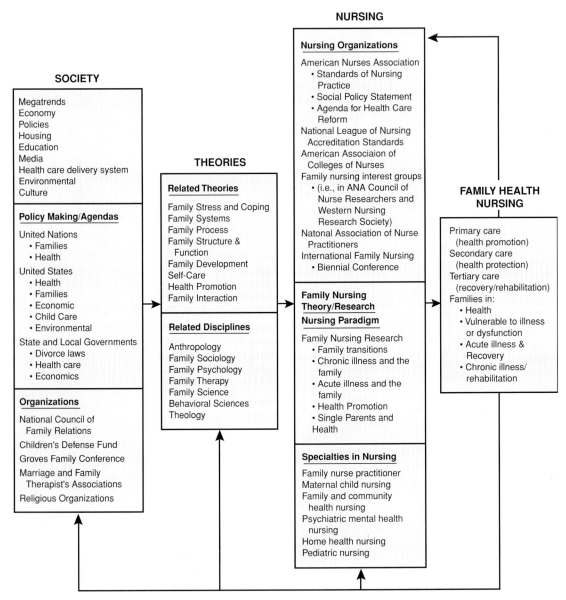

FIGURE 1–5. Variables Influencing Contemporary Family Health Nursing.

Questions regarding this paradigm remain: What is the family health nursing paradigm? Is it family, family health, family environment, and family nursing? Or is the family simply the environment for individual health?

Loveland-Cherry in Chapter 2 of this text discusses the contributions of nurse theorists to family health promotion. The writings of nursing theorists and scholars (Friedman, 1992; Friedemann, 1989; Newman, 1986; Pender, 1987; Schlotfeldt, 1987) clearly indicate that the goal of family health nursing is to enhance the well-being of the family unit.

NURSING EDUCATION. A number of crucial factors influence the shaping of the conceptual frame-

works of programs of study. These variables include the use of the nursing paradigm (human beings, nursing, health, and environment) as the basis for curricular planning; recommendations given in the National League of Nursing accreditation standards, the American Nurses' Association's *Social Policy Statement* (1980), and the ANA's *Standards of Nursing Practice* for over six specialties; consumer demands and changing societal norms; and the national policy agenda for health promotion and prevention. As a consequence of these factors, family nursing graduate programs have been developed to prepare specialists to care for families at the various types of family nursing practice, and undergraduate curricula have been strengthened to prepare a family nurse generalist (Hanson & Heims, 1992). There is lack of consistency in curricular design, content, theorist, organization of curricula, titles of graduates, and conceptual frameworks used.

FAMILY NURSING RESEARCH. Although complex and sometimes flawed, family-focused research in nursing has evolved as the result of a nursing and interdisciplinary interest in families (Gillis & Davis, 1993; Murphy, 1986). Family nursing research has progressed in the past 20 years from a focus on family dyads of mother and infant or husband and wife to a focus on the family as the unit of analysis. The focus has progressed to include the impact of chronic illness on families (Hymovich & Hoagopian, 1992; McCubbin, 1993) and the effects of transitions across the life span on family health. Commitment to family nursing research is shown by the planning and initiation of the *Journal of Family Nursing* in 1995 (Bell, 1995).

Related Disciplines

Theoretical advances in related disciplines such as anthropology, family life education, family ecology, psychology, sociology, health promotion, and family counseling/therapy have contributed to family nursing science. In addition, the research of family scientists such as David Olson and colleagues, Hamilton McCubbin and colleagues, and Kay Paisley have provided frameworks and assessment measures for understanding and assessing family health. These disciplines continue to provide rich resources and a network of colleagues for family nurses.

Family Organizations

A variety of organizations have contributed to the evolution of family nursing. Interdisciplinary organizations such as the National Council of Family Relations (NCFR), the Children's Defense Fund, and others provide publications on the status of families and children, disseminate research on family issues across the life span and the health/illness cycle, and serve as a vehicle to facilitate networking and collaboration. Although there is no formal family nursing organization, family nurses have formal interest groups within a number of interdisciplinary organizations such as the NCFR, the American Public Health Association, and national groups of marriage and family counselors and therapists. Since 1983, within NCFR there has been a Family Nursing Focus Group that meets at the annual meeting. Approximately 75 family nurses from the United States and Canada are members of this focus group. Other sections in NCFR to which nurses belong include those on single-parent families, remarriage and step-parenting, farm families, ethnic minority families, family and health, theory construction, research methodology, family life

education and enrichment, family therapy, and family action sections.

National and International Agendas for Family Health

There is national and international concern for health and the quality of life in families. For example, the Canadian government places a major emphasis on improving family health and the United Kingdom has "health visitors" who focus primarily on the individual in the family context but who are increasingly focusing on the family as the unit of care.

1994 International Agenda for Families

Internationally, the United Nations is concerned about the health of individual family members and the family unit. For example, 1994 was designated "The International Year of the Family" (IYF) (United Nations, 1991). The key goals of the International Year of the Family were to (1) provide information at national, state, and local levels; (2) communicate and encourage dialogue with and between local governments and people at the grass-roots level; (3) support active partnerships between governments, volunteer organizations, business, and labor; (4) review legislation relevant to the health of families; and (5) encourage research on family issues.

The agenda included goals for governments, voluntary organizations, national governmental organizations, the media, opinion leaders, social services, family organizations, education, research, and families. Selected educational goals included (1) the use of educational networks to discuss family needs; (2) the encouragement of family-centered activities in health and education, taking into account the variety of family types; (3) the provision of special education sessions for families with special needs; and (4) further encouragement of research on the role of families in various cultural and social contexts.

The IYF Agenda for Families aimed to (1) develop family councils to make decisions and respect the capabilities, dignity, and needs of all family members; (2) stress the responsibilities of all with regard to children and disadvantaged members; (3) enhance the feeling of family togetherness through gatherings, shared meals, and leisure activities; and (4) motivate all family members to share effectively all household and other responsibilities.

The national focus on the "Health of the Nation 2000" and the rhetoric of many public leaders about the concern for "family values" substantiate the need for family nurses to work in partnership with other professionals and with families to enhance the quality of family life. These agendas will significantly affect family nursing practice, research, and education.

Objectives for the Health of the Nation

A crucial factor that renewed the interest of many health professionals in health promotion was the Surgeon General's landmark report, *Healthy People* (U.S. Public Health Service, 1979) and a companion report, *Promoting Health/ Preventing Disease: Objectives for the Nation* (U.S. Public Health Service, 1980). These documents set goals for 1990 to improve the health of Americans across the life span in 15 priority areas. Although some improvement was noted during the 1980s, in 1990 most categories still existed and other health problems (such as HIV infections) emerged. In 1990, the Department of Health and Human Services (DHHS) report *Healthy People 2000* identified new goals for the nation's health:

- Increase the span of healthy life for Americans.
- Reduce health disparities among Americans.
- Achieve access to preventive services for all Americans.

The objectives for health promotion, health protection, and prevention for the United States in the decade from 1990 to 2000 are shown in Table 1–2. Other areas of concern identified were the health status of children, adolescents, young adults, older adults, and minorities.

Health professionals at many levels and in many settings have adopted these objectives as models for intervention with clients. Although many of the priorities are individually focused, it would be nearly impossible to succeed in making significant changes unless the family unit is a focus of care. The saliency of this is best stated by David Olson, 1990 President of NCFR, in the NCFR Presidential Report *2001: Preparing Families for the Future.* He states that "The family must be a national priority if we are to effectively deal with the multitude of problems in our society today. Most of the problems with individuals and society either begin or end up in the family" (1990, p.1). This document will be the basis for many health promotion, health maintenance, and prevention programs for family nursing practice with individuals, families, and aggregates in the coming years.

SOCIETAL CHANGES. Contemporary families live in a rapidly changing society. As the reader will note in Chapter 3, the structure of families has changed. In addition, a number of trends are significantly influencing family life and family nursing. These trends include a high information society, high touch, increasing emphasis on self-help and self-care, consumer demand for participation in decision making, more complex and increasing technology, and changes in the types of and age configuration of families (Naisbitt, 1982). Dynamic changes in the economy, increases in

TABLE 1–2. PRIORITIES IDENTIFIED FOR U.S. HEALTH PROTECTION AND PREVENTION FOR THE YEAR 2000

HEALTH PROMOTION
Reduction in use of tobacco
Reduction in alcohol and drug abuse
Improved nutrition
Increased exercise and physical fitness
Improved control of stress and violence
Improved mental health
Improved family planning
Reduction of the incidence of chronic diseases
Elimination of violent and abusive behaviors
Educational and community-based programs

HEALTH PROTECTION
Increased control environmental hazards
Improved occupational safety and health
Reduction of unintentional injuries
Improved oral health
Food and drug safety

PREVENTIVE HEALTH SERVICES
Improved maternal and infant health
Reduction of heart disease and stroke
Prevention of cancer
Reduction of sexually transmitted diseases
Reduction of HIV infection
Control and reduction of diabetes and chronic
    disabling conditions
Increase in clinical preventative services

SURVEILLANCE AND DATA SYSTEMS
Surveillance and data systems

From *Healthy People 2000: National Health Promotion and Disease Prevention Objectives.* (1990). Available from the Superintendent of Documents, Washington, D.C., U.S. Government Printing Office, DHHS Publications No. PHS 91-5213.

health care costs, reduction of the size of the military, changes in family size and structure, the increasing number of homeless families, and the decreasing value placed on family life are dynamic forces affecting family nursing practice, education, and research.

THE CHANGING FAMILY. The family continues to experience dramatic shifts and families are becoming more diverse and complex in structure and lifestyle than families of the past (Skolnick, 1993). Examples of these diversities, family structures, and complexities include more blended families, more cohabitation, more single-parent and dual-earner families, more aged family members, decreasing fertility rates, increased urbanization, and so on. In addition, families of the late 1990s and the 21st century will be coping with increasing upheavals such as poverty, increasing chronic illness, HIV infections of family members across the life span, and a myriad of other health problems, which will force health care system changes to provide relevant and adequate health care to all citizens. Chapter 3 discusses changing family demographics. As families realize that they must assume more responsibility for their health, an increasing number are joining in partnership with professionals to improve the health status of individual family members and the family unit.

In response to numerous developments in theory and research and changes in the family's ecosystem, a new specialty called Family Science emerged (Burr & Leigh, 1983). Phenomena of interest include such topics as family interaction, family patterns, family health, value placed on family, diverse family types and issues, culture and ethnicity, family preservation, and strategies useful in assisting families to lead healthier lives.

FAMILY HEALTH NURSING PRACTICE

Family health nursing has many of the characteristics of family-centered community nursing as described by Barkauskas (1986) and family nursing (Clements & Roberts, 1983; Friedman, 1992; Gillis et al., 1989; Hymovich & Barnard, 1979). It is based on many of the theories and skills from nursing specialties, primary health care, family science, family therapy, and behavioral health.

The terms "family nursing," "family health nursing," "family and community health nursing," "family nurse practitioner," and "family clinical nurse specialist" are often used interchangeably. This contributes to the confusion about whether or not there is an actual difference in the roles. In some instances, it seems that the term chosen is merely a matter of preference of the faculty in graduate programs. For example, some schools that have graduate family health nursing programs deliberately use the concept "health" to denote the focus on the care of well or "worried well" family units. However, according to ANA the term *specialist* does indicate graduate preparation. Hanson (1987) stated that this specialty "is both old and new, and has always been an integral part of American nursing. It is simultaneously innovative and conservative" (p. 4). Perhaps the difference in the titles "Family Nurse" and "Family Health Nurse" is merely semantics.

If the nurse defines health as encompassing illness and wellness, as Brubaker (1983) suggests, then all nurses who provide care to families as a unit are family health nurses. Family health nurses may desire to direct their practice toward a specific area on the health continuum such as illness care, prevention, or health promotion. In addition, some may choose to provide nursing care to families in specific settings, such as the community, and to families at particular stages in family development, such as childbearing families, families with an acute or chronic ill member, families experiencing transitions, and families

seeking approaches to improve the level of their well-being as a unit. However, the ultimate goal with all clients (individual or family units) would be to assist them to achieve optimal levels of health.

As shown in Figure 1–1, the family is multifaceted and nurses providing care to family systems need to be cognizant of the realms of family experience. Table 1–3 further elaborates on the key concepts in each of five realms. These realms can be used to guide systematic assessment and intervention with family systems to promote family health. Chapter 11 in particular and many other chapters in this book provide the reader with lists of measures and offer examples of measures to assess family health.

Family nursing, like community health nursing, provides its practitioners with "challenges to apply multiple skills in especially creative and independent ways . . . with clients to maintain health and promote wellness in the client's natural environment" (Barkauskas, 1986, p. 5). Family health nurses also collaborate with professionals from a variety of disciplines in the promotion of family health and well-being.

TABLE 1–3. REALMS OF THE FAMILY HEALTH EXPERIENCE FOR FAMILY HEALTH NURSING PRACTICE

FAMILY INTERACTION
Family relationships
Communication
Nurturance
Intimacy
Social Support

DEVELOPMENTAL TRANSITIONS
Family development
Individual development

FAMILY HEALTH PROCESSES
Family health beliefs
Health status of members
Health responses and practices
Lifestyle (health promotion/prevention)
Health care during illness and wellness

COPING PROCESSES
Management of resource
Problem solving
Adaptation to stressors and crises

INTEGRITY PROCESSES
Shared meanings
Family history
Family boundary maintenance
Family identity and commitment
Family values
Family rituals

Data from Anderson, K. & Tomlinson, P. (1992). The family health system as an emerging paradigmatic view for nursing. Image, 24(1), 57–63.

TABLE 1–4. ROLES OF SPECIALIST IN FAMILY HEALTH NURSING

Family advocate	Health care planner
Caregiver	Case manager
Collaborator	Consultant
Coordinator	Facilitator
Family health educator	Leader
Role model	Researcher
Supervisor	

Roles of the Family Health Nurse

Family health nursing roles vary depending on the setting in which the family nurse practices and the type of client (individual or family unit) (Table 1–4). Nursing care ranges from primary care to tertiary care. Most family nurses choose a specific area of interest such as (1) a particular developmental stage of the family, (2) developmental transitions such as retirement or parenting, (3) families with acute care needs or chronic illness of a member, (4) stress management, (5) fitness, or (6) nutrition. It is beyond the scope of this text to include the endless possibilities of current and future innovative roles of family health nurses. The area of practice is limited only by the creativity of the nurse. See Table 1–5 for a description of family nursing practice.

Chapter 2 of this book addresses the role of the family nurse in family health promotion, and Chapter 19 focuses on the nurse's role in preventing disease in family members. Chapter 12 applies Neuman's Systems Model to family nursing process and family assessment. Unit 3 discusses the role of family nurses in the assessment of family health, nutrition, recreation and exercise, environmental health, sleep, stress management, and family transitions.

Settings for Family Health Nursing Practice

Family nurses may practice in any setting where there are families. These include, but are not limited to, hospital units, home health care settings, schools, physicians' offices, clinics, health education centers, occupational health centers, marriage and family counseling clinics, private practice offices, maternal and child settings, wellness centers, and hospices. Family health nurses may also be independent entrepreneurs, and may practice in settings such as:

- Anticipatory guidance groups, addressing major life events such as pregnancy, the climacteric, grief, and divorce
- Church health ministries
- Community health education centers
- Day-care centers for children and the aging
- Diabetes education groups

TABLE 1–5. DESCRIPTION OF FAMILY HEALTH NURSING PRACTICE

Sites of family health nursing practice are located in a variety of settings where individuals, families, and groups have health concerns within the realm of family health promotion and prevention
The focus of nursing practice is individuals in the family context, family unit, and groups of families (aggregates)
The major goal is assistance to families to achieve higher levels of health and to prevent ill health or family dysfunction
The family health nurse assists families in adjusting to acute and chronic illnesses and changes in family structure and function
Family health nursing practice is likely to be autonomous, independent, and/or entrepreneurial
Relationships with families usually last for a longer term then in acute care settings
Assessment may include not only individual assessment but also a holistic assessment of family structure, function, developmental tasks, health behavior patterns and health status, lifestyle, and pyschosocial variables
Families are partners in planning interventions and decision making

Adapted from Barkauskas, V.H. (1986). Community health nursing. In B.B. Logan & C.E. Dawkins (Eds.), *Family-Centered Nursing in the Community* (pp. 4–30). Reading, MA: Addison-Wesley.

- Family and marital counseling clinics
- Family life education groups, focusing on areas such as parenting, communication, and sexuality
- Lactation counseling groups
- Support groups for families experiencing the care of chronically ill family members (AIDS, Alzheimer's, or cancer)
- University health centers

Although the focus of this book is on family health promotion, this is not to say that acute care and rehabilitative nursing are not also legitimate foci of family nursing. Providing nursing care to individuals and families in all states of their health, whether illness or wellness, is within the realm of family nursing practice because family health encompasses both illness/dysfunctional and wellness/functional (Danielson, Hamel-Bissel, & Winstead-Fry, 1993).

However, if nurses do not respond to changes in clients' needs for health promotion and disease prevention, other professionals with skills in health teaching and anticipatory guidance will assume nursing's role in family health promotion and health protection. For example, on one occasion, the author visited a clinic where family nurse practitioners were providing physical assessment, diagnosing, and prescribing treatment. At the same time, health educators were delegated major responsibility for anticipatory guidance and health teaching such as appropriate use of family planning methods, explanation of the birth process, and directions for taking prescribed medication. In the past both these activities (health teaching and primary care) were considered the responsibility of the nurse.

Beliefs about Families

Assumptions and beliefs about families influence a family nurse's practice. Each nurse must therefore examine his or her own assumptions and beliefs about families. A proposed philosophy of family health nurse practice might include the following assumptions:

- Individuals and families are unique.
- Family decisions about their health are influenced by many psychological, social, cultural, orientation to life, and spiritual variables.
- Family decisions about health are made independent of the nurse.
- Success in attaining a goal is best achieved when the family determines the goal.
- Family health is a dynamic, multidimensional concept, and what is correct today may be incorrect tomorrow.
- Families will engage in health behaviors that are relevant and pertinent to their family life career and social context.

- Family health is more than the health of the individual members.
- All families have the potential for growth in their level of health, which can be facilitated by a nurse who is caring, comforting, and nurturing.
- The family nurse's role is to appraise and enhance the health status, health assets, and health potentials of individuals in the family context, families, and aggregates.

Family Health Nursing Education

Although education about family health is believed to be essential content to professional curricula, family nursing curricula are diverse and range from undergraduate to doctoral programs. Many have a limited family focus. Some emphasize the family and community health aspect or the individual in the family context, while others focus on family therapy (Hanson & Heims, 1992; Wright & Leahey, 1984). Hanson (1987) stated that the "placement of family content may be serendipitous" and "in graduate education is equally elusive." Other curricula focus on individual family members or families at different levels of the family life cycle; nurse practitioner skills; well families; and primary, secondary, or tertiary care. The level of sophistication of family health nursing practice depends on the academic preparation a nurse receives. Table 1–6 suggests the levels of family health nursing practice.

TABLE 1–6. LEVELS OF FAMILY NURSING PRACTICE

LEVEL OF PRACTICE	GENERALIST/ SPECIALIST	EDUCATION	CLIENT
Expert	Advanced Specialist	Doctorate	All Levels Family Nursing Theory Development Family Nursing Research
Proficient	Advanced Specialist	Masters With Added Experience	All Levels Beginning Family Nursing Research
Competent	Beginning Specialist	Masters	Individual in the Family Context Interpersonal Family Nursing Family Unit as Client Family Aggregates
Advanced Beginner	Generalist	Bachelors With Experience	Individual in the Family Context Interpersonal Family Nursing (Family Systems Nursing) Family Unit as Client
Novice	Generalist	Bachelors	Individual in the Family Context

Data from Friedemann, M.L. (1989). The concept of family nursing. *Journal of Advanced Nursing.* 14, pp. 211–221; and Benner, P. (1984). *From Novice to Expert: Excellence and Power in Clinical Nursing Practice.* Menlo Park, CA: Addison-Wesley.

Graduates from baccalaureate programs are prepared as generalists and to assume positions as staff nurses in hospitals and community health agencies. Their expertise is the individual in the family context. Graduates of master's degree programs are specialists who may practice more independently and collaboratively. Graduate nurses intervene with the individuals and also with the family as client and depending on their preparation, with family interactions. See Table 1–4 for a list of the roles of the family nurse clinical specialist. A number of graduate schools have doctoral programs in family nursing and a few provide opportunities for postdoctoral study in family nursing.

THE FUTURE AND FAMILY HEALTH NURSING

From the first three international family nursing conferences (1988, 1991, 1994), a collection of articles on family nursing research, theory, and practice have been published. The first, *The Cutting Edge of Family Nursing* (Bell, Watson, & Wright, 1989) focused on family nursing, family nursing theory, family policy, and family research (conceptual and methodological issues). The second, *The Nursing of Families* (Feetham et al., 1993) is a collection of invited papers presented by family nurse scholars at the Second International Family Nursing Conference. In addition to these, a third book, *Family Theory Development in Nursing* (Whall & Fawcett, 1991), discusses the science and art of family nursing. These three volumes will provide a basis for continued development of family nursing theory, concept clarification in family nursing, and family nursing research methodologies.

A number of variables will shape the nursing profession and ultimately family health nursing in the 21st century (Bezold & Carlson, 1986; Skolnick, 1993). Although the future is uncertain, change will be unavoidable. Family nurses are encouraged to be cognizant of three major dynamics in society and health care that affect nursing and health care. The first dynamic is *institutional* changes that include decreased census in acute care settings, increased census in home health care, changes in the management of health care institutions, changes in financing health care, and escalating costs. The second dynamic is *societal* changes which include the following:

- More assertive and knowledgeable consumers with interest in health promotion
- Changes in individual and family lifestyles
- More vulnerable families (single parent, chronic illness, low income, uninsured, underinsured, homeless)

- Legislative and regulatory changes in health policy
- Concern for quality and equality in health care
- Changes in the demographics proportions to include more aged and varied cultural groups (legal and illegal immigrants)

Lastly, the *professional* variables are (1) higher levels of educational preparation for nurses in leadership positions and for all professional staffs in hospitals; (2) higher levels of academic requirements for professional nurses; and (3) increased entrepreneurial opportunities in health care.

As the locus of health care shifts to the community, family nurses will assume leadership in an assortment of roles. Family health nurses will be in more entrepreneurial positions, for example, managing wellness institutes and community health promotion programs; owning home health agencies and family consulting firms and a variety of organizations; and operating managed care organizations. Family research will be more focused on the family as a unit and on all aspects of family health, particularly health risk behaviors, health promotion, and health protection.

Family health nurses also need to assume leadership roles in the political arena. The range of participation will include (1) being informed about the issues relevant to health promotion, families, and the delivery of care; (2) networking within nursing organizations; (3) testifying at hearings; (4) supporting candidates who draft legislation to improve health of individuals and families; (5) running for public office: and (6) conducting research on the effects of public policy on family health (see Chapter 21).

Curricula at the undergraduate and graduate levels should be designed to include more family theory and greater depth regarding the role of the nurse in all aspects of the individual client in the family context and all aspects of family health. In addition, more emphasis will be placed on primary care, vulnerable families, and family nursing research (Taylor, 1995). Doctoral programs in nursing will offer specialization in family nursing research. Theory development in family nursing will uncover new relationships and add to the clarity of understanding family nursing theory. According to Artinian (1991), much of family nursing theory is implicit. However, as the current family nursing scientists test and develop family nursing theory, more clarity will be achieved in family nursing concepts.

As nursing enters the 21st century, the family health nursing role will become more actualized as the myriad of social, political, economic, health care, and consumer demands and lifestyle changes affect nursing practice. Then family health nurses will be closer to "being" than "becoming."

CHAPTER HIGHLIGHTS

The family has been idealized as the client of the nursing profession since the pre-Nightingale era; however, in reality the client is the individual within the family context and not the family unit.

In the 1970s, the family unit as the client became a focus of concern for assessment and intervention for an emerging nursing specialty—family health/family nursing.

Many social, political, professional, behavioral, and interdisciplinary variables influenced the development of contemporary family health nursing practice.

Family nursing assessment and enhancement occurs at four levels of practice: individual within the family as context, the family as client, family as client with family interactions as focus, and family aggregates.

The family health nurse's practice occurs in any setting where there are families or individuals within a family context.

The future of family health nursing will be influenced by health policy, health promotion agendas, economics, changes in the nursing profession, consumer demands, and health promotion lifestyle changes, and the growing concern for the quality of family health.

REFERENCES

American Nurses' Association. (1991). *Nursing's Agenda for Health Care Reform.* (ANA Publication No. PR-12-91). Washington, DC: American Nurses' Association.

American Nurses' Association. *Social Policy Statement.* (1980). Nursing: A social policy statement (Ana Publication No.-NP6335-M) Kansas City, MO: American Nurses' Association.

American Nurses' Association. (1986). *Standards of Community Health Nursing Practice.* Washington, DC: American Nurses' Association.

American Nurses' Association. (1978). *Standards of Pediatric Oncology Nursing Practice.* Kansas City, MO: American Nurses' Association.

American Nurses' Association. (1973a). *Standards of Nursing Practice.* Kansas City, MO: American Nurses' Association.

American Nurses' Association. (1973b). *Standards of Community Health Nursing Practice.* Kansas City, MO: American Nurses' Association.

American Nurses' Association. (1973c). *Standards of Maternal-Child Nursing Practice.* Kansas City, MO: American Nurses' Association.

American Nurses' Association. (1973d). *Standards of Psychiatric Mental Health Nursing Practice.* Kansas City, MO: American Nurses' Association.

American Nurses' Association. (1973d). Why standards of practice? *Standards of Nursing Practice* (ANA Pub. No. NP-41). Kansas City, MO: American Nurses' Association.

Anderson, K.H., & Tomlinson, P.S. (1992). The family health system as an emerging paradigmatic view for nursing. *Image,* 24, 57–63.

Archer, S.E. (1982). Synthesis of public health science and nursing science. *Nursing Outlook,* 30(8), 442–446.

Artinian, N.T. (1991). Philosophy of science and family nursing theory development. In A.L. Whall & J. Fawcett (Eds.), *Family Theory Development Nursing: State of the Science and Art* (pp. 43–53.) Philadelphia: Davis.

Austin, A.L. (1975). Nurses in American history: Wartime volunteers—1861–1865. *American Journal of Nursing,* 75(5), 816–818.

Barkauskas, V.H. (1986). Community health nursing. In B.B. Logan & C.E. Dawkins (Eds.), *Family-centered Nursing in the Community* (pp. 4–30). Reading, MA: Addison-Wesley.

Barnard, K.E. (1984). The family as a unit of measurement. *The American Journal of Maternal Child Nursing,* 9(1), 21.

Benner, P. (1984). *From Novice to Expert: Excellence and Power in Clinical Nursing Practice.* Menlo Park, CA: Addison-Wesley.

Bell, J.M. (1995). Avoiding isomorphism. A call for a different view. *Journal of Family Nursing.* 1(1), 5–7.

Bell, J.M., Watson, W.L., & Wright, L.M. (1989). *The Cutting Edge of Family Nursing.* Calgary, Alberta: Family Nursing Unit Publications.

Bezold, C., & Carlson, R. (1986). Nursing in the 21st century. *Journal of Professional Nursing,* 2(1), 69–71.

Brubaker, B.H. (1983). Health promotion: A linguistic analysis. *Advances in Nursing Science,* 5(3), 1–14.

Burr, W.R., & Leigh, G.K. (1983). A new discipline. *Journal of Marriage and the Family,* 45, 467–480.

Chavigny, K.H., & Kroske, M. (1983). Public health nursing in crisis. *Nursing Outlook,* 31(6), 312–316.

Christy, T.E. (1970). Portrait of a leader: Lillian D. Wald. *Nursing Outlook,* 18(3), 50–54.

Clements, I.W., & Roberts, F.B. (Eds.). (1983). *Family Health: A Theoretical Approach to Nursing Care.* New York: Wiley & Sons.

Clements-Stone, S., Eigisti, D.G., & McGuire, S.L. (1987). *Comprehensive Family and Community Health Nursing.* New York: McGraw-Hill.

Cummingham, R. (1978). Family-Centered care. *Canadian Nurse,* 2, 34–37.

Danielson, C.B., Hamel-Bissel, B., Winstead-Fry, P. (1993). *Families, Health and Illness.* St. Louis: Mosby.

DeYoung, L., Sifferlin, K., & Mitzel, A. (1983). The family health nurse in a leadership role. *Nursing Administration Quarterly,* 7(2), 50–56.

Feetham, S.L., Meiser, S.B., Bell, J.M., & C.L. Gillis (Eds.) *The Nursing of Families* (pp. 259–265). Newbury Park, CA: Sage.

Fitzpatrick, M.L. (1975). Nursing and the Great Depression. *American Journal of Nursing,* 75(12), 2188–2190.

Ford, L.C. (1979). The development of family nursing. In D.P. Hymovich & M.W. Barnard, (Eds.), *Family Health Care: General Perspectives* (Vol. 1). (2nd ed.). (pp. 88–105). New York: McGraw-Hill.

Forster, M. (1984). *Significant Sisters.* New York: Knopf.

Friedemann, M.L. (1989). The concept of family nursing. *Journal of Advanced Nursing,* 14, 211–216.

Friedman, M.M. (1992). *Family Nursing: Theory and Assessment* (2nd ed.). Norwalk, CT: Appleton-Lange.

Gillis, C.L., & Davis. L. (1993). Does family interventions make a difference? An integrative review and meta-analysis. In S.L. Feetham, S.B. Meiser, J.M. Bell, & C.L. Gillis (Eds.), *The Nursing of Families* (pp. 259–265). Newbury Park, CA: Sage.

Gillis, C.L. (1983). The family as a unit of analysis: Strategies for the nurse researcher. *Advances in Nursing Science,* 5(3), 50–59.

Gillis, C.L., Higley, B.L., Roberts, B.M., & Martinson, I.M. (1989). *Toward a Science of Family Nursing.* Reading, MA: Addison-Wesley.

Hall, B.A., & Allan, J.D. (1986). Sharpening nursing's focus by focusing on health. *Nursing and Health Care,* 7, 315–320.

Ham, L.M., & Chamings, P.A. (1983). Family nursing: Historical perspectives. In I.W. Clements & F.B. Roberts (Eds.), *Family Health: A Theoretical Approach to Nursing Care* (pp. 33–43). New York: Wiley.

Hanson, S.M., & Heims, M.L. (1992). Family nursing curricula in U.S. schools of nursing. *Journal of Nursing Education,* 31(7), 303–308.

Hanson, S.M. (1987). Family nursing and chronic illness. In L.M. Wright & M.L. Leahey (Eds.), *Families and Chronic Illness* (pp. 1–31). Springhouse, PA: Springhouse.

Heinrich, J. (1983). Historical perspectives on public health nursing. *Nursing Outlook,* 31(12), 317–320.

Hill, L., & Smith N. (1990). *Self-Care Nursing: Promoting Health.* Englewood Cliffs, NJ: Prentice-Hall.

Hymovich, D.P., & Barnard, M.U. (Eds.). (1979). *Family Health Care: General Perspectives* (Vol. 1). (2nd ed). New York: McGraw-Hill.

Hymovich, D.P., & Hoagopian, G.A. (1992). *Chronic Illness in Children and Adults. A Psychosocial Approach.* Philadelphia: Saunders.

Janosik, E.H., & Miller, J.R. (1980). *Family Focused Care.* New York: McGraw-Hill.

Kalisch, P.A., & Kalisch, B.J. (1986). *The Advance of American Nursing* (2nd ed.). Boston: Little, Brown.

Kandzari, J.H., & Howard, J.R. (1981). *The Well Family: A Developmental Approach.* Boston: Little, Brown.

King, I. (1981). *A Theory of Nursing.* New York: Wiley.

Logan, B.B., & Dawkins, C.E. (Eds.). (1986). *Family Centered Nursing in the Community.* Menlo Park, CA: Addison-Wesley.

Matejski, M.P. (1986). Ladies' aid societies and the nurses of Lincoln's army. *Journal of Nursing History,* 1(2), 35–51.

McCubbin, M.A. (1993). Family stress theory and development of nursing knowledge about family adaptation. In S.B Feetham, S.B. Meister, J.M. Bell, & C.L. Gillis (Eds.), *The Nursing of Families* (pp. 46–58). Newbury Park, CA: Sage.

Mischke-Berkey, K., Warner, P., & Hanson, S. (1994). In P.J. Bomar (Ed.), *Nurses and Family Health Promotion.* Philadelphia: Saunders.

Murphy, S. (1986). Family study and nursing research. *Image: Journal of Nursing Scholarship,* 18(4), 170–174.

National Council on Family Relations. (1995). *Initiatives for Families: Research, Policy, Practice and Education.* Minneapolis, MN: National Council on Family Relations.

Naisbitt, J. (1982). *Megatrends—Ten New Directions for Transforming Lives.* New York: Warner Books.

Neuman, B. (1982). *The Neuman Systems Model: Application to Nursing Education and Practice.* Norwark, CT: Appleton-Century-Crofts.

Newman, M.A. (1994). *Health as Expanding Consciousness* (2nd ed.). New York: National League for Nursing.

Nightingale, F. (1946). *Notes on Nursing: What It Is and What It Is Not.* Philadelphia: Lippincott. (Original work published in 1859.)

Nightingale, F. (1949). Sick nursing and health nursing. In I.A. Hampton (Ed.), *Nursing of the Sick—1893* (pp. 24–43). New York: McGraw-Hill. (Original paper presented in 1893.)

Olson, D.H. (1990). NCFR Presidential Report: *2001: Preparing Families for the Future.* Minneapolis, MN: National Council on Family Relations.

Orem, D.E. (1980). *Nursing: Concepts of Practice.* New York: McGraw-Hill.

Paradis, L.F., Schultz, J., Hollers, K., & Marstrom, K. (1987). Home health agencies and hospices—stronger together or alone? *Nursing and Health Care,* 8(3), 167–172.

Pender, N.J. (1986). Health promotion: Implementing strategies. In B.B. Logan & C.E. Dawkins (Eds.), *Family Centered Nursing in the Community* (pp. 295–334). Menlo Park, CA: Addison-Wesley.

Pender, N.J. (1987). *Health Promotion in Nursing Practice* (2nd ed.). Norwalk, CT: Appleton & Lange.

Pletsch, P.K. (1981). Mary Breckinridge: A pioneer who made her mark. *American Journal of Nursing,* 81(12), 2188–2190.

Roberts, F.B. (1983). An interaction model for family assessment. In I.W. Clements and F.B. Roberts (Eds.), *Family Health* (pp. 189–204). New York: Wiley.

Rogers, M.E. (1980). Nursing: A science of unitary man. In J.P. Riehl & C. Roy, *Conceptual Models for Nursing Practice* (2nd ed., pp. 329–337). New York: Appleton-Century-Crofts.

Roy, C. (1976). *Introduction to Nursing: An Adaptation Model* (2nd ed.). Englewood Cliffs, NJ: Prentice-Hall.

Schlotfeldt, R.M. (1987). Defining nursing: A historic controversy. *Nursing Research,* 36(1), 64–67.

Skolnick, A. (1993). Families in transition: America's and the World. In K. Altergott (Ed.), *One World, Many Families* (pp. 8–11). Minneapolis: National Council on Family Relations.

Selavan, I.C. (1975). Nurses in American history: The Revolution. *American Journal of Nursing,* 75(4), 592–594.

Smith, J.A. (1983). *The Idea of Health: Implications for Nursing Practice.* New York: Teachers College Press.

Spradley, B.W. (1985). *Community Health Nursing: Concepts and Practice* (2nd ed.). Boston: Little, Brown.

Steiger, N.J., & Lipson, J.G. (1985). *Self-Care Nursing: Theory and Practice.* Bowie, MD: Brady.

Swanson, J.M., & Albrecht, M. (1993). *Community Health Nursing.* Philadelphia: Saunders.

Taylor, C. (1995). Social threats to family health: Redefining nursing's roles. *Journal of Family Nursing.* 1(1), 30–40.

Teachman, I.D., Polonko, K.A., Scanzoni, J. (1987). Demography of the family. In M.B. Sussman & S.K. Steinmetz (Eds.), *Handbook of Marriage and the Family* (pp. 3–58). New York: Plenum.

Ten trends to watch. (1986). *Nursing and Health Care,* 1(1). 17–19.

Tinkham, C.W., Voorhies, E.F., & McCarthy, N.C. (1984). *Community Health Nursing: Evolution and Process in the Family and Community* (3rd ed.). Norwalk, CT: Appleton-Century-Crofts.

United Nations. (1991). *1994 International Year of the Family.* Vienna: United Nations.

U.S. Department of Health and Human Services. (1990). *Healthy People 2000: National Health Promotion and Disease Prevention Objectives* (Pub. No. PHS 915213). Washington, DC: U.S. Government Printing Office.

U.S. Public Health Service. (1980). *Healthy People: The Surgeon General's report on Health Promotion and Disease Prevention* (DHEW Pub. No. PHS 79-55071). Washington, DC: U.S. Government Printing Office.

U.S. Department of Health and Human Services. (1980). *Promoting Health/Preventing Disease: Objectives for the Nation.* Washington, DC: U.S. Government Printing Office.

U.S. Department of Health and Human Services. (1979). *Healthy People: The Surgeon General's Report on Health Promotion and Disease Prevention* (U.S. Public Health Service, Pub. No. PHS 79-55071) U.S. Department of Health, Education and Welfare. Washington, DC: U.S. Government Printing Office.

Whall, A.L., & Fawcett, J. (1991). *Family Theory Development in Nursing. State of the Science and Art.* Philadelphia: Davis.

Whall, A.L. (1986). The family as the unit of care in nursing: A historical review. *Public Health Nursing,* 3(4), 240–249.

Williams, C.A. (1977). Community health nursing—What is it? *Nursing Outlook,* 25(4), 250–254.

William, C.A. (1983). Making things happen: Community health nursing and the policy arena. *Nursing Outlook,* 31(4), 225–228.

Wong, D.L. (1995). Whaley and Wong's *Nursing Care of Infants and Children* (5th ed.). St. Louis: Mosby.

Wright, L., & Leahey, M. (1990). Trends in nursing of families. In J.M. Bell; W.L. Watson; & L.M. Wright (Eds.), *The Cutting Edge of Family Nursing* (pp. 5–15). Calgary, Alberta: The University of Calgary.

Wright, L., & Leahey, M. (1994). *Nurses and Families: A Guide to Family Assessment and Intervention* (2nd ed). Philadelphia: Davis.

FAMILY HEALTH PROMOTION AND HEALTH PROTECTION

CAROL J. LOVELAND-CHERRY

Look to your health; and if you have it praise God, and value it next to a good conscience; for health is the second blessing that we mortals are capable of; a blessing that money cannot buy.

IZAAK WALTON

OBJECTIVES

On completion of this chapter, the reader will be able to:

1. Examine the critical dimensions of family health
2. Compare and contrast health promotion and health protection relative to the American family
3. Identify the current status of health promotion and health protection activities in the American family
4. Analyze the current knowledge base regarding health promotion and health protection in the American family
5. Analyze major factors that influence family health
6. Examine the role of the nurse in family health promotion

INTRODUCTION

Although the major emphasis in this country continues to be on illness, a shift toward health promotion and health protection has been evident throughout the last decade in both the United States and Canada (Ferguson, 1980; Laffrey et al., 1986; Stacctchenko & Jenicek, 1990; Green & Kreuter, 1991). The Surgeon General's report (U.S. Department of Health, Education & Welfare, 1979) was a major turning point that emphasized the need to focus on the avoidable aspects of morbidity and mortality. The focus on health promotion is especially evident in the wellness movement (Dunn, 1961, 1975). A concomitant move has been the recognition of the interrelationships between health and the family (Litman, 1974; Mauksch, 1974; Baranowski & Nader, 1985; Doherty & McCubbin, 1985; Turk & Kerns, 1985; Gilliss, 1989; Bomar, 1990; Fisher, Terry, & Ransom, 1990). The need to examine the interplay of family, social, and economic environments related to health promotion is a priority in the effort to improve the health status of the population of the United States (Nightingale et al., 1980; Duffy, 1988).

An understanding of both the critical dimensions of health promotion and the factors that contribute to this goal remains in germinal stages and is more evident for individuals than for families. Advances in public health and medical technology provide a physiologic base for disease prevention, but psychosocial aspects are not as clearly understood. Thus, although there is growing knowledge of the physiologic factors that contribute to health promotion and health protection, this knowledge is incomplete without a similar understanding of the interplay of environmental factors. Mauksch (1974) maintains that "the most challenging although least studied area in which the family concept could be a significant addition to health care is in the tasks of health maintenance and health maximization" (p. 526).

This chapter will focus on the examination of the current knowledge available to understand health promotion, and health protection in the American family. The family has been viewed from two different perspectives relative to health.

First, the family has been identified as a basic unit within which health behavior, health values, and health risk perceptions are developed, organized, and performed. Thus, the family is an important environment for health promotion and health protection for individual family members.

Second, the health of the family system itself is of concern relative to its ability to fulfill vital functions and tasks. In reality, it is difficult to separate these two perspectives when working with families. A healthy family system is usually necessary to produce healthy family members and to meet their health-related needs. Conversely, healthy family members are usually prerequisite to a healthy family system.

DIMENSIONS OF FAMILY HEALTH

Family Health as a Concept

Family health is a concept that is often referred to in the literature and is identified as a goal of nursing intervention; however, it is seldom defined. Definitions of family health can be derived from theoretical perspectives, from clinical perspectives, and from families themselves. In the first instance, dimensions of family health can be inferred from both family theory and nursing theoretical models.

Walsh (1982) identifies four perspectives for defining "normal" (or healthy) families: (1) asymptomatic family functioning characterized by an absence of any symptoms of dysfunction or psychopathology in individual members; (2) optimal family functioning as evidenced by an ideal family having the characteristics defined as optimal by a particular model or paradigm; (3) average family functioning determined by a family falling within the range of the usual or prevalent existing mode; and (4) transactional family processes based on the integration, maintenance, and growth of the family system relevant to internal and external demands within societal and temporal contexts. A model for defining family health could be developed within any one of these four views. For example, the Timberlawn studies originally viewed a healthy family as one not having an adolescent in psychiatric treatment but moved to defining optimal, midrange, and dysfunctional families based on dimensions identified within a systems framework (Lewis et al., 1976; Beavers, 1982; Walsh, 1982). The first three categories define family health as a state; the fourth views family health as a process.

Additional dimensions of family health can be elaborated from Smith's (1983) models of health. Smith (1983) identified four models of health: *clinical, role-performance, adaptive,* and *eudaimonistic.* The first is similar to the first perspective described by Walsh; health is viewed as the absence of disease. Within the role-performance model, health is defined as effective performance of roles. Elements of Walsh's second and fourth categories are found in the adaptive and eudaimonistic models. Health in the adaptive model is viewed as effective, productive interaction with the physical and social environment, with the emphasis on flexible adaptation. Within the eudaimonistic model, health is viewed as self-actualization derived from complete development of the potential for general well-being and self-realization. The clinical and role-performance models focus on maintaining stability and thus health protection. The adaptive and eudaimonistic models focus on growth and change and are consistent with health promotion.

Although Smith discusses the four models primarily in terms of individuals, they could be extended to describe family health (Table 2–1). In the clinical model, family health would be considered as lack of evidence of physical, mental, or social disease in family members or lack of deterioration or dysfunction of the family system. Family health in the role performance model could be defined as the ability of the family system to carry on family functions effectively and achieve family developmental tasks. Adaptive family health would be defined as family patterns of interaction with the environment, characterized by flexible, effective adaptation or ability

TABLE 2–1. FOUR MODELS OF FAMILY HEALTH

Family health: Clinical model	Lack of evidence of physical, mental, or social disease or deterioration or dysfunction of family system
Family health: Role-performance model	Ability of the family system to carry on family functions effectively and to achieve family developmental tasks
Family health: Adaptive model	Family patterns of interaction with the environment characterized by flexible, effective adaptation or ability to change and grow
Family health: Eudaimonistic model	Ongoing provision of resouces, guidance, and support for realization of family's maximum well-being and potential throughout the family life span

to change and grow. Family health in the eudai-monistic model is characterized as the ongoing provision of resources, guidance, and support for the realization of family members' maximum well-being and potential throughout the family life span. These definitions of family health within the four models are not mutually exclusive. Smith (1983) suggests that the four models can be viewed as forming a scale, progressing along an expanding conception of health.

Anderson and Tomlinson (1992) identify "conceptual and paradigmatic ambiguity" in current definitions of family health in nursing (p. 61) and conclude that the emerging definitions of family may be more complex than those evident in other disciplines. They suggest that a definition of family health should include five "realms of family experience": interactive, developmental, coping, integrity, and health processes. These processes constitute a proposed "family health system."

The idea of family health being more than the sum of the health of individual family members and not being ascertainable merely through assessment of individuals is clearly presented in Mauksch's (1974) concept of the "family health estate." The family health estate reflects a pattern characteristic of the family unit, not individual family members, which is developed within the emerging family and involves knowledge, attitudes, values, behaviors, and allocation of tasks and roles. Thus, the importance of looking beyond individuals' behaviors, attitudes, beliefs, and values to family system patterns in determining family health is emphasized.

Family Theories

Family theories developed in disciplines other than nursing provide direction for identifying characteristics of optimal families. For example, the developmental framework (Aldous, 1978; Duvall & Miller, 1985; Hill & Mattessich, 1979; McGoldrick & Carter, 1982) identifies family life-cycle stages with defined developmental tasks to be accomplished. A family that is able to meet stage-specific developmental tasks both of family members and of the family unit could be defined as optimal and, therefore, healthy. This definition is consistent with the role-performance model of health. Other frameworks that have been used by nurses include the structural-functional framework (Eshleman, 1981; Broderick, 1971), systems models (Kantor & Lehr, 1975; Beavers, 1977, 1982; Beavers & Voeller, 1983; Hill & Mattessich, 1979; Lewis et al., 1976), the Circumplex Model of Family Functioning (Olson et al., 1979; Olson, 1989), the Double ABCX Models (Hill, 1958; McCubbin & Patterson, 1982; McCubbin, 1989; Burr, Klein et al., 1994), the family environment (Moos & Moos, 1976), and the family ecology model (Hook & Paolucci, 1970; Roberts & Feetham, 1982).

Pratt (1976) identified the "energized family" as an ideal family form. This type of family is characterized by promotion of freedom and change, varied and active contact with other groups and organizations, flexible role relationships, egalitarian power structure, and a high degree of autonomy in family members. Pratt proposes that this family form and the consequent functioning are associated with the development of self-esteem and self-efficacy, resulting in personal competence. Personal competence is necessary for active participation in health promotion. An energized family form would be consistent with a eudaimonistic model of health.

Nursing Theoretical Models

A number of theoretical models have been developed within nursing (Rogers, 1970; Orem, 1995; Roy, 1984; King, 1981; Neuman, 1982, 1989; Erickson et al., 1983) that examine the phenomena central to the discipline of nursing—client/person, health, environment, and nursing—from various philosophical and conceptual perspectives. For the most part, these models were originally developed to focus on individuals. A few (such as Rogers, 1970) did not limit the concept of person to individuals and were considered to be applicable to families (Fawcett, 1975; Whall, 1980). Others (such as Orem, 1985) considered the family to be an important influence or environment for the individual. Recently, expansion of the models relevant to consideration of families as clients has been evident (Clements & Roberts, 1983; Hanson, 1984; Tadych, 1985; Chin, 1985; Johnston, 1986; Gonot, 1986). Consequently, beginning definitions of family health have been developed. Johnston (1986) notes that within Rogers's model, health is viewed as an ambiguous, value-laden, changing concept; therefore, family health can only be defined with a specific family at any one point in time. Each family is identified by its own unique pattern, which must be determined at the current time. Within King's (1981) model, Gonot (1986) defines family health as "dynamic life experiences through which the family adjusts to environmental stressors to achieve maximum potential for daily living" (p. 47). He states that family health is "reflected in the members' abilities to function in social roles" (p. 47).

Other definitions of family health can be inferred from the definitions of health presented within each of the nursing models. For example, consistent with Roy's (1984) definition of health, family health could be viewed as a state and a process of being and becoming an integrated and whole family system.

The idea of competence has been expanded to apply to families (Boardman, 1973; Petze, 1984; Pridham & Hansen, 1977). The characteristics of family competency are similar to those described as ideals by family theorists and include effective communication patterns, cohesiveness, capacity for change, support for family members, fostering of autonomy in family members, shared rules and norms, shared power, and skillful negotiation.

Family Cycle of Health and Illness

Family life is dynamic and during its life cycle the family experiences both periods of wellness and illness. Danielson, Hamel-Bissell, & Winsted-Fry (1993) developed a model of the Family Cycle of Health and Illness. They suggest the family's experience of health and illness is cyclical and progresses through the following eight phases:

1. Family and family member health
2. Family vulnerability and symptom experience
3. The sick role and family appraisal
4. Medical contact-diagnosis
5. Illness career and family adjustment/adaptation
6. Recovery and rehabilitation
7. Chronic adjustment/adaptation
8. Death and family reorganization (p. 71)

This book focuses on the first two phases, which are actually primary care. During the first phase, the members are well and there is no identifiable health problem or family dysfunction. The nurse's role in this phase is health education and anticipatory guidance that would help the family and its members remain well and functional. The family actively participates in activities that promote the health of its unit and the members. In the second phase, the family is vulnerable to dysfunction and/or a member may be vulnerable to illness or display symptoms of an illness. In this phase, family or folk remedies and previous patterns of adjusting and adapting are often used. During the remaining phases, the family makes adjustments and adaptations to the illness and either recovers and returns to phase one, or progresses on to the chronic illness while coping as a unit to the multiple family stressors and needed adaptations. Lastly, in some cases the disease progresses to the eighth phase, which may mean death of a family member or, in the case of unresolved dysfunction, dissolution of the family (Danielson et al., 1993; Doherty & Campbell, 1989). The family nurse nursing assessment and intervention should include knowledge of the family resources, perception of the health and vulnerability to illness family meaning of the illness, family and community resources, number of family stressors, the type of family and their problem solving abilities (McCubbin & McCubbin, 1993).

Evaluation of Family Health Status

Determination of family health status clinically is an ongoing effort of family scholars and family nurses. In an attempt to identify traits of healthy families, Curran (1983) surveyed 551 professionals who work with families. The 15 most frequently identified traits indicated that the healthy family:

1. Communicates and listens
2. Affirms and supports one another
3. Teaches respect for others
4. Develops a sense of trust
5. Has a sense of play and humor
6. Exhibits a sense of shared responsibility
7. Teaches a sense of right and wrong
8. Has a strong sense of family in which rituals and traditions abound
9. Has a balance of interaction among members
10. Has a shared religious core
11. Respects the privacy of one another
12. Values service to others
13. Fosters family table time and conversation
14. Shares leisure time
15. Admits to and seeks help with problems (pp. 24–25)

Clinical measures have been developed to evaluate dimensions of family interaction or functioning, which are indirect measures of family clinical health. The Family Function Index (FFI) (Pless & Satterwhite, 1973), the Family APGAR (Smilkstein, 1978), and the Calgary Family Assessment Model (CFAM) (Wright & Leahey, 1994) are examples of clinical assessment models. For a more extensive description and list of assessment measures the reader is encouraged to see Chapter 12.

Although nursing diagnoses, especially the North American Nursing Diagnosis Association (NANDA) system, are increasingly being used in the practice arena, family and health promotion have not been adequately addressed by these systems (Donnelly, 1990). Donnelly identified only one NANDA diagnosis that is appropriate to family health promotion—Family Coping: Potential for Growth. The diagnosis has been defined as pertaining to the family's potential to change and grow related to adapting to a family member's health challenge. Indeed, the diagnosis can be interpreted as encompassing family health promotion, but it does so only in terms of responding to the needs of an individual member. Nursing diagnosis is an area that clearly requires additional development if family health promotion is to be adequately addressed.

In a less frequent approach, families (both parents and children) were asked to explain what they thought were characteristics of family health (Loveland-Cherry, 1985). Seven major categories of responses were identified. Fifty-five percent of the respondents identified participation in health behaviors—eating healthy foods, getting enough rest, exercising regularly, wearing proper clothing, and avoiding risk behaviors such as smoking or taking drugs; 22% identified indicators of absence of illness—very little sickness, no chronic illness, healthy bodies, mental and emotional health; 8% stated characteristics of a feeling of well-being—feeling good, having a high energy level, living enthusiastically; 6% described elements that contributed to well-being—happy home, positive atmosphere, supportive and nurturing environment, mutual respect, love, fun together; 4% identified use of health services—having regular checkups, seeing a dentist regularly, and receiving good preventive care; 3% related to abilities to function in usual roles; and 1% indicated genetic background and luck. These findings indicate that although families have varied perceptions of family health, their perceptions are not that different from those proposed by professionals. Other approaches to assess family health status in selected areas are presented in Units 2 and 3 of this text.

In summary, family health has a number of dimensions and can be defined within various contexts and from a number of theoretical and clinical viewpoints. It is essential that the specific understanding of family health be clarified both by the nurse and with the family in order to have a shared goal and to design appropriate interventions. For the purpose of this book, family health is considered to be a dynamic process that includes the activities a family uses to promote and protect the well-being of the family as a unit and individual family members.

HEALTH PROMOTION AND TODAY'S FAMILY

Historically, the focus of health professionals' work with families has been in the areas of medical care and disease treatment. Only recently has increased attention been allocated to health promotion. Although health promotion may be the most complex and difficult area in which to intervene, the potential benefits are thought to justify the necessary efforts (U.S. Department of Health, Education & Welfare, 1979). The Surgeon General's report (U.S. Department of Health, Education & Welfare, 1979) delineated three groups of behaviors that would improve the health of the population: (1) preventive health services, including family planning, pregnancy and infant care, immunizations, sexually transmissible disease services and high blood pressure control; (2) health protection actions, including toxic agent control, occupational safety and health, accidental injury control, fluoridation of community water supplies, and infectious agent control; and (3) health promotion behaviors, including smoking cessation, reduction in misuse of alcohol and drugs, improved nutrition, exercise and fitness, and stress control. Health promotion is different from disease prevention; the focus is not on avoiding any one specific disease or health problem

(Laffrey et al., 1986; Pender, 1987). Rather, the concern is with increasing well-being and quality of life relative to self-identified goals. Brubaker (1983) defines health promotion as:

. . . health care directed toward high-level wellness through processes that encourage alteration of personal habits or the environment in which people live. It occurs after health stability is present and assumes disease prevention and health maintenance as prerequisites or byproducts (p. 12).

Similarly, Pender (1987) states:

Health promotion consists of activities directed toward increasing the level of well being and actualizing the health potential of individuals, families, communities, and society (p. 4).

Families perform a number of functions that contribute directly and indirectly to health promotion. Affection among family members provides a nurturing emotional climate that contributes to healthy growth and development and growth of personal competence. A sense of cohesiveness and nurturance in families has been found to be related to health promotion behaviors and healthy outcomes (Loveland-Cherry, 1983; Beavers, 1977). Maintaining morale and motivation are related aspects of this function that have obvious implications for health promotion.

Families also provide for socialization of family members and subsequent placement within the society in which they live. In this way families transmit their cultural heritage, goals, values, attitudes, and patterns of behavior, including those relevant to health. Both the definitions of and the value placed on health and well-being are developed largely within the context of the family, beginning early in childhood. Both definitions of health and the importance, or value, of health have been identified as important variables related to participation in health-promoting behaviors (Laffrey, 1985; Pender, 1987; Wallston et al., 1976). The type of family socialization practices, specifically the type of childrearing methods, has been demonstrated to be related not only to children's health promoting behaviors but also to those of parents (Loveland-Cherry, 1986; Pratt, 1976; Baranowski & Nader, 1985). Positive relationships between supportive child-rearing methods and health-promoting personal health practices have been found (Pratt, 1976), as well as a negative relationship between mothers' use of aversive control and children's, mothers', and total family health practices (Loveland-Cherry, 1986). Further, Pratt (1976) found positive relationships between health training efforts by parents and family members' health-promoting personal health practices. Families also monitor and provide information from a variety of media that relates to health promotion knowledge.

The function of physical maintenance includes the provision of shelter, food, clothing, and health care. The family is largely responsible for the nutritional habits and status of family members. Adequate shelter influences the comfort, opportunities for privacy and interaction, and rest and relaxation of family members. Having these needs met, in turn, influences the energy levels available for meeting self-actualizing goals.

The family both provides and regulates economic resources required to meet basic needs and support activities that foster health promotion and health protection. Family decisions on resource allocation are based both on necessity and on values. Expenditures on certain activities or purchases that might at first seem frivolous may contribute to the overall well-being of the family by providing for aesthetic needs.

Families function to monitor not only internal interactions but also interactions with social, cultural, political, educational, and other systems. The extent of participation in organizations and activities outside the family, especially for children, has been demonstrated to be related positively to health-promoting behaviors (Loveland-Cherry, 1986; Pratt, 1976).

Models for Family Health Promotion

Models for health promotion have been developed primarily with the focus on individuals, as have definitions of health. The knowledge base for understanding family health promotion is still in the formative stage. A preliminary model based on Pender's revised model for health-promoting behavior and family theory and research is presented in Figure 2–1. It is offered as a beginning point for articulating an understanding of family health promotion.

Although the importance of family health promotion has been emphasized, little documentation of intervention strategies or their effectiveness is evident. Pender (1986, 1987) proposes a series of strategies that are consistent with family theory and knowledge regarding healthy families and health promotion. These strategies offer a beginning point from which to implement and evaluate family health promotion strategies. They include value clarification, enhancement of interpersonal relationships and support systems, lifestyle review, and development of a family health promotion-protection plan. As the format in Figure 2–2 illustrates, the family health promotion-protection plan provides a method for identifying family health goals and monitoring progress toward meeting them. Reports of family interventions to promote diet and exercise behavior indicate some limited success (Simons-Morton et al., 1986; Sunseri et al., 1984; Allendorf et al., 1985; Johnson et al., 1987; Nader et al., 1992). This is an area with tremendous opportunities for the development and testing of nursing interventions.

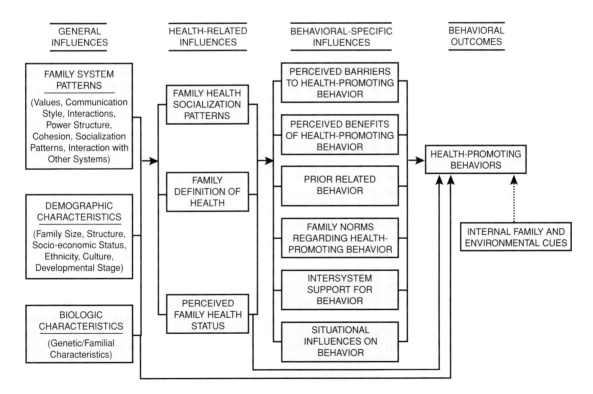

FIGURE 2–1. Family health promotion model.

Designed for (Family Name) _____

Family Form: _____

Family Members:

NAME	SEX	POSITION IN FAMILY	BIRTH DATE	OCCUPATION (IF EMPLOYED)
_____	__	_____	____	_____
_____	__	_____	____	_____
_____	__	_____	____	_____
_____	__	_____	____	_____
_____	__	_____	____	_____

Home Address: _____

Home Telephone: _____

Work Telephone Number: _____

Cultural Background: _____

Spiritual–Religious Orientation: _____

Type of Housing: _____

Major Formal Roles of Family Members: _____

_____

Community Affiliations of Family: _____

_____

Communication Patterns (Verbal and nonverbal, including expression of caring/affection):

Family Decision-Making Patterns

Family Values with Highest Rank:

1. _____
2. _____
3. _____
4. _____
5. _____

Rank Order of Health as a Value (if not listed above):

_____

Value Conflicts in Family (if any):

Goals Important to Family:

MUTUAL GOAL OR SPECIFIC TO DYAD (D) OR TRIAD (T)

_____	_____
_____	_____
_____	_____
_____	_____

Family Strengths:

Major Sources of Stress for Family and Perceived Ability to Deal with Stressors:

Current or Recent Family Developmental or Situational Transitions:

Family Concerns or Challenges:

Family Self-Care Patterns

Current Health Protecting or Preventive Behaviors (e.g., immunization, self-examination, periodic screening/examination by health professionals, avoidance of toxic exposure, use of seat belts):

Current Health-Promoting Behaviors (Life Style Review):
Nutritional Practices:

Physical–Recreational Activities:

Sleep–Relaxation Patterns:

Stress Management:

Family Sense of Purpose:

Family Actualization Efforts:

Relationships in Family and with Others:

Environmental Control:

Information-Seeking Patterns of Family in Relation to Health Promotion:

Use of Health-Promotion Facilities or Services by Family:

Other Behaviors:

Consistency Among Family Values, Goals, and Health Actions:

Family Health Goals

GOALS	FAMILY PRIORITY (1 = MOST IMPORTANT)

Areas for Improvement in Family Health

Target Health Goal:

AREA OF CHANGE (SEE CATEGORIES UNDER FAMILY SELF-CARE PATTERNS)	SPECIFIC BEHAVIOR CHANGE	FAMILY PRIORITY (1 = MOST DESIRABLE)	APPROACHES SELECTED TO FACILITATE FAMILY CHANGE

Evaluation of Progress Toward Change in Family Life Style

Two weeks:

One month:

Three months:

Six months:

One year:

FIGURE 2–2. Format for a family health promotion-protection plan. (Reprinted with permission from Pender N.J. (1987). *Health Promotion in Nursing Practice* (2nd ed.) Norwalk, CT: Appleton & Lange.)

HEALTH PROTECTION AND THE FAMILY

In contrast to health promotion, health protection emphasizes maintaining a state of wellness or health by decreasing the risks of specific conditions. Thus, activities in this arena are disease or condition specific. Pender (1986), who prefers the use of "health protecting" behaviors, offers the following definition:

The primary goal of health protection is the removal or avoidance of encumbrances throughout the life cycle that may prevent the emergence of optimum health. . . .

Prevention is a defensive posture or set of actions that ward off specific illness conditions or their sequelae that threaten the quality of life or longevity" (p. 38).

All of the family functions examined relative to health promotion are also relevant to health protection. Families provide information and resources, make decisions, set goals and priorities, and develop attitudes and behaviors regarding health protection. Content on specific family protective health behaviors is presented in Chapter 18.

Use of Professional Services

An important aspect of health care for which the family has primary responsibility is the use of professional services aimed toward maintaining health and preventing disease or debilitating conditions. These services include family planning, prenatal care, well-child care, immunizations, dental care, routine physical examinations, mammograms and pap tests for women, and rehabilitative care. The family makes and implements decisions regarding not only the use of economic resources but also those of time and effort. The role of the family in the use of services has been studied extensively, but the use of preventive services is somewhat more limited. The most well-developed and widely used model for examining families' use of services was developed by Andersen and his colleagues (Andersen, 1968; Andersen & Newman, 1973; Andersen & Aday, 1978). Andersen (1968) delineated three major categories of variables that contribute to the use of health services. The first category, labeled *predisposing conditions,* includes family composition (age, sex, and marital status of head of the family; family size (and ages of the youngest and oldest members of the family); family social structure (employment, education, social class, and occupation of wage earner; race; and ethnicity); and family health beliefs. *Enabling factors,* the second component, include family resources (family income, family savings, health insurance, regular source of care, and welfare care) and community resources (availability of services in the community in which the family lives). The final component, *need factors,* includes the amount of illness perceived by the family (health level, symptoms, disability days) and response (seeking care for symptoms and regular physical examinations).

Results of a study to test the model (Andersen, 1968) indicate that larger, younger families and families with a well-educated main wage earner employed full time in a high prestige occupation tend to use more services. Health beliefs, such as the value of health services, were also related to service use but not as strongly as other predispos-

ing variables. Further, families with higher income, health insurance, a regular source of care, or access to welfare care used more services. However, the need component (the family's perception of symptoms, disability days, and health level) was a major correlate of service use. The model continues to be used and modified by researchers in the area (Bass & Noelker, 1987; Wolinsky et al., 1983). Use of preventive services has also been linked to family social networks, stage in the family life cycle, the mother's education, parents' health training efforts, parents' health status, and family interaction patterns (Litman, 1974; Pratt, 1976). In a comparison of high and low clinic care use (Weimer et al., 1983), high-use families characterized themselves as being less expressive, being more achievement oriented, having more parental control, and having less social activity than low-use families. In addition, children in high-use families reported greater moral and religious concern and less independence.

Risk Behaviors

The family plays an important role in the participation or nonparticipation in risk behaviors. There is evidence that both perceived and received support from the family is positively related to pregnant women's nonparticipation in smoking, alcohol consumption, and caffeine consumption (Aaronson, 1989). Adolescents' participation in the risk behaviors of cigarette, alcohol, and marijuana use also has been examined from the perspective of the family (McCubbin et al., 1985). Interestingly, parents may underestimate the percentage of adolescents who smoke cigarettes (Cohen, Felix, & Brownell, 1989). Family problem solving was negatively related to adolescent health risk behaviors, and family stressors and strains were positively related to adolescent health risk behaviors. Adolescent health risk behaviors also have been related to parents' education, occupation, and religious group; to home climate—maternal affection and control; to parental beliefs, supports, and controls; to parental approval; to family closeness; to parental monitoring and enforcement of rules; to parental involvement in the child's activities; and to parental substance use (Jessor, 1984; Dielman et al., 1990–1991).

Self-Care in Chronic Illness

Another area of health protection is the self-care responsibility needed by families to carry out treatment regimens for chronic illness in order to prevent further disability. Family characteristics influence how individuals view their health, including chronic conditions, and how competent they view themselves to be in caring for their health. In a study of home treatment for children with cystic fibrosis (Patterson, 1985), family stress was not significantly related to compliance; family expressiveness was positively related to family compliance; and active recreation orientation was negatively related to family compliance. A family emphasis on independence, participation in social/recreational activities, and organization were positively related to perceived competence by children with diabetes (Hauser et al., 1985). Further, children's adjustment to diabetes was related to a family emphasis on independence, achievement, intellectual/cultural orientation, religious/moral orientation, recreational activities, cohesion, and organization (Hauser et al., 1985). In another study of adolescents with diabetes, adolescents with good metabolic control reported more cohesion and less conflict among family members, and their parents reported more encouragement of independence (Anderson et al., 1981). Good metabolic control in adults with diabetes was associated with reports of families low in conflict and organization and oriented toward achievement (Edelstein & Linn, 1985). The effects of family organization may differ for individuals at different developmental stages. More positive outcomes have been associated with higher levels for adolescents but with lower levels for adults. Thus, it would appear that families characterized by flexibility, cohesion, support, goal direction, independence, and low levels of conflict may be more effective in dealing with the experience of chronic disease.

Lifestyle Changes

Lifestyles are important factors that contribute to health protection. Family influences on eating and exercise patterns are related to the avoidance of specific conditions, such as cardiovascular disease, as well as to health promotion. African-American women with hypertension report family barriers to adherence to lifestyle changes that control and reduce hypertension include: stressors of care giving of children, ill parents, and/or spouses; worry about adolescent and adult children; finances; family eating patterns; and lack of social support for lifestyle changes (Bomar, 1995). Positive diet and exercise behaviors have been related to other family members' behaviors in these areas, health training efforts by parents, promotion of autonomy, cohesiveness, participation in the community, and family interactions (Loveland-Cherry, 1982; Pratt, 1976).

The documented relationship between diet and exercise and cardiovascular health/disease has led to a variety of prevention interventions directed at changing these behaviors through the family unit (Simons-Morton et al., 1986; Perry et al., 1988; Perry et al., 1989). Baranowski et al. (1985) found that behaviors can be changed through family communication and support; however, families need assistance in learning these

supportive behaviors. Chapters 13–16 discuss family lifestyles that influence family health protection as well as family health promotion.

The importance of families in health protection is well established. Historically, nursing, especially community health nursing, has intervened with families in this arena, using such techniques as anticipatory guidance and health education. Unfortunately, the efficacy of these interventions has not been systematically documented nor communicated.

INFLUENCES ON FAMILY HEALTH

A number of factors influence family health and the actions families take to promote and maintain health and to prevent disease. Families do not exist in isolation; they interact with an array of religious, cultural, social, political, and scientific systems. An understanding of the implications of these interactions for family health is critical to planning effective interventions.

Religious Influences

Religion affects family health by providing an important source of social support, both tangible and intangible; by shaping family values, goals, and socialization practices; and by influencing health-related behaviors (Bringman, 1992). A number of religions, such as the Jewish, Mormon and Muslim faiths, have dietary restrictions that need to be considered in working with families to plan nutritious and therapeutic diets that will be acceptable. Religious beliefs will also influence not only how family planning is viewed but also behavior during pregnancy and childbearing and childrearing practices, including seeking preventive health care. The belief that a higher being is in control may negatively influence a family's participation in a variety of health promotion and health protection practices. For example, some religions discourage the use of medications. It is important to determine the nature and extent of religious involvement with the family and not to assume that identification with a specific faith has the same implications for all families. Chapter 11 in this text explores in more depth family religion and the influence on family health.

Cultural Influences

The American population is a mix of racial and ethnic groups. Major ethnic family subgroups include Native-American, African-American, Asian-American, Mexican-American, Hispanic, and Middle Eastern. This is not to discount the numerous European groups who constituted the early major immigrations to the United States.

These groups are based on common beliefs, values, norms, ancestry, language, nationality, and behaviors. Definitions of health, health values, attitudes, and practices vary among cultural groups. Cultural norms and values influence all spheres of family life. An assessment and understanding of the cultural and ethnic background of families is a critical element of health intervention. It is important, however, to be aware that acculturation does occur and that there is diversity within subgroups. Therefore, it is important that generalizations from one family to another within any cultural group be done with caution in order to avoid stereotyping and making inappropriate assumptions. The potential conflict of the formal health care systems and folk medicine is well recognized; how these two systems can complement each other to provide holistic health care is still in preliminary stages. The reader is referred to Chapter 5 for a more in-depth discussion of family culture and ethnicity.

Social Influences

A number of social changes have had significant impact on the family and family health. The very structure of families has changed: The variations in family form include single-parent families, dual-career families, blended families, lesbian and gay domestic partners with and without children, unmarried and married couples with and without children, multigeneration families, and traditional nuclear families. As societal values and norms change, so do the dominant family forms. Increasingly, it is recognized and acknowledged that no one family form is "good" or "bad," "better" or "worse," "functional" or "dysfunctional"; they are different and unique. Although the United States is a rich country with a high standard of living, tremendous inequalities continue to exist. A two-tiered health care system is increasingly evident, with one set of resources available to those who can afford them and another to those who cannot. Within the latter group, one subgroup qualifies for subsidized services and a second does not. This last group has increased in numbers and is of increasing concern.

Our society has grown smaller, in one sense, because of the impact of the media. Now, as never before, families are exposed to a barrage of information on alternative lifestyles, health practices and products, health care options, and divergent opinions and attitudes. Other social groups, formal and informal, perform functions previously designated to the family, such as health education, sexuality information, and socialization. Chapter 9 discusses the various dimensions of internal and external family social support. The increase in the longevity in the population has created both advantages and burdens for families. The increase in multigeneration families has in-

creased social support available to families on the one hand and has increased the burden of caring for elderly family members on the other. The negative effect of some of these social changes is evident in increased levels of substance abuse, adolescent pregnancy, homelessness, family violence, and divorce. Dealing with the stress and frustration of social changes presents challenges to both families and health professionals in promoting and maintaining family health. Chapters 10 and 14 present information on stress theory and family stress management.

Political Influences

Although the United States has no national policy related to families, family health is affected by the numerous policy and funding decisions made at local, state, and national levels (see Chap. 21). For example, the shift to increased home health care with increased levels of acuity has placed tremendous burdens on families who provide this care. Part of this shift is accounted for by the institution of a prospective reimbursement system for hospital care based on diagnostic related groups (DRGs). Changes in government programs providing support to families, such as nutritional supplements or medical care, in conjunction with the fluctuating economy, present uncertainty and concern for the health of a growing number of families. Although increasing recognition is given to the importance of health promotion and health protection, commitment of government programs continues to be primarily reactionary, with the emphasis on illness care.

Until recently, government programs were primarily reactionary, with the emphasis on illness care. Although attempts at legislative action to bring about national health care reform during the early stages (1994) of the Clinton administration failed, major shifts in resources from illness care to primary care are occurring. There are national priorities for preparation of primary health providers versus specialists. Increasingly, health promotion/risk reduction services and programs are available through managed care systems. The viability of these changes and their impact on the health of the population are yet to be determined.

Scientific Influences

Sanitary, medical, and technologic advances have decreased morbidity and mortality from communicable and infectious diseases. Consequently, the major causes of morbidity and mortality in this country are related chronic diseases and lifestyle-related conditions. Furthermore, infants are now surviving premature birth and its consequences and congenital and birth-related conditions. Coupled with increasing life expectancy, the dependent portion of the population is increasing. Families continue to provide care to these segments of the population. These demands compete with responsibilities for promoting and maintaining family health. However, the increasing knowledge regarding health promotion and health protection provides increasing options to families for promoting and maintaining their health.

THE ROLE OF THE NURSE IN FAMILY HEALTH PROMOTION

Nursing has a long, rich history both of working with families and of promoting and maintaining health. As a professional group, nursing has accumulated considerable experience with and knowledge about families and health promotion. However, the profession has been slow in articulating and communicating that knowledge to other nurses, other professionals, and consumers.

Family health promotion requires a *collaborative* effort on the part of the family and the nurses. This means that the responsibility is shared and that competencies of both families and nurses are recognized and used. The nurse may function in a number of roles. First, families often need assistance in *assessing* their current health status and appropriate health goals. This can and should be done collaboratively with the family and any other appropriate professionals. The assessment should include a review of family lifestyle, identifying both strengths in family patterns and areas for modification.

Second, the nurse can function as a *client advocate* to assist families to deal with complex systems, to assist families to identify and use community resources, and to act as a liaison between families and community systems. Additionally, this advocacy can be expanded to include working for social and policy change that will support and promote family health.

Health education is another important role; however, to be effective, it must entail more than "information giving." It implies a role in assisting families to identify and evaluate options, as well as assisting families to use health knowledge effectively. Health education areas in which nurses can work with families to promote health include teaching risk behaviors, developing parenting skills with children of different ages, teaching developmental milestones across the life span, developing coping strategies, and facilitating communication patterns to improve marital health and family interaction.

Rankin and Duffy (1983) have developed a comprehensive approach to patient-family education that emphasizes the importance of including the family in all phases of the educational process. The approach is based in a systems theory framework and assesses four aspects of the "family profile": (1) family education, lifestyles, and beliefs;

(2) family understanding of actual or potential health problems; (3) family functioning; and (4) resources available to the family (p. 21).

Other nursing roles include intervening by assisting families to identify their strengths and self-care competencies; working with families to establish goals and priorities for change and growth; and formulating with families plans for lifestyle modification. Pender's (1987) family health promotion-protection plan provides a format for reviewing family lifestyle as well as for planning lifestyle modification and monitoring progress toward identified goals. Just as in working with individuals, it is important that nurses use a systematic approach in intervening with families for health promotion. The family nursing process, which is discussed in detail in Chapter 12, provides an organizing framework for assessing family health and planning and for implementing and evaluating health promotion interventions. Based on the conceptualization of family health estate described earlier, it is important that the entire family be involved at all stages of the health promotion plan.

Family health promotion both continues and varies over the life span. Much of the interest in family health promotion has focused on the growing family with considerable attention given to childbearing and parenting skills with children of various ages. Indeed, the early stages of family development are crucial to the formation of family patterns that affect health attitudes, values, and behaviors. However, recognition of the continuing need for and changing nature of family health promotion has prompted increased attention to families in the child-launching, empty nest, and aging stages. Nursing intervention for family health promotion in the later stages of the family life span are not as well defined as those for earlier stages and warrant increased attention.

In addition to the intervention role, nurses have a role in conducting *research* in family health promotion, which will contribute to building a sound knowledge base for developing interventions and influencing policy formation. Examples of potential areas for research include delineating specific health promotion tasks and needs for families at various points in the family life span and evaluating the impact of nursing interventions for family health promotion. The nurse knowledgeable in family health promotion can also function as a consultant to community groups, other professionals, and legislators. As important is the need for nursing to articulate the resulting knowledge and communicate it (Gillis & Davis, 1993). Last, the family nurse must be a role model in the area of health promotion and health protection.

Nursing has an important role in health promotion across the life span of the family. The remaining chapters in this book offer both the theoretical bases and the nursing processes for effective family health promotion.

CHAPTER HIGHLIGHTS

The health of the family is influenced by the health of its members and influences the health of the members.

Conceptual definitions of family health are varied (theoretical, clinical, and family).

Key ideas from definitions indicate that family health is greater than the sum of the health of its members; a systems process that is dynamic, ranging from functional to dysfunctional; and influenced by multiple and complex variables.

Family health is defined as a dynamic process that includes the activities a family uses to promote and protect the well-being of the family as a unit and the individual family members.

Promoting and protecting the health of the family unit is in the formative stages; therefore, health professionals have challenging opportunities to develop and test interventions in family health promotion.

The Family Health Promotion Model illustrates that complex multiple factors influence a family's health promoting outcomes.

The role of the nurse in family health promotion includes assessment and intervention with families, collaboration with other families and other professionals, anticipatory guidance and family education, researching and building a knowledge base for family health promotion, and dissemination of family nursing outcomes and research findings.

REFERENCES

Aaronson, L.S. (1989). Perceived and received support: Effects on health behavior during pregnancy. *Nursing Research,* 38(1), 4–9.

Aldous, J. (1978). *Family Careers: Developmental Change in Families.* New York: Wiley.

Allendorff, S., Sunseri, A.J., Cullinan, J., & Oman, J.K. (1985). Student heart health knowledge, smoking attitudes, and self-esteem. *Journal of School Health,* 55(5), 196–199.

Andersen, R. (1968). *A Behavioral Model of Families' Use of Health Services.* Center for Health Administration Studies, Graduate School of Business, The University of Chicago, Research Series 25.

Andersen, R. & Aday, L.A. (1978). Access to medical care in the U.S.: Realized and potential. *Medical Care,* 16, 533–546.

Andersen, R., & Kasper, J.D. (1973). The structural influence of family size on children's use of physician services. *Journal of Comparative Family Studies,* 4, 116–130.

Andersen, R., & Newman, J.F. (1973). Societal and individual determinants of medical care utilization in the United States. *The Milbank Quarterly,* 51, 95–124.

Anderson, B.J., Miller, J.P., Auslander, W.F., & Santiago, J.V. (1981). Family characteristics of diabetic adolescents: Relationship to metabolic control. *Diabetes Care,* 4(6), 586–594.

Anderson, K.H. & Tomlinson, P.S. (1992). The family health system as an emerging paradigmatic view of nursing. *Image,* 24(1), 57–63.

Baranowski, T. & Nader, P.R. (1985). Family health behavior. In D.C. Turk & R.D. Kerns (Eds.), *Health, Illness, and Families* (51–77). New York: Wiley.

Bass, D.M., & Noelker, L.S. (1987). The influence of family caregivers on elder's use of in-home services: An expanded conceptual framework. *Journal of Health and Social Behavior,* 28, 184–196.

Beavers, W.R. (1977). *Psychotherapy and Growth: A Family Systems Perspective.* New York: Brunner/Mazel.

Beavers, W.R. (1982). Healthy, midrange and severely dysfunctional families. In F. Walsh (Ed.), *Normal Family Processes.* New York: Guilford Press.

Beavers, W.R., & Voeller, M.N. (1983). Family models: Comparing and contrasting the Olson circumplex model with the Beavers systems model. *Family Process,* 22(1), 85–98.

Boardman, V. (1973). School absence, illness, and family competence (Doctoral dissertation, Department of Epidemiology, University of North Carolina, Chapel Hill, 1972). *Dissertation Abstracts International,* 33, 3748B. (University Microfilms No. 73-4802).

Bomar, P.J. (1995). Barriers to health regimens for African-American with hypertension. In J.F. Wang (Ed.), *Proceedings of the Second International and Interdisciplinary Health Research Symposium: Health Care and Culture* (pp. 197–205). Morgantown, WV: Department of Health Systems, School of Nursing, West Virginia University.

Bomar, P. (1990). Perspectives on family health promotion. *Family & Community Health,* 12(4), 1–11.

Bringman, K.M.L. (1992). Religion and family strengths: Implications for mental health professionals. *Topics in Family Psychology and Counseling.* 1(1), 39–52.

Broderick, C.B. (1971). Beyond the five conceptual frameworks: A decade of development in family theory. *Journal of Marriage and the Family,* 33, 139–159.

Brubaker, B.H. (1983). Health promotion: A linguistic analysis. *Advances in Nursing Science,* 5(3), 1–14.

Burr, W.R., Klein, S.K. et al. (1994). *Reexamining Family Stress: New Theory and Research.* Thousand Oaks, CA: Sage.

Chin, S. (1985). Can self-care theory be applied to families? In J. Riehl-Sisca (Ed.), *The Science and Art of Self-Care.* Norwalk, CT: Appleton-Century-Crofts.

Clements, I.W., & Roberts, F.B. (Eds.). (1983). *Family Health: A Theoretical Approach to Nursing Care.* New York: Wiley.

Cohen, R.Y., Felix, M.R.J., & Brownell, K.D. (1989). The role of parents and older peers in school-based cardiovascular prevention programs: Implications for program development. *Health Education Quarterly,* 16(2), 245–253.

Curran, D. (1983). *Traits of a Healthy Family.* Minneapolis: Winston.

Danielson, C.B., Hamel-Bissell, B., & Winsted-Fry, P. (Eds.) (1993). *Families, Health, and Illness. Perspec-*

tives on Coping and Intervention. St. Louis, MO: Mosby.

Dielman, T.E., Butchart, A.T., Shope, J.T., & Miller, M. (1990–1991). Environmental correlates of adolescent substance use and misuse: Implications for prevention programs. *Journal of the Addictions,* 25(7A & 8A), 855–880.

Doherty, W.J. & Campbell, T.J. (1989). *Families and Health.* Newbury Park, CA: Sage.

Doherty, W.J. & McCubbin, H.I. (1985). Families and health care: An emerging arena of theory, research, and clinical intervention. *Family Relations,* 34, 5–11.

Donnelly, E. (1990). Health promotion, families, and the diagnostic process. *Family & Community Health,* 12(4), 12–20.

Duffy, M.E. (1988). Health promotion in the family: Current findings and directives for nursing research. *Journal of Advanced Nursing,* 13, 109–117.

Dunn, H.L. (1961). *High-Level Wellness.* Arlington, VA: R.W. Beatty.

Dunn, H.L. (1975). Points of attack for raising the level of wellness. *Journal of the National Medical Association,* 49, 223–235.

Duvall, E.M., & Miller, B.C. (1985). *Marriage and Family Development* (6th ed). New York: Harper & Row.

Edelstein, J., & Linn, M.W. (1985). The influence of the family on control of diabetes. *Social Science and Medicine,* 21(5), 541–544.

Erickson, H.C., Tomlin, E.M., & Swain, M.A. (1983). *Modeling and Role-Modeling: A Theory and Paradigm for Nursing.* Englewood Cliffs, NJ: Prentice-Hall.

Eshleman, J.R. (1981). *The Family: An Introduction* (3rd ed.). Boston: Allyn & Bacon.

Fawcett, J. (1975). The family as a living open system: An emerging conceptual framework for nursing. *International Nursing Review,* 22, 113–116.

Ferguson, M. (1980). *The Aquarian Conspiracy: Personal and Social Transformation in the 1980s.* Los Angeles: J.P. Tarcher.

Fisher, L., Terry, H.E., & Ransom, D.C. (1990). Advancing a family perspective in health research: Models and methods. *Family Process,* 29, 177–189.

Gillis, C.L., & Davis, L.L. (1993). Does family intervention make a difference? An intergrative review and meta-analysis. In S.L. Feetam, S.B. Meister, J.M. Bell, & C.L. Gillis (Eds.), *The Nursing of Families: Theory, Research, Education, and Practice* (pp. 259–265). Newbury Park, CA: Sage.

Gilliss, C.L. (1989). Why family health care? In C.L. Gilliss, B.L. Highley, B.M. Roberts, & I.M. Martinson (Eds.), *Toward a Science of Family Nursing* (pp. 3–8), Menlo Park, CA: Addison-Wesley.

Gonot, P.W. (1986). Family therapy as derived from King's conceptual model. In A.L. Whall (Ed.), *Family Therapy Theory for Nursing: Four Approaches.* Norwalk, CT: Appleton-Century-Crofts.

Green, L.W., & Kreuter, M.W. (1991). *Health Promotion Planning: An Education and Environmental Approach* (2nd ed., pp. 1–43). Mountain View, CA: Mayfield.

Hanson, J. (1984). The family. In C. Roy (Ed.), *Introduction to Nursing: An Adaptation Model* (2nd ed.). Englewood Cliffs, NJ: Prentice-Hall.

Hauser, S.T., Jacobson, A.M., Wertlieb, D., Brink, S., & Wentworth, S. (1985). The contribution of family environment to perceived competence and illness adjustment in diabetic and acutely ill adolescents. *Family Relations,* 34, 99–108.

Hill, R. (1958). Generic features of families under stress. *Social Casework,* 39, 139–156.

Hill, R., & Mattessich, P. (1979). Family development theory and life span development. In P.B. Baltes & O.G. Brim, Jr. (Eds.), *Life Span Development and Behavior* (Vol. 2). New York: Academic Press.

Hook, N.C., & Paolucci, B. (1970). The family as an ecosystem. *Journal of Home Economics,* 62(5), 315–318.

Jessor, R. (1984). Adolescent development and behavioral health. In J.D. Matarazzo, S.M. Weiss, J.A. Herd, N.E. Miller, & S.M. Weiss (Eds.), *Behavioral Health: A Handbook of Health Enhancement and Disease Prevention.* New York: Wiley.

Johnson, C.C., Nicklas, T.A., Arbeit, M.L., Franklin, F.A., Cresanta, J.L., Harsha, D.W., & Berenson, G.S. (1987). Cardiovascular risk in parents of children with elevated blood pressure. *Journal of Clinical Hypertension,* 3, 559–566.

Johnston, R.L. (1986). Approaching family intervention through Rogers' conceptual model. In A.L. Whall (Ed.), *Family Therapy Theory for Nursing: Four Approaches.* Norwalk, CT: Appleton-Century-Crofts.

Kantor, D.H., & Lehr, W. (1975). *Inside the Family: Toward a Theory of Family Process.* San Francisco: Jossey-Bass.

King, I.M. (1981). *A Theory for Nursing.* New York: Wiley.

Laffrey, S.C. (1985). Health promotion: Relevance for nursing. *Topics in Clinical Nursing,* 7(2), 29–38.

Laffrey, S.C., Loveland-Cherry, C.J., & Winkler, S.J. (1986). Health behavior: Evolution of two paradigms. *Public Health Nursing,* 3(2), 92–100.

Lewis, J.M., Beavers, W.R., Gossett, J.T., & Phillips, V.A. (1976). *No Single Thread: Psychological Health in Family Systems.* New York: Brunner/Mazel.

Litman, T.J. (1974). The family as a basic unit in health and medical care: A social behavioral overview. *Social Science and Medicine,* 8, 495–519.

Loveland-Cherry, C.J. (1983). Family system patterns of cohesiveness and autonomy: Relationship to family members' health behavior. (Doctoral dissertation, Wayne State University, 1982). *Dissertation Abstracts International,* 43, 43–11B, 35–37.

Loveland-Cherry, C.J. (1985, April). Toward a definition of family health. Paper presented at the meeting of the Midwest Nursing Research Society, Minneapolis, MN.

Loveland-Cherry, C.J. (1986). Personal health practices in single parent and two parent families. *Family Relations,* 35(1), 133–139.

Mauksch, H.O. (1974). A social science basis for conceptualizing family health. *Social Science and Medicine,* 8, 521–528.

McCubbin, M. (1989). Family stress and family strengths: A comparison of single- and two-parent families with handicapped children. *Research in Nursing and Health,* 12, 101–110.

McCubbin, H.I. & M.A. (1993). Families coping with illness: The resiliency model of family stress adjustment and adaptation. In C.B. Danielson, B. Hamel-Bissell & P. Winsted-Fry (Eds.), *Families, Health, and Illness. Perspectives on Coping and Intervention* (pp. 21–63). St. Louis, MO: Mosby.

McCubbin, H.I., Needle, R.H., & Wilson, M. (1985). Adolescent health risk behaviors: Family stress and adolescent coping as critical factors. *Family Relations,* 34, 51–62.

McCubbin, H.I., & Patterson, J.M. (1982). Family adaptation to crises. In H.I. McCubbin, A.E. Cauble, & J.M. Patterson (Eds.), *Family Stress, Coping, and Social Support*. Springfield, IL: Charles C. Thomas.

McGoldrick, M., & Carter, E.A. (1982). The family life cycle. In F. Walsh (Ed.), *Normal Family Processes*. New York: Guilford Press.

Moos, R.H., & Moos, B.S.A. (1976). A typology of family social environments. *Family Process*, 15, 357–371.

Nader, P.R., Sallis, J.F., Abramson, I.S., Broyles, S.L., Patterson, T.L., Senn, K., Rupp, J.W., Nelson, J.A. (1992). Family-based cardiovascular risk reduction among Mexican- and Anglo-Americans. *Family and Community Health*, 15(1), 57–74.

Nader, P.R., Sallis, J.F., Patterson, T.L., Abramson, I.S., Rupp, J.W., Senn, K.L., Atkins, C.J., Roppe, B.E., Morris, J.A., Wallace, J.P., & Vega, W.A. (1989). A family approach to cardiovascular risk reduction: Results from the San Diego Family Health Project. *Health Education Quarterly*, 16(2), 229–244.

Neuman, B. (1989). *The Neuman Systems Model. Application to Nursing Education and Practice* (2nd ed.). Norwalk, CT: Appleton & Lange.

Neuman, B. (1982). *The Neuman Systems Model: Applications to Nursing Education and Practice*. New York: Appleton-Century-Crofts.

Nightingale, E., Cureton, M., Kalmar, V., & Trudeau, M. (1980). *Perspectives on Health Promotion and Disease: Prevention in the United States*. Ann Arbor, MI: University Microfilms International.

Olson, D. (1989). Circumplex model and family health. In C.N. Ramsey Jr. (Ed.), *The Science of Family Medicine* (pp. 75–94) New York: The Guilford Press.

Olson, D., Sprenkle, D., & Russell, C. (1979). Circumplex model of marital and family systems: 1. Cohesion and adaptability dimensions, family types, and clinical applications. *Family Process*, 18, 3–28.

Orem, D.E. (1995). *Nursing: Concepts of Practice* (5th ed.). New York: McGraw-Hill.

Patterson, J. (1985). Critical factors affecting family compliance with home treatment for children with cystic fibrosis. *Family Relations*, 34, 79–89.

Pender, N.J. (1986). Health promotion: Implementing strategies. In B.B. Logan and C.E. Dawkins (Eds.), *Family-Centered Nursing in the Community*. Menlo Park, CA: Addison-Wesley.

Pender, N.J. (1987). *Health Promotion in Nursing Practice* (2nd ed.). Norwalk, CT: Appleton & Lange.

Perry, C.L., Luepker, R.V., Murray, D.M., Hearn, M.D., Halper, A., Dudovitz, B., Maile, M.C., & Smyth, M. (1989). Parent involvement with children's health promotion: A one-year follow-up of the Minnesota Home Team. *Health Education Quarterly*, 16(2), 171–180.

Perry, C.L., Luepker, R.V., Murray, D.M., Kurth, C., Mullis, R., Crockett, S., & Jacobs, D.R. (1988). Parent involvement with children's health promotion: The Minnesota Home Team. *American Journal of Public Health*, 78(9), 1156–1160.

Petze, C.F. (1984). Health promotion for the well family. *Nursing Clinics of North America*, 19(2), 229–237.

Pless, I.B., & Satterwhite, B. (1973). A measure of family functioning and its application. *Social Science and Medicine*, 7, 613–621.

Pratt, L. (1976). *Family Structure and Effective Health Behavior*. Boston: Houghton-Mifflin.

Pridham, K.F., & Hansen, M. (1977). Anticipatory care as problem solving in family medicine and nursing. *Journal of Family Practice*, 4, 1077–1081.

Rankin, S.H., & Duffy, K.L. (1983). *Patient Education: Issues, Principles and Guidelines*. Philadelphia: Lippincott.

Roberts, C.S., & Feetham, S.L. (1983). Assessing family functioning across three areas of relationship. *Nursing Research*, 31, 231–235.

Rogers, M.E. (1970). *An Introduction to the Theoretical Basis of Nursing*. Philadelphia: F.A. Davis.

Roy, C. (1984). *Introduction to Nursing: An Adaptation Model* (2nd ed.). Englewood Cliffs, NJ: Prentice-Hall.

Simons-Morton, B.G., O'Hara, N.M., & Simons-Morton, D.G. (1986). Promoting healthful diet and exercise behaviors in communities, schools, and families. *Family and Community Health*, 9(3), 1–13.

Smilkstein, G. (1978). The family APGAR: A proposal for a family function test and its use by physicians. *The Journal of Family Practice*, 6(6), 1231–1239.

Smith, J.A. (1983). *The Idea of Health: Implications for the Nursing Professional*. New York: Teachers College Press, Columbia University.

Stacctchenko, S., & Jenicek, M. (1990). Conceptual differences between prevention and health promotion: Research implications for community health programs. *Canadian Journal of Public Health*, 81, 53–59.

Sunseri, A.J., Alberti, J.M., Kent, N.D., Schoenberger, J.A., & Dolecek, T.A. (1984). Ingredients in nutrition education: Family involvement, reading and race. *Journal of Occupational Safety and Health*, 54(5), 192–196.

Tadych, R. (1985). Nursing in multiperson units: The family. In J. Riehl-Sisca (Ed.), *The Science and Art of Self-care*. Norwalk, CT: Appleton-Century-Crofts.

Turk, D.C., & Kerns, R.D. (1985). The family in health and illness. In D.C. Turk & R.D. Kerns (Eds.), *Health, Illness, and Families* (pp. 1–22). New York: Wiley.

U.S. Department of Health, Education and Welfare. (1979). *Healthy People: The Surgeon General's Report on Health Promotion and Disease Prevention* (DHEW [PHS] Publication No. 79-55071). Washington, DC: U.S. Government Printing Office.

Wallston, K.A., Maides, S., & Wallston, B.S. (1976). Health-related information seeking as a function of health-related locus of control and health value. *Journal of Research in Personality*, 10, 215–222.

Walsh, F. (1982). Conceptualizations of normal family functioning. In F. Walsh (Ed.), *Normal Family Processes*. New York: Guilford Press.

Weimer, S.R., Hatcher, C., & Gould, E. (1983). Family characteristics in high and low health care utilization. *General Hospital Psychiatry*, 5(1), 55–61.

Whall, A.L. (1980). Congruence between existing theories of family functioning and nursing theories. *Advances in Nursing Science*, 3, 59–67.

Wolinsky, F.D., Coe, R.M., Miller, D.K., Prendergast, J.M., Creel, M.J., & Chevez, M.N. (1983). Health services utilization among the noninstitutionalized elderly. *Journal of Health and Social Behavior*, 24, 325–337.

Wright, L.M., & Leahey, M. (1994). *Nurses and Families* (2nd ed.). Philadelphia: F.A. Davis.

3

THE AMERICAN FAMILY: HISTORY AND DEVELOPMENT

KATHLEEN A. GROVE

A family is a link to the past, a bridge to the future.

ALEX HALEY

OBJECTIVES

On completion of this chapter, the reader will be able to:
1. Understand the premises of defining the family
2. Describe historical changes in the American family
3. Discuss how changing demographics will shape future families
4. Explain the dynamics of the stages of family development
5. Recognize nursing implications of current family styles

INTRODUCTION

An understanding of the historical evolvement of the American family is crucial to the examination of the family health nursing role in health promotion and health protection. There are similarities in families; however, nurses working with families must recognize that families also have unique differences in characteristics such as lifestyle, health behaviors, roles, interaction, power, social and kin networks, and financial management. Many disciplines such as sociology, psychology, anthropology, history, biology, ecology, behavioral health, religion, philosophy, nursing, and medicine have contributed to the knowledge base of the family as a unit. Family health nurses contribute to the understanding of families in their health behaviors through nursing research and application of nursing theories and related theories to nursing practice.

This chapter has three major sections. The first is a definition of family that reflects contemporary family types. The second section is a brief description of the historical changes that have affected American families, such as immigration, urbaniza-

tion, and industrialization. Modern American families are profoundly more diverse than in colonial times, and family roles have been shaped by changing demographics and advanced industrialization. In the third section, family developmental theory is highlighted. This chapter will enhance the reader's understanding of the dynamic American family as a health-promoting unit.

DEFINITION OF FAMILY

The term "family" has been variously defined. The federal government, through the Bureau of the Census publications, defines family as a "householder and one or more other persons living in the same household who are related to the householder by birth, marriage or adoption" (U.S. Bureau of the Census, 1990).

Friedman (1992) defines family as "two or more persons who are joined together by bonds of sharing and emotional closeness and who identify themselves as being a part of the family" (p. 9). Clements and Roberts (1983) consider a family to be "people related by blood or marriage, whether they reside in the same household or not" (p. 8). Strong and DeVault (1992) add that a family cooperates economically, may share a

In the first edition, this chapter was contributed by Kathleen Murphy Mallinger and revised for this second edition by Kathleen Grove.

36

common dwelling place, and may rear children (p. 7).

Throughout this book, the term "family" is defined as one or more individuals closely related by blood, marriage, or friendship. This definition is obviously broad: It would include cohabiting people of either sex, single parents and their children, and blended (step) families, as well as the stereotypical nuclear family. In addition, this definition is bound neither by residence (household) nor by age cohort (generation). Thus, "family" can refer to one's extended family of origin as well as to one's close friends. By using this broad definition of family, the family system becomes a dynamic, interrelated concept, not restricted by artificial legal or residential boundaries.

To restrict the definition of "family" to a legal (marriage), residential, or blood-related base would eliminate many of the different kinds of relatedness that actually exist. Legal bases for describing or defining the family are limited in at least two ways. First, there are legal gray areas for the family, such as surrogate mothering or "black market" adoption. Second, the legal system is an institution created for imposing order or settling disputes. With these political goals, the legal system doesn't necessarily correspond to the behaviors, affections, and relationships of many people in their definition of family.

Residential bases for defining the family are also inadequate. The term "household" is the appropriate term to define who lives with whom, not who is in one's family. Household composition is an important description long used by the Bureau of the Census and historical researchers. Studies of household changes may be used to describe social and economic trends. However, one's household is not one's family, just as one's brain is not one's mind.

There are inherent exclusions in legal, residential, or simple blood kin descriptions of "family." The blood or biologic base of family doesn't of necessity correspond to a person's affective ties. The definition of a family as one or more individuals closely related by blood, marriage, or friendship, although broad, is accurate because it takes into account the possible human matrices of relationships. Using this definition, the nurse would get a more accurate assessment of family interaction by asking the patient (client), "Who are you close to?" rather than "Who lives with you?" or "Who are your relatives?"

Family types and compositions are shown in Table 3–1.

As indicated in Table 3–1 and throughout this book, there is an effort to avoid biased terminology. In describing family types, certain words demonstrate what Roberts (Clements & Roberts, 1983, p. 6) calls "unexamined conceptions of an ideal family." For example, to describe a child living with a single parent as coming from a "broken" home infers that single-parent homes are not whole but inadequate or deviant. Idealization of a certain type of family may present problems in nursing practice. Being aware of one's own biases may permit a more thorough assessment of the actual advantages and disadvantages of a particular family situation.

HISTORY OF THE AMERICAN FAMILY

Social history focuses on the experiences, values, and daily living patterns of ordinary people. As nursing has expanded from a narrow interest in illness behavior to examine how family systems function to promote or diminish health, social history has turned from interest in wars, royalty, and epic events to examine how people live and how families experience and enact economic and cultural changes.

As there are preconceived and possibly negative perceptions of family styles, the term "American" is also one that has gathered many assumptions in its meaning. Although geographically incorrect, the term "American" in this chapter refers to those people who lived or live within the current boundaries of the United States. For the purposes

TABLE 3–1. FAMILY TYPES

FAMILY TYPE	COMPOSITION
Nuclear dyad	Married couple, no children
Nuclear	Husband, wife, and children (may or may not be legally married)
Binuclear	Two post-divorce families with children as members of both
Extended	Nuclear plus blood relatives
Blended	Husband, wife, and children of previous relationships
Single parent	One parent and child(ren)
Commune	Group of men, women, and children
Cohabitation (Domestic Partners)	Unmarried man and woman sharing a household
Homosexual couple	Same-gender couple
Single person (adult)	One person in a household

Data from Goldenberg, I. & Goldenberg, H. (1985). *Family Therapy: An Overview*. (p. 13). Monterey, CA: Brooks/Cole; and Rice, F.P. (1990). *Intimate Relationships, Marriages and Families*. (pp. 5–6). Mountain View, CA: Mayfield.

of this chapter, the author will use "American" to refer only to geographic locale, not to citizenship or to political attributes of people.

Early Americans: Precolonial and Colonial

Details of the family interactions and dynamics of the first "Americans" before the European invasion are limited by the lack of written records. There is, however, more detailed knowledge of European families since the Middle Ages. Stone (1975) describes the changes in European families that affected the first precolonial and colonial immigrants to the New World. From 1450 to 1630, the European family's loyalty was to the extended kin network, and privacy and individual autonomy were not important in daily family life. With the rise of kings and the nation-state, there was a gradual decline in kinship loyalties and an increase in individual (and family) privacy and geographic mobility, shown by the marked growth of the cities. Stone believes that by 1800 a more compassionate and egalitarian nuclear family was the dominant European family style.

Although this was the family style transferred to the New World, the new settlements were more isolated and vulnerable. Demos (1970) studied the records of the Plymouth Colony, including wills, court documents, and the census of 1698. He found that the nuclear family, with parents and children living together, was the dominant type. Although this settlement was united by a common religion, there were records of variations or disputes within norms. Divorces were granted for bigamy, willful desertion, and adultery. In addition, because the settlement was small, there was little privacy. But the small size of the community had its advantages, as families had a unified educational, religious, and economic welfare system.

It is likely that other homogeneous frontier communities were similar in family style. There was a sense of community welfare because the labor of every person was needed for survival; thus large families were valued. In these agricultural preindustrial communities, where the "workplace" was not widely separated from the residence, "housework" was an industry that was of primary importance for the economic functioning of the family. As bought goods were likely to be unavailable to preindustrial communities, the family "homework" of growing and preserving food; cooking; weaving; and making clothes, candles, and soap was a necessity.

The northeastern colonial records include a number of moral precepts or prescriptions for good family life, the most common found in sermons. Rothman and Rothman (1972) assembled a collection of these early American moral precepts for the family. There was controversy about the appropriateness of divorce, which was legal in some areas. There were guidelines for treating servants and educating children. Childrearing rules were promoted, and women were admonished, by Cotton Mather, in 1710, to breast-feed their children. This evidence indicates a preoccupation with manners and morality. Although these behavioral guidelines appear rigid, there were indications that the small homogeneous communities were changing. One change was the westward migration of families and communities.

Rutman's (1977) study of New Hampshire towns of the mid- and late-1700s describes a pattern of expanding communities. This pattern was marked by husbands leaving their wives and children and traveling to a newer, less populated area, usually in search of more or better farm land. Wives and children were likely to follow their husbands and fathers in a year or two and establish residence in the new town.

This pattern was similar to the later immigrant style of migrating fathers from Europe who were joined later by their spouses and children. It is likely that an extended absence of the father caused a shift in family dynamics as the mother assumed a larger parental role. After an extended paternal absence, the move from a known community with established friendships and routines may have caused further stress within the family. A similar process of extended paternal absence and frequent geographic moves affects our present day corporate executives, military families, and migrant laborers.

Hall (1977) describes the rise of related family members in business firms in Massachusetts in 1700–1850. When there were limited banking resources, extended family members (blood or marriage kin) were used to expand business. These relatives were used to provide investment capital and trustworthy associates. In the growing business sector, this arrangement provided financial support for business expansion and career training for those who supplied labor. Extended kin networks in businesses may be found in modern families. This dual relationship, family and business, may have financial and cultural advantages, particularly for new immigrant groups. However, this mix of family and business may also present greater strains if either component is stressed by other factors.

Family life changed as the economic base of the country moved from an agrarian base to an industrial one. However, this process was slow, as early industrialization in the United States began in the countryside, not in urban centers. At first, the early mills attracted young single women who had grown up on farms as workers (Dublin, 1979). Although industrialization began in the early 1800s, by the 1860s 80% of the population still lived on farms or in small towns (Blumin, 1977).

Blumin (1977) studied the demographics of three New York state towns, for the period 1800–1860. The three towns had different economic bases: early industrial, commercial, and agricultural. Blumin found that nuclear families made up the vast majority of family styles, comprising over 80% in all three areas. Rural agricultural areas tended to have large families. Some families, 13% to 15%, also lived with another relative, but a larger portion, 30% to 40%, were likely to have a nonrelated lodger or boarder living in their household. In rural areas, the boarders were likely to be foreign-born hired hands. The urban boarders were a more transient group, from lawyers to laborers, and a mix of foreign and native born. All boarders were likely to be men. The concept of boarders or lodgers may become popular today in areas with either limited housing or very expensive housing. The pattern of young adults sharing housing (roommates) is a modern example of the 19th-century lodgers.

Glasco's (1977) study of Buffalo in 1855 adds to the picture of the nuclear family as the dominant type, with about 20% of families having a live-in boarder or relative. Glasco describes slightly different patterns of family styles for German, Irish, and native-born families.

Gutman (1976) studied black family life in slavery and freedom from plantation records, letters, and Freedman's Bureau registration. He found evidence of long-term stable extended kin relationships, even when marriage partners were separated by choice, slave trades, or death. Premarital pregnancies were encouraged by slave owners because they represented an increased investment. About 75% of slave households studied by Gutman consisted of two-parent families. With emancipation, mobility, especially to northern cities, increased and extended networks of relatives, and lodger systems assisted this mobility. Gutman's demonstration of strong kin attachments indicates the adaptive response of black families living under severe economic and cultural pressures. Chapter 5, in this text, addresses current issues of family health and ethnicity.

During the last quarter of the 19th century and continuing until 1924 when the immigration laws changed to impose quotas, large numbers of Italian, Irish, and Eastern European immigrants came to the United States. These immigrants settled primarily in eastern cities and worked in the growing manufacturing industries. With changes such as the liberation of black families, the immigration of southern and eastern Europeans, and the annexation of western lands with large Spanish and Indian populations, the term "American" encompassed diverse regional, ethnic, and occupational variations.

The growth of the cities and the waves of non-English-speaking immigrants caused several social movements. One notable reaction was the effort to improve the social welfare of urban immigrant families through settlement houses. In addition, the public education movement gathered much support as non-English-speaking children crowded into urban schools. Jackson (1986) describes how child welfare agencies of the period ferried orphaned and abandoned street kids to midwest farm families for adoption. Public health movements mobilized in response to epidemics and perceived needs of maternal and child health. Social reformers of the day worked to enact child labor, public education, and public health laws (Rosen, 1958; Rosenkrantz, 1972; Wiebe, 1967).

There were multiple and substantive changes in American families from the mid-19th century to the mid-20th century. These changes included an increasing ethnic diversity, the separation of the workplace from the home, urbanization and suburbanization, and changes in family styles or constellations produced by changing fertility and mortality rates. With the additional population and the growth of industrialization, differences in socioeconomic strata also became more pronounced.

Despite nostalgia for the mythical preindustrial extended family, the most profound shift in family life caused by industrialization was the separation of workplace from home. In the preindustrial United States, the family unit was responsible for producing almost all of what it consumed, so "housework" was of primary economic importance, and the nuclear household filled many functions. The family acted as a workshop, reformatory, asylum, school, church, and hospital. According to Hareven (1986), when housework lost its productive value—that is, it no longer produced goods important for family functioning—it lost status.

Another significant change in family life resulted from changing birth and mortality rates. Hareven (1986) also describes how 19th-century demographics affected family life. Although both adults and children were not as likely to live as long as during the 20th century, women married later and had more children in the 19th century. The high fertility rate as well as a high mortality rate meant that child-care responsibilities lasted almost to the end of the parents' lives. Parents were likely to be widowed while their children were still young. The larger number of children and the higher mortality rates meant that many younger children in a family were raised by their older siblings, a pattern that is unusual in the 20th century.

American Families in the 20th Century

Currie and Skolnick (1988) are among the many authors who have described the economic shift from agriculture to industry to the present-day service-based economy. This service economy is marked by few people employed in a primary food-producing activity, the decline of blue collar industrial employment, and an increase in service employment (areas such as finance, health, and education). While some of these jobs are well paying and challenging, others (such as dishwasher and sales clerk) offer few rewards.

Kuttner (1983) argues that in the post-industrial economy more families are pushed out of the middle class. Increasingly, people work in jobs that are low paying, precarious, and offer few benefits (such as health care insurance).

As the economy has changed, so have the characteristics of the workforce, with more women employed outside the home. In 1960, only 35% of American women worked outside the home, and only 19% of married women were in the paid labor force. (Hacker, 1986). By 1989, 57.8% of married women were in paid employment (U.S. Bureau of the Census, 1991).

Another trend that began in the 1970s and has continued to be a pattern is a relatively high divorce rate. Divorce rates reflect higher expectations for marriage, greater societal tolerance for divorce, and the increased financial independence of women. Bane (1976) demonstrates that the falling death rates have somewhat balanced the rising divorce rates, so the total number of marital disruptions (either by the death of a parent or divorce) affecting children did not increase. The majority of divorced people remarry. Table 3–2 presents a summary of 1990 census data.

The census data also describe, by 1990, a fertility rate that has been relatively stable since the early 1970s. From 1973 to 1990, the fertility rate has remained between 65 and 70 births per 1000 women from ages 18 to 44 (U.S. Bureau of the Census, 1991). This translates to an average number of children per women ranging from 1.6 to 1.9.

And although the fertility rate has remained stable, the number of women in paid employment continues to increase. Census studies (U.S. Bureau of the Census, 1991) indicate that 53.1% of the women who gave birth in the year preceding June 1990 were in the labor force, compared to 38% in 1980 and 31% in 1976.

These demographic changes were accompanied by cultural and intrafamily changes. As women entered the labor force in larger numbers, issues of child care and responsibility for household tasks became salient. Moral arguments about the appropriateness and adequacy of child care abound. At the same time, housework has suffered a loss of social standing, so many people regard it as distasteful. Hochschild (1989) cites evidence that husbands of working wives do not routinely help with the "second shift" of housework and child care duties and that this can become a significant source of strain in a marriage.

Although most women are in the labor force and appear to want to be there, a substantial gap between the earnings of women and men remains. Many of these demographic changes are played out as issues in family dynamics, as spouses may not clarify their differing values of work, income, child care, and household tasks. In addition, the service economy seems to have produced extremes in income and economic depressions for agricultural and industrial areas, and as a result, increased numbers of both homeless and hungry families exist.

In addition to the increasing participation of women in paid employment, the other major demographic implication for the future is the growth in the number of elderly people. Those over 65 years of age increased from 9.9% of the population in 1970 to 12.5% in 1989 (U.S. Bureau of the Census, 1989). With the current low mortality rates and stable fertility rates, the elderly section of the population is expected to have the greatest increase in size in the future. Kart (1990) is one of the many gerontologists that believe the elderly will continue to be involved in their families and communities. Designated communities may market services and security to the wealthy elderly in the future but present no advantages for the larger number of elderly on minimum fixed incomes. This may be an exciting time for nurse clinicians to focus on the elderly, as their increasing numbers may promote changes in the health care service structure.

FAMILY DEVELOPMENT THEORY

Developmental theories have long been popular with nursing and other social sciences. Theories provide a framework to interpret what we are trying to understand and assess in our work. Before beginning this section in which theories of development will be reviewed, one important caution should guide the knowledgeable clinician: Be critical. Rather than shaping assessment of family dynamics and behaviors into any rigid theory, a thorough evaluation of family inter-

TABLE 3–2. MARITAL STATUS BY PERCENT OF POPULATION

	NEVER MARRIED	CURRENTLY MARRIED	DIVORCED & SEPARATED	WIDOWED
Male	25.9%	64.4%	7.0%	2.7%
Female	18.9%	59.8%	9.1%	12.2%

(1990 Census of the Population)

actions may present elaborations of or contradictions to existing theory.

Before stages of family development are reviewed, it is crucial to reflect on how one's definition of the family will affect what theoretical frameworks are useful in understanding the dynamics in the family. Given that the definition of the term "family" is not exclusively related to a married couple, both individual and family developmental theories can be valuable to understand family dynamics and behavior.

Psychological and psychoanalytical theories of individual development abound in the literature. Theorists such as Freud, Jung, Adler, Piaget, Mahler, and Erikson describe the stages of growth of the individual in different ways and with different therapeutic implications. A working familiarity with the ideas of the dominant psychological theorists is a valuable investment for the skilled nurse clinician. However, because most of their theories are more appropriate to studies on individual development, they will not be reviewed in this chapter as they fail to capture the interactive dynamics of the family.

Perhaps the most comprehensive description of family development is that of Okun (1984). Okun's description of family developmental tasks and issues presents a well-organized theory. Carter and McGoldrick (1988) also present a similar organization of stages in family life development.

Okun recognizes that the developmental tasks and issues she describes relate to middle-class America (p. 88). She elaborates on Duvall's (1977) theory of family development, and her definition of "family" appears to be a heterosexual couple with children. Although Okun is careful to avoid a prescriptive bias, the reader should be aware that Okun's developmental tasks and issues may not easily extend to nonnuclear families or families that are pressed by extreme economic need. Chapter 20, in this text, more completely describes diversity in family life development. Carter and McGoldrick (1988) also provide a description of developmental tasks of other types of families.

However, Okun's work provides a comprehensive interpretation of family development theory. Okun describes the development tasks that face the family as they move through developmental stages in their life span. Table 3–3 summarizes the stages of family development.

Although this model of stages applies to those families who are composed of a married couple with a child or children, a family can be in several stages, such as a child born to a family that has adolescents or a postparental family that cares for an infant or preschool child.

Beginning Family

In the beginning family, partners deal with issues such as separation from their families of origin, management of a household, and dissolution of the idealized images of their mates. Although the partners may be fairly young adults, the decision to have children is an issue in this family. The three-person family (husband, wife, and child) creates the infant family, which is faced with issues such as time and energy management, decisions (implicit or explicit) about parenting styles, reactions to grandparental styles, and career decisions. Carter and McGoldrick (1988) divide this period into two separate stages of family development: leaving home (which involves the differentiation of self and the establishment of financial and emotional independence) and the formation of the couple.

TABLE 3–3. STAGES OF FAMILY DEVELOPMENT AND TASKS

DEVELOPMENTAL STAGE	AGE OF MEMBERS	CRITICAL TASKS
Beginning	Parents usually young adults, can be a remarriage	Separating from family of origin Managing a household Deciding to have children
Infant	Newborn child added	Managing time, energy Developing parenting skills
Preschool	Child is ages 3 to 5	Making employment decisions Deciding to have more children
School Age	Child is in school full time	Developing parental identity
Adolescent	Child is adolescent, parents are in middle adulthood	Evolving independence of child Facing economic issues
Launching	Child leaves home after high school	Disengaging Reestablishing marital bond
Postparental	Parents at or near retirement	Deciding on and dealing with retirement
Aging	Parents in late adulthood	Dealing with loss of function, dependency

Data from Okun, B. (1984). *Working with Adults: Individuals, Family, and Career Development.* Monterey, CA: Brooks/Cole; and Carter, E. & McGoldrick, M. (1988). *The Family Life Cycle: A Framework for Family Therapy* (2nd ed.). New York: Gardner Press.

Preschool Family

The preschool family, when the child is between three and five years of age, has continuing issues of parental discipline styles, decisions to have more children, and career and economic pressures. Okun (1984) recognizes increased stress in the single-parent family. If the single parent lives alone with the child, issues dealing with custody decisions and heightened economic pressure may exist (p. 108).

School-Age Family

The next stage, the school-age family, is when the child enters school full-time until he or she reaches puberty. As the more intense childrearing tasks decrease, parents may experience individual identity crises. Mothers may reassess time management and career goals. This may relate to school institutions serving both educational and day-care or babysitting functions. If both parents work outside the home (as is the most likely case), issues of child care on school vacations may arise. Families with young children have to make adjustments within the marriage and realign their relationships with the extended family to include parenting and grandparenting roles (Carter and McGoldrick, 1988). A central struggle for couples with young children is the division of childcare and household responsibilities. Hochschild (1989) finds that marital conflict often centers on these problems and their resolution is important for marital stability.

Okun cites evidence of increased divorce at this stage in the family life cycle. The effects of divorce on children are extremely individualized. A divorce may relieve or increase fears and insecurities of children, which may result in physical or behavioral symptoms at home or at school. Both parents usually have significant, stressful issues to resolve during a divorce: child custody, establishment of another household, readjustment to a role as newly single, and increased financial demands.

Remarried families, according to Carter and McGoldrick (1980, p. 206), "carry the scars of the first families." For the parents, the first family may have unresolved issues, as well as issues arising from the family of origin. Children may have difficulty with multiple family roles, such as a lingering sense of guilt about the divorce and fantasies about their biologic parents, which may delay adjustment. Carter and McGoldrick (1988, p. 23), suggest that step-family integration seems to "require a minimum of two or three years before a workable new structure permits family members to move on emotionally." In any event, a divorce/remarriage situation presents more complex family dynamics, which require both adaptation and renegotiation.

Adolescent Family

As children reach adolescence, new issues arise within the family that relate to the growing power of the child. Issues include parental authority and the freedom and/or responsibility of the adolescent child. Parental reaction to the beginning sexuality of the child may relate to issues from the parent's family of origin. This may also be a time for increasing costs of childrearing, as an adolescent child may react to peer pressures by wanting more consumer goods. There may be struggles over dependence versus independence of the child and the child not performing household tasks. In addition, Okun feels that a divorce during this stage may be more threatening to the parents' self-concepts, as they have had a "married" identity for a long time. Single parents may have more potential for difficulty at this stage than a married couple with an adolescent child as issues of parental authority arise.

Launching

The launching stage refers to a period of disengagement of parents from children as the children physically distance themselves through college, the military service, or a move to a different residence. Duvall and Miller (1985) call this the beginning of a contracting phase of the family life cycle. Okun sees this as an irreversible change and describes studies that indicate marital satisfaction is lowest at this stage of family life. She relates this to the uneven nature of the disengagement. Sussman and Steinmetz (1987) also describe the possibility that the almost-adult child will return home several times after launching. Young adult children may return home just when the family system has adjusted to their absence. The returning young adult children find the family changed, and both parents and children experience ambivalent feelings for each other. The launching stage may be seen as a process of letting go rather than binding, and the primary developmental issue is dealing with the changed family composition.

Rubin (1979) finds that fathers have more difficulty than mothers with this stage. He believes that fathers who were more distant during childrearing perceive a distinct and severe loss when children leave home. From Rubin's study, the "empty nest syndrome" (feelings of loss and sadness when a child leaves home) occurs more frequently with fathers than with mothers. By having a closer involvement in their children's daily lives, mothers have perceived more gradual separation and independence of their children, and are more prepared for the readjustment to daily living without them.

Carter and McGoldrick (1988) add that at the same time their children are leaving, a couple's parents are often becoming ill or dying, creating considerable responsibilities. Caregivers are overwhelmingly women and most provide care for 1 to 4 years. This can be a demanding job and many caregivers report high levels of stress. (Foster & Brizius, 1991).

For other families, especially those with adequate finances, the launching stage is a liberating time, with the potential for travel and hobbies. Those women who postponed their occupational plans may now decide to enter or reenter a career. The mother's health and age may be critical factors in this decision.

Postparental Parents

Although Okun describes the next stage as postparental, parents are truly never finished being parents, even when children are firmly established in separate residences. Okun terms this stage "one of rediscovery or disappointment" (p. 238) as parents have more time for each other. This stage may include negotiating the grandparental role and style. As people live longer, the grandparental function may move from a more conventional, distant role to a more informal, active one in which a grandparent may be a partner in play and fun with the grandchild. The active grandparental relationship may become more difficult or painful when that role is diminished by a divorce and custody changes for the grandchild.

Retirement

Another important issue at this stage is retirement, which presents a major change in daily living patterns. Families at the postparental stage are also likely to experience the death of significant others. Older adults may experience a dovetailing of loss as family and friends die, careers end, and financial resources diminish. The grandparenting role may help replace other lost roles, offering the older adult the opportunity for closeness without the responsibilities of parenthood. (Carter & McGoldrick, 1988).

Reactions to illness, medical treatment, and functional and physical losses at this developmental stage relate to the family position of the affected member, the established patterns of communication and dependencies, and past experiences of family coping. When a family member dies, the remaining members may not have similar patterns of grieving or adjustment. This may be a period of shifting power alliances as adult children reenter as decision makers for their aging parents. As Sussman and Steinmetz (1986) indicate, this may mean a 60- or 70-year-old "child" making disposition decisions or being asked to care for a 90-year-old parent. When a spouse dies, the widow or widower may move toward dependency on other family members. However, the loss of a spouse may also promote new independent

functioning in new friendships, a remarriage, or increased communication with children or other relatives.

Aging Family

The final development stage is termed the aging family. If couples survive into late adulthood, the major task facing them is dealing with their inevitable deaths, a final letting go of each other. Because of increased curative technologies, it is likely that an elderly couple will go through a period of physical and mental dependency and gradual loss of function. Families may react to health care institutions such as hospitals and skilled nursing facilities with various levels of competence and communication. The imposition of illness is an additional and usually stressful variable added to the constellation of family styles, dependencies, and communication patterns.

This caretaking period can present a timely opportunity to resolve previous difficulties, clarify and communicate affection and concern, and prepare for the grief and bereavement process. Couples who have never established the foundations of support and affection (although they have lived together and had children) may be unable to adapt to change and crisis. Death is a normal family experience, but Okun feels that if a family did not successfully manage developmental stages, illness and dying may present unmanageable crises.

This description of family stages and developmental issues that arise at different stages is helpful to understand the interactional tasks in process when variables such as financial stress or illness are added to a family at any stage.

But what of families that are not nuclear? According to census studies (U.S. Bureau of the Census, 1990), in 1990, 28.1% of families were single-parent ones. In addition, as elderly families become more numerous, do they have different stages? Does living alone mean that the elderly are socially isolated, as Hareven (1986) fears? The increase in life expectancy has created a group of people who will live in extended widowhood periods, yet their developmental issues are not well studied.

Sussman and Steinmetz (1987) suggest the need to redefine the use of traditional terms to describe American families. The "nontraditional" forms of single-parent, dual-income, separated, remarried, voluntarily childless, homosexual, cohabitating, and never-married families actually comprise more of the population than the married couple with father working and mother remaining at home with the kids. Therefore, we need to rethink the meaning of "different" in families. "Nontraditional" family styles are more frequent, and thus are more "normal" than the stereotypical family composition. Chapter 20 will discuss in detail the common diversities in family life.

IMPLICATIONS FOR FAMILY HEALTH NURSING

This review of the history of the American family demonstrates that the nuclear form (parents and children composing the immediate family) has persisted as the dominant family style. However, it is now more likely that this family will be blended, that both parents will work outside the home, and that there are more older families, whose children have established separate house-holds. In addition, the issues at each stage of family development may be pressured from outside, larger economic trends as the nation moves further from its industrial and agricultural bases.

Because of the diversity in family styles, developmental stages, ethnic groups, and socioeconomic strata, the clinician cannot use personal frames of reference when understanding and assessing families. By considering the individual client within his or her family system, the family nurse can recognize the stages of family development and the family system interactions that affect health behavior and promotion.

CHAPTER HIGHLIGHTS

Family nurses must be cognizant of the fact that although families have many similarities, each family is unique.

The modern American family is different in structure and size due to historical changes such as immigration, urbanization, and industrialization.

Family is defined in various ways. The family is more than household members and those related by blood or law. A more broad definition of family describes family as one or more individuals closely related by blood, marriage, or friendship.

To determine the family of a client, the nurse might ask "Who you are close to?" in addition to "Who lives with you?"

The most profound change in family structure and type was caused by the industrial revolution when the home was no longer the workplace, the school, the church, and the hospital.

The family of the 20th century is diverse and has many types, such as nuclear families, dual earner/dual career, single-parent, blended families, multiple generations, and domestic partners (heterosexual and homosexual), to name a few. Changes in the modern family include increases in single-parent families, women in the workforce, homelessness, remarriage, aging family members, and domestic partners. There is a slight decrease in the divorce rate in the past decade.

The family across the life span experiences change and has developmental tasks to accomplish in each stage of the family life cycle.

Because of the diversity of family types, lifestyles, developmental stages, ethnic groups, and socioeconomic status, the family health nurse is encouraged to evaluate his or her personal frame of reference when assessing and intervening with families.

REFERENCES

Bane, M.J. (1976). *Here to Stay: American Families in the Twentieth Century.* New York: Basic Books.

Baxandall, R., Gordon, L., & Reverby, S. (Eds.). (1976). *America's Working Women: A Documentary History—1600 to the Present.* New York: Vintage Books.

Blumin, S.M. (1977). Rip Van Winkle's grandchildren: Family and Household in the Hudson Valley, 1800–1860. In T.K. Hareven (Ed.), *Family and Kin in Urban Communities, 1700–1930* (pp. 100–121). New York: New Viewpoints.

Carter, E.A., & McGoldrick, M. (1980). *The Family Life Cycle: A Framework for Family Therapy.* New York: Gardner Press.

Carter, E.A., & McGoldrick, M. (1988). *The Family Life Cycle: A Framework for Family Therapy* (2nd ed.). New York: Gardner Press.

Claiborne, R. (1973). *The First Americans.* New York: Time-Life Books.

Clements, I.W., & Roberts, F.B. (1983). *Family Health: A Theoretical Approach to Nursing Care.* New York: Wiley.

Currie, E., & Skolnick, J. (1988). *America's Problems: Social Issues and Public Policy* (2nd ed.). Glenview, Illinois: Scott, Foresman.

Davis, M.R. (1982). *Families in a Working World: The Impact of Organizations on Domestic Life.* New York: Praeger.

Demos, J. (1970). *A Little Commonwealth: Family Life in Plymouth Colony.* New York: Oxford University Press.

Dublin, T. (1979). Women at Work: The Transformation of Work and Community in Lowell, Massachusetts, 1826–1860. New York: Columbia University Press.

Duvall, E.M. (1977). *Marriage and Family Development* (5th ed.). Philadelphia: J.B. Lippincott.

Duvall, E.M., & Miller, B.C. (1985). *Marriage and Family Development.* (6th ed.). New York: Harper & Row.

Foster, S.E., & Brizius, J.A. (1991). *Caring Too Much? American Women and the Nation's Caregiving Crisis.* Southport, CT: Southport Institute for Policy Analysis.

Friedman, M.M. (1992). *Family Nursing: Theory and Assessment* (3rd ed.). Norwalk, CT: Appleton-Century-Crofts.

Gilligan, C. (1982). *In a Different Voice.* Cambridge, MA: Harvard University Press.

Glasco, L.A. (1977). The life cycles and household structure of American ethnic groups: Irish, German and native born whites in Buffalo, N.Y., 1855. In T.K. Hareven (Ed.), *Family and Kin in Urban Communities,*

1700–1930 (pp. 122–143). New York: New Viewpoints.

Goldenberg, I., & Goldenberg, H. (1985). *Family Therapy: An Overview* (2nd ed.). Monterey, CA: Brooks/Cole.

Gordon, M. (Ed.). (1978). *The American Family in Social-Historical Perspective* (2nd ed.). New York: St. Martin's Press.

Gutman, H.G. (1976). *The Black Family in Slavery and Freedom, 1750–1925.* New York: Pantheon Books.

Hacker, A. (1986, August). Women and work. *The New York Review of Books, 26–33.*

Hall, P.D. (1977). Family structure and economic organization: Massachusetts merchants, 1700–1850. In T.K. Hareven, *Family and Kin in Urban Communities, 1700–1930* (pp. 38–61). New York: New Viewpoints.

Hareven, T.K. (1986). American families in transition: Historical perspectives on change. In A.S. Skolnick & J.H. Skolnick, *Family in Transition* (5th ed.) (pp. 40–56). Boston, MA: Little, Brown.

Hareven, T.K. (Ed.). (1977). *Family and Kin in Urban Communities, 1700–1930.* New York: New Viewpoints.

Hochschild, A. (1989). *The Second Shift: Working Parents and the Revolution at Home.* New York: Harper & Row.

Jackson, D.D. (1986, August). It took trains to put street kids on the right track out of the slums. *Smithsonian Magazine,* 95–103.

Kahne, H., with Kohen, A. (1975, December). Economic perspectives on the roles of women in the American economy. *Journal of Economic Literature,* 1249–1292.

Kart, C.S. (1990). *The Realities of Aging: An Introduction to Gerontology* (3rd ed.). Boston: Allyn & Bacon.

Kuttner, B. (1983). "The declining middle". *Atlantic Monthly* 252 (July), 60–63.

Luker, K. (1984). *Abortion and the Politics of Motherhood.* Berkeley, CA: University of California Press.

Masnick, G., & Bane, M.J. (1980). *The Nation's Families, 1960–1990.* Boston, MA: Auburn House.

McGoldrick, M. (1982). Irish families. In M. McGoldrick, J.K. Pearce, & J. Giordino (Eds.), *Ethnicity and Family Therapy* (pp. 310–339). New York: Guilford Press.

Moch, L.P., & Stark, G.D. (1983). *Essays on the Family and Historical Change.* College Station, TX: Texas A&M University Press.

Newsweek. (1986, March). p. 47.

Okun, B.F. (1984). *Working with Adults: Individuals, Family, and Career Development.* Monterey, CA: Brooks/Cole.

Olson, D.H., & McCubbin, H. (1983). *Families: What Makes them Work.* Beverly Hills, CA: Sage.

Oppenheimer, V.K. (1970). *The Female Labor Force in the U.S.* Berkeley, CA: University of California Press.

Rabb, T.K., Rotberg, R.I. (Eds.). (1973). *The Family in History: Interdisciplinary Essays.* New York: Harper & Row.

Rice, F.P. (1990). *Intimate Relationships, Marriages and Families.* Mountain View, CA: Mayfield.

Rosen, G. (1958). *A History of Public Health.* New York: MD Publications.

Rosenberg, C.E. (Ed.). (1975). *The Family in History.* Philadelphia, PA: University of Pennsylvania Press.

Rosenkrantz, B.G. (1972). *Public Health and the State: Changing Views in Massachusetts, 1842–1936.* Cambridge, MA: Harvard University Press.

Rothman, D.J., & Rothman, S.M. (Eds.). (1972). *Family in America: Collected Essays.* New York: Arno Press and the *New York Times.*

Rubin, L.B. (1979). *Women of a Certain Age: The Midlife Search for Self.* New York: Harper & Row.

Rutman, D.B. (1977). People in process: The New Hampshire towns of the 18th Century. In T.K. Hareven (Ed.), *Family and Kin in Urban Communities, 1700–1930* (pp. 16–37). New York: New Viewpoints.

Seward, R.R. (1978). *The American Family: A Demographic History.* Beverly Hills, CA: Sage.

Singelmann, J. (1978). *From Agriculture to Services: The Transformation of Industrial Employment.* Beverly Hills, CA: Sage.

Skolnick, A.S., & Skolnick, J.H. (1992). *Family in Transition* (8th ed.). New York: HarperCollins.

Stack, C.B. (1974). *All Our Kin: Strategies for Survival in a Black Community.* New York: Harper & Row.

Stone, L. (1975). The rise of the nuclear family in early modern England. In C.E. Rosenberg (Ed.), *The Family in History* (pp. 13–57). Philadelphia, PA: University of Pennsylvania Press.

Stromberg, A.H., & Harkness, S. (Eds.). (1978). *Women Working: Theories and Facts in Perspective.* Palo Alto, CA: Mayfield.

Strong, B., & DeVault, C. (1992). *The Marriage and Family Experience* (5th ed.). St. Paul, MN: West.

Sussman, M.B., & Steinmetz, S.K. (Eds.). (1987). *Handbook of Marriage and the Family.* New York: Plenum Press.

U.S. Bureau of the Census. (1991). *Fertility of American Women: June, 1990* (Current Population Reports, Series P-20, No. 454). Washington, DC: U.S. Government Printing Office.

U.S. Bureau of the Census. (1990). *Household and Family Characteristics March 1990 & 1989* (Current Population Reports, Series P-20, No. 447). Washington, DC: U.S. Government Printing Office.

U.S. Bureau of the Census. (1989). *Resident Population, by Age and Stage* (Current Population Reports, Series P-20, No. 1058). Washington, DC: U.S. Government Printing Office.

Wiebe, R.H. (1967). *The Search for Order, 1877–1920.* New York: Hill and Wang.

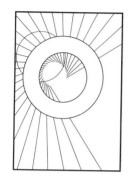

UNIT II

Concepts and Frameworks for Family Health Nursing Practice

THE FAMILY AS A SYSTEM

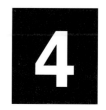

BARBARA A. CASEY

> ... Each individual family member is a subsystem and a system.
> An individual system is both a part and a whole as in a family.
>
> LORRAINE WRIGHT
> MAUREEN LEAHEY

OBJECTIVES

On completion of this chapter, the reader will be able to:

1. Discuss the types of systems frameworks and the major concepts defined by systems theorists
2. Relate systems theories to families
3. Discuss the application of family systems theory to nursing practice
4. Analyze the use of a nursing conceptual model with a systems perspective

The systems view of families provides a method for understanding the interaction and interdependence of individuals within a family, as well as the family's interaction with other systems. The assessment of the family from a systems perspective can allow nurses to conceptualize the interrelatedness of components in the family system and determine areas for change, particularly in the area of health promotion.

As Barkauskas (1986) has noted, systems are defined in terms of their structure, the relationship of the parts of the system, the processes in which the system engages, and the interaction between the system and its environment. These major concepts will be discussed from the point of view of several leading family system theorists. In addition, the use of a holistic, systems-oriented nursing perspective will be discussed as it relates to family health nursing.

As Wright and Leahey (1994) have pointed out, the most significant variable that promotes or impedes family-centered care is how a nurse conceptualizes problems. If nurses use conceptual frameworks that go beyond the "individual perspective" and include the family as a "system," data can be organized and intervention planned that promotes family-centered care.

Theories of family functioning are usually divided into three types: (1) psychoanalytic, (2) behavioral, and (3) systems-interactional.

EVOLUTION OF FAMILY SYSTEMS THEORY

Friedman (1992) has noted the growth in the use of systems theory in the health care field. The family movement, which began in the late 1940s and early 1950s, has contributed significantly to the body of knowledge of systems theory and to the shift from an individualistic orientation to a family orientation. Many of the pioneers in family therapy were conducting research with schizophrenic families and with behavior difficulties and delinquency in children. These investigators were confronted with conceptualizing a family relationship system.

Nathan Ackerman is most frequently considered the founding father of family-centered therapy (Guerin, 1976). In his individual work with children, he recognized that healthy family relationships were needed for improvement with the child. This was an innovative, tradition-breaking concept at the time, but soon other therapists began to recognize the complexities of the family and the need for intervention geared toward this social system.

In the middle 1950s, Gregory Bateson, Jay Haley, John Weakland, and Don Jackson initiated a 10-year research project to learn the etiology and nature of schizophrenia. With the idea that the family contributed to the etiology of the patient's pathology, their work was central to the development of systems thinking in relation to human behavior (Guerin, 1976).

Bowen's (1976) shift to the family also originated with his individual therapy with schizophrenic patients and their mothers. Observation of family relationships at the National Institute of Mental Health in Bethesda, Maryland, where he hospitalized whole families, led him to believe that the family was the unit of illness. This work led to prolific writing, including what is referred to today as Bowen's family systems theory.

In the late 1960s and early 1970s, Salvador Minuchin was working with families of the urban poor. Influenced by Haley's contributions, he developed a systems-based view known as structural family therapy (Gurman & Kniskern, 1991).

The family therapy movement has progressed through several stages, influenced by research and theory building, psychosocial changes in the family and society, and expansion of training programs across the country. It has not been the scope of this historical review to note all the important contributors of the past several decades, but rather to highlight the work of several important pioneers and how their ground-breaking systems view of families evolved.

Within systems orientations there are five generally accepted frameworks: (1) general systems theory, (2) Bowen's family systems theory, (3) Minuchin's structural paradigm, (4) interactional or communication theory, and (5) the Circumplex model. In addition, family developmental theory and selected nursing models view families as possessing characteristics of systems. Each of these will be considered separately, illuminating the central concepts of each framework.

General Systems Theory

General systems theory has been adopted as the most commonly used framework in the family movement. Von Bertalanffy (1968), a biologist, sought to find those principles that would be valid for all systems. Subsequently, he described several properties that apply to systems: wholeness, openness, feedback, homeostasis, equifinality, boundaries, and environment. He believed it was useful to understand phenomena in their wholeness and complexity, rather than dividing them into smaller and smaller elements to find a cause-and-effect relationship. The latter view, a mechanistic perspective, is consistent with the medical

model. Von Bertalanffy was concerned with wholeness and organization rather than with reduction. In the general systems view, the pieces of the picture are the same, but the way in which they are seen is different. One of the central propositions of general systems theory is the view that the system is not the total sum of its parts but is characterized by *wholeness* and unity: "The whole is greater than the sum of its parts."

Hall and Fagen (1956) defined a system as "a set of objects together with relationships between the objects and between their attributes" (p. 18). Relationships tie the parts of a system together and make them interdependent. Systems have both structural properties and functional properties.

Von Bertalanffy (1968) stated that there are two kinds of systems: *open systems* and *closed systems*. Open systems, such as living or organismic systems, are characterized by wholeness, feedback, and equifinality. In closed systems, there is no exchange of information or energy with the environment.

Wholeness refers to the organization and complexity of a system by stressing the relationship of the parts to the whole. Watzlawick et al. (1967) contend that "every part of a system is so related to its fellow parts that a change in one part will cause a change in all of them and in the total system" (p. 123).

Feedback is the process through which the system's parts (or subsystems) relate to each other and maintain the system's functioning (self-regulation). Systems can embody many complex feedback loops that impinge on one another. Feedback is also described as positive or negative. *Positive feedback* is part of a system's output that is returned to the system as information about the output and moves the system away from homeostasis. It changes the pattern of how the system operates. *Negative feedback,* on the other hand, maintains the system within its homeostatic limits. Negative feedback is returned to the system to correct alterations or deviations from the steady state. The concept of *homeostasis,* particularly as it applies to human relationships, will be explored in more detail later. Systems with feedback loops, output leaving the system and reentering the system, are also characterized by the notion of *circular causality.* Circular causality does not have a beginning or end in the circle. The response of B is also a stimulus for the next event in this interdependent chain, A>B>A. *Linear causality,* on the other hand, suggests that A occurs and B is caused by A's occurrence—a cause-and-effect relationship (Watzlawick et al., 1967).

The principle of *equifinality* of systems suggests that the same results may come from different origins (Watzlawick et al., 1967, p. 127). Results are determined by the nature of the process or the system parameters. Von Bertalanffy (1968) also describes equifinality by suggesting that the final state or goal can be achieved from different initial conditions. Galvin and Brommel (1986) conclude that adaptive family systems demonstrate equifinality; that is, they have the capacity to accomplish goals from many different starting points. Equifinality is not present in closed systems.

It is also important to consider the concept of environment when examining systems. Every system is part of a larger system referred to as environment and continually interacts with its environment. Hall and Fagen (1956) define environment as "the set of all objects a change in whose attributes affect the system and also those objects whose attributes are changed by the behavior of the system" (p. 20).

Any given system can be further subdivided into subsystems. The separation of a system from its subsystem or from its environment can be an arbitrary one. Boundaries of a system, separating a system from its environment, are also referred to as open or closed, depending on the degree of permeability. The permeability of the system's boundaries controls the exchange of energy and information.

The concept of *hierarchies* also applies to living systems, with lower-level systems and higher-level systems. Each system has a subsystem(s) and a suprasystem. A system's capacity to monitor its own progress toward a goal and to correct and elaborate its response depends on the complexity of its feedback structure (Burr et al., 1979). At the highest order of complexity are the psychologic, family, social, or cultural systems. These systems must be capable of changing their basic structure, organization, and values in order to remain viable (Hill, 1971; Speer, 1970).

A systems view applied to families suggests that families are goal-directed, self-maintaining, and constantly evolving. Families have multiple subsystems such as dyads, triads, sibling subsystems, marital subsystems, and parental subsystems that are constantly interacting with other systems (i.e., school, work, extended family, church).

These parts or subsystems are interrelated, and one part cannot be understood in isolation from the rest of the system. The family system is part of a larger suprasystem. To fully understand family functioning and family health patterns, each part must be viewed as it relates and interacts with other parts of the system. The interactional patterns of the family system shape the behavior of family members.

Understanding the boundaries of the family's systems is also essential to making a thorough assessment of family health care needs. Determining the degree of permeability of the boundaries in the family system and how much information and energy are exchanged can determine areas for intervention. For example, are the boundaries of the parental system intact or so weak that parental functions with children are ineffective? Does the

family allow adequate information regarding health practices? Are the sibling subsystems so isolated from parental dyads that socialization is impaired?

Assessing what suprasystems the family is a part of can also enable the nurse to influence environmental variables that affect family health functioning. Are appropriate community resources used? Does the family have adequate interaction with other social systems such as neighborhoods, schools, social groups, or churches?

Wright and Leahey (1994) contend that the family is able to create a balance between change and stability. They are suggesting that families are capable of much more than maintaining homeostasis. Several authors applying systems theory to complex units such as families or social systems have challenged the concept of homeostasis (Hill, 1971; Speer, 1970; Olson et al., 1979). They have suggested that the family is not principally an equilibrium-seeking or homeostatic system but is a complex, adaptive, and ever-changing system.

The family, as an example of a social system, is viewed at the highest order of complexity of systems. Speer (1970) maintains that, along with the positive feedback principle previously described, the "organization of social systems tends to increase in complexity and flexibility with increased viability, variability or change with the system" (p. 268). Thus, homeostasis characterizes lower-level living systems, and viability with the capacity for growth and self-directed change characterizes the family. This view suggests that families are constantly evolving toward more complexity rather than attempting to achieve a homeostatic, steady state. Friedman (1992) describes this process as differentiation. She contends that families grow and evolve so that the system becomes increasingly more discriminate, articulate, and complex

Bowen's Family Systems Theory

The family systems theory developed primarily by Bowen (1976) originally centered around concepts related to psychoanalysis and schizophrenia. He has since developed a more comprehensive systems-based theory of emotional dysfunction, with several well-defined concepts.

From his extensive work with families, Bowen observed several phenomena. One of the core concepts of Bowen's theory is the *differentiation of self*. This concept refers to the degree to which individuals are able to distinguish between the feeling process (emotional system) and the intellectual process (intellectual system). Individuals on the low end of the scale of differentiation are more controlled by emotions, particularly anxiety, directing their decisions and behavior. They are less adaptable and are usually more prone to physical or emotional illness. Bowen further suggests that individuals with a low level of differentiation and a weak sense of self tend to form highly dependent and emotionally fused relationships. Their ability to recover from the stress that leads to dysfunction is also impaired (Bowen, 1976). Bowen uses a scale from 0 to 100 to rate the level of differentiation. At the high end of the scale are individuals who have a more differentiated sense of self. That is, they are more guided by reason and rational decision making and are less instinctive or impulsive in their behavior. The more functional the intellectual system, the greater the sense of self. The level of differentiation in an individual reflects the degree to which the intellectual system has guidance over and directs the emotional system.

Bowen proposes that partners seek out partners with similar levels of differentiation and that the level of differentiation is passed from one generation to the next. The level of differentiation of self is determined in the family of origin, and this influences the nuclear family that they will create, as well as future generations. Bowen refers to this phenomenon as the *multigeneration transmission process*. If the most impaired child in a family is followed through successive generations, one will see lower and lower levels of differentiation (Bowen, 1976, p. 87).

The level of differentiation is operationalized by *triangles* set up within families. When a dyad in a system experiences increasing levels of anxiety, a third person is triangled in to decrease the level of discomfort and anxiety. The more uncomfortable person attempts to decrease the level of anxiety by moving toward fusion with a third person. For example, in the mother-father dyad, a child is often triangled in to diffuse the anxiety between mother and father. At lower levels of differentiation, there is more anxiety in families, and triangles are commonly formed to bind the anxiety (Bowen, 1976). When available family triangles are exhausted, the family triangles in persons or systems from outside the family system, such as nurses, police, school, or social agencies. One of the keys to understanding triangles is keeping in mind the force of emotionality that drives them (Kerr, 1981).

Family projection process refers to Bowen's description of how parental lack of differentiation impairs one or more children and is used to stabilize the system. The process can focus first on one child and then select others for lesser degrees of involvement. The process usually begins with anxiety in the mother who establishes a pattern of infantilizing the child. The emotional fusion between mother and child can lead to symptoms in the child. This type of family is often referred to as the child-focused family. The mother's (or parent's) emotionality defines what the child is like, which may have little to do with what the child is really like. The mother projects attributes on to the child. Eventually what the mother projects on to the child is what he becomes (i.e., rebellious, loner, overachiever) (Kerr, 1981).

Sibling position can often determine which child is selected as the object of the family projection process. Sibling position can also determine certain personality characteristics. For example, the eldest sibling may be overly responsible, or the youngest may be more dependent. The level of differentiation in the family and the triangles operating within the family system also influence the behaviors associated with sibling positions.

Nuclear family emotional system refers to emotional functioning of a family in a single generation. Knowledge of details of family functioning in the present generation can allow one to reconstruct the family processes of past generations. Intense emotional fusion in a marriage can characterize a present generation but have its origins in the families of both spouses. Bowen (1976) maintains that this undifferentiation in a marriage results in marital conflict, dysfunction in one of the spouses, or projection of the problems onto the children.

Emotional cutoff describes the methods an individual uses to deal with unresolved fusion in families of origin. These individuals cut themselves off from the parental family. The more differentiation of self there is, the less cutoff that exists. The degree of unresolved emotional attachment to the parents is related to the degree of differentiation that has to be handled over the course of a person's life.

Observing the family interactional style over a period of time allows the nurse to assess the relationship system in a family. Bowen's systems theory suggests that less differentiated families are more prone to illness, both physical and emotional. For this reason, nurses may come in frequent contact with families with problems of differentiation. The structure of the family should be assessed before intervention is planned. It is important not only to take into account the marital interaction but to observe the interaction between parents and children. Family members' illnesses may be perpetuated by the interaction of the family. For example, an ill child may continue with symptoms to maintain the overinvolvement of mother as a mechanism to keep the triangling process going.

Nurses have often been instrumental in helping individuals and families deal with the anxiety of illness. When nurses work with families to reduce anxiety, there may be less dysfunctional triangling. Nurses can assist families with healthier ways of relating that may influence what is passed on to the next generation.

Bowen's family systems theory is particularly useful for viewing family processes over several generations. The use of a family genogram can aid nurses in collecting and analyzing generational data. (The reader is referred to Chapter 9 for a discussion of genograms.) The influence of grand-parents and extended family on the level of a family's functioning can be put in a new perspective with possible opportunities for intervention. For example, in work with the elderly, the isolation from their children may be related to the emotional cutoff process. Using Bowen's family systems theory and the related dynamics of the family system can allow nurses to conceptualize problems from a systems view and plan care that is family centered.

Minuchin's Structural Paradigm

Minuchin and several coworkers (1967) developed a framework for family intervention known as structural family therapy. This view, consistent with systems theory, sees the individual in an interdependent relationship with his or her social system. Because the family is considered the basis of the individual's socialization, structural therapy has been conducted primarily through family intervention. However, other social systems are seen as contributing to the development of the individual and the family, and all of the social systems of the family are considered in the change process. In addition, the structure of the family system as well as its functions are assessed as parameters of family functioning (Aponte & Van-Deusen, 1981).

The family is seen as a system that operates through transactional patterns, which, when repeated, define the structure of how, when, and to whom to relate. Individual family members' behavior is regulated by these transactional patterns. The structural dimensions are referred to as boundary, alignment, and power (Minuchin, 1974).

Subsystems allow the family functions to be carried out. Minuchin describes the parental subsystem functions as nurturance and socialization of children. The spouse subsystem functions include providing emotional support to one another and engaging in mutual accommodation. The sibling subsystem teaches the children how to negotiate and cooperate (Minuchin, 1974).

Boundaries direct participation in subsystems and allow contact with other members of the system. Clarity of boundaries is essential to proper functioning of the subsystem. At one extreme are boundaries that are blurred and diffused with a high degree of permeability. Minuchin describes these systems as *enmeshed,* and they are characterized by overinvolvement and lack of autonomy in the members. At the other extreme are rigid boundaries that inhibit contact and communication and lead to *disengagement* (Minuchin, 1974). He suggests that enmeshed and disengaged systems are present to some degree in most families, but operating at either extreme leads to dysfunction in families.

Alignment, a structural dimension of families, refers to patterns of members working together or in opposition to one member of the system. Functioning families have flexible alignments that allow the functions of the family to be carried out. A *coalition* is an example of alignment where mother and child may act together opposing father.

Power in family systems also influences how family functions are carried out. Power relates to the degree of influence one member has on another. Decision making is one component of power. How decisions are made in families and who makes them certainly has an effect on families' ability to carry out their functions. Power as a structural dimension has also been referred to by structural therapists as force (Aponte & VanDeusen, 1981).

Underorganization is a concept that originated from the work of Minuchin and coworkers (1967) with families from low socioeconomic backgrounds. Underorganization refers to families' inability to develop effective structural dimensions. These families are characterized by limited abilities to organize themselves to solve problems. They also may be rigid in how they employ the structures they have and inconsistent in the use of those structures (Aponte & VanDeusen, 1981).

Minuchin has also described an elaborate set of strategies and techniques for intervening in family systems. Those techniques are most appropriately applied in formal family therapy and will not be described here. However, the structural family paradigm based on systems theory concepts is useful for nurses in assessing family problems and influencing family transactions.

Knowledge of family subsystems and the functions of those subsystems can guide nurses in intervening where boundaries are poorly defined or too rigid. An example may be parental and sibling subsystems with diffuse boundaries that allow children to assume parental functions. Intervention may be directed at the parental subsystem, such as information/education on limit setting, or intervention may be directed at the sibling subsystem. For example, the nurse may suggest age-appropriate activities for the children to enable them to work on the tasks of cooperation and negotiation with their peers. Nurses may also intervene when a parent, frequently the father, is excluded from the parent-child subsystem.

Nurses can be instrumental in restructuring the boundaries of the subsystems. Often the assignment of tasks is beneficial. Where the boundaries lead to disengaged subsystems, nurses can be facilitators of more open communication or more support and involvement among family members.

Interactional Family Theory

Don Jackson, Gregory Bateson, Jay Haley, and John Weakland are often considered together, not only for their joint association at the Mental Research Institute in Palo Alto, California but also because of the similarity of their theoretical conceptions about communication. For an in-depth review of communication theory and its application to work with families, the reader is referred to Chapter 8 of this text. Jackson was influenced by Von Bertalanffy's (1968) approach to systems theory and emphasized the cognitive aspects of communication. Haley placed an emphasis on the question of who is in control of a relationship. Bateson, who was trained as an anthropologist, studied communication levels and channels and how one message changed or was significant in understanding another (Gurman & Kniskern, 1991).

Jackson, together with Watzlawick and Beavin (1967), developed axioms of communication as aids to understand how family relationships are established and as an approach to examine family communication styles. These principles of communication highlight the interdependent nature of the systems' parts and the interactional nature of communication in a family.

One of the primary feedback mechanisms in family subsystems is the communication process. How this process occurs and its effectiveness is an important aspect of family functioning. Poor boundary maintenance may result in decreased communication and isolation with family subsystems or with the whole family system.

Communication serves many functions in a family system. The Circumplex Model described below stresses how communication influences the family system's ability to maintain cohesion and adaptability. Nurses working with family systems need to assess the effectiveness of communication in the family, as well as to establish communication with the family. Important areas to consider in this assessment include how clear and concise messages are and how congruent they are with nonverbal behavior. Also, are the messages free of contradictory information or do they contain many levels of meaning that are difficult to interpret? The directness of messages also facilitates the communication process.

Circumplex Model

Olson et al. (1979) note the abundance of concepts in the literature that attempt to describe the phenomena of family dynamics. They have integrated these concepts in a model that uses general systems theory as an underlying framework. The Circumplex Model of marital and family systems is a model developed to locate families in a circumplex matrix created by the two central dimensions of family cohesion and family adaptability. The third dimension, *communication,* facilitates families in cohesion and adaptability (Olson, 1986). The central area of the matrix, where a balance of cohesion and adaptability occurs, is viewed as the area of op-

timal family functioning. There are 16 types of marital and family systems, which are broken down into three major types: balanced, midrange, and extreme (see Fig. 4–1). Families in the center of the matrix show flexible separateness, flexible togetherness, structured separateness, and structured togetherness (Russell, 1979).

Olson et al. (1979) suggest that at least 40 concepts previously described relate conceptually to their definition of cohesion. Included in their cluster of concepts is Minuchin's (1974) description of enmeshed or disengaged boundaries and Bowen's (1976) level of differentiation. Olson et al. (1979) have defined cohesion as "the emotional bonding members have with one another and the degree of individual autonomy a person experiences in the family system" (p. 5). They further suggest that a balanced degree of family cohesion allows for optimum individual development and effective family functioning.

Variables influencing family cohesion include emotional bonding, boundaries, independence, coalitions, time, space, friends, decision making, and interests (Olson et al., 1979, p. 5). The assessment of these variables will then allow one to place a family under one of the four levels of cohesion: disengaged, separated, connected, or enmeshed.

Olson et al. (1989) agree with several other theorists that viewing the family as primarily homeostasis oriented is limiting and does not allow for the view of families changing and evolving to more complex systems. They view families as capable of adapting and changing to meet the needs of the family and the demands of developmental transitions. The second dimension of the Circumplex Model is adaptability (or change). Adaptability is defined as "the ability of a marital/family system to change its power structure, role relationships and relationship rules in response to situational and developmental stress" (Olson et al., 1979, p. 12).

In order to assess a family's capacity for adaptability, the specific variables to be reviewed include the family's power structure, negotiation styles, role relationships, relationship rules, and feedback. Again, a family can be placed on a continuum of adaptability ranging from chaotic to flexible to structured and then to rigid. Families who are able to be structured and show stability yet at the same time allow for change and flexibility are seen to have the most effective functioning.

The process of communication facilitates family change and cohesion. Families with a flexible level of adaptability and cohesion will likely be more successful in problem solving and negotiating. Communication will be more open and family rules more explicit. Positive communication will be more frequent, and members will feel freer to communicate their needs to the family (Olson, 1986).

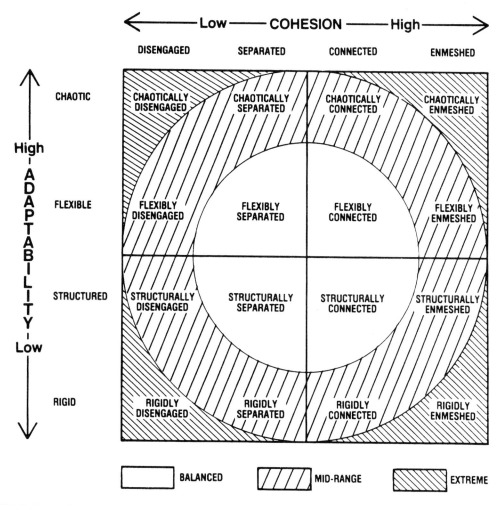

FIGURE 4–1. Circumplex model: Sixteen types of marital and family systems. (From Olson, D.H. (1986). Circumplex Model VII: Validation studies and FACES III. *Family Process,* 25, 339. Copyright 1986 by *Family Process.* Reprinted with permission.

To develop further the theoretical framework of family systems and to assist professionals to determine family functioning and family systems, Olson et al. (1985) developed the *Family Adaptability and Cohesion Evaluation Scales III* (FACES III).* The scale is a self-report instrument that assesses a family's perception of their family system and their ideal descriptions. It is a 20-item scale that has evolved as FACES I and FACES II have been modified. FACES IV was developed in 1991 (Olson, 1991). The instrument has been used as a framework for studies to test hypotheses about functioning of balanced, midrange, and ex-

*FACES III can be obtained by writing:
Family Social Science
University of Minnesota
290 McNeal Hall
St. Paul, MN 55108

treme families (Olson, 1986). To determine family communication, the *Marital Communication Scale* and/or the *Parent-Adolescent Communications Scale* are suggested (Barnes & Olson, 1982).

Olson and colleagues (1989) have attempted to bridge the gap between existing systems frameworks and have provided valid and reliable tools to assess family functioning. The Circumplex Model proposes a dynamic view of family systems adapting to developmental changes over the life cycle.

Developmental Framework

In addition to understanding the family as a system, it is necessary to understand the phases of family development through the life cycle. Mattessich and Hill (1987) describe family development as "an underlying, regular process of differentiation and transformation over the family's history" (p. 437). Consistent with the view of the family as a living system is the conception of its capacity for maintenance and for evolution. Phases of family development place demands for change on a family inasmuch as individual growth and development of members affects the family system. Families may have to deal with many different progressions at once. Carter and McGoldrick (1988) highlight the changing patterns of the family life cycle in today's world and emphasize viewing the family with at least a three-generational view.

Solomon (1973) reminds us that each stage of development in the family is a crisis, and there can be disorganization of the system at each stage. Also, the family can restructure its patterns of relating and communicating and create new structures in the adaptation process. Olson et al. (1989) emphasize this capacity in their Circumplex Model. Minuchin and Fishman (1981) also suggest that family development moves in stages that follow a progression of increasing complexity, with periods of balance and adaptation alternating with periods of disequilibrium.

Although many authors have described functions of the family system through the life cycle, Ackerman's succinct description is used here for its inclusiveness. The functions of the family system involve five areas:

1. The family as a survival and growth unit
2. Affectional needs of family members
3. The balance between autonomy and dependency
4. Social and sexual training
5. Growth and development of each member (Bloch & Simon, 1982, p. 210)

These functions constitute one of the regularities of the family as a system. The functions of a family give it direction and encourage interdependence of family members. These functions also set the family apart from other systems (Hill, 1971).

No assessment of family functions would be complete without attention to the function of health promotion in the family system. Family behaviors that enhance or diminish health status of individuals or the family unit must be considered.

Forrest (1981) suggests that the family, as the unit of socialization, promotes what health values are to be adopted by the family. How much value a family places on health and the level of information a family system accepts determines the family's health functioning.

Areas for assessment by nurses include how receptive a family system is for health knowledge and how well families are capable of using this information. Understanding the value a family places on health behavior and health promotion may lead to areas for intervention.

Nursing Models

Adopting existing theories of family functioning from disciplines other than nursing can be beneficial if the central concepts of nursing theory (person, man, environment, and nursing) are also incorporated (Whall, 1980, 1991). Fawcett (1975), Johnston (1986), and Friedemann (1989) present conceptual frameworks of the family as a living system, integrating concepts from the Rogerian model. Roger's (1970) conceptual framework has been selected for its similarities to the family systems approach.

Examining each of Rogers's basic assumptions in her science of unitary beings will enable integration of both frameworks. The first of these assumptions is that "man is a unified whole possessing his own integrity and manifesting characteristics that are more than and different from the sum of his parts" (Rogers, 1970, p. 47). As has been previously discussed, the family unit is also viewed in its wholeness; it is composed of subsystems that are interdependent and that together form a unity that is different than the sum of the family subsystems. This view of wholeness is central to family theorists who subscribe to systems theory.

The second assumption on which nursing science builds is "Man and environment are continuously exchanging matter and energy with one another" (Rogers, 1970, p. 54). To understand, family system nursing also needs to examine the environment of which the family is a part. Families are continuously influenced by information within the environment, and depending on the degree of permeability of the boundaries, they are constantly responding to this input. Fawcett (1975) also stresses this view of the family as a dynamic whole engaged in mutual simultaneous interaction with the environment.

The third assumption that Rogers delineates states that "the life process evolves irreversibly and unidirectionally along the space-time continuum" (Rogers, 1970, p. 59). The family system is also subject to change, which takes place along the space-time axis. The family moves through stages of development in a sequential, unidirectional manner. "Irreversibly" refers to the concept of not returning to a previous state. The movement is forward when one examines family development. A family cannot return to the same previous stage of development. Stages do not repeat themselves, even though there may be similarities in each new stage or crisis.

The fourth assumption described by Rogers is particularly important in viewing the family as a complex system, which has been stressed throughout this chapter. Rogers (1970) states "Pattern and organization identify man and reflect his innovative wholeness" (p. 65). The family as an open system, in constant interaction with the environment through exchange of matter and energy, evolves toward a growing level of complexity. Patterning that takes place over time can be observed in families. Homeostasis implies returning to the previous state in the family system. Organization, on the other hand, implies a dynamic movement forward toward greater complexity.

The last assumption that Rogers describes is what makes humankind unique among other living systems. "Man is characterized by the capacity for abstraction and imagery, language and thought, sensation and emotion" (Rogers, 1970, p. 73). The family also has the capacity for feeling, for knowing, for comprehending, and for using these processes to determine patterns, make choices, and recognize its environment.

FAMILIES AS HEALTH-PROMOTING SYSTEMS

Several of the theorists previously discussed have acknowledged that health and illness behaviors are learned within the context of the family system (Bloch & Simon, 1982; Bowen, 1976; Guerin, 1976; Minuchin & Fishman, 1981). Family functions include health care and health promotion. Each family will define for itself what it perceives to be adequate functioning with regard to health.

How the family organizes itself to meet the basic needs of its members for health is an important area for nursing assessment. Individual health and family health greatly influence each other and contribute to the family's total level of health, as suggested by systems principles. The family as a system generates, prevents, or corrects health problems. Anderson and Tomlinson (1992) propose a holistic definition of family health that includes five realms of family experience, which comprise the family health system.

Marie Friedemann (1992) advocates working with families as a unit; this includes encouraging them to work together to foster family togetherness and time for family members to actualize themselves individually. Family health promotion can be enhanced by empowering members to work together to create harmony as they make changes and adapt to environmental and family demands. The family nurse assists the family system in taking control to protect them from harm through family maintenance (including the acceptance of family rules, roles, decision making, sharing tasks, and consensus). Readers are encouraged to consult Dr. Friedeman's *Enhancing*

Families: A Counseling/Education Model: Field Training Manual for Counselors (1992).

The family's environmental system also has an influence on family health. The physical environment of the family and the social and interpersonal environments interact to influence the health of family members and the health of the family unit. How families establish and maintain linkage with community systems (and community subsystems such as health care systems) is important to determine. Are the exchanges of information adequate for the family in coping with and managing their specific developmental issues and crises? Are resources for health promotion appropriately used? Families must also prioritize the health-promoting tasks to be carried out within the family system. Forrest (1981) encourages health practitioners to allow families to be more active participants in their own health behaviors.

IMPLICATIONS AND DIRECTIONS FOR FAMILY HEALTH NURSING

The family as the client continues to receive emphasis in nursing. Family-centered nursing recognizes that the family system must be a target of service and that family health and individual health strongly influence each other. Furthermore, the health of the family system affects the health of the community.

CHAPTER HIGHLIGHTS

Theorists have developed models to understand the types of family systems and assessment measures to determine the family type.

Families are units of individuals that are interdependently interrelated and one part cannot be understood in isolation from the rest of the system.

Conceptualization of families as interrelated components assists the nurse to understand the impact of change in family members on family health, and vice versa.

Change is constant at the individual, intrafamily, and supra-system levels; therefore, assessment systems boundaries and interactions are crucial to determining a family's health and areas for growth.

Each family is a health-promoting system and develops unique health-promoting patterns as a system.

Knowledge of the type of family system is crucial to planning interventions with families. Use of tools such as FACES III to assess the family system might be useful in some situations. In addition, relating concepts from Bowen's family systems theory, from interactional communication theory, from general systems theory, and from Minuchin's structural theory to families will assist in understanding families as unique yet similar systems.

As nursing continues to expand its knowledge base through integration of nursing models with existing conceptual frameworks tested by research, nurses will become more prepared to deal with the complexities of family health care. Theorists across several disciplines have continued to describe similar phenomena in their observations of families. Nursing has been associated with family health care for a long time, and nurses are in a unique position to continue adding to the body of knowledge about family functioning through nursing research. Nursing can make significant contributions by further examining how families achieve and maintain wellness.

REFERENCES

Anderson, K.H., & Tomlinson, P.M. (1992). The family health system as an emerging paradigmatic view for nursing. *IMAGE*, 24(1), 57–63.

Aponte, H.J., & VanDeusen, J.M. (1981). Structural family therapy. In A.S. Gurman & D.P. Kniskern (Eds.), *Handbook of Family Therapy* (pp. 310–360). New York: Brunner/Mazel.

Barkauskas, V.H. (1986). Community health nursing. In B.B. Logan & C.E. Dawkins (Eds.), *Family-Centered Nursing in the Community* (pp. 39–44). Menlo Park, CA: Addison-Wesley.

Barnes, H., & Olson, D.H. (1982). Parent adolescent communication scale. In D.H. Olson et al. (Eds.), *Family Inventories*. St. Paul, MN: Family Social Science, University of Minnesota.

Bateson, G., Jackson, D., Haley, J. & Weakland, J. (1956). Toward a theory of schizophrenia. *Behavioral Science*, 1, 251–264.

Bloch, D., & Simon R. (Eds.). (1982). *The Strength of Family Therapy: Selected Papers of Nathan Ackerman*. New York: Brunner/Mazel.

Bowen, M. (1976). Theory in the practice of psychotherapy. In P.J. Guerin (Ed.), *Family Therapy Theory and Practice* (pp. 42–89). New York: Gardner Press.

Burr, W.R., Hill, R., Nye, F.I., & Reiss I.L. (1979). *Contemporary Theories about the Family* (Vol. 2). New York & London: Free Press.

Carter, B., & McGoldbrick, M. (Eds.). (1988). *The Changing Family Life Cycle: A Framework for Family Therapy*. New York & London: Gardner Press.

Duvall, E.M., & Miller, B.C. (1985). *Marriage and Family Development*. New York: Harper & Row, Publishers.

Fawcett, J. (1975). The family as a living open system: An emerging conceptual framework for nursing. *International Nursing Review*, 22, 113–116.

Forrest, J. (1981). The Family: The focus for health behavior generation. *Health Values: Achieving High Level Wellness*, 5(4), 138–144.

Friedemann, M.L. (1992). *Enhancing Families: A Counseling/Education Model: Field Training Manual for Counselors*. Detroit, MI: Wayne State University.

Friedemann, M.L. (1989). Closing the gap between theory and mental health practice with families. Part 1: The framework of systematic organization for nursing of families and family members. *Archives of Psychiatric Nursing*, 3(1), 10–19.

Friedemann, M.L. (1989). Closing the Gap Between Grand Theory and Mental Health Practice with Families. Part 2: The Control Congruence Model for Mental Health Nursing of Families. *Archives of Psychiatric Nursing*, 3(1), 20–28.

Friedman, M.M. (1992). *Family Nursing: Theory and Assessment* (3rd ed.). Norwalk, CT: Appleton & Lange.

Galvin, K.M., & Brommel, B.J. (1986). *Family Communication: Cohesion and Change*. Glenview, IL & London, England: Scott, Foresman.

Guerin, P.J. (1976). *Family Therapy: Theory and Practice*. New York, Toronto, Sydney, & London: Gardner Press.

Gurman, A.S., & Kniskern, D.P. (Eds.). (1981). *Handbook of Family Therapy*. New York: Brunner/Mazel.

Gurman, A.S., & Kniskern, D.P. (Eds.). (1991). *Handbook of Family Therapy Volume II*. New York: Brunner/Mazel.

Hall, A.D., & Fagen, R.E. (1956). Definition of systems. *General Systems Yearbook*, 1, 18–28.

Hill, R. (1971). Modern systems theory and the family: A confrontation. *Social Science Information*, 10(5), 7–26.

Johnston, R. (1986). Approaching family intervention through Roger's conceptual model. In A. Whall (Ed.), *Family Therapy Theory for Nursing* (pp. 11–32). Norwalk, CT: Appleton-Century-Crofts.

Kerr, M. (1981). Family systems theory and therapy. In A.S. Gurman & D.P. Kniskern (Eds.), *Handbook of Family Therapy* (pp. 226–264). New York: Brunner/Mazel.

Mattessich, P., & Hill, R. (1987). Life cycle and development. In M.B. Sussman & S.K. Steinmetz (Eds.), *Handbook of Marriage and the Family* (pp. 437–469). New York & London: Plenum Press.

Minuchin, S. (1974). *Families and Family Therapy*. Cambridge, MA: Harvard University Press.

Minuchin, S., & Fishman, R. (1981). *Family Therapy Techniques*. Cambridge, MA & London, England: Harvard University Press.

Minuchin, S., Montalvo, B., Guerney, B., Rosman, B., & Schumer, F. (1967). *Families of the Slums*. New York: Basic Books.

Olson, D. (1986). Circumplex model VII: Validation studies and FACES III. *Family Process*, 25, 337–351.

Olson, D.H. (1991). Commentary: Three-dimensional (3-D) Circumplex Model and revised scoring of FACES III. *Family Process*, 30, 74–79.

Olson, D., Portner, J., & Lavee, Y. (1985). FACES III. St. Paul, MN: Family Social Science, University of Minnesota.

Olson, D., Sprenkle, D., & Russell, C. (1979). Circumplex Model of marital and family systems: I. Cohesion and adaptability dimensions, family types, and clinical applications. *Family Process*, 18, 3–28.

Olson, D., Sprenkle, D., & Russell, C. (Eds.). (1989). *Circumplex Model: Systematic Assessment and Treatment of Families*. New York: Hawthorn Press.

Rogers, M. (1970). *An Introduction to the Theoretical Basis of Nursing*. Philadelphia: F.A. Davis.

Russell, C.S. (1979). Circumplex Model of marital and family systems: III. Empirical evaluation with families. *Family Process,* 18, 29–45.

Solomon, M. (1973). A developmental, conceptual premise for family therapy. *Family Process,* 12, 179–188.

Speer, D. (1970). Family systems: Morphostasis and morphogenesis, or is family homeostasis enough? *Family Process,* 9(3), 259–278.

Von Bertalanffy, L. (1968). *General System Theory.* New York: Braziller.

Watzlawick, P., Beavin, J., & Jackson, D. (1967). *Pragmatics of Human Communication.* New York & London: W.W. Norton.

Whall, A. (1980). Congruence between existing theories of family functioning and nursing theory. *Advances in Nursing Science,* 3, 59–67.

Whall, A. (1986). The Family as the Unit of Care in Nursing: A Historical Review. *Public Health Nursing,* 3(4), 240–249.

Whall, A., & Fawcett, J. (1991). *Family Theory Development in Nursing: A State of the Science and Art.* Philadelphia: F.A. Davis.

Wright, L., & Leahey, M. (1994). *Nurses and Families: A Guide to Family Assessment and Intervention* (2nd ed.). Philadelphia: F.A. Davis.

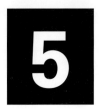

FAMILY CULTURE AND ETHNICITY

JOHN M. LANTZ

If we are to achieve a richer culture, rich in contrasting values, we must recognize the whole gamut of human potentialities, and so weave a less arbitrary social fabric, one in which each diverse human gift will find a fitting place.

MARGARET MEAD, 1935

The ultimate goal of a professional nurse scientist and humanist is to discover, know, and creatively use culturally based knowledge with its fullest meanings, expressions, symbols, and functions for healing, and to promote or maintain well-being (or health) with people of diverse cultures in the world.

MADELEINE M. LEININGER

OBJECTIVES

On completion of this chapter, the reader will be able to:

1. Define culture and ethnicity
2. Explain the components of culture and ethnicity
3. Describe the impact of family culture and ethnicity and beliefs about health and illness on family health promotion and disease prevention
4. Identify the impact of family culture and ethnicity on a health-promoting lifestyle
5. Identify the relevance of culture, ethnicity, and social class to family health nursing practice when collaborating with families to use health-promoting behaviors
6. Collaborate with families of varied cultural and ethnic backgrounds to implement health-promoting behaviors through health teaching and anticipatory guidance

Annually, an estimated one million individuals legally and illegally enter the United States in search of economic security, freedoms, and safety. With current trends, America will be a land with no single ethnic majority population by the year 2080. In such a pluralistic society, the nation's systems of service and its professions will be challenged to consider the uniqueness of these parts that compose the whole.

Historically, America was viewed as a multicultural "melting pot." This view assumes that group ethnicity and cultural uniqueness is unimportant; instead, an amalgamation into a single group is stressed, and a national allegiance and identity is primary. One becomes an American, with American beliefs, values, attitudes, and life patterns. To become part of this homogeneous entity, one's heritage is put aside, and a new culture is assimilated. In this process, individuals gradually conform to the standards of life of the dominant group. The process of assimilation is considered complete when all previous cultural dimensions are fully merged into the dominant cultural group (McLemore, 1980).

Such a cultural or behavioral assimilation may be referred to as *acculturation* (Spector, 1991). The degree to which this process occurs is influenced by age, ability to speak the language of the dominant culture, and amount of contact with the original or dominant culture (Lee, 1976; Keefe, 1981). The political, educational, and health care delivery systems support and endorse this process. Little recognition is given to the fact that acculturation occurs to varying degrees. As a society, we have consistently failed to accept the reality that different cultures coexist within our national boundaries (Staples & Mirandé, 1986). However, these differences provide richness and diversity; they are the essence of humankind in America, and as such can and should be seen as a national strength.

Nursing is concerned with humankind's most valuable asset—health. Nursing is unique among the health professions in that its approach is holistic, and consideration is given to the individuality of the client. These two foundations of nursing practice reflect a transcultural approach to health care, in which the nurse attempts to recognize and transcend barriers and obstacles established by cultural uniqueness. The nurse considers both the common threads that are held by all cultures and the elements that are maintained from a particular group. Only through an approach that combines both can effective, quality, culturally sensitive nursing occur (Leininger, 1978, 1991).

Culturally sensitive nursing is translated into action by respect for people as unique individuals and by exhibiting an understanding that culture is a major force that contributed to this uniqueness (Fong 1985). In a culturally sensitive approach to nursing care, a number of elements are included. These elements are especially important in addressing the health promotion and health maintenance needs of the "well" family. Emphasis is placed on family and human values; concern for a total approach to care; achievement of one's maximum level of well-being; and therapeutic partnership with the individual, family, and nurse. A recognition of the indirect and direct impact of the family on health status is essential.

The notion of family exists as an important unit in all cultures. How a culture defines "family" may vary, but the contribution to the individual remains the same. Through this basic unit of society, an individual learns about himself or herself and about his or her culture. This process is called *enculturation.* It is a process whereby future generations are provided cultural values, beliefs, and attitudes. Included in such a process are basic elements about health and health promotion. The child learns a meaning for health, a meaning for illness, strategies to ensure and maintain health status, and attitudes about health care services. This process is greatly influenced by the family's acculturation status. The focus of this book is to provide the nurse with those common threads useful in intervening with families in an effort to improve their health status. This chapter provides a foundation for a better understanding of those cultural elements not reflected in the dominant culture. This includes the elements gained and maintained through the cultural heritage of the family.

CULTURE

Culture is a universal experience and represents the assumptions we make about life (Leininger, 1989; Lynam, 1992). "Humans do not exist without culture" (Boyle & Andrews, 1989, p. 12). It is a multifaceted, complex, dynamic construct composed of numerous components or concepts. It refers to the sum total of acquired values, beliefs, practices, laws, customs, traditions, artifacts, knowledge, language, and patterns of behavior that permit people to interact effectively with their environment (Leininger, 1989; Branch & Paxton, 1976; Hartog & Hartog, 1983). It is the expression of the essence of a people (Deloria, 1969) and a learned "design for living" (Murray & Zentner, 1985). "Culture is characterized by universality, uniqueness, stability, changeability, unconscious influence and variability" (Clark, 1992, p. 335). Cultures are not static (Mandelbaum, 1991). Culture is learned not only through formal education but also through a process of "cultural osmosis." This process begins in the family and expands into the community as a whole (Boyle & Andrews, 1989). According to Ogburn and Nimkoff (1950), certain components exist in all cultures. The components include:

- A communication system
- Means for physical welfare
- Means for travel
- Exchange of goods for service
- Forms of property
- Sexual and family patterns
- Societal controls—mores, customs, and laws
- Artistic expression
- Leisure-time interests and activities
- Religious and magical beliefs
- Basic knowledge for survival
- Basic human patterns (i.e., competition, conflict, cooperation)

These components provide us with an understanding of the universality of culture, and many of these components are family system patterns basic to health promotion. One can also conclude from these components how culture structures the development of health beliefs, attitudes, and practices. It is crucial to consider cultural variables when providing health care to clients (Leininger, 1978, 1991).

Values

Values are standards that people use to assess themselves and others. Values are essential to one's culture. A number of authors have identified areas that differentiate culture (Brink, 1984; Hartog & Hartog, 1983; Paul, 1955). This differentiation explores human values and common human problems. Five common areas are included: *man nature, human nature, relational, time,* and *activity.* These areas can form barriers that prevent families from seeking health care, using health resources, complying with both preventive and therapeutic regimens, and becoming actively involved in health promotion strategies. The nurse who understands these variant value orientations can compare and contrast various cultures.

Man nature is the basic relationship that humans have with nature. This relationship may be subjugating, submitting, or in harmony. Its effect on health status is related to man's attitude to illness. This attitude determines if a family will become actively involved in health promotion activities in an attempt to prevent illness or whether one fatalistically accepts illness as inevitable.

Human nature is how one views people—the innate human characteristics of good or evil. Some see humans as basically evil, and illness becomes a punishment for unacceptable behavior.

The third element is *relational,* or the impact of people's relationship to each other. Differing values concerning interpersonal relationships cause the individual to follow authoritarian, horizontal, egalitarian, or individualistic patterns of relating. The nurse-client relationship is greatly influenced by the preferred style. It affects how decisions will be made and how health care issues will be resolved.

Time orientation, whether toward the past, present, or future, determines what an individual will do about health problems. Those who are future oriented will not hesitate to choose health promotion measures. Present-oriented persons tend not to choose health promotion. This is why many elderly tend not to become actively involved in health promotion. Present-oriented individuals do not adhere strictly to a time-structured schedule and because they may be frequently late for appointments are considered disrespectful and noninterested. Patterns reflective of this orientation need to be assessed and should not become a barrier to care (Giger & Davidhizar, 1991).

The final value orientation, or common human problem is *activity.* This orientation is toward "doing" versus "being." A "doing" person is an individual who assesses health status and defines

appropriate health promotion strategies based on this assessment (Hartog & Hartog, 1983).

Ethnicity (Social Structure Component)

Ethnicity describes a sense of community transmitted over generations by families. It provides an individual the basis by which "self" can be defined (Rampusheski, 1989). Ethnicity commonly is reinforced by the surrounding community. It is one of a number of social structure components of culture. Ethnicity is part of the essence of humankind "derived from membership, usually through birth in a racial, religious or subgroup with its associated culture" (Hartog & Hartog, 1983, p. 911). It involves a conscious and unconscious association that provides identity and historical continuity (Giordano & Giordano, 1977). Ethnicity is a major determinant of family patterns and belief systems.

Although the concept of ethnicity is complex and somewhat abstract, it is an integral part of health care activities and rituals (Rampusheski, 1989). Primary and secondary characteristics indicative of ethnicity have been identified. They include:

Primary

- Common geographic origin
- Race
- Language
- Religion

Secondary

- Ties to neighborhood or a specific community
- Food preference
- Literature
- Art
- Music
- Employment
- Traditions

(Thernstrom, 1980)

Ethnicity is often viewed interchangeably with the primary characteristic of race. Race is a nonscientific classification of human beings and is based on physiological characteristics such as skin color, eye shape, or texture of hair (Melville, 1988).

Ethnic identification may be seen through one of these primary or secondary characteristics or through a combination. Both an internal sense of distinctiveness and an external perception of distinctiveness are factors for consideration. Currently over 100 ethnic groups, representing all the countries of the world, reside in the United States (Thernstrom, 1980). Each brings ethnic characteristics that need to be considered by the nurse. In addition, Tripp-Reimer and Lauer (1987) emphasize that there is intraethnic diversity within groups and between groups. Knowledge of the heterogeneity of Americans can assist the nurse to avoid stereotyping individuals of ethnic groups.

Family Culture

Family culture is another concept related to the social structure component of culture. "Family culture consists of ways of living and thinking that constitute the family and sexual aspects of group life" (Murray & Zentner, 1985, p. 146). Through the family unit, culture is learned, and through culture, the unit provides individual identity and a sense of responsibility toward others. Family culture provides the following:

- A definition of family
- Roles of family members
- Status of family members
- Communication patterns
- A decision-making process
- Rituals and rites

The elements listed provide both a general framework and a framework for health promotion and health care expectations. Family focused nursing must consider that while the family is the basic unit of society, its elements are dynamic. For example, one family structure change has been the number of female-headed households. Currently women comprise 19% of heads of households. Within this group, another related factor that impacts health status and health promotion activities has been called the "feminization of poverty." Female heads of households as a group comprise 61% of those below the poverty level (Radecki, 1991).

Beliefs

Although it often appears to individuals that their beliefs are a product of a unique psychic experience, the reality is that beliefs are convictions that certain things are true or real based on life experience (Harris, 1975). Belief implies mental acceptance of truths learned through family and community. As an element of culture, beliefs are the feeling dimensions that are translated into actions. "It includes the beliefs men hold about themselves, and the social, biological, and physical world in which they live, and about their relations to one another, to society and nature, and to such other beings as they discover, accept or conjure up" (Chinoy, 1967, p. 32). Some elements included in the domain of beliefs are:

- Faith
- Trust
- Confidence
- Credence
- Opinions
- Judgments

Health-focused beliefs may be prescriptive, restrictive, or taboos. Prescriptive beliefs are positively stated, describing expective behaviors, while restrictive beliefs are negatively phrased and limit choices and behaviors. Taboos are restrictive in nature but identify potential supernatural consequences. Two examples of taboos during pregnancy are (1) avoiding moonlight or lunar eclipses so that the baby will not be born with a deformity (Latino), and (2) not having your picture taken during pregnancy because it may cause a stillbirth (African American) (Boyles & Andrews, 1989).

Customs

Customs are usual practices or habits carried out by a defined population. They are orderly, comprehensive, and standardized expectations, specifying ways in which things are and should be done and the rights and obligations of individuals. Customs are sanctioned by tradition and sustained by the pressures of group opinion. A group tends to resist changes in customs both overtly and covertly. The following three evaluative criteria can be considered in identifying a custom:

1. Custom establishes the "norm" or "ideal" form of behavior in a given situation.
2. Custom embodies a force to constrain individuals to conform.
3. Custom reveals group judgments about preference through actions and behavior (Parsons, 1970).

Such actions and behaviors include communication, decision making, roles, rituals, etiquette, and routines. Of these actions, communication can be an insurmountable problem in providing family-focused, culturally sensitive care. If clients speak a different language it should not be seen as a client problem, but a mutually shared problem. Elements to consider as aspects of communication include dialect, style, volume, use of touch, context of speech, and kinesics (Giger, 1990).

The major concepts developed as part of the construct of culture are *values, social structure, beliefs,* and *customs.* All elements are socially created, shared, and transmitted as a way of life. A cultural approach to health promotion involves a consideration of these interrelated, interdependent concepts.

CULTURAL ASSESSMENT

A variety of culturally focused assessment tools have been developed to assist health care providers. Such cultural assessments provide meaning to patterns of behavior that might otherwise be judged unimportant, inappropriate, or in conflict with the beliefs and values of the provider or the delivery system. Leininger (1978) defined a cultural assessment as a systematic appraisal of cultural beliefs, values, and practices within the cultural context of the individual being evaluated.

Most cultural assessment tools include basic cultural data such as:

- Ethnic affiliation
- Family patterns
- Religion
- Nutrition/food patterns
- Ethnic health care practices
- Family health promoting life-style

Lipson and Meleis (1985) developed a list of items essential for a minimum cultural assessment. This tool included information on length of time in the host country, role of the family, language spoken, religion, and ethnic affiliation. Bloch (1983) Brownlee (1978), and Friedman (1992) developed comprehensive, community-focused cultural assessment tools. The tools serve as comprehensive guides that are useful in identifying cultural domains that are important in working with culturally distinct communities. Elements included in this type of assessment are communication, language, family, politics, economics, education, and religion. This provides a systems analysis of culture and considers its relationship to health.

Tripp-Reimer et al. (1984) and Louie (1985) believe that a cultural assessment should begin with a general impression of individuals and their family unit. Next, the nurse should solicit problem-specific information. Clients are asked to give reasons why they feel health care is needed. A health-focused cultural assessment cannot and does not require information on every element of culture. The assessment must occur openly, without judgments, conclusions, or generalizations. Unlike biologic and psychologic data, which attempt to identify deviations from the norm, cultural assessments are done "to identify deviations in cultural parameters with the goal of modifying the client's system or modifying the health care professional's system in order to increase congruence between them" (Tripp-Reimer et al., 1984, p. 81). Response to this assessment allows the nurse an opportunity to categorize and analyze culturally specific directives and interventions.

A primary concern in cultural assessment is to determine the place and role of the family with respect to health and illness (Clark, 1992). Culturally specific directives that are family focused and aimed at health promotion and disease prevention should consider four domains: values, social structure, beliefs, and customs. Attitudes and responses to health-promoting behaviors are based

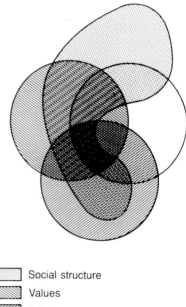

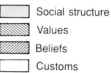
- Social structure
- Values
- Beliefs
- Customs

FIGURE 5–1. Four domains that compose culture and health culture.

on the interrelationship of these elements. Any attempts, however sound, are liable to fail unless the nurse takes into consideration his or her own culture and the family's culture, to bridge the cultural gap between the nurse and the family unit. Because there are an infinite variety of cultures, the nurse is advised to acknowledge these varieties and their unique health practices rather than attempt to be an expert in all cultures (Tripp-Reimer & Lauer, 1987). Figure 5–1 shows how all four domains interrelate and affect health.

HEALTH CULTURE

In the simplest of societies, values, societal components, beliefs, and customs are interrelated, thereby providing a foundation for well-being and self-preservation. Every society, therefore, has its own health culture. This health culture is identified as the traditional way a society copes with illness and maintains well-being. Individuals and families tend to feel more comfortable with their own health culture because it reflects their own values and views of life. Health culture defines the following:

1. Health
2. Illness
3. Disease causation
4. Healer's role
5. Sick role
6. Acceptable treatment modalities
7. System of services

The American health culture is based primarily on a Western medicine system. This system tends to be illness focused with a defined cause for disease. The system stresses the use of scientific methods of diagnosis and treatment. This system often does not meet the health care expectations of different cultural groups (Branch & Paxton, 1976; Scott, 1974). The gap may be due to language barriers, economic problems, or a lack of "cultural fit" with the culturally pluralistic society. Other cultural barriers to delivery of services include the fee-for-service system, depersonalization by providers, and fragmentation of services. Whether real or perceived, these barriers have to be considered by the provider.

Illness Behavior and Culture

Illness introduces a new dimension into any family. It is an unwelcome intruder: a threat that may lead to death. Culture influences how illness events are perceived and managed (Lynman, 1992). A cultural determinant of a reaction to illness is reflective of an understanding and interpretation of the cause of disease. In some societies, ill persons are isolated, and no care is given to them. This practice probably originated with group fear of infectious diseases. In other societies, a constant massive family vigil is important during illness. Many families initiate treatment before seeking medical care (Kleinman, 1978).

Families tend to approach illness from a holistic perspective. Their life patterns and beliefs about illness also influence their approach and behaviors toward health promotion (Tripp-Reimer & Lauer, 1987). Beliefs also define conditions under which a "sick role" may be legitimately assumed. The sick role is an undesirable state with the following expectations:

1. A sick person cannot be held responsible for the illness because he or she cannot overcome it by desire or willpower.
2. It is expected that the sick person wants to get well
3. While sick, a person may be exempt from carrying out his or her usual roles and tasks.
4. If attempts made by the family are unsuccessful, the individual must seek competent help and is obliged to comply with the caregiver in getting well (Parsons, 1970).

Culture, therefore, defines illness and the conditions under which the sick role may be assumed. It establishes expected behavior for that role and a support system to meet the needs of the individual.

Social Class and Health

One barrier to involvement in health promotion relates to economics. It is estimated that 1 of every 8 American families has an income below the federal poverty level (*Healthy People 2000*, 1992). Poverty is a major obstacle for families in their efforts to maintain and promote their health state (Bauwens & Anderson, 1992). Poverty makes the family less capable to seek care and accounts for greater susceptibility to illness. Poverty cuts across ethnic and racial lines. Like other elements of culture, "it can be passed on, it can be cyclic, be self-perpetuating, and is assumed to be reinforced in the next generation" (Spector, 1979, p. 106).

The relationship of poverty and death is a direct one. The poor have a higher incidence of disease and death rates twice the rates of people with incomes above the poverty level. (Bauwens & Anderson, 1992). A cultural relationship to poverty exists, with poverty higher in people of color. One-third of Black Americans live below the poverty level, a rate three times greater than the White population (*Healthy People 2000*, 1992). Despite a philosophy that health is a "right of all persons," the poor prioritize food, adequate shelter, and clothing as more important. Health promotion is often abstract and a nonreality to the poor. According to Koos (1954), the poor are not likely to make use of available preventive health care because of personal conflicts and other priorities, whereas the more affluent have their basic needs met and have the resources to participate in health promotion and health protection.

Health promotion efforts by nurses are usually aimed at white, middle-class Americans, the healthiest segment of the population. Strategies for minorities, older individuals, or low-income population segments need to be adapted (Freudenberg, 1985).

HEALTH PROMOTION AND CULTURE

Before asking a group of people to assume new health habits, it is wise to ascertain the existing habits, how these habits are linked to one another, what function they perform, and what they mean to those who practice them.

BENJAMIN PAUL, 1935

Impact of Culture and Ethnicity on Health Promotion

"Culture, learned and transmitted from one generation to another, may be viewed as a blueprint for living which guides a group's thoughts, actions and sentiments" (Reinhardt & Quinn, 1973, p. 47). Such a blueprint includes a multitude of intercultural beliefs and practices that provide the family unit direction for health-promoting behaviors. It is composed of those things the family does to maintain its highest level of functioning. The nurse needs to build on these existing resources and strengths and include these cultural variables that influence decisions, actions, and behaviors. Health promotion is the actualization of health potential. It occurs through processes that encourage alteration or reinforcement of personal habits or changes in the environment in which the family lives (Brubecker, 1983; Pender, 1987).

Among all people there is generally agreement that good health is essential for survival and well-being (Spector, 1991). Health is a socially interpreted phenomenon, and health behaviors are not individually determined (Clinton, 1986). People in various cultural groups tend to be *ethnocentric* in that they believe their own view of the world is desirable and actually superior to others (Levine & Campbell, 1972). These beliefs and attitudes affect a family's approach to health promotion.

Families learn from their cultures and ethnic backgrounds how to be healthy. An awareness, respect, sensitivity, and acceptance of the existence of cultural differences are essential to effective nursing. Through review of cultural differences, one may conclude that intragroup differences may exceed intergroup differences. Through analysis of such differences, nurses can identify their own misconceptions and base health promotion strategies on those cultural elements of the family unit.

In addition to this professional dimension, "each individual can find fulfillment and can experience new dimensions of living by expanding beyond his or her boundaries and exploring the personal meaning of the experiences they have with people of different lifestyles and different world views" (Branch & Paxton, 1976, p. 8). "A major obstacle in providing culturally relevant nursing care is that nurses rarely question the validity of their own beliefs and values, which have been shaped by the professional health culture" (Clinton, 1986, p. 579). Self-awareness as a nurse and as a member of a culture is essential.

It is important for nurses to remember the following words of caution as they work with individuals and families in planning culturally sensitive health promotion strategies:

> We should not exaggerate the extent of cultural pluralism in the United States and should realize that widespread cultural assimilation has taken place in America. To try to perceive cultural differences where none exist may be as detrimental as ignoring those which are real.
> J. BANKS, 1978

Impact of Family Culture and Ethnicity on Health-Promoting Lifestyle

Respect for cultural differences and a nonintrusive and collaborative perspective is fundamental in the nurse's approach in family health promotion. Family culture is a way of life for its members, and it provides the basis for health-promoting lifestyle strategies. The best source of information about the families health promoting

lifestyle is the family unit itself. To determine the baseline for practice, these nurses must begin with two basic questions. First, "How do people stay healthy?" and second, "How do members of your family stay healthy?" Direct your questioning from broad to specific.

The mother tends to be the primary care provider during illness and the one who shares her knowledge and experiences regarding ways to stay healthy (Clinton, 1986). The nurse may begin here and validate beliefs through observations of behaviors reflective of those beliefs. The nurse should be alert to the possibility that the family unit may express what they believe the nurse wants to hear. The nurse will encounter health problems that are culturally defined, understood, and expressed differently than he or she is accustomed to. The nurse's approach must be based on the client's perception and definition of health status. The formulation of outcomes must be in the client's terminology (Clinton, 1986).

Family recreation, exercise and fitness, risk reduction, proper nutrition, stress management, and functional communication are just a few health-promoting lifestyle strategies included in this text–none of which can be incorporated into the family unit's lifestyle unless they are nonconflicting or nonthreatening to the family's culture. Exercise may be seen as "menial labor," resulting in perspiration and a state of degradation. Relaxation techniques may be seen as "hocus-pocus" or mystical, where possible loss of control can occur. Overeating may be seen as a symbol of prosperity and success, and gifts of food may be symbols of love, support, comfort, and concern (Fong, 1985). For example, the American Indian family drinks specific teas and eats certain foods at certain times of the year to assure future good health. Lice may be a symbol of life and purposely placed on a child's head while the child is hospitalized. Traditionally, roots, herbs, potions, oils, powders, rituals, or ceremonies may be used to stay healthy. These mystical practices and procedures develop to fill a void when a desire exists and means are not defined. Such customs translate beliefs and values into practice in a family unit.

Although all four elements of culture (social structure, values, beliefs, and customs) are important in implementing health-promoting strategies, values are the standards used to assess importance of new behaviors by the family. Values dictate directly or indirectly whether a family unit will become actively involved. Values seen by one family as negative, inferior, undesirable, or threatening may be the foundation of practice for another family unit. The nurse, simply by exposing the family to a new idea or practice, must recognize that it will not automatically result in inclusion in lifestyle. Such values must be translated into beliefs that become "truths." These truths then become actions and practices. They become a way of life.

Implications for Nursing Practice and Research

Culture is the "set of perceptions, technologies, and survival systems used by members of a specified group to ensure the acquisition and perception of what they consider to be a high quality of life" (Taylor, 1986, p. 2). These perceptions, technologies, and survival systems must then be considered by the nurse as the basis for health promotion behaviors.

Leininger (1977) discusses nurses who are culturally blind and behave as if cultural differences are nonexistent. These individuals often believe that everyone should conform to the majority's practices. Such beliefs are referred to as *cultural imposition.* These responses are an extension of ethnocentrism. "To understand transcultural nursing and implications for nursing practice, one must have a basic understanding of culture, cultural values, and culturally diverse nursing care" (Giger & Davidhizar, 1991, p. 4).

One cannot begin any interventions until common culturally prescribed beliefs and practices are identified (Bauwens & Anderson, 1992; Friedman, 1992; Tripp-Reimer & Lauer, 1987). The nurse cannot begin the family nursing process until completing an assessment of the family's beliefs about the future and their beliefs about their control over their destiny. If the family believes that "whatever will be, will be," what value are the nurse's interventions? The nurse must know these beliefs and begin there. Only by using this approach can effective integration of the cultural uniqueness of the family occur. The fundamental approach must be the family, and the major nursing strategy is communication. The interrelationship between communication and culture is very important. Communication is the vehicle by which culture is transmitted and expressed (Giger & Davidhizar, 1991).

Leininger (1978) stated that in order to provide culturally meaningful health services to patients, the client's view concerning health and illness must be systematically studied by nurses. Four research methods can be used to accomplish this: (1) emic, (2) etic, (3) synchronic, and (4) diachronic. *Emic* methodology is an in-depth qualitative analysis of the cultural meaning and origins of health promotion behaviors. Through interviewing methods, those behaviors deemed culturally appropriate are identified. *Etic* methodology studies those beliefs, values, customs, and social structures of culture from the outside. One analyzes such universals by observation (Leininger, 1985b, 1991). *Synchronic* methods analyze those fixed elements of structure, function, and meaning of culture, and *diachronic* methods study the historical developments and influences of a changing culture. A combination of these approaches will assist researchers and practitioners in identifying the ideal, *what ought to be;* the real, *what is;* the explicit, *the concrete observable;* and the implicit, *the invisible, silent* dimensions of health promotion.

When recruiting ethnically diverse research subjects, researchers should explore the intricate differences of each group by learning more about the group through an ethnohistory. An ethnohistory is the cultural history of a specific culture (Leininger, 1991). In addition, particularly in qualitative research, Hautman and Bomar (1995) recommend that researchers be cognizant of the four key figures in the research process: community, participant, researcher, and the setting. Success in the recruitment and retention of culturally and ethically diverse research samples is enhanced by considering the interactional dimensions of (1) caring about the dignity and respect of research subjects; (2) a non-hierarchical reciprocal relationship between the researcher and subjects; (3) developing trust between the researcher and subjects, (4) sensitivity of the researcher about subjects' culture ethnicity and environment and so on; and (5) involvement of the researcher in the community to facilitate understanding the emic view of the culture (Hautman & Bomar, 1995).

By considering these elements the nurse is better able to provide culturally congruent nursing

---

CHAPTER HIGHLIGHTS

Culture is a universal, multifaced, complex, and dynamic concept that represents the assumptions one makes about life. It refers to the sum of acquired values, beliefs, practices, laws, customs, and so forth.

Culture is a significant force that contributes to the uniqueness of individuals, families, and communities.

Culturally sensitive nursing provides nursing care to individuals, families, and communities with respect for their cultural uniqueness.

There are a variety of cultures, and the nurse is advised to assess each family's culture and acknowledge their unique health practices.

The health status and health patterns of the family and its members is significantly influenced by family culture.

Health and illness beliefs and behaviors are learned and transmitted from one generation to another.

care. Such care is "cognitively based assistive, supportive, facilitative, or enabling acts or decisions that are tailor-made to fit with individual, group, or institutional cultural values, beliefs, and lifeways" (Leininger, 1991, p. 40).

REFERENCES

Bauwens, E., & Anderson, S. (1992). Social and cultural influences on health care. In M. Stanhope & J. Lancaster (Eds.), *Community Health Nursing: Process and Practice for Promoting Health* (3rd ed.) (pp. 91–108). St. Louis: Mosby.

Bloch, B. (1983). Bloch's assessment guide for ethnic/culture variations. In M.S. Orque & B. Bloch (Eds.), *Ethnic Nursing Care: A Multi-Cultural Approach* (pp. 49–75). St. Louis: C.V. Mosby.

Boyle, J.S., & Andrews, M.M. (1989). *Transcultural Concepts in Nursing Care.* Glenview, IL: Scott, Foresman.

Branch, M., & Paxton, P. (1976). *Providing Safe Nursing Care for Ethnic People of Color.* New York: Appleton-Century-Crofts.

Brink, P. (1984). Value orientations as an assessment tool in cultural diversity. *Nursing Research,* 4, 198–203.

Brownlee, A.T. (1978). *Community, Culture, and Care: A Cross-Cultural Guide for Health Workers.* St. Louis: C.V. Mosby.

Brubacker, B.H. (1983). Health promotion: A linguistic analysis. *Advances in Nursing Science,* 5(3), 1–14.

Chinoy, E. (1967). *Society: An Introduction to Sociology.* New York: Random House.

Clark, M.J. (1992). *Nursing in the Community.* Norwalk, CT: Appleton & Lange.

Clinton, J. (1986). In C. Edelman & C. Mandle (Eds.), *Health Promotion Throughout the Lifespan* (pp. 570–583). St. Louis: C.V. Mosby.

Deloria, V. (1969). *Custer Died for Your Sins.* New York: Avon.

Fong, C.M. (1985). Ethnicity and nursing practice. *Topics in Clinical Nursing,* 1(3), 1–10.

Freudenberg, M. (1985). Health promotion and class. *Health/PAC Bulletin,* 16(11), 24, 31.

Friedman, M.M. (1992). *Family Nursing: Theory and Practice* (3rd ed.). Norwalk, CT: Appleton Lange.

Giger, J.N., & Davidhizar, R.E. (1991). *Transcultural Nursing: Assessment and Interventions.* St. Louis: Mosby-YearBook.

Giger, J.N. (1990). Transcultural nursing assessment: A model for advancing nursing practice. *International Nursing Review,* 37(1), 199–202.

Giordano, J., & Giordano, G. (1977). *The Ethno-Cultural Factor in Mental Health.* New York: Institute on Pluralism and Group Identity of the American Jewish Community.

Harris, M. (1975). *Culture, People, Natives* (2nd ed.). New York: Thomas Y. Crowell.

Harris, M. (1975). *Culture, People, Nature: An Introduction to General Anthropology.* New York: Thomas Y. Crowell.

Hartog, J., & Hartog, E. (1983). Cultural aspects of health and illness behavior in hospitals. *Western Journal of Medicine,* 139, 910–916.

Hautman, M.A., & Bomar, P.J. (1995). Interactional model for recruiting ethnically diverse research participants. *Journal of Multicultural Nursing and Health,* 1(4), 8–15.

Healthy People 2000 (1992). U.S. Department of Health and Human Services, Public Health Services (Pub. No. PHS 91-50212). Boston: Jones and Bartlett.

Keefe, S.E. (1981). Folk medicine among urban Mexican-Americans: Cultural persistence, change, and displacement. *Hispanic Journal of Behavioral Science,* 2(3), 41–58.

Kleinman, A. (1978). International health care planning from an ethnomedical perspective: Critique and recommendations for change. *Medical Anthropology,* 2, 71–94.

Koos, E.L. (1954). *Health in Regionville.* New York: Columbia University Press.

Lee, I. (1976). *Medical Care in a Mexican-American Community.* Los Alamitos, CA: Hwong Pub. Co.

Leininger, M. (1991). *Culture Care Diversity and Universality: A Theory for Nursing.* New York: National League for Nursing.

Leininger, M. (1977). Cultural diversities of health and nursing care. *Nursing Clinics of North America,* 12, 5–18.

Leininger, M. (1978). Culturological assessment domains for nursing practices. In M. Leininger (Ed.), *Transcultural Nursing: Concepts, Theories and Practices* (pp. 85–106). New York: Wiley.

Leininger, M. (1989). A new generation of nurses discovers transcultural nursing. *Nursing & Healthcare,* 8, 38–45.

Leininger, M. (1985a). *Qualitative Research Methods in Nursing.* Orlando, FL: Grune & Stratton.

Leininger, M. (1985b). Transcultural care diversity and universality: A theory for nursing. *Nursing and Health Care* 4, 209–212.

Leininger, M. (1978). *Transcultural Nursing: Concepts, Theories, and Practices.* New York: Wiley.

Levine, R., & Campbell, D. (1972). Ethnocentrism. *Theories in Conflict, Ethnic attitudes, and Group Behavior.* New York: Wiley.

Lipson, J., & Meleis, A. (1985). Culturally appropriate care: The case of immigrants. *Topics in Clinical Nursing,* 3(10), 48–56.

Louie, K. (1985). Transcending cultural bias: The literature speaks. *Topics in Clinical Nursing,* 3(10), 78–83.

Lynam, M.J. (1992). Toward the goal of providing culturally sensitive care: Principles upon which to build nursing curricula. *Journal of Advanced Nursing,* 17, 149–157.

Mandelbaum, J.L. (1991). Why there cannot be an international theory of nursing. *International Nursing Review,* 38(2), 51–55.

McLemore, D. (1980). *Racial and Ethnic Relations in America.* Boston: Allyn and Bacon.

Melville, M.B. (1988). Hispanics: Race, class, or ethnicity? *The Journal of Ethnic Studies,* 16(1), 67–83.

Murdock, G. (1971). *Outline of Cultural Materials* (4th ed.). New Haven, CT: Human Relations Area Files.

Murray, R., & Zentner, S. (1985). *Nursing Concerns for Health Promotion* (3rd ed.). Englewood Cliffs, NJ: Prentice-Hall.

Ogburn, W., & Nimkoff, M. (1950). *Sociology* (2nd ed.). Boston: Houghton-Mifflin.

Parry, E.H.O. (1984). People and health: The influence of culture. *World Health Forum,* 5(1), 49–58.

Parsons, T. (1970). *Social Structure and Personality.* London: Free Press.

Paul, B. (1955). *Health Culture and Community*. New York: Russell Sage Foundation.

Pender, N.J. (1987). *Health Promotion in Nursing Practice* (2nd ed.). Norwalk, CT: Appleton & Lange.

Radecki, S.E. (1991). A racial and ethnic comparison of family formation and contraceptive practices among low-income women. *Public Health Reports,* 106(5), 494–502.

Rampusheski, V.F. (1989). The role of ethnicity in elder care. *Nursing Clinics of North America* 24(3), 717–724.

Reinhardt, A.M., & Quinn, M.D. (1973). *Family-Centered Community Nursing*. St. Louis: C.V. Mosby.

Scott, C.S. (1974). Health and healing practices among five ethnic groups in Miami, Florida. *Public Health Report,* 89(6), 524–532.

Spector, R. (1991). *Cultural Diversity in Health and Illness*. New York: Appleton-Century-Crofts.

Spector, R. (1979). *Cultural Diversity in Health and Illness*. New York: Appleton-Century-Crofts.

Staples, R., & Mirandé, A. (1986). Racial and cultural variations among American families: A decennial review of the literature on minority families. In A.S. Skolnick & J.H. Skolnick (Eds.), *Families in Transition* (pp. 474–497). Boston: Little, Brown.

Taylor, O. (1986). *Treatment of Communication Disorders in Culturally and Linguistically Diverse Populations*. San Diego, CA: College Hill Press.

Thernstrom, S. (Ed.). (1980). *Harvard Encyclopedia of American Ethnic Groups*. Cambridge: Harvard University Press.

Tripp-Reimer, T., Brink, P., & Saunders, J. (1984). Cultural assessment: Content and process. *Nursing Outlook,* 2, 78–82.

Tripp-Reimer, T., & Lauer, G.M. (1987). Ethnicity and families with chronic illness. In L.M. Wright & M. Leahey (Eds.), *Families and Chronic Illness* (pp. 77–100). Springhouse, PA: Springhouse.

6

FAMILY ROLES

EVELYN ANDERSON

All the world is a stage
And all men and women are merely players;
They have their exits and entrances
And one man in his time plays many parts.

WILLIAM SHAKESPEARE

OBJECTIVES

On completion of this chapter, the reader will be able to:

1. Describe role theory
2. Define role expectation, role incongruence, role conflict, role overload, role stress, and role strain
3. Describe family roles in relationship to role theory
4. Identify traditional and nontraditional families by structure and function
5. Discuss the role of the family in health promotion and disease prevention
6. Apply family assessment strategies using family role concepts
7. Synthesize role theory and family concepts with assessment data to develop a meaningful application for family health nursing

The study of family health promotion requires an understanding of the family and its roles. The roles and functions assumed and enacted by family members are multiple and complex. Through research and theory development, the nurse gains important information that supports efforts toward promoting family health.

Role theory is a science concerned with the study of behaviors that are characteristic of persons within contexts and with various processes that presume to produce, explain, or affect those behaviors (Biddle, 1979). Role theory represents a collection of concepts and a variety of hypotheti-

cal formulations that predict how actors will perform in a given role or under what circumstances certain types of behaviors can be expected. Family health nurses can offer clients important insight regarding their health status by developing a holistic family assessment that includes evaluation of family roles. As professionals, nurses are aware of the need to understand their role in health promotion and protection. Similar importance should be assigned to understanding the roles of families in their quest for optimal health.

This chapter will begin with a review of role theory and a clarification of the associated terms. The second section will introduce the reader to family roles and the characteristics of these roles as they affect the American family today. The third section will discuss variables affecting

---

This chapter was originally written by Kathleen O'Grady Winston and was revised by Evelyn Anderson.

family roles. Assessment of family roles in health promotion using family role theory data will follow. And last, implications for family health nursing will be emphasized. The reader will be provided with an understanding of the concepts associated with family roles and a framework for assessment of family roles.

ROLE THEORY

Concepts critical to understanding role theory include role expectation, stress, strain, conflict, incongruence, ambiguity, overload, sharing, negotiation, modeling, complementary roles, and transitions. Definition and application of these terms will be included in this section as a basis for understanding family role theory. There are many additional terms associated with role theory found in the literature. This chapter will discuss those that are most critical to understanding family role theory and family health nursing.

George Herbert Mead (1934) pointed out the importance of our role-taking ability to see ourselves as others see us as the major difference between humans and primates. His concept of self, role-taking, and symbolic interaction formed the basis of social psychology. Sarbin (1954) clearly describes social role theory and its dimensions. This classic body of work has been evaluated, criticized, and tested over the past 30 years. Since Sarbin's early work, role theory has evolved from several of the social science disciplines that have related interests in the study of the human condition.

Multiple philosophies exist regarding the study of social role theory (Sarbin, 1954; Hardy & Conway, 1978; Biddle, 1979). First, many social scientists view role theory as simply a subfield of psychology, sociology, or anthropology. Others suggest that rather then a subfield, role theory should be interpreted as a single discipline that combines the core concepts of psychology, sociology, and anthropology. This approach supports a framework that allows the researcher to examine role theory from an individualistic, collective, and cultural perspective. A third orientation for the discussion of role theory emerges from a concern that other social sciences consider role theory as central to their disciplines' conceptualization. Specifically, the helping professions are well equipped to incorporate role theory into their core concepts. Nursing, with its emphasis on care of the family and its biopsychosocial definition of humankind, applies role theory to its theoretical development. The role-function mode of Roy's (1976) adaptation model uses role concepts in its theory development. Roy describes the development of roles as expected behaviors that a person should perform to maintain a title. Role theorists contend that individuals and groups have shared *role expectations* regarding their behavior and the behavior of others (Smith & Reid, 1986; Biddle, 1979). For example, family members may expect the father to leave home for work each morning and the mother to get the children off to school. The idea of expectation presumes that individuals are aware of the experiences and the environment. It implies that people will conform their behavior to meet the behavioral expectations held for them based on their role (i.e., status, or position). The importance of shared expectations is evidenced by the implication that there are common experiences among those who exhibit the same roles.

Like the field of role theory itself, the concepts or components of the theory, such as expectation, evolve from theatrical usage. Shakespearean literature clearly describes the expectations for the characters in Hamlet and Romeo and Juliet. In nursing we can extend the dramatic metaphor and apply the concept of expectation to real-life experience in the family.

Role Stress

As life in American society has become more complex, theorists have come to recognize that the field of role analysis is not simply the examination of one's performance of expected behaviors. Many people hold a number of roles requiring intense demands. It is the intensity of these demands on the expected or prescribed roles of the individual, combined with the playing of several roles at the same time, that produces *role stress.* This condition is generally perceived as external to the role occupant, but it generates a condition of role strain for the individual. *Role strain,* as defined by Goode (1960), is the difficulty felt in fulfilling role obligations; role relations were seen as a sequence of role bargains by which an individual seeks to reduce role strain. Role stress and the potential for subsequent role strain is the focus of this chapter. Family nurses must be able to interpret the meaning of family role stress by determining the various sources. It is important to remember that role stress and strain are outcomes of other role experiences. It is a family's conflict, incongruence, and overload experiences that create the stress, which when prolonged is manifested as role strain. Family nurses should also understand the meaning of role theory terms that can be applied to protect families from developing role stress and strain. Family nurses can use their knowledge about role sharing, role negotiation, role modeling, complementary roles, and role transitions to prevent or ameliorate family role stress.

Role Conflict

Role conflict becomes another source of role strain experienced by the individual when multiple roles, with their intense demands, become viewed as competitive with their expectations. For example, the expectation for women in business includes demonstrating strong leadership qualities while continuing to subscribe to an ethic of caring. If a business decision requires the occupant to behave in an insensitive manner, conflict may follow. The concept of conflict stems from external issues, as does the concept of role stress.

Role Incongruity

Role incongruity emerges when expectations are in disagreement with the individual's self-perception or values (Hardy & Conway, 1978). Role conflict and incongruity are similar in their production of role strain but differ in their source of stress. The stress and subsequent strain that results from role conflict is due to competition between role behaviors, and the source of role stress and strain due to incongruity reflects an incompatibility between the role and the role incumbent.

Role Ambiguity

Often the term "role incongruity" is used synonymously with "role ambiguity." Both terms suggest that the family is at risk for role stress and role strain experiences, but their meanings are distinctly different. Role ambiguity occurs when the expected role is undefined or incomplete. The insufficiency of the expectation leads to vagueness and ambiguity. Role ambiguity produces disharmony due to the incompleteness of the role expectation, and role incongruity produces disharmony due to the individual's values.

Role Overload

Role demands are also perceived as difficult to fulfill when the role incumbent (actor) experiences role overload. Role overload produces role strain due to the incumbent's inability to complete the role obligations or to meet the role expectations within the prescribed amount of time. In studies of families (Barnett, 1982; Beutell & Greenhaus, 1983; Freudiger, 1983), role overload appears to be a significant source of role stress. Many families participate in multiple roles, often while experiencing incongruity, conflict, and stress. These role experiences combined with the issue of overload seem to produce the greatest amount of role strain. Little empirical research exists to support this notion, yet the data that describe role conflict and role strain generally include examples of role overload (Barnett, 1982; Beutell & Greenhaus, 1983; Freudiger, 1983; Gray, 1983).

It is beyond the scope of this chapter to discuss the myriad of role theory terms that are in the literature. There are several terms, however, that

for the purpose of this chapter should be explained.

Role Sharing

Role sharing is a concept that will be presented as a method of reducing role strain later in the chapter. Smith and Reid's (1986) case study research defined the notion of role sharing as the implementation of family activities by members without regard for gender identity. The stereotypical jobs belonging to a husband or wife had no relevance in the role-sharing marriage. The presumption of an egalitarian partnership is made in a role-sharing environment, and each member has claims for home and nonhome roles. This approach to role enactment was introduced by Rapoport and Rapoport (1969, 1976) and was later followed by the investigations of Scanzoni and Fox (1980).

Role Negotiation

Like role sharing, role negotiation is a method that can reduce the role strain in a family situation. Clements and Roberts (1983) define "role negotiation" as the agreement among members regarding the appropriate behaviors associated with a role. In essence, role negotiation permits mutual acceptance of role expectations. The role negotiation process may be implicit, as in the case where a teacher encourages students to question and challenge. This freedom to explore disagreement infuses the student with a sense that negotiation is an acceptable alternative. Explicitly, role negotiation might be seen in a discussion delineating employment responsibilities.

Role Modeling

Role modeling is a third concept that the family health nurse can use to help a family achieve optimal health. Defined, role modeling is the patterning of behaviors. It provides a standard by which others can measure their progress. In the family, parents are often role models for children in learning health-promoting and health-protecting behaviors.

Complementary Roles

The concept of complementary roles is important in social role theory because the existence of these roles supports the function of other roles (Nye, 1976). For example, the child nurturance/socialization role is enacted most effectively when the mother and father roles are intact. The absence or diminished effectiveness of the mother or father role causes an incompleteness that decreases the function of the child nurturance/socialization role. In complementary roles, one or more roles fit together so that other role activities are able to be accomplished. The complementary roles of nurse, client, physician, and health professional work together to achieve specific functions.

Role Transition

"Role transition" is the last role theory term that has relevance for family roles. Transition simply means to change from one place or state to another (Duval & Miller, 1985; Gray, 1983; Nye, 1976; Smith & Reid, 1986). In families, role transitions or changes occur regularly and throughout the life cycle. In addition to maturational transitions, such as singlehood to marriage, to parenthood, and so on, there are situational role transitions that also occur. The multiple and complex roles enacted by all family members today represent these situational role transitions. In both examples, actual and potential stress is evident. The family health nurse's role is to assist the family in identifying role transitions and to facilitate the prevention of role strain. Coping strategies can be introduced, and future role transitions can be anticipated.

Role theory is still a young field of study with a complexity of questions waiting to be answered. Currently it does offer social scientists and helping professionals a framework for understanding human behavior. This field of work is not limited to the use of one social science discipline but affords family nurses the opportunity to examine the human situation from a holistic approach with significant behavioral meanings. In the next section, an analysis of the family using role theory will demonstrate the applicability of these concepts to family nursing practice.

FAMILY ROLES

The Family as a Social Unit

Social behavior is an acquired phenomenon. Individuals are not born with characteristics of social behavior. Such behavior is developed over time and through the life cycle of social interaction. People adjust their behaviors depending on the prescriptions outlined for them as they interact within their social environment. In addition to the response we receive from others, our own perceptions alter our behavioral prescriptions and expectations. Socialization refers to the process by which an individual acquires skills, knowledge, attitudes, values, and motives necessary for the performance of social roles (Brim, 1968). Roles are constantly changing due to the individual's movement through the developmental life cycle, environmental influences, self-perception, and life experiences. The individual's first social unit of interaction is the family. It is this social structure that introduces the person to expected and accepted behaviors for their prescribed roles. Early in these family experiences, children are taught the appropriate roles for girls and boys and for good and bad. It is through this life process of intentional or incidental role modeling that children learn the expected roles for father, mother, sister, brother, friend, neighbor, man, woman, and so on (Robischon & Scott, 1969).

Gender Roles in the Family

Gender issues are significant for professionals working with families, and the research findings regarding gender roles and gender identity have tremendous social relevance (Losh-Hesslebart, 1987). *Gender identity* is the experience of knowing that one is male or female and occurs as a learned behavior in early childhood. Research has shown that by age two, children recognize their own gender and can differentiate between males and females. The development of gender identity occurs through the socialization process. Often this process, which occurs both in the family and in the larger society, is a direct effort toward shaping a child's gender identity. In addition to conscious efforts, the process includes role modeling, imitation of same-sex adults, and the influence of biologic differences (Losh-Hesslebart, 1987). Gender identity becomes the basis for gender role development. *Gender role recognition* evolves from the socialization process and extends beyond knowing that one is a male or a female. *Gender roles* (sex roles) are the behaviors assigned to males and females by society. Within a family, the social interaction that occurs helps the child develop as a social being and introduces him or her to expected and accepted societal roles. Beliefs about gender role behavior emerge from the process of children watching adult behaviors and attitudes and embracing pieces of these as they grow and develop. Through the discovery of what Mom and Dad do and what boys and girls can do, the child begins to develop an understanding about gender roles.

Gender role development is an important component of the adult role function in a family. The process begins at birth with sex-appropriate toys, rough versus gentle play, and sex-related behaviors. Assisting the child in developing a sense of maleness and femaleness is a function of the child nurturance/socialization role. Gender roles are established on the basis of sex and on the basis of society's acceptance that men enact instrumental roles and women enact expressive roles. In other words, men perform tasks that represent assertive, controlled behaviors, and women perform tasks that represent nurturing behaviors. Gender roles (sex roles) are society's acceptance of standards of behavior as belonging to men or women, therefore making them masculine or feminine (McCubbin & Dahl, 1985).

The impact of gender roles on family health is recognized by its potential for producing role strain. Like other role issues mentioned in this chapter, the stress associated with gender roles can precipitate family role conflict. If a woman fails to fit into the accepted expressive dimension traditionally prescribed for women, the potential for conflict within herself and with her significant others increases. Though traditional gender stereotyping diminishes as women's numbers continue to increase in the labor force, as they continue to choose unmarried status, and as they choose to bear fewer children, there continues to be a potential for stress associated with the gender role transition. Stressful gender role transitions are shared by men and children as well. Contemporary male gender roles are enmeshed in parenthood and family. Because children develop attitudes toward gender roles through their observations of adult behaviors, they witness unprecedented diversity. Huber (1993) states that gender role change is widely documented, and has been caused by factors such as industrialization, mass education, women's labor force participation, the decline of marriage as a social institution, and below-replacement fertility. Future family roles will respond to such factors as the need for grown children to care for their older parents, the division of household and child-care labor, the effects of remarriage on step-siblings, and the effects of single parenthood on children.

Recent literature suggests that gender roles in the modern family are primarily androgynous (Galvin & Brommel, 1986). Androgyny means "the human capacity for members of both sexes to be masculine and feminine in their behaviors—both dominant and submissive, active and passive, tough and tender (DeFrain, 1979, p. 237). The transition from traditional gender stereotyping toward the more androgynous approach of gender identity may also produce stress associated with the transition. Little preparation has been made for these gender role transitions, and limited experience with these new role behaviors can prove stressful. The family health nurse can intercede with the family and assist them through the stressful adjustments associated with such role transitions. Teaching families about androgyny will help to reduce the stress associated with lack of knowledge. Education will provide the family with the skills to make a sound choice regarding acceptance or rejection of the androgynous approach. Theoretically, androgyny sounds like the best of all worlds for both men and women. However, a tremendous amount of controversy surrounds the subject. Families should be taught about both the concept and its controversies. Heightened awareness regarding actual and potential role stress and strain due to the transition toward androgyny will strengthen a family's health-promoting behaviors. With increased awareness, self-responsibility for developing healthy attitudes about gender roles will be encouraged. The combined efforts of the family and the family nurse can develop the awareness and self-responsibility into health-promoting behaviors.

Formal and Informal Family Roles

There are numerous family types, as discussed in Chapters 3 and 20. Although families are distinct in their structural composition, there is an overlap when categorization is attempted to include role and function. Family roles are defined as "repetitive patterns of behavior by which family members fulfill family functions" (Epstein et al., 1982, p. 124). Friedman (1992) has described family function through formal and informal roles. The formal roles include the behaviors associated with the role position of mother, father, sister, brother, or grandparent. Informal roles include encourager initiator-contributor, compromiser, blocker, dominator, the blamer, recognition seeker, the great stone face, the pal, the family scapegoat, the placator, the pioneer, the distractor, the family go-between, and the bystander (Friedeman, 1992). Selected examples of other covert roles are presented in Table 6–1 and are a reflection of the work of Satir (1972); Hartman and Laird (1983); and Kantor and Lehr (1975). The examples serve only as a sampling of the number of informal roles that have been identified in the literature. Knowledge about both formal and informal roles enacted by the family will prove essential to the development of effective nursing strategies. For example, it is crucial to know which family member has the role of health teacher and health care provider in the family.

Traditional Role Performance and Contemporary Role Sharing

Traditionally in American society, family roles have been relatively clear. Until the age of industrialization, family roles, though clear, more closely resembled nontraditional family roles as they are defined today. Families worked collabo-

TABLE 6–1. INFORMAL ROLES

Harmonizer is responsible for mediating among family members. Using all skills available, this individual seeks to smooth over family disagreements.
Opposer is described as negative to all family suggestions, ideas, and activities.
Martyr sacrifices everything, including self, for the sake of the family.
Follower goes along with all decisions made by the family and passively accepts the ideas of others in the family.
Coordinator organizes and plans family activities and serves to bring the family closer together.

ratively in the home and at work; many of the family roles were shared. Though men and women often had separate and distinct types of work, this occurred because of practical necessity rather than from gender differences or stereotypes. Role sharing is again surfacing in the American family. During the preindustrial era, role sharing simply represented an economic and philosophical reality. It appears that the resurgence of this concept may once again reflect an economic and philosophical reality of society. A *role-sharing* marriage is defined as both partners having equal claim to the breadwinning role, the domestic care role, and the child nurturance/socialization role (Smith & Reid, 1986). A role-sharing family expands the concept to include the children, as well as others considered family members, in family decision making and domestic care responsibilities. Though these role-sharing marriages and families continue to be in the minority, many modern family functions resemble the characteristics of the role-sharing family. The idea of role sharing extends beyond the division of formal roles and tasks to include new egalitarian values that will also influence the informal roles enacted by the family. Role sharing is not simply the notion of partnership, although partnership is a crucial component. Role sharing strives to reject the traditional role performance that has become comfortable for many American families. Admittedly, efforts toward the achievement of a role-sharing marriage or family often result in a compromise between the contemporary and the old-fashioned experience.

The concept of traditional family roles, in contrast, emerged from the growth of the United States as an industrialized nation. This definition of family includes a mother who serves as primary caretaker of the children and household and who generally does not work outside the home; a father whose primary role is that of economic provider and decision maker for all other family members; and children who clearly are recipients of parental caregiving.

Today, families are highly diverse, as discussed in Chapters 3 and 20 of this text. Dietz (1991) looked at couple adaptation in stepfamilies and traditional nuclear families in pregnancy. Stepfamilies emerged as evolving families whereas traditional nuclear families manifested themselves as established families. The roles of all family members today are multiple and complex, both in scope and in nature. An understanding of family roles is essential to the development of effective nursing care for families in need of intervention.

A review of the family literature suggests that there are three primary roles within a family: the breadwinner role, the domestic care role, and the nurturance/socialization role. As previously mentioned, in a traditionally structured family, the father typically was the breadwinner, the mother was the domestic caregiver, and both participated in the nurturance/socialization roles. Today, though the family may be traditional in structure (i.e., a nuclear family), it most likely is nontraditional in its enactment of family roles.

A number of investigations have examined the impact of new and multiple roles on women (Woods, 1980, 1984; Vanfossen, 1981; Verbrugge, 1983; Rendely & Holmstom, 1984). Other studies have explored the role conflicts experienced by women in multiple roles and have examined coping strategies and life satisfaction (Beutell & Greenhaus, 1983; Facione, 1994; Protrkowski, 1983; Holahan & Gilbert, 1979). Mothers have been targeted by family health nurses for the implementation of health promotion because of their actual or potential health problems resulting from the strain of role overload. Research has shown that the number of women in the workplace has increased but that these working women continue to maintain primary responsibility for the housekeeping, home management, and child-nurturing roles (Barnett, 1982; Nye, 1976; Smith & Reid, 1986; Geerken & Gove, 1983). Fathers continue to perform the traditional role of provider and to do household maintenance, while attempting to learn new roles associated with child nurturing and housekeeping. Beutell and Greenhaus (1983) found in an investigation of home and nonhome roles among married women that the husband's and wife's sex role attitudes were associated with the wife's coping strategies when role conflicts occurred. In other words, the reduction of role strain as experienced by the female was dependent on the perception and expectations associated with male and female roles. The potential for role conflict and role stress is tremendous. With such impressive data supporting the potential for family role strain, it is understandable why the concept of role sharing has gained new strength. Smith and Reid (1986) examined the concept of tradition and change, the extent of role sharing within a marriage, and issues associated with role sharing. The case studies presented reflected a reduction in role conflict, in stress, and therefore in role strain when role sharing was present.

Today both spouses often contribute to the economic success of the family, and more men participate in domestic responsibilities than in the past. However, Horchschild (1989), in a study of working women, reported that women experience greater role strain/stress than men. The roles of nurturer and socializer were primarily the female's responsibility. Women were described as having a "second shift." Despite the fact that more men participated in child care and household tasks than in the past, women reported more hours spend in child care and domestic responsibilities after a full day of work outside the home.

Children also participate in the family today, which was not acceptable in former traditional settings. Children are no longer simply the recipients of parental care but serve to nurture siblings and parents in the family system. With improved treatment in modern medicine, for example, more people with chronic illness are marrying and attaining parenthood. A family program to address the needs of children whose parents have seizures because of epilepsy (Lannon, 1992) looks at changing family roles. It is common for children to participate in family decision-making activities. The literature is limited in the study of children and role sharing. Further research is needed to investigate the impact of all family member roles on the family's health status.

Each role held by a family member significantly influences the behavior of the entire family, therefore it is essential for family health nurses to recognize that nontraditional roles performed by the modern family can easily be the source of role stress. If the role stress is manifested as role strain, the family unit suffers from family role strain. It is this dysfunction that the family health nurse should seek to prevent. One successful method of prevention appears to be the introduction of role-sharing concepts.

Member Influence on a Family's Health

The formal and informal roles performed by the family members are defined as intrarole activities, and interrole activities represent those role performances that occur outside the family system. Interrole activity includes the ability of the family to link its members to the larger society. In the case of the children, this linkage occurs through the nurturance and socialization process. All other family members, however, must also be prepared for the movement of the family unit into the greater community of life. In the area of health care, this becomes an essential part of the family's ability to function. When the family is unable to meet the needs of a family member, linkage with outside resources becomes necessary. Families make decisions regarding its members' health promotion behaviors. If parents value the idea of health prevention activities, such as yearly physicals, then children will most likely receive this kind of health care. Children also influence their parents' lifestyle by bringing from the larger society (i.e., school) information that supports health promotion activities. Families have the primary responsibility for meeting the health needs of its members, therefore it is essential that the family be provided wellness opportunities.

The importance of one family member's behavioral influence on the entire family cannot be overstated. Hanson (1986) found that single-parent families were as competent as other family configurations in their enactment of family roles. More important, this study developed the notion that parents need to understand the impact that

their health status has on the health status of their children. Galvin and Brommel (1986), Losh-Hesselbart (1987), and Forrest (1981) also described the significance of the parents' health in relationship to the health of the family system.

Illness can have a dramatic impact on family roles (Lannon, 1992). Northouse et al. (1991) discussed the psychological consequences of breast cancer, and the supportive roles maintained by both husband and children for the patient. Warda (1992) used a role theory approach to look at chronic sorrow for the family with ill children. Payne (1988) did a case study of role changes in a family whose father suffered a cerebrovascular accident, while Killen (1990) investigated how kinship functioning changed after spinal cord injury. Yang and Kirschling (1992) studied the role of caregiving experienced by family members of terminally ill older persons.

Mothers are particularly meritorious regarding the family's health. In most American homes, the mother has been identified formally with the role of nurse when the family requires health-related interventions. Linguistically, the word "nurse" implies a female activity or person. Traditionally, the expectation for practicing nurses has been that they be nurturing females. The strong association between femininity and the practicing nurse supported the appropriateness of mother serving as health leader within the family. This seems to be a continuing role assignment in modern families. During childhood illnesses, the mother is often the caregiver, and at other times she is the decision-maker regarding health checkups. This is a powerful role that must not be overlooked by the family health nurse. Health promotion activities will include the entire family, but the mother's acceptance or rejection of health promotion behaviors will prove decisive.

Though the mother's influence on the family's health appears to be the most distinctive, client behavior is influenced by the entire family's perception of wellness and illness. In nursing, the inhibitors we often associate with the individual's behavior becomes manageable when family health nurses acknowledge the family's influence.

Families today could be compromised by the existence of nontraditional and androgynous family roles. Each family member is involved in multiple roles requiring intense demands. As noted, the father no longer concerns himself simply with the economic needs of the family but today actively participates in the growth and development of the children and of his spouse. The wife no longer participates simply as a nurturing mother but contributes to the financial success of the family. The family also participates in interrole activities that help to link the family to the larger society. Other family roles include social roles such as a commitment to friendships, extended family, church, and community. The pressures of a complex, highly technologic society are intense, and the potential for conflict follows (Losh-Hesselbart, 1987).

In addition to the role conflicts that can ensue from interrole activities, there exists the possibility for intrarole conflict. Families, though moving toward this contemporary picture of roles, have not quite settled into these behaviors as the societal norm. The overload, conflict, and incongruity of the multiple roles cause role stress in families today, but it is the subsequent family role strain that is experienced by the members themselves that poses health risks for the group. The family's role in minimizing role strain for its members is significant, but few families have developed the skills necessary for creating a balance in family roles. The "superwoman syndrome" has transcended to include the "superfamily syndrome," where all members are perceived to be able to do all things for all people without succumbing to the maladaptive consequences of such physical and psychologic strain.

VARIABLES AFFECTING FAMILY ROLES

Cultural Considerations

Expectations regarding the role performance of a mother, even in contemporary America, will look very different in a first-generation Hispanic family than in a Caucasian family. Ethnicity has been established as a significant variable in the development of sex role attitudes and family role performance (Garcia-Preto, 1982). Specific examples can be found in the community health nursing literature regarding domestic care, socialization/nurturance, and breadwinner roles (Stanhope & Lancaster, 1992; Clements & Roberts, 1983; Leininger, 1976). As discussed in Chapter 5, nurses must explore the cultural background of a family with whom they plan interventions. The insight gained regarding cultural values, beliefs, and experiences will assist in health promotion efforts. For example, if the father in a home is culturally recognized as the decision-maker, and this has been established as a formal role in the family's heritage, then the nurse should be certain to include the father in decisions about the family's health. He becomes an important target for education and intervention.

Socioeconomic Considerations

Socioeconomic variables are also considerations regarding the assignment, expectation, and performance of family roles. Often the need for economic survival forces a family with traditional beliefs about the mother's role into a contempo-

rary role enactment situation. In this example, the mother might be employed outside the home, although the family believes that her roles of domestic care and nurturance/socialization are paramount. Great potential for conflict, stress, and strain exists in such families. Common role issues include role stress/strain, role ambiguities, role conflict, and role induction. Stress is often reduced by role sharing.

Another example of socioeconomic impact on roles is the family that expects traditional role behaviors of the mother who seeks a more contemporary performance of her roles. Both cultural and socioeconomic factors will influence formal and informal roles. Informally, a family member may assume the role of martyr due to the financial stress in the home. Under other circumstances, this member might be the family harmonizer. These informal roles are more flexible and mobile then the formal roles discussed in this chapter. A family member may enact a variety of informal roles and quickly change to perform only one. Informal roles are highly susceptible to situation. Less conflict and stress is generally associated with these role transitions unless, like changes in formal role performance, the variation creates disequilibrium, conflict, and stress.

Developmental Considerations

Developmental influences are a final consideration for the reader. Duvall and Miller (1985) described the family in terms of life span. Families will enact different roles as they travel through the life span. As a childless couple, the formal roles of domestic care and provider might easily be shared roles. Once the family enters the developmental phase of the childbearing family, new role considerations arise. Suddenly there are nurturance and socialization roles that must be performed, and the socioeconomic status of the family may change, causing the breadwinner role to take on new meaning. As families complete the life cycle, even greater changes in their formal roles occur. As older adults, the parenting roles are no longer appropriate and are replaced with the role of grandparent. The role of grandparent has been one that society has traditionally taken for granted. Along the life span, individuals who have been parents will very often become grandparents. Little research has been done on the role of grandparents, and only recently has the concept of the grandparent role emerged as a significant social phenomenon (Bengtson, 1985).

Because of the increasing life span and the aging of the baby boomer generation, grandparents will have increased relevance to family health nursing. Currently, grandparents have been identified as a highly diverse group with more differences in their role enactment as grandparents than most other social or family roles. Expectations regarding the role are unclear because the phenomenon is new. Several roles within the family have been established. For example, the grandparents are often identified as negotiators between parents and children. They serve as arbitrators, helping to maintain family continuity between the generations. Grandparents are historical links between the past and the future and provide family biography; their presence protects the family from the realities of their mortality. Though grandparents differ in age, acceptance of the role, interpretation of the role behaviors, cultural backgrounds, and gender identities, they are a social force whose impact on the family can be positive or negative but at the very least significant. Once children have been launched into society, the couple once again lives together as they did during the childless phase of the life cycle, but those role behaviors no longer apply. The individual maturation that has occurred over the years alters the role of childless couple as they experience that role in their older years. As mentioned earlier, the subsequent transition into grandparenthood may affect the couple.

Family roles are tremendously influenced by life cycle changes that occur in families. In addition to this life span influence on family roles, another developmental consideration has been described by Tapia (1975) in studying families during the 1970s. Tapia developed a schema that described the family developmentally as infant, childhood, adolescent, young adulthood, or mature. During each of these phases, the family was described in terms of behaviors, and family nurse interventions were essentially dependent on the developmental level of the family. The roles that families enacted, both formal and informal, varied according to the level of development. An infant family, for example, was void of a responsible adult able to effectively enact the role of decision-maker. Adult families were generally characterized by trust and an ability to enact formal and informal roles successfully. This theoretical approach to assessing families is suitable to the discussion of family roles because it provides the family health nurse with information about a family's ability to enact roles.

Family roles change as members experience acute and chronic illness and varied life transitions. Chapter 20 discusses the impact of transitions on family roles. With this information about contemporary family roles, the nurse must begin to examine methods of assessment and intervention that will meet the needs of these modern families.

ASSESSMENT OF FAMILY ROLES

The family health nurse can facilitate achievement of family health by including an assessment of family roles in the holistic family assessment process. By doing so, the nurse will then be able to provide the family with information, resources, and strengths to achieve family wellness. The family health nurse serves as a resource person, providing clarification about the formal and informal roles and the meanings attached to these performances and strengthening the problem-solving skills of the family. The nurse assists the family in identifying its current and previous coping strategies and encourages the exploration of feelings and impressions. Meleis & Swendsen (1978) tested the effect of role supplementation as a preventive nursing intervention on families who were experiencing a transition because of the birth of a first child. Role modeling and role rehearsal were strategies used to develop role-clarity and role-taking skills for their clients.

As a teacher, the family nurse supports the family in its efforts to find new identities. Specifically, the family nurse shares role assessment data with the family as the educational approach develops. Employing teaching strategies, the nurse may offer a historical review of families in American society. This enables the family to discover possible sources of their feelings, beliefs, and family role practices. In addition to historical review, the nurse will direct her teaching toward role sharing as a method of reducing role strain and will explore family perceptions of such a change.

The scope of family health nursing practice includes understanding the family structure and its family role functions. It is essential that the nurse first examine the inter- and intraroles of the family. Assessment of family roles is best achieved by family assessment tools that facilitate the gathering of data by exploring major areas of family role function and providing clues regarding potential health problems of the family. Information can be obtained through both interview and observation. A suggested model for assessing family roles is shown in Table 6–2.

Identifying the family type is the first step in completing a family role assessment. In other words, is the family blended or nuclear? In addition to gaining appropriate data regarding family structure, specific identifying information should be gathered regarding roles of family members. The nurse assesses the family according to its formal interrole behaviors. This simply means that the roles, described in this chapter for mother, father, and so on, are identified. After the assessment questions regarding these roles have been considered, the nurse explores the informal interrole behaviors unique to the family. The assessment questions search for meanings attached to behavior as perceived by the family. The interview and observation should also include clarification regarding the family's culture, socioeconomic status, and placement in the life cycle. Finally, the nurse examines the intrarole

TABLE 6–2. GUIDELINES FOR FAMILY ROLE ASSESSMENT

Family Structure
1. How would the family be structurally defined?
   A. Traditional   B. Nontraditional

Family Function (Formal Interrole)
1. What are the formal interroles in the family?

   A. Father   F. Child
   B. Mother   G. Breadwinner
   C. Brother   H. Domestic caregiver
   D. Sister   I. Nurturer/Socializer
   E. Spouse   J. Health Leader

2. Describe how each member enacts his or her formal roles.
3. What are the multiple roles enacted by the family?
4. How does the family support its members in their multiple roles?
5. Which of the following do family members experience regarding their formal roles?
   A. Role incongruence   C. Role conflict
   B. Role overload   D. Role stress
6. Do these experiences further manifest themselves as role strain?
7. How effectively do family members enact their formal interroles?
8. How have the family roles changed from the roles enacted previously?
9. What kind of preparation did the family have for the role changes it has experienced?
10. What are the response patterns of the family to these role changes?

Family Function (Informal Interrole)
1. What are the informal interroles in the family?
   A. Harmonizer   D. Follower
   B. Opposer   E. Organizer
   C. Martyr   F. Other
2. Describe who enacts these informal roles.
3. Identify if these informal roles are healthy or dysfunctional to the family unit.
4. How do these informal role enactments facilitate or inhibit the formal role behaviors?
5. Do these informal role enactments create role incongruency, role overload, role conflict, and/or role stress in family members?
6. Do these role stresses manifest themselves as role strain in the family?
7. How have these informal roles changed from previous informal role enactments?
8. What are the family response patterns to these informal roles?
9. What purpose do these informal role behaviors serve for the family?
10. How were these informal role behaviors learned by the family members?

Intrarole Function
1. What are the intrarole functions of the family members?
   A. Friend   C. Community participant
   B. Kinship   D. Church participant
2. Describe how each family member enacts his or her nonhome roles.
3. What are the family's multiple nonhome roles?
4. How do these nonhome roles influence the formal interroles enacted by the family?
5. Does the family support its members in their multiple nonhome roles?
6. Do family members experience role incongruency, conflict, overload, and/or stress regarding these nonhome roles?
7. Do these experiences further manifest themselves as role strain?
8. How do informal interroles affect the intraroles of the family?
9. How have these roles changed from previously enacted nonhome roles?
10. What kind of preparation did the family have for the role changes it has experienced?

behaviors, or the nonhome roles, enacted by the family. Here the impact of school, friends, relatives, church, and so on are explored. All the categories combined will provide the nurse with a clear, but unique, picture of family roles. Health promotion activities as well as protective strategies can be employed by the family unit to meet the needs of the family. Unit III of this text presents intervention strategies. Role theory, family role theory, and the variables of culture, socioeconomic status, and life span development combine to form a salient component of the holistic family health assessment process.

IMPLICATIONS FOR FAMILY NURSING

Anderson (1973) suggested that the position of "nurse" identifies a particular body of expected behavior that is relational; the nurse plays the role in relation to the counter-position of the pa-

TABLE 6–3. NANDA NURSING DIAGNOSES RELEVANT TO ROLE TRANSITIONS*

Altered Role Performance
Altered Parenting
Risk for Altered Parenting
Altered Family Processes
Caregiver Role Strain
Risk for Caregiver Role Strain
Parental Role Conflict
Family Coping: Potential for Growth

*These are a sample of role categories in NANDA Nursing Diagnoses: Definitions and Classification 1995–1996. Philadelphia: NANDA, 1994.

tient. What is expected of the nurse are "role obligations"; the "role set" are the relevant others of doctor, ancillary personnel, and the patient's family.

The importance of assessing family roles cannot be overemphasized. Appropriate role assessment provides the nurse and the family with insight regarding current and potential health problems and aids in identifying the family's level of wellness (see Table 6–3 for NANDA Nursing Diagnoses related to family roles). Changes in family role structure magnify the potential for family stress. A variety of these role transitions are discussed at length in Chapter 20. With the changing structure of the family, for example, a single-parent family is faced with intense demands for breadwinning, nurturing/socializing, and domestic care, often without adequate support. The potential for role stress and strain leading to physical and psychologic health problems is tremendous. Even in the traditionally structured family, there is a tremendous change in the formal role functions of the family members. Today the multiple roles held by all members may place the family system in emotional and physical jeopardy. The informal roles acquired by family members also serve to support or suppress a family's wellness. In each family, the informal roles will add to or reduce the stress associated with formal family roles.

An important nursing role is teaching the family how to anticipate conflict as new developmental stages are approached, as situational experiences create sudden changes in the family norm, and as individual members experience changes in development. Family nurses are charged with teaching families how to adapt, cope, and grow with role changes that occur. Strategies such as role sharing and role negotiation help to reduce stress. Families will benefit from instruction about the development of gender identity and techniques that will help children clarify their gender roles. Assisting families in recognizing the impact of values and beliefs on family interaction and family health is another important role for family nurses. Role

CHAPTER HIGHLIGHTS

The roles and functions of family members are complex and multifaceted.

The family nurse needs to be cognizant of formal and informal family roles in health promotion, prevention, and illness to assist families in improving, maintaining, or regaining their level of health.

A holistic assessment of family roles helps the nurse to gain insight about multiple roles and their unique functions in each family.

An understanding of the definitions of such role terms as role stress, role conflict, role incongruity, role ambiguity, role overload, role sharing, role negotiation, role modeling, complementary roles, role transition, gender roles, and formal and informal family roles will assist the professional to comprehend family dynamics and to develop effective nursing strategies.

Formal and informal roles of health teacher and care giver significantly influence the health behaviors of family members during illness and health promotion and prevention.

Family roles are influenced by culture, family structure, developmental stage of the family unit and its members, education level, and economic status.

Assessment of family roles includes observation and interview of multifaceted family overt and covert roles.

modeling healthy interactions and clearly defined role behaviors for the family will provide a standard for families to follow. Finally, the implications of changing family roles in the American culture include the activation of self-care behaviors. Family members must be instructed and encouraged to develop strategies that will support the family unit and its members.

Nursing is offered a unique challenge in working with families today. The discipline is presented with a complex social unit whose health or illness will affect the individual's health as well as the health of the larger society.

REFERENCES

Anderson, E.R. (1973). *The Role of the Nurse.* United Kingdom: Royal College of Nursing and National Council of Nurses of the United Kingdom.

Barnett, R. (1982). Multiple roles and well being. A study of mothers of preschool age children. *Psychology of Women Quarterly,* 7(2), 175–178.

Bengston, V. (Ed.). (1985). *Grandparenthood.* Beverly Hills: Sage.

Beutell, N.J., & Greenhaus, J.H. (1983). Integration of home and non-home roles: Women's conflict and coping behavior. *Journal of Applied Psychology,* 68, 43–48.

Biddle, B.J. (1979). *Role Theory: Expectations, Identities, and Behaviors.* New York: Academic Press.

Brim, O.G. (1968). Adult socialization. In J.A. Clausen (Ed.), *Socialization and Society* (pp. 182–226). Boston: Little, Brown.

Clements, I.W., & Roberts, F.B. (Eds.). (1983). *Family Health: A Theoretical Approach to Nursing Care.* New York: Wiley.

DeFrain, J. (1979). Androgynous parents tell who they are and what they need. *The Family Coordinator,* 28, 237–243.

Dietz, O.M. (1991). Couple adaptation in stepfamilies and traditional nuclear families during pregnancy. *Nursing Practice,* 4(3), 6–10.

Duvall, E.M., & Miller, B.C. (1985). *Family Development* (6th ed.). New York: Harper & Row.

Epstein, N.J., Bishop, D.S., & Baldwin, K.N. (1982). McMasters model of family functioning: A view of the normal family. In F. Walsh (Ed.), *Normal Family Processes* (pp. 115–154). New York: Guilford.

Facione, N.C. (1994). Role overload and health: The married mother in the waged labor force. *Health Care for Women Int.,* 15(2):157–167.

Forrest, J. (1981). The family: The focus for health behavior generation. *Health Values: Achieving High Level Wellness,* 5, 138–144.

Freudiger, P. (1983). A life satisfaction among three categories of married women. *Marriage and Family,* 45, 213–219.

Friedman, M.M. (1992). *Family Nursing: Theory and Assessment* (2nd ed.). Norwalk, CT: Appleton-Lange.

Galvin, M.K., & Brommel, B.J. (1986). *Family Communication: A Cohesion and Change.* Glenview, IL: Scott, Foresman.

Garcia-Preto, N. (1982). Puerto Rican families. In M. McGoldrick, J. Pearce, & J. Giordano (Eds.), *Ethnicity and Family Therapy.* New York: Guilford.

Geerken, M., & Gove, W. (1983). *At Home and At Work.* Beverely Hills: Sage.

Goode, W.J. (1960). A theory of role strain. *American Sociological Review,* 25, 483–496.

Gray, J.D. (1983). Married professional women: An examination of her role conflicts and coping strategies. *Psychological Women's Quarterly,* 7, 235–243.

Hanson, S. (1986). Healthy single-parent families. *Family Relations,* 35(1), 125–132.

Hardy, M., & Conway, M. (1978). *Role Theory Perspective for Health Professionals.* Norwalk, CT: Appleton-Century-Crofts.

Hartman, A., & Laird, J. (1983). *Family-Centered Social Work Practice.* New York: Free Press.

Hochschild, A. (1989). *The Second Shift: Working Parents and the Revolution at Home.* New York: Viking.

Holahan, C., & Gilbert, L. (1979). Interrole conflict for working women: Career vs. jobs. *Journal of Applied Psychology,* 64, 86–90.

Huber, J. (1993). Gender role change in families. In T.H. Brubaker (Ed.), *Family Relations: Challenges for the Future.* (Vol. 1. Current Issues in the Family). Newbury Park, CA: Sage.

Kantor, D., & Lehr, W. (1975). *Inside the Family.* San Francisco: Jossey-Bass.

Killen, J.M. (1990). Role stabilization in families after spinal cord injury. *Rehabilitation Nursing,* 15(1), 19–21.

Lannon, S.L. (1992). Meeting the needs of children whose parents have epilepsy. *Journal of Neuroscience Nursing,* 24(1), 14–18.

Leininger, M. (1976). *Transcultural Health Care Issues and Conditions.* Philadelphia: F.A. Davis.

Losh-Hesselbart, S. (1987). Development of gender roles. In M.B. Sussman & S.K. Steinmetz (Eds.), *Handbook of Marriage and Family* (pp. 535–563). New York: Plenum.

McCubbin, H., & Dahl, B.B. (1985). *Marriage and Family Individual Life Cycles.* New York: Wiley.

Mead, G.H. (1934). *Mind, Self and Society.* Chicago: University of Chicago Press.

Meleis, A.I., & Swendsen, L.A. (1978). Role supplementation: An empirical test of a nursing intervention. *Nursing Research,* 27(1), 11–17.

North American Nursing Diagnosis Association. (1994). Nursing Diagnosis: Definitions and Classifications 1995–1996. Philadelphia: NANDA.

Northouse, L.L., Cracchiolo-Caraway, A., & Appel, C.P. (1991). Psychologic consequences of breast cancer on partner and family. *Seminars in Oncology Nursing,* 7(3), 216–223.

Nye, F.I. (1976). Role Structure and Analysis of the Family. Beverly Hills: Sage.

Payne, M.B. (1988). Utilizing role theory to assist the family with sudden disability. *Rehabilitation Nursing,* 13(4), 191–194.

Protrkowski, C.S. (1983). Young women at work: Implications for individual and family functioning. *Occupational Health Nursing,* 31, 24–29.

Rapoport, R., & Rapoport, R.N. (1969). The dual-career family: A variant pattern of social change. *Human Relations,* 22, 3–30.

Rapoport, R., & Rapoport, R.N. (1976). *Dual Career Families Reexamined.* New York: Harper Colophon.

Rendely, J., & Holmstom, R. (1984). The relationship of sex role identity, lifestyle, and mental health in suburban American homemakers: Sex role, employment, and adjustment. *Sex Roles,* 11, 839–846.

Robischon, P. & Scott, D. (1969). Role theory and its application to family nursing. *Nursing Outlook, 17,* 52–57.

Roy, C. (1976). *Introduction to Nursing: An Adaptation.* Englewood Cliffs, NJ: Prentice-Hall.

Sarbin, T.R. (1954). Role theory. In G. Lindzey (Ed.), *Handbook of Social Psychology* (pp. 488–567). Reading, MA: Addison-Wesley.

Satir, V. (1972). *Peoplemaking.* Palo Alto, CA: Science and Behavior Books.

Scanzoni, J., & Fox, G.L. (1980). Sex roles, family and society: The seventies and beyond. *Journal of Marriage and Family,* 42, 743–756.

Smith, A.D., & Reid, W.J. (1986). *Role-Sharing Marriage.* New York: Columbia University Press.

Stanhope, M., & Lancaster, J. (1992). *Community Health Nursing: Process and Practice for Promoting Health.* St. Louis: C.V. Mosby.

Tapia, J.A. (1975). Nursing process in family health. In B.W. Spradley (Ed.), *Contemporary Community Health* (pp. 252–258). Boston: Little, Brown.

Vanfossen, B. (1981). Sex differences in the mental health effects of spouse support and equity. *Journal of Health and Social Behavior, 22,* 130–143.

Verbrugge, L.M. (1983). Multiple roles and physical health of women and men. *Journal of Health and Social Behavior, 24,* 16–30.

Warda, M. (1992). The family and chronic sorrow: role theory approach. *Journal of Pediatric Nursing, 7*(3), 205–210.

Woods, N.F. (1980). Women's roles and illness episodes: A prospective study. *Research in Nursing and Health, 3,* 137–145.

Woods, N.F. (1984). Employment, family roles and mental ill health in young married women. *Nursing Research, 34,* 4–10.

Yang, C., & Kirschling, J.M. (1992). Exploration of factors related to direct care and outcomes of caregiving: Caregivers of terminally ill older persons. *Cancer Nursing, 15*(3), 173–181.

FAMILY SELF-CARE

7

V. RUTH GRAY

The main responsibility for health of families rests with the adults in each family, who have joint responsibilities for themselves and their children.

RAY MARSHALL

OBJECTIVES

On completion of this chapter, the reader will be able to:

1. Define the concept of self-care as it relates to the individual and the family
2. Identify theories from other disciplines that provide a framework for family self-care nursing theory
3. Discuss family self-care nursing theory derived from the nursing model of Orem and general systems theory
4. Use types of family self-care specific to health promotion and health protection
5. Examine factors that influence the family's ability to exercise self-care
6. Promote family self-care contracting using the theory and principles of behavior modification
7. Assess family self-care effectiveness through the role of follow-up to determine improved health behaviors
8. Visualize family health nursing as the vital link for promoting the concept of family self-care

INTRODUCTION

For centuries, the majority of health care occurred within the context of the family. Health practices were passed down through the generations in all societies, and among these were specific care practices, especially in the area of health promotion. However, history tells us little about what most deeply concerned ordinary people and their ideas about health and healing (Steiger & Lipson, 1985, p. 5).

Several centuries after Hippocrates was born (406 B.C.), the early European church had an im-

pact on the concept of self-care. It was during this time that illness was regarded as punishment for sin, and prayer became the only appropriate measure to be used for the prevention and treatment of disease. In the 14th and 16th centuries, knowledge of human anatomy increased, and the body came to be regarded as a human machine. Engle (1977, p. 131) describes the perspective of disease at this time as "the breakdown of the machine"; the doctor's task was the repair of the machine. Additionally, the "positivist" view of disease as a deviation from a biochemical norm reached its peak in Europe in the 19th century, when the germ theory was formulated and advances in immunology, pathology, and surgical techniques

The contribution of James S. Sergi to this chapter as it appeared in the first edition is acknowledged.

became a reality (Ahmed et al., 1979, p. 8). This was the evolution of the medical model as we know it today, which merited the approval of the church, encouraged physicians to be educated in universities, and resulted in the improvement of sanitation with concomitant reduction in communicable disease.

These advances, however, did not reach all the families needing assistance. Many were still subject to ineffective 19th-century practices such as purging and blood letting. There was little individual and family access to the educated physician. Only lay practitioners could be sought for care. Many were forced to use their own self-assessment, self-diagnosis, and self-treatment in order to prevent and/or solve their health care problems. The record of these health-seeking behaviors gives evidence that the self-care concept was coming into vogue.

At the beginning of the 20th century, communicable disease accounted for most illnesses in the United States. Once again, individuals and families had to rely on self-care measures to prevent and/or fight these diseases. As antibiotics and vaccines became available in the 1930s and 1940s and the incidence of communicable diseases decreased, the emphasis on self-care declined again. It is interesting to note that as the incidence of communicable disease declined, there was a concomitant increase in diseases linked to lifestyle, such as hypertension, cardiovascular disease, ulcers, and diabetes.

By 1960, emphasis on self-care for individuals, families, and communities was on the rise again. Attention focused on learning and practicing self-care skills that would promote health. It was believed that human beings could control their own destinies, including no longer tolerating sickness. This thinking, along with an increased standard of living and technologic advancement, stressed health as each individual's responsibility.

Ensuing years brought further shifts in perceptions of health and illness and of locus of responsibility for health care practices. Although self-care and prevention of communicable and other diseases and conditions were encouraged, there was an increasing emphasis on diagnosis and treatment of disease. These shifts, closely related to the philosophy of health in our multicultural, pluralistic society, may have negated the effective use of self-care.

In the mid-1970s the federal government played a key role in promoting the concept of self-care. There was a major attempt to define the health needs of the people of the United States, and this was paramount to their self-care practices. In 1975, the Department of Health, Education and Welfare published a "Forward Plan for Health: 1977–1981." The report identified lifestyle and psychosocial factors as having the greatest influence on the reduction of morbidity and mortality rates. Self-care topics such as diet, obesity, exercise, alcohol consumption, smoking, and environmental factors were discussed.

In 1979, the Surgeon General's report acknowledged that an emphasis on prevention of disease had enabled individuals, families, and communities to experience an increased standard of health. *Healthy People: The Surgeon General's Report on Health Promotion and Disease Prevention* predicted that a reduction of 20%–35% in morbidity and mortality in the American population could be achieved through use of self-care practices (U.S. Department of Health, Education and Welfare, 1979).

Naisbitt (1982, p. 131) referred to this self-care emphasis as a megatrend that moves health care from institutional help of the medical establishment to self-help or personal responsibility for health. He identified three trends that will influence the self-care tide for individuals and families. These include (1) new self-care habits that actualize our newfound responsibility for health, (2) self-care that illustrates our self-reliance in areas not genuinely requiring professional help, and (3) the triumph of the new paradigm of wellness, preventive medicine, and holistic care over the old model of illness, drugs, surgery, and treating symptoms rather than the whole person.

The author believes that the emergence of self-care in the 1980s can be viewed as a reflection of the increased commitment of health professionals to education for individuals and families; of growing consumer awareness that individuals are capable of sophisticated self-care; and of a variety of social, economic, and technologic movements toward assuming responsibility for self-care. In the 1980s there were major declines in death rates for many diseases including heart disease, stroke, and unintentional injuries. This was greatly due to reduction in risk factors, such as cigarette smoking, blood cholesterol, and dietary fats, as well as early detectors and control of high blood pressure. In the 1990s and beyond, the focus is shifting from decreasing death rates to improving the quality of life by reducing unnecessary suffering, illness, and disability. To meet this objective, the U.S. Department of Human Health and Services (DHHS) proposes goals to (1) increase the span of health life for all Americans, (2) reduce health disparities among Americans, and (3) achieve access to preventative services for all families. The increased rate of syphilis and HIV infection, continued aging of the American population, the cost of health care, and the need for health care insurance reform are trends that require attention when considering family self-care and health promotion and protection (DHHS, 1991, p. 6).

Emphasis on self-care practices today has prompted family health nurses to expand and directly relate that concept to family self-care. Hence, family self-care encompasses principles and practices, tools and techniques that enable families to pursue self-care. The concept of family self-care is interwoven with the importance of the family's responsibility in health promotion and health protection. This emphasis is intricately related to society's view of humankind and its relationship to the world, as well as its view of health and illness.

This chapter will present the concept of self-care as it relates to individuals and families and will review the theories of self-care nursing. It will discuss types of family self-care specific to health promotion and health protection and factors that may influence self-care. Useful tools for promoting family self-care, such as contracting and family assessment, will be incorporated. And last, the important role of family health nursing in promoting family self-care will be emphasized.

SELF-CARE DEFINED

Individual self-care as a framework for nursing is defined as a specific approach to clinical practice that places primary emphasis on the individual's ability to promote and protect health. Orem (1985, p. 31) defined self-care as "the production of actions directed to self or to the environment in order to regulate one's functioning in the interests of one's life, integrated functioning, and well-being." The basic premise of Orem's concept is the individual's personal responsibility to take action for self-care. A major outcome of effective self-care is that the individual is able to perform self-care with only minimal contact with health care services. The conceptual relationship in this design permits the family to exert control over the environment and work toward predetermined health behaviors. These behaviors are deliberate and transcend through the action-oriented self-care process. The realm of self-care encompasses (1) cognitive activities, (2) social activities, (3) psychologic activities, and (4) physical activities (Sullivan, 1980, p. 59). Each of these activities is interrelated and enmeshed within the family milieu. Self-care, then, is a complex mixture of activities directing the family toward being, behaving, and becoming.

Family self-care as a framework for nursing is defined as a specific approach to clinical practice that recognizes the uniqueness and strength of the family constellation and places primary emphasis on the family's ability to promote and protect health. This definition is preferred to a broader one because it paves the way for accepting the family's self-care behaviors in the promotion and protection of health. This is not to say, however, that accepting this definition is without intellectual difficulty. If this narrow definition is accepted, then the decision to engage in self-care behaviors and the effectiveness of the actions are always the responsibility of the family. Taylor (1989) states that nursing the family as a unit requires different considerations from nurs-

ing the individual within the context of the family. This is because the family has a "nonmaterial unity which leads to structure and functions that are substantially different from those of the individual" (p. 135). It is within the family that members learn self-care and dependent care agency, as well as strategies for meeting the goals of health promotion and protection. Therefore, a major outcome of effective family self-care is that the family is able to perform self-care with only minimal contact with health care services. Those who value their health will engage in self-care behaviors. Additionally, family health nurses acknowledge that members of a family are interdependent, and when assessing the needs of one family member, it is necessary to determine the needs and effects of a possible change in the whole family.

Specific criteria for making these simple definitions of individual self-care and family self-care operational can be found in comparing the role of the decision maker in the self-care and medical model frameworks. According to McIntyre (1980, p. 34), the medical model suggests that the professional has the knowledge, skill, and expertise necessary to make decisions concerning causes of symptoms and courses of action. The client provides the professional with the information necessary to make judgments and then cooperates with the professional by carrying out the prescribed therapeutic plan. In contrast, the self-care model suggests that individuals and families, when assisted by the professional, have the knowledge and ability to analyze their present situation and make decisions about what needs to be done. This implies a personal awareness of the factors involved in one's health and a personal "ownership" of the right and responsibility to manipulate those factors in a pattern congruent with personal values and beliefs.

The self-care model allows clients to be involved in the decision making specific to their plan of health care. Therefore, the personal value system and beliefs of professionals within the health delivery system can no longer be used to label the client as "noncompliant." Traditionally, health care professionals have behaved as if they were the only resource for health care. More and more, individuals and families are challenging this practice. They are viewing themselves as competent, responsible, and motivated for maintaining their own health, either independently or by contracting with professionals. By assuming less control, the family health nurse facilitates clients' assumption of more control of their health care situation.

Family health nurses, working in concert with families within this self-care model framework, concentrate on the concept of health and assist individuals and families to keep in touch or to get in touch with what promotes health for them. In other words, nurses assist families to exercise their rights and responsibilities in decision making, regarding health and health care for themselves and their significant others. This approach to health care differs from the episodic solution-oriented care axiomatic in the literature. The family health nurse facilitates the families' appraisal of their health by assisting them to define concerns rather than just offering solutions (Chalmers & Farrell, 1983, pp. 62–64).

SELF-CARE THEORY

The basic premise of nursing theory is that concepts are developed that will guide nursing practice in a manner congruent with the health promotion of individuals, families, and communities. Nursing theory specific to the concept of family self-care can take many directions. Orem's model of self-care is the basis for this discussion.

The conceptual basis of self-care evolved from Orem's (1959, 1971, 1979, 1980, 1985, 1990) model of nursing, which encompasses rudiments from general systems theory, which is also philosophically congruent with the perceptual theory of behavior (Combs & Snygg, 1959) and the constructivist method of behavior (Magoon, 1977).

From perceptual theory, Orem focused on the effects of variation in perception and the personal meaning attached to that perception (Combs & Snygg, 1959). The perceptions are the phenomena of personal meaning. Derived from this theory is that humans are in constant interaction with the environment and purposefully respond to stimuli to which there is personal meaning.

Orem's self-care model uses constructivist theory as a descriptive quantitative method that examines how individuals construct and interpret the meaning of their circumstance (Magoon, 1977). The basic tenant of the constructivist method is that individual behavior is a result of personal meanings and purposes constructed by individuals themselves.

By observing the family as a self-care system as presented in Chapter 4, the author defines the *family self-care system* as one in which selective family boundaries filter matter, energy, and information into and out of the system in a manner that directs the family to promote and protect health. Within the family self-care system, the members are in constant and continuous motion that maintains homeostasis or health through the feedback scheme of input, throughput, and output (Clements, 1983, pp. 64–67).

For example, the self-care system can be directly applied to a family that has just had a member diagnosed with cancer. Many therapeutic self-care demands are placed on the individual and the family by the cancer diagnosis and the chemotherapy regimen. Self-care systems result from the family's knowledge and use of behaviors known to meet self-care requisites that may result from chemotherapy. The family must also exert deliberate and personal control over illness and its symptoms by participating in the therapeutic regimen. Through the design of the nursing system, the family health nurse assesses and diagnoses the family's self-care system. On completing the assessment or input phase, goals and objectives are planned that assist the family in meeting their self-care deficits. The next phase involves implementing the co-created plan or throughput, followed by an evaluation of the nursing system to determine if the family self-care system is again functional. This output is returned to the origin of the system as feedback, and the system self-regulates.

Orem's self-care model therefore encompasses perceptual theory, constructivist methods, and general systems theory; these are symbolically interrelated. This allows family health nurses to view families as purposive, cognitive agents whose behavior is a result of their perception. The basic premise of self-care theory is that all families require self-care in order to promote health, maintain their quality of life, and prevent ill health. The ability of the family to mobilize health actions within the self-care domain through interaction with the environment is the self-care system.

A threat to the integrity of the self-care system may result when the family is confronted with a new health care experience requiring the family to be engaged in different self-care behaviors. Self-care behaviors are responses by the family when they acknowledge the need to initiate self-care. Therefore, family health nursing interventions are required when the family is unable to meet health care demands imposed on the self-care system.

Returning to the family with cancer, the knowledge and skills necessary to meet therapeutic self-care demands related to chemotherapy are complex. The knowledge and skills necessary for self-care of the family may include basic knowledge about the drugs, the side effects, the management of side effects, and when to request reevaluation of the chemotherapy. The family may draw on family health nurses as resources to facilitate family self-care abilities. Nurses will examine the family and assist them in achieving the necessary knowledge and skills to meet self-care deficits.

The design of the self-care system, when operationalized by family health nurses, supports families to exert control over their environment and works toward predetermined health behaviors. Such an approach recognizes that potential self-care behaviors can be evaluated by families in relation to their personal value and belief system. Three general requisites are essential for self-care and basic to the framework: knowledge about health, motivation for health, and ability to initiate and perform self-care behaviors (Orem, 1971, pp. 31–36).

In seeking knowledge about health, the family recognizes that the development of self-care agency is a personal, purposive psychologic human sense that evolves from the joint presence of input and the existent environment to validate the meaning and value of self-care behaviors (Orem, 1985, p. 130). The family's ability to engage and sustain self-care behaviors is a learned response that requires motivation to initiate and sustain the behaviors necessary to satisfy the demands for family care as these demands are known and understood. The inability of the family to meet these demands may result in a demand for family health nursing intervention (Orem, 1971, p. 76).

Self-care abilities and the family's concepts of self influence the uniqueness with which each of the requisites are actualized by the family. These requisites are mediated by specific characteristics inherent within each family constellation and are identified in Table 7–1.

The view of self-care is often confined to an individual or a family providing care for themselves. However, in reality, self-care encompasses care provided to families, groups, or communities with the potential to engage in the operations required for self-care. These may be referred to as a self-care agent. The empirically manifested demands of self-care agents are to maintain life, health, and well-being. These have become known as therapeutic self-care demands. These demands refer to the totality of requirements established specifically for self-care. Self-care agents, therefore, engage in self-care actions to meet family health care needs of a (1) universal, (2) health-deviated, and (3) developmental nature.

Universal self-care requisites are purposive actions required by all self-care agents to meet their basic needs. Orem (1971, pp. 21–28) identified six categories of universal self-care requisites as (1) air, food, water; (2) excrements; (3) activity and rest; (4) solitude and social interaction; (5) hazards to life and well-being; and (6) human normalcy. Orem's (1971) universal requisites to the family represent the totality with which the family interacts and coexists with its environment. Universal self-care requisites foster positive health of the family and supports the family's development and maturation (Orem, 1985, p. 91). *Health deviation requisites* are associated with conditions of diminished health that may necessitate changes of a self-care practice (Orem, 1971, pp. 29–30). The health deviation self-care system transcends the family to participate as a receiver of care to maintain or restore normalcy in the family unit. The family's acceptance and participation in care is self-care. *Developmental self-care requisites* are associated with processes and events specific to family developmental stages (Orem, 1980, p. 47). Orem (1985, pp. 95–97) describes two categories of health deviation self-care requisites that (1) prevent developmental deficits and promote development in accordance with the

TABLE 7–1. MEDIATING FACTORS AFFECTING FAMILY SELF-CARE

Age of Family Members
Sex of Family Members
Education of Family Members
Sociocultural Orientation of the Family
Developmental State of the Family
Roles Family Members Play
The Family System
Health Status of Family Members
Health Situation of the Family
Life Cycle Event of Family Members
Pathologic Disorders of Family Members
Other Mediating Factors

Adapted from Orem, D. E. (1971). *Nursing: Concepts of Practice* (pp. 13–14). New York: McGraw-Hill.

family's potential (e.g., pregnancy) and (2) prevent the occurrence of deleterious effects of conditions (e.g., terminal cancer) that can affect family development or mitigate the effects from a particular condition (e.g., impending death).

As mentioned earlier, the self-care system used by Orem evolved from an interaction-oriented, general systems approach. The self-care system can be described by dynamic interaction within the family of the therapeutic self-care demand and the self-care agent. Self-care deficits result when families are unable to meet therapeutic self-care demands. When this occurs, the self-care agents require family health nursing interventions. The nurse uses the nursing process to design a nursing system through which the exercise of self-care is regulated and families' therapeutic self-care demands are estimated and met (Orem, 1980, p. 29).

Orem's self-care system has been furthered by Harper (1984). According to Harper, the self-care system is composed of throughput subsystems that bridge the system (pp. 31–32). Harper (1984) used the earlier work by Backscheider (1974) and the Nursing Development Conference Group (1979) to postulate that the self-care throughput system operated because of specific human capabilities that include cognitive, psychologic, and physical factors (pp. 31–32). Therapeutic self-care demands are met through interaction and processing by the family within the throughput system. Throughput results become assets or deficits of the family after the system inputs are processed. The balance between these assets and deficits determines the family's decision to engage in self-care activities and the quality of these health behaviors. Therapeutic self-care demands are met when input and processed throughput elements are regulated to meet therapeutic self-care output (Harper, 1984, p. 32). The system is self-regulated via a feedback loop. If however, the input and throughput elements are not self-regulated, then therapeutic self-care demands are not able to be met, and the family requires family health nursing interventions. The family health nurse becomes the self-care agency until the family self-care system is functional.

The family self-care system strives to meet its self-care demands through the openness of its boundaries, which allow for change and growth. It is the interaction and interdependence of the family as a whole, and not as separate individuals, that allows families to process throughput received from the environment and within the family itself in order to establish a personal self-care system.

Central to Orem's theory is the concept of *nursing systems,* referring to a set of concrete actions produced from the deliberate action of nurses and families, through which the family's ability for self-care is regulated. This system serves as the thread that joins the nurse agency to the family self-care system. Orem (1985, pp. 152–157) describes three possible variations in nursing systems that are reflective of three levels of self-care agents' abilities to meet self-care requisites. These are described as (1) the wholly compensatory system, (2) the partly compensatory system, and (3) the supportive-educative system. The family health nurse assists families by designing a nursing system that follows prescribed methods: acting for, guiding, supporting, and providing an environment that promotes personal development and education (Rosenbaum, 1986, p. 415).

The family health nurse moves the family through one or more of the hierarchical nursing systems to meet family self-care requisites. The *supportive-educative* nursing system is a system where the family is able, or can and should learn, to perform self-care behaviors but requires nursing assistance (Orem, 1985, pp. 156–157). The *partly compensatory* nursing system is a system in which both the nurse and the family perform self-care measures or other activities that involve manipulative activities or behaviors (Orem, 1985, p. 156). The *wholly compensatory* nursing system is characterized by the family's total inability to engage in self-care behaviors (Orem, 1985, pp. 154–156). For example, the family with a member receiving palliative chemotherapy for cancer may progress from a supportive-educative system to a partly compensatory system just prior to death of the family member, then back to a partly compensatory system, and finally to a supportive-educative system before being discharged from family health nursing care. Synthesizing the triad of nursing systems assists family health nurses to increase family self-care agency with the ultimate goal of structural and functional integrity of the family self-care system.

In summary, the paradigm provided by Orem offers the family health nurse the following set of assumptions for self-care:

1. Self-care can be evaluated by families in a variety of situations. Orem's theory permits the assessment of families in relation to their self-care potential as it relates to health promotion and health protection. Each individual family member is viewed as a self-care agent who makes a personal continuous contribution to his or her own health.

2. Self-care relates to the personal values and health beliefs of the family. This allows the family's self-care behavior to evolve through a combination of social and cognitive experiences that have been learned through interpersonal relationships, communication, and culture that are unique to each family.

3. Self-care can be administered to families by self-care agents. Specifically, this allows the family members, either individually or collectively, to initiate and perform self-care derived from knowledge about their self-care requisites. This includes attitudes about their health and their ability to perform self-care behaviors.

4. Self-care can be used to foster the promotion of health in families and to recognize and evaluate areas of diminished health that may exist.

Steiger and Lipson (1985, p. 5) use Orem's theory to stress that self-care ability in families is demonstrated in their power to perform self-care actions. If self-care limitations exist in families, then certain limitations in the areas of knowledge, skill, and motivation are present. These constitute self-care deficits and result in an inability to engage in self-care. Such self-care deficits in families pose challenges for the family health nurse whose objective becomes assisting the family with self-care actions they are unable to perform for themselves.

The self-care model with its underlying need for family integrity has as its basis many biologic, psychologic, and sociologic-cultural theories that provide direction through the family health nurse to promote family self-care. Accepting and using the eclectic theoretical framework of self-care is not a new method but a process that promotes family self-care and family health nursing.

TYPES OF SELF-CARE

In attempts to understand the nature of self-care, one central issue has been the distinct differences among self-care behaviors. Self-care behaviors can be described in terms of three categories: promotion, protection, and prevention. The family serves as an important source of motivation, reward, and reinforcement for health promotion, health protection, and preventive health behaviors.

Health promotion begins with the basic assumption that individuals and families are healthy and encourages the development of lifestyles that maintain and support their wellness. The family's perception of control over health behaviors forces identification and augmentation of movement toward health (Chalmers & Farrell, 1983, p. 62). The idea of health promotion is based on a philosophy of holism. This includes a belief in the interactive effects of the mind, body, spirit, and environment. The concept of health promotion differs from disease prevention, which focuses on protecting the family from harm. For example, behaviors that families engage in to prevent ill health usually maintain or promote health, and health promotion should be incorporated into disease management (Steiger & Lipson, 1985, p. 14).

Family health nurses assist families to develop self-care resources. Examples include (1) developing an exercise program as part of the family's physical fitness plan, (2) developing a stress-coping program as part of the family members' daily lives, and (3) developing effective communication patterns in family relationships.

Health promotion and health protection are often used interchangeably. However, as illustrated in Chapter 2, they are not the same, nor are they mutually exclusive. The objective of health protection is for the family to develop and maintain a sense of control over health or ill health rather than to feel that their health deficits have control over them. Self-care activities families employ to maintain health may include getting enough rest and activity, learning to cope with stressors inherent in the family's environment, meeting the extra demands during pregnancy, and coping with various developmental changes of the family.

Leavell and Clark (1965) describe three assumptions essential to preventive health care: (1) knowledge of the natural history of human disorders, (2) knowledge of the combination of etiologies that are actualized when specific disorders of human structure and functioning occur, and (3) an identified rational basis for methods of intercepting etiologic factors prior to the onset of a disorder or at some time point after its inception (pp. 14–38). Preventive self-care thus requires knowledge of specific therapeutic self-care behaviors with normal family structure and functioning at various life stages in particular environments (Orem, 1971, p. 134).

FAMILY SELF-CARE CONTRACTING

Through the use of family self-care contracting, the family health nurse can assist the family to gain control over identified health problems and to increase the overall family health status. The use of contracts between the nurse and the family can set up a working relationship or agreement that can be continuously renegotiated to promote health (Hill & Smith, 1990; Spradley, 1990; Steiger

& Lipson, 1985). The contract is developed in mutual agreement with the family and provides direction for the family through the identification of objectives and responsibilities. "Without mutual participation, clients (families) cannot develop self-care abilities. Contracting makes the goal of self-care explicit" (Spradley, 1990, p. 282). Furthermore, the contract allows the family to participate actively in self-care by choosing those goals that are realistic and measurable.

There are different types of self-care contracting. The three primary types are self-contracting, nurse-client contracting, and contingency contracting. Specifically, *self-care contracting* as described by Hill and Smith (1990) has four major steps: assessment, problem identification, goal setting with environmental planning and reinforcement choice, and reevaluation. Advantages of this type of contracting are that it reduces client passivity and dependency, parallels the nursing process, provides a direct and simple approach to self-care, focuses on specific objectives, facilitates open communication, uses the influence of modeling, and facilitates personal experimentation by nurses (Zangari & Duffy, 1980, p. 454). In simpler terms, the self-contract is an agreement that an individual personally initiates with or without the assistance of a support person. It is designed to improve self-care behavior and builds on the value society places on self-control and self-management (Hill & Smith, 1990).

Nurse-client contracting is any working agreement continuously renegotiated between nurse and client (Sloan & Schommer, 1975, pp. 224–225). The contract provides direction through identification of mutual objectives and responsibilities of both the client and the family health nurse. The contract also allows clients to participate actively in their own care by choosing goals that can be realistically achieved.

Contingency contracting, on the other hand, is an intervention strategy that evolved from reinforcement theory as an applied behavior modification program. There is a systematic arrangement for the reception of a reinforcer in return for performance of a specific behavior (Steckel, 1982). This type of contract is discussed in more depth later.

Of the contracts listed above, the self-contract and the nurse-client contract may be oral or written, formal or informal. The contingency contract is a duplicate, formal written contract, signed by both the nurse and the client.

Major components of nurse-client contracting as described by Sloan and Schommer (1975) can be applied to family self-care contracting. These include (1) mutual exploration of family health problems, concerns, and goals; (2) establishment of agreeable health goals; (3) exploration of resources available to accomplish goals; (4) development of a plan to specify the steps and methods for achieving the goals; (5) negotiation of responsibilities between the nurse and the family; (6) agreement of the time modification of the contract to accomplish contract goals; and finally (7) modification, renegotiation, or termination of the contract to meet the needs of the individual or family (pp. 224–225).

Certain characteristics are essential for all contracts. These characteristics (Herge, 1980, pp. 30–34) include the following:

1. Contract goals should be realistic.
2. Contract behavior for achievement for the goals must be measurable.
3. Contract goals should be stated in positive terms.
4. Behavior indicating goals that have been attained must be measurable.
5. Behavior indicating goals that have been attained must be rewarded.

The authors feel the contingency contract is the most suitable for promoting the family self-care contract. Contingency contracting is essentially a plan for systematic reinforcement of a desired behavior. It is a written or implied agreement between the nurse and the family that a reward will be received in return for the performance of a specific behavior (Steckel, 1982).

The contingency contract provides incentives for achieving the desired behavior change that will promote family health. The rewards agreed on should be immediate and given as often as possible. Likewise, rewards should be withheld when the terms of the contract are not met. The nurse needs, however, to encourage the terms of the contract and not impose penalties. Even small penalties might create an atmosphere of resentment and negate the integrity of the contract.

Family self-care contingency contracting infers that family health nurses work in concert with families to write the contract. The contract must clearly define the responsibilities of the family and those of the family health nurse. It must focus on the behaviors that the family members agree to assume responsibility for and on the behaviors that the nurse agrees to assume responsibility for, such as giving information, providing training and counseling, and giving the specific reinforcement or reward when the contract goals are achieved.

Contingency contracting can be used with the family who has a member on chemotherapy for cancer. In the family member mentioned previously, a major reaction to the chemotherapy was loss of appetite, including no desire for necessary fluids. The family member receiving therapy became extremely weak, dehydrated, and lethargic. A health visit revealed a low white count and dehydration. Other family members, all employed and out of the home at varying times during the day, felt responsible for the situation. They knew that the chemotherapy would produce loss of appetite, but they had hoped their provision of necessary food and fluids would have been sufficient to negate such a situation. Although they were caring, they had little time for this additional responsibility.

It was important for the family health nurse in this situation to remember that it is easier to increase or learn a designed behavior than it is to decrease or eliminate a behavior that is currently being practiced and could be an established habit (Steckel, 1982). The contingency contract with this family focused on successfully increasing participation of each of the family members in planning and implementing a nutrition plan for their family member. There was negotiation and discussion with each member when the contract was being developed. One member agreed to prepare food that appeared most palatable; another agreed to come home during an office break to assist with a feeding; and another agreed to come home at noon to serve lunch. At least one member would be present each evening to ensure proper intake at the dinner hour. There was agreement in determining a way to make certain that the necessary food and fluids were available at all times. Within the contract, the method for observing, measuring, and recording the intake was included. The reinforcers, established by the family members were also recorded; they included eventually restoring the family member to a state of nutrition and hydration, knowing how to plan adequately for future chemotherapy should it be necessary, sharing in this family endeavor yet not having to assume full responsibility, and encouraging their family member to resume the previous self-care pattern once strength and usual vigor was restored. A major reinforcer they all agreed on was avoiding the expense of hiring an outsider to do in the home what they were able to do with a little direction and encouragement from the family health nurse.

FACTORS INFLUENCING FAMILY SELF-CARE

Factors or variables that may influence family self-care can be described from two basic approaches: first, individual characteristics of the family and, second, processes of the suprasystem or system above the family system. The individual characteristics of families and environments that interact with families influence the kinds of self-care behaviors families engage in. The type and amount of self-care behaviors that families engage in are subject to environmental and familial constraints.

Family self-care is influenced by factors unique to the family system. The author listed factors Orem (1971) identified that may contribute to the family's ability to engage in self-care (see Table 7–1). The scope of self-care behaviors a family can engage in is generally determined by individual factors of age, sex, values, beliefs, life cycle events, education, and health and family factors of ethnicity, developmental stage, and general health status. In addition, each family's established pattern of responding to external and internal stimuli will influence its decision to engage in self-care activities. The family's decision to engage in self-care is a complex process. It is formed in part by the network of social exchanges that result in a family theme or value system. The interplay between individual self-care needs, values, and beliefs results in the family value orientation and influences the selection as well as the perception and ranking of alternative means for achieving self-care. Furthermore, family role patterns are the result of interactions, over time, of family members and environments that determine the content and process of family self-care. Self-care practice, however, is dependent on the health status of the family. Infants, children, adolescents, the aged, the ill, and disabled family members may require assistance to meet their therapeutic self-care demands. Self-care of other family members facilitates the health of dependent members of the family structure.

The emergence of family self-care is mediated in part by input from the suprasystem. The seemingly infinite and multifactorial variables that bombard the system are the result of contact between the self-care family agency and the environment. What one needs to realize is that there are broad issues in self-care that need to be considered before one suggests self-care as a panacea for all the ills of the family.

Traditionally, self-care has been indigenous and organized around traditional family and cultural-social values. However, the structure and patterns of social organization within the family are in a state of rapid flux, and the impact these trends will have on self-care development is yet to be seen.

Family self-care is also subject to consequences of its primary goal: personal control over one's health. Although families appear to recognize the need to assume strong management of their own health care, the question is whether or not they will be successful in this endeavor. For example, when families are responsible for self-monitoring of bodily functions such as blood pressure, ear oximetry, and pregnancy tests, are the consequences accurate or are there false positives or false negatives? In addition, what is the quality and reliability of durable medical equipment and instruments marketed for home use by families (e.g., ear oximeters, home pregnancy test kits, and blood glucose monitors)? Furthermore, who is responsible for assisting the family when self-care monitoring goes astray?

Concurrent with, and inseparable from, the above self-care behaviors is a rising tide of popu-lism in which families are seeking more personal control over their health care. This is evident from the literature designed to help individuals and families enhance self-care behaviors (e.g., *Self-Health, Family Health, COPING,* and *Harvard Medical School Health Letter*). However, although self-care is promoted as being effective in maintaining and promoting health, there is little empirical data to support this claim.

Levin (1977) theorized that a self-care competent society would affect the medical-economic monopolies. Such an impact, however, would result in a redistribution of the economic benefits to be gained by self-care to families and society as a whole. Health care industries, health care institutions, and nurses themselves place constraints on the implementation of family self-care. Mullin (1982) outlined five constraints imposed by the health care and nursing systems on the implementation of self-care: (1) a focus on illnesses, not on individuals or families; (2) a focus on tasks, not on mutually identified needs; (3) an identification of care by the type of task; (4) a conflict between meeting the needs of the system and meeting the needs of the family; and (5) a misconception of the autonomy and accountability of nurses and families. Only by expanding our consciousness of these constraints and their effects on health care can family health nurses modify the effect these constraints have on the family self-care model.

Structural factors also influence family health care. Kronenfeld (1979) felt that a lack of a structural analysis of self-care ignored the realistic possibilities of self-care among families from different social strata. The potential for "blaming the victim" for personal poor health when in fact structural issues are more to blame than family values and beliefs must be avoided. In addition, insofar as self-care emphasizes attending classes or reading health literature and acquiring sophisticated knowledge of one's body, there is both an educational bias and a time bias. Such bias limits movement of the self-care model to reach large numbers of families and to significantly affect their behavior.

Families exist in a given time and space, surrounded by, and inextricably linked to, an environment that provides an infinite number of intervening influences. The capacity of the family to identify and filter these influences is constrained or enhanced by the degree to which the environment is perceived as generating possible influencing factors. No one factor mediates in isolation; each is interactive and at times synergistic. The family self-care system is a set of interacting components that co-vary, with each member dependent on the state of functions of each other member with whom it has a relationship. To a large extent, family self-care is rooted in an understanding of how family and environment influence family self-care behaviors.

ASSESSMENT OF FAMILY SELF-CARE

Family self-care is multifaceted, and therefore its assessment is complex. If one looks at family self-care and applies Orem's theory, then assessment would evolve from the framework of the nursing process. Within that context, the steps consist of assessing why families need nursing, designing a nursing system, implementing the delivery of the nursing system, and evaluating and controlling the delivery of nursing.

The phases of the Nursing Process are assessment, diagnosis, plan, and evaluation. Taylor (1989, p. 25) states that nurses practicing within any theoretical perspective may use similar assessment techniques. She emphasized that the substance of the data gathered and its interpretation will vary depending on the philosophical and theoretical perspective. Self-Care Deficit Nursing Theory (SCDNT) (Orem, 1985) provides a structure and language for the use of nursing diagnosis as process and label. The individual's demand for care can be calculated, the capabilities and limitations for providing care according to the calculated demand can be determined, and the relationship between the demand and capability can be identified. Assessment then, pertaining to family self-care, is the deliberate, systematic collection of data, together with the assignment of meaning to the input received. Emphasis is placed on the educational needs of the family as well as specified assets and limitations related to self-care skills. A statement of family self-care needs could be made following a comprehensive assessment. That statement should include a specific set of self-care actions needing to be performed in order to meet human needs.

Orem (1980, p. 203) describes a set of five crucial questions that family health nurses might employ while assessing the educational needs of individuals and families. These questions include:

1. What are the family self-care needs?
2. Does the family have a self-care deficit?
3. What is the nature and reason for that self-care deficit?
4. Should the family be assisted to refrain from self-care or to protect self-care capabilities that already exist?
5. What is the family's potential for learning new self-care behaviors?

Family health nurses in concert with families need to assess the families' self-care abilities. This assessment should focus on the families' knowledge about self-care, their motivation to perform self-care, and the presence of an overall evidence of self-care skills.

Another assessment approach is to consider the family self-care practices in light of the families' knowledge, motivation, and skills. Pender (1987, p. 198) states that knowledge can be assessed in a variety of ways, including informal discussion, health knowledge checklists, and structured tests of knowledge in specific content areas. Furthermore, motivation to engage in health education activities in order to develop greater expertise in self-care is critical to assess. The motivated family member will aggressively seek health information that will assist in self-care activities.

The family health nurse needs also to assess the psychomotor skills of the family to determine if fine and gross motor coordination is available to carry out the physical aspect of self-care (Pender, 1987, p. 200). This assessment is beneficial for both the nurse and the family member. It enables the nurse to evaluate where each family member is and what can be expected in the area of physical care. It enables each family member to recognize personal strengths as well as goals to work toward.

FAMILY SELF-CARE IMPLEMENTATION

Interventions involve the interaction and throughput of the nurse-family system to achieve mutually acceptable goals. Goals should be both short-term and long-term, and they should be established and approved by all members of the

---

CHAPTER HIGHLIGHTS

Family self-care encompasses principles and practices, tools and techniques that enable families to assume self-responsibility for the health of its members and the family as a unit.

It is within the family that members learn self-care, health promotion and health protection, and disease prevention activities.

Family health nurses work in cooperation with families to assess their self-care needs, to assist in the identification of areas of concern, and co-create problem-solving approaches.

The family's ability to begin and sustain self-care activities is influenced by the level of family motivation and the family health nurse's ability to facilitate family participation.

A family self-care contract is a strategy that may be used to facilitate the negotiation of family commitment to reaching a health-promoting, health protection or prevention goal.

Environmental, individual, and family characteristics may influence the ability to engage in self-care behaviors.

family. For example, a family with a background of cardiovascular disease might wish to have a goal of increased physical fitness. The long-term goal to work toward walking two miles per day could be established. Short-term activities might include checking pulse rate; finding different, yet convenient, areas to walk; and developing a chart to record walking achievements.

Accurate family self-care implementation is a goal to be achieved by the family health nurse. If families are involved in the self-care system, they will more readily achieve their maximum health potential. Self-care practices will enable families to be ultimately responsible for their own health, and this will include areas of health promotion and health protection.

REFERENCES

Ahmed, P.I., Rolker, A., & Coehio, G.V. (1979). Toward a new definition of health: An overview. In P.I. Ahmed & G.V. Coehio (Eds.), *Toward a New Definition of Health*. New York: Plenum Press.

Chalmers, K., & Farrell, P. (1983). Nursing interventions for health promotion. *Nurse Practitioner,* 8(10), 62–64.

Clements, I.W. (1983). Elements of a living system. In I.W. Clements & F.B. Roberts (Eds.), *Family Health: A Theoretical Approach to Nursing Care* (pp. 61–70). New York: Wiley.

Combs, A.W., & Snygg, D. (1959). *Individual Behavior.* New York: Harper & Row.

Engle, G.E. (1977). The need for a new medical model: A challenge for biomedicine. *Science,* 196(4286), 129–136.

Harper, D.C. (1984). Application of Orem's theoretical constructs to self-care medication behaviors in the elderly. *Advances in Nursing Science,* 6(3), 29–46.

Herge, P.A. (1980). Hows and whys of patient contracting. *Nurse Education,* 5(1), 30–34.

Hill, L., & Smith, N. (1990). Self-care in perspective. In L. Hill & N. Smith (Eds.), *Self-Care* Norwalk, CT: Appleton & Lange.

Kronenfeld, J.J. (1979). Self-care as a panacea for the ills of the health care systems: An assessment. *Social Science and Medicine,* 13A, 263–267.

Leavell, R.H., & Clark, G.E. (1965). *Preventive Medicine for the Doctor in His Community* (3rd ed.) (pp. 14–38). New York: McGraw-Hill.

Levin, L.S. (1977). Forces and issues in the revival of interest in self-care: Impetus for redirection in health. *Health Education Monographs,* 5(2), 115–120.

Magoon, A.J. (1977). Constructivist approaches in educational research. *Review of Educational Research,* 47(4), 651–693.

McIntyre, K. (1980, November/December). The Perry Model as a framework for self-care. *Nurse Practitioner,* pp. 34–38.

Mullin, V.I. (1982). Implementing the self-care concept in the acute care setting. *Nursing Clinics of North America,* 15(1), 177–190.

Naisbitt, J. (1982). *Megatrends* (pp. 131, 134). New York: Warner Books.

Nursing Development Conference Group. (1979). *Concept Formalization in Nursing: Process and Product.* Boston: Little, Brown.

Orem, D.E. (1959). *Guides for Developing Curricula for the Education of Practical Nurses.* Washington, D.C.: Government Printing Office.

Orem, D.E. (1971). *Nursing: Concepts of Practice.* New York: McGraw-Hill.

Orem, D.E. (Ed.). (1979). *Concept Formalization in Nursing Process and Product.* Boston: Little, Brown.

Orem, D.E. (1980). *Nursing: Concepts of Practice* (2nd ed.). New York: McGraw-Hill.

Orem, D.E. (1985). *Nursing: Concepts of Practice* (3rd ed.). New York: McGraw-Hill.

Orem, D.E. (1990). *Nursing: Concepts of Practice* (4th ed.). St. Louis: Mosby.

Pender, N.J. (1987). *Health Promotion in Nursing Practice.* Norwalk CT: Appleton & Lange.

Rosenbaum, J.N. (1986). Comparison of two theorists on care: Orem and Leininger. *Journal of Advanced Nursing,* 11, 409–419.

Spradley, B.W. (1990). *Community Health Nursing: Concepts and Practice* (3rd ed.). Glenview, IL: Scott, Foresman.

Sloan, M.R., & Schommer, B.T. (1975). The process of contracting in community nursing. In B.W. Spradley (Ed.), *Contemporary Community Nursing* (pp. 224–225). Boston: Little, Brown.

Steckel, S. (1982). *Patient Contracting.* Norwalk, CT: Appleton-Century-Crofts.

Steiger, N.J., & Lipson, J.C. (1985). *Self-Care Nursing: Theory and Practice.* Bowie, MD: Brady Communications.

Sullivan, T.J. (1980). Self-care model for nursing. *ANA Publication,* G-147, pp. 57–68.

Taylor, S.C. (1989). An interpretation of family within Orem's general theory of nursing. *Nursing Science Quarterly,* 2(3), 131–137.

U.S. Department of Health and Human Services. (1991). Healthy People 2000: National Health Promotion and Disease Prevention Objectives. (DHHS Pub. No. PHS 91-50213). Washington, DC: U.S. Government Printing Office.

U.S. Department of Health, Education and Welfare. (1979). *Healthy People: The Surgeon General's Report on Health Promotion and Disease Prevention.* (DHEW Pub. No. 79-55071). Washington, DC: U.S. Government Printing Office.

Zangari, M., & Duffy, P. (1980). Contracting with patients in day to day practice. *American Journal of Nursing,* 80, 451–455.

8

FAMILY COMMUNICATION

JEANNE HOFFER

Once a human being has arrived on this earth, communication is the largest single factor determining what kinds of relationships he makes with others and what happens to him in the world about him. How he manages his survival, how he develops intimacy, . . . are largely dependent on his communication skills.

VIRGINIA SATIR

OBJECTIVES

On completion of this chapter, the reader will be able to:

1. Summarize transactional processes that occur in family communication
2. Distinguish between growth-producing and status quo family communication
3. Analyze the changing communication processes that occur at various stages of family development
4. Formulate appropriate nursing interventions applicable in diminished family communication settings

INTRODUCTION

The method of transferring information, knowledge, values, customs, and understanding from one family member to another is known as communication. One of the most important factors in an interactional relationship is communication. Many theorists view interaction as a transactional phenomenon because people who communicate with one another have an impact on one another (Watzlawick et al., 1967; Galvin & Brommel, 1986; Whall, 1986).

Family communications are complex, dynamic processes that involve many variables. Power, cohesion, adaptability, rules, networks, environment, socioeconomic status, political viewpoints, developmental stages, and cultural background are but a few of the variables that influence the communication patterns in families.

This chapter will discuss the definitions and theories of communication, the variables that affect communication, family communication patterns, the effects communication has on family health, and nursing interventions to improve family communications and family health. A healthy marriage and family life require skill in communication (Miller et al., 1988; Olson et al., 1983b).

COMMUNICATION THEORY

Many definitions of communication exist. In the formal sense, communication means the transferring of information from one system to another. Webster gives several definitions of communication:

1. Act or fact of communicating
2. Intercourse by words, letters, or messages; interchange of thoughts and opinions
3. That which is communicated; a verbal or written message
4. Act, power, or means of communicating or passing from place to place
5. A system, as of telephone, telegraph, and so on, for communicating.

From these definitions, communication is viewed as a process. The process consists of transmitting information from a person (the source) to another person (the receiver). The information transmitted is the message. The message must be clearly stated in order to be effective.

When the communication process is viewed as a systems process, the source sends a message and this is considered *output.* The reception by the receiver is the *input.* The response by the receiver to the message (in this case the input) results in a response by the receiver. Initiation of the response and the response itself results in feedback to the source.

The source of the original message knows the receiver obtained a message, and in return, the receiver initiates a response or feedback. The response becomes a message to the source, who in turn provides feedback to the receiver. This process, then, is cyclic.

Many factors affect the communication of one person to another. The source may have a poor day and as a result not send the message intended. The receiver may also have a poor day or be preoccupied and thus not receive the messages accurately. Perceptions held by both the receiver or the source can interfere with the actual meaning of the message.

Communication, then, is something that happens between two or more individuals. Interactions are the actions or processes between people. When a message is the source of action between individuals, the process is considered a *transaction.* Family members involved in transactions with one another over a period of time develop a pattern for communicating.

Watzlawick et al. (1967, p. 21) suggested that human communication consists of three areas: semantics, syntactics, and pragmatics. *Semantics* is concerned with meanings; that is, the individuals involved in the human communication know the words used to connote specific meanings. *Syntactics* refers to "the problems of coding, channels, capacity, noise, redundancy, and other statistical properties of language" (p. 21). *Pragmatics* refers to the behavior affected by communication. Pragmatics includes semantic and syntactics as well as verbal and nonverbal communication.

The relationship between the source and the receiver, then, is the area of interest for the study of pragmatics. This relationship between the two individuals is also a focus for the field of psychology. Pragmatics means the study of the behavior found during communication between individuals. Watzlawick et al. (1967) reported multiple communication channels. One channel contains the information found in the content of the message. He called this channel the report aspect of the communication. The second channel was called the command aspect and was considered the relational channel of the message. A simple message might contain both content and relations.

For instance, the message "see that Mr. Brown, in room 234, and his family receive discharge planning" provides the content to give discharge planning to Mr. Brown. If the person making the statement is the head nurse, the relationship between the head nurse and the staff nurse is established. Such simple communications contain both content and relationships.

Formal communication theory is concerned with transmission of informational content; communication theory as an approach to couples and families is primarily concerned with relationships among participants. It is this difference in interest that directs family researchers and clinicians toward command rather than report aspects of communications (Rausch et al., 1979, p. 473).

Therefore, the command (relationship) aspect of communication is of vital importance to family health nurses.

Family Homeostasis

Families have an interplay of forces within the membership that seeks to maintain an equilibrium in the family system. Communication is one force that helps families maintain homeostasis. When the balance in the family system is threatened by either external or internal forces, the mechanism known as feedback signals a change, and the family reacts to the change in order to maintain homeostasis. Negative feedback results in the maintenance of the status quo. Furthermore, Miller (1965) proposed that all living systems are maintained by negative feedback mechanisms.

Positive feedback is as an amplifying process causing constructive growth within the family system. Positive feedback causes a change in form or structure, which results in feedback leading to temporary uncertainty and confusion. Uncertainty and confusion open the door to change, which leads to growth in the system. Morphogenesis is the term used to describe the process leading to family growth as a result of positive feedback (Olson et al., 1979). Communication by family members promotes sharing as individual and family growth occurs.

Metacommunications

Family members frequently discuss the meanings of their communications to one another. When both verbal and nonverbal communications are discussed, metacommunication occurs. *Metacommunication* is defined as people discussing the meanings attached to communications, clarifying communications, and discussing ways to improve future communications. Metacommunication leads to improvement in the relationships between family members. Metacommunication among family members helps to shape family structure and offers a mechanism for the family to set unique family meanings (Galvin & Brommel, 1986, p. 13). The following example illustrates the metacommunication process.

Tom and Sue Jay, a newly married couple, have had a major disagreement about spending money. While discussing the current management of their money, the discussion turns toward former conversations about the use of their combined salaries. They review the previous conversations and their individual interpretations of those conversations. To their surprise, both Tom and Sue discovered misunderstandings in those conversations. Because Sue's mother had always handled the money, she assumed she would also handle the family finances. Tom had assumed he would handle the finances because that was his area of expertise. The couple had never decided exactly how they would handle the checking account nor who would actually pay the bills. Sue was astonished when Tom discussed his need to handle the money. The couple established a way to handle their finances to the satisfaction of both. In later years this discussion becomes known to the couple as the "balance of power" conversation. This discussion of previous communications is known as a metacommunication. The Jay family was engaged in communication about their communication.

Family Transactions

Communication is an action that goes on between individuals, groups, and families. A message is delivered, feedback occurs, and an interaction develops. This interaction causes individuals to become involved in repeated exchanges. The exchanges offer revealing definitions of one person to another person, and the cycle continues as the other person, in turn, reveals definition of himself or herself, thus initiating further communication. Stewart (1977) terms this process a transaction. Transaction events impact family members and help establish individual identities (Stewart, 1977; Galvin & Brommel, 1986). Family theorists view communication within families as transactional communication. Galvin and Brommel (1986) further state:

A transactional view of communication and systems perspective of the family complement each other, since both focus on relationships, which take precedence over individuals. A communication perspective focuses on the interaction of two or more persons. Accordingly, from a systems perspective it is nonproductive to analyze each individual separately because of the integrative nature of the system (p. 9).

The establishment of communications within a family is not a simple undertaking. When a young couple enters a marriage, they must learn and know the meanings attached to specific symbols. Each person brings rules and meanings from the family of origin. The couple must negotiate and establish family meanings for the newly established family. Meanings are not established quickly. Some families struggle for years to establish a common understanding (Galvin & Brommel, 1986).

The process families establish to learn communication frequently results in making specific rules for communicating within that specific family. The rules force a certain family pattern, and within the patterns, a redundancy in communications occurs. It is crucial for health professionals interacting with families to be cognizant of family communication patterns. This includes rules about who talks to whom, what subjects are taboo, and how family members talk with each other. Infrequent and redundant communication causes confusion and chaos, and excessive redundancy contributes to inefficiency and boredom (Kantor & Lehr, 1976). The redundancy that occurs in families provides the individual communication styles of each family.

AXIOMS OF COMMUNICATION

Watzlawick (1967) developed some tentative axioms for human communications. The first axiom was based on the belief that all interaction resulted from a behavior found in a communication situation. The behavior demonstrated may be active or passive, with no movement nor acknowledgment to another individual. Words, silence, ignoring, or arguments are all messages and carry message value. Therefore, the first axiom was stated as *"one cannot not communicate"* (p. 49).

The second axiom referred to the relationship between the individuals communicating as well as to the content of the communication. Family members recognize the relationship prior to hearing the content. Thus, the second axiom proposed was that all *communication has both content and relationship aspects.* The relationship dictates how the content is to be understood, thus a metacommunication occurs.

The exchanges of messages between family members occurs in patterns, and as a result, sequences are developed. The term "punctuation" refers to the sequencing in a communication. Therefore, the third axiom proposed that the *nature of a relationship defined by command messages depends on the punctuation of the communication between the family members involved in the communication exchange.*

Family communication theorists recognize two categories of communication (Ruesch, 1954). "Analogic" communication (which is primarily nonverbal) and "digital" communication (primarily verbal). Both verbal and nonverbal communication can be found in any family interaction. Verbal and non verbal communication occur with either report or command messages. The total transaction must be examined to determine the identity of the speaker or the listener within the family. The fourth axiom focused on *individuals who communicate both analogically and digitally.* Digital communication is complex and logical but lacks semantics to reveal the relationship, and analogic communication possesses semantics but lacks syntax for defining the nature of a relationship.

Bateson et al. (1963) described two different patterns of communication within families: symmetrical and complementary. *Symmetrical patterns* are patterns that exist when one partner's behavior mirrors the other partner's behavior. *Complementary patterns* exist when one partner's behavior supplements the behavior of the other. For instance, one partner may be loud, aggressive, and bossy while the other is quiet, submissive, and obedient. Both patterns, symmetrical and complementary, are present in healthy families (Watzlawick et al., 1967).

Watzlawick et al. (1967) described competitiveness between partners as a danger in symmetrical relationships. Competitiveness often leads to arguments and fighting in a marriage. Eventually, competitive relationships result in some type of rejection, either in the relationship or of a partner. Rejection in a symmetrical relationship produces destructiveness to the self or one partner and possibly to both partners. Rejection negates the personhood of one or both partners.

Even more destructive in the symmetrical relationship than rejection is disconfirmation. Disconfirmation in a relationship denies existence or acceptance of the other as a reality. (Watzlawick et al., 1967). Therefore, the fifth and last axiom stated that *all communicational interactions are symmetrical or complementary, depending on the basis of equality or difference of the relationship.*

LEVELS OF COMMUNICATION

Powell (1977) maintains that there are five levels of communication. The levels represent willingness to communicate. The lowest level of communication is called "cliche conversation." This type of communication allows for little personal disclosure.

The second level for communication is reporting facts about others. This level allows for little self disclosure; in fact, it is often thought of as gossip. The third level of communicating is reporting ideals and judgments. In this case, the speaker takes some risk in disclosure but remains cautious. The fourth level of communication reveals emotions. Powell (1977) referred to this as the gut level. The speaker discloses emotions in the conversation, thus opening the door to a personal encounter. Peak communication is the fifth and highest level of communication. This level allows for openness and honesty. Peak communi-

cations are necessary in a marriage and in healthy family communications.

FAMILY COMMUNICATION PATTERNS

Miller et al. (1988) identified four patterns of communication in their book *Connecting with Self and Others,* which is based on an international couples communication program. The four patterns of communication are (1) small talk, (2) control talk, (3) search talk, and (4) straight talk. "Small talk," which is similar to cliche conversation, is described as shallow, relaxed, and chatty. Little is accomplished with small talk.

"Control talk" has two levels: light control and heavy control. Light control talk is natural and may alter the status quo by directing, advising, cautioning, praising, instructing, giving expectations, and stating concerns. Heavy control talk is the communication pattern used when a person's primary goal is getting his or her own way through the use of an aggressive and harsh conversational tone. In heavy control talk, the person is often ordering, name calling, labeling, nagging, accusing, blaming, sarcastic, and complaining (pp. 52–56).

"Search talk" is the approach used to explore or gather information without accusing. It is used to ascertain the facts without making decisions or judging. An example of search talk is "You seem down in the dumps. Anything happen to you today?"

The last pattern is "straight talk." This is the communication pattern most effective in problem solving, sharing, handling tensions, expressing feelings, discussing anticipated change, and asking forgiveness (pp. 68–75). This approach attempts to speak to the behavior rather than to attack the person's self-esteem, and it does not blame or use sarcasm. It uses "I messages." An example of straight talk is "I worry when you are late. It would relieve my anxiety if you would call when you are going to be late." Search talk, light control talk, and straight talk are used in varied situations, but heavy control talk is discouraged because it causes anger and hurts others.

Gender Styles

Tannen (1990) described the different focuses reflected by the communication styles of men and women. Men tend to view status as independence and as being important, while women seek intimacy through a complex network of friendships and connections. The different focuses of men and women make communication a continuous juggling act. Each has a style, but the styles are different and misunderstandings occur because of these gender differences.

Tannen (1990) coined knowledge of the gender differences in communication as *genderlect*. She encourages increased understanding of genderlect to improve relationships between men and women. Nurses who understand and can counsel families about the different gender styles can offer a fresh perspective to interactions.

Communication Across the Family Life Cycle

Different stages of family development entail new family dynamics and communication patterns for the family members. Dynamics of families change as a marriage matures. The evolving family dynamics also cause communication alterations.

Young Adult

McGoldrick and Carter (1980) suggest that unattached young adults separate themselves from the family of origin to achieve autonomy and recognize the desire to begin a new family. Communication is a key factor in the completion of the task of separation. The use of communication at this time prevents problems later. The young adult needs to gain the independence of living his or her own life while remaining close to the family of origin (Bowen, 1978; Galvin & Brommel, 1986).

Engagement

The second stage, the "engagement" period, sets the stage for the development of communication patterns by the young couple. At the announcement of a formal engagement, the young couple communicates their intention to form a new family. Issues such as children, religion, friends, family, money management, sexual needs, where to live, careers, dreams, and aspirations become the focus of discussions. Open, honest, in-depth communication during the engagement period helps set the stage for a lasting marital relationship. Role definition and expectations are communicated to one another during the self-disclosure process of engagement. In-depth communication during the engagement period increases the likelihood of healthy family communications later in the marriage. Navran (1967) proposed that the communication history of the couple reflects the nature and duration of the relationship during the engagement period.

Couples define themselves to one another during the engagement period. Each individual in the dyad has experiences that are different. These experiences help to shape the self. As the couple discusses past individual experiences, they may discover similarities, but because each person perceives experiences differently, meanings and differences occur. Often one person interprets the words of the other to mean that the experiences are perceived exactly the same by both. This causes misdefinitions of self as contrasted to the other. Misdefinitions cause disruptions, pain, and frequently miscommunication (Liss, 1972, p. 132). The engagement period allows time for the couple to honestly define themselves to one another.

Beginning Marriage

In the beginning marriage, the dreams and aspiration voiced during the engagement period start becoming a reality. Role responsibilities are assumed; the balance of power is established. Communication patterns are established and redundancy occurs. Partners openly discuss issues or ignore differences. Open discussions lead to successfully handling conflict. Couples who refuse to discuss differences set the stage for future communication problems (Galvin & Brommel, 1986).

Beginning marriage is the time to develop intimacy in a marriage. Navran (1967) found that happy couples differ from unhappy couples because they talk more to one another. They let their partner know they understand what is being said, talk about a wider range of topics, maintain communication channels, show sensitivity to one another's feelings, develop family language symbols, and use nonverbal techniques in their communication.

In all families, communication styles between spouses make a difference in marital satisfaction. Hawkins et al. (1980) studied the preferred style in emotional family events. Four styles of communication behavior were identified: conventional, controlling, speculative, and contactful. Controlling style halts verbalization of thoughts by giving a closed, even rejecting, manner toward further conversation. Conventional style permits avoiding or refusing to discuss the issues. Speculative style is open to thoughts about an issue; the speaker is willing to discuss issues. Contactful style attempts to elicit further communication.

Conventional and controlling communication style are considered closed, and speculative and contactful are open. The closed styles are defensive communication behaviors, and the open are supportive.

In the study, women were found to want less controlling communication behavior styles from the husband. Men perceived themselves as controlling communicators. Women also wanted more contactful styles from their husbands. Again, men preferred to give less contact communication than women wanted. Men were found to have less potential for marital dissatisfaction from the perceived communication styles in the marriage than women.

Communication is significantly related to family cohesion and adaptability (Olson et al., 1983b). Other studies suggest that positive regard may be more important than communication in marital adjustment (Barnes et al., 1984). Jorgensen and Gaudy (1980) found that self disclosure—that is, discussing personal and intimate matters—increased marital satisfaction.

Wynne et al. (1982) view "healthy communication" on the part of the parents as important in promoting healthy adjustment in the offspring by providing children with a model for communicating ideas and feelings clearly and directly. Healthy communication in families is clear in meaning, with behavior congruent to the interaction. The birth of a child causes the need for new and demanding communication patterns in marriages (Galvin & Brommel, 1986).

Childbearing

During the first pregnancy, couples spend time discussing the changes that will occur in their daily life after the birth of the child. Decisions about infant care must be made. If the mother is working, will she resign her job and stay home to care for the child? Can adequate child care be obtained so that the mother and father may continue their careers? These and many other decisions must be reached. Naming the child becomes very important. The couple must decide on the relationship to be established with both sets of their parents. The birth of a child may complicate relationships with parents. Families are drawn closer together, or there may be a need for more independence for the new parents from their parents. Communications with parents may become more difficult if the new parents insist on maintaining independence when the grandparents are not ready to allow increased independence.

Teaching the infant to communicate is also a task for the parents. Brazelton (1991) reported that an infant can distinguish its mother's voice from other women's voices at seven days and will choose his mother's silent face before choosing another woman's face at ten days. In addition, the infant will choose his father's voice and face instead of another man's voice or face at fourteen days.

This recognition by the infant produces an excited response from the parents that increases attention, cuddling, and vocalizing to the infant. At about one month the infant responds with an audible babble. Parents and infant develop a rhythm of smiling or vocalizing back and forth. This cycle continuously repeats itself as the parents encourage the infant to respond. Thus, the family begins to establish communication patterns of responding to one another.

Parents and infant master four kinds of learning to successfully communicate: (1) control over autonomic and central nervous system, (2) development of patterns of attention and withdrawal, (3) recognition and use of signals, and (4) enlarging upon the signals (Brazelton, 1981).

Childrearing

As the child (or children) grow older, communication patterns within the family change. An infant is taught communication by the constant talking and sharing and by the parent's interaction with the child. As the child grows older, imitation and sharing offers the child increased opportunity to develop skills in verbal and nonverbal communication.

In Hubbell et al.'s (1974) investigation of communication in a four-member family, age and sex of the children were found to result in different interactions with parents. In the study, one child family member was three or four, and the second child was six or seven years old. The focus of the study was on verbal communication of the children and on how the parents interacted with the children. Findings indicated that parents talked more to the younger children than to the older children but that parents used a greater variety of words when talking with the older children. Another finding indicated that parents offered twice the amount of positive feedback rather than negative feedback to girls than to boys, even though the language skills of boys and girls were the same. In the study, fathers interacted more with sons and mothers interacted more with daughters.

Parents find increasing need to communicate with more and more people involved with their children. Teachers, scout leaders, parents of the children's friends, and church members all become important to the child. Parents have the responsibility of knowing all these people and their child's relationship with each. The increasing circle of people involved with the children of a family encourage socialization into community social life.

The incentives, status, and roles of family members within the social system are provided by the family (Lidz, 1963). The community recognizes this group of individuals as a family entity. Family entities are thought to help stabilize the community. Families interact with and change the community and society in which the family lives (Zuzich & Boyd, 1986).

ADOLESCENCE. A particularly turbulent time for family life occurs when the children reach adolescence. Family beliefs and values are questioned by the adolescent. Peer pressure heightens conflicts of beliefs and values already present. The adolescent displays frequent mood changes, varying from dependence to independence. Parents are no longer considered all knowing and all wise. Parents may have difficulty allowing the adolescent to move away from the family. Some parents encourage independence, and others discourage it. Parental anger and frustration are frequently verbalized as a result of the adolescent's questioning.

Adolescents test family adaptability. Communication patterns offer one essential tool to help families negotiate increased family adaptability (Barnes & Olson, 1982). Adolescents value parental respect for their opinions and expressions of confidence. When respect and confidence are provided to the adolescents by the parents, better family communications are enjoyed (Bienvenu, 1969). Additionally, congruent communication, honesty, love, and growth-producing activities are needed by adolescents to develop high self-esteem (Satir, 1988).

Launching

During launching, as adult children strive to become independent from the family of origin, communication is a key factor to a smooth and functional separation. Negotiations between parents and adult children are required in regard to career selection, living arrangements, money independence, selection of mates, and so on. Conflicts may arise when adult children remain in the home longer than parents anticipate. This period can be tumultuous at times, as the parents attempt to increase intimacy but deal with the myriad of conflicts and changing relationships during the launching stage (Galvin & Brommel, 1986 pp. 215–217).

The Empty Nest

The "empty nest" syndrome, when all children are grown and have left home, presents a difficult time for some couples. Many couples report lack of topics to discuss. In these families, past communications have centered around the children and the children's activities. The more fortunate couples have formed a friendship relationship with their adult children. Friendship with the adult children allows continued conversation and close contact for the grandparents.

During this period, many couples become grandparents. Neugarten and Weinstein (1964) suggested a reconceptualization of the grandparent role. Communication between the parents and the adult children results in a new relationship with the grandchildren. The traditional grandparenting role included the "formal" grandparent, the "surrogate parent," and the "reservoir of family wisdom" grandparent. The "funseeker" and the "distant figure" grandparent are more common today.

Retirement

As couples mature, retirement plans are needed. Communication and negotiation are in-creased as couples make plans for retirement and spend more time together. Frequently, retirement presents opportunities for second careers or increased opportunities to spend time with children and grandchildren. Retired grandparents have time to listen and encourage children, especially adolescents. Grandparents frequently verbally review their lives, offering valuable history lessons to those taking the time to listen.

Intrapersonal communication about life and meaning from that life offers perspective to older individuals. Reminiscing is important for both interpersonal and intrapersonal communication in the older adult (Galvin & Brommel, 1986).

Satir (1988) discussed the aging process in healthy people. Factors important in healthy aging include successful transition into the later years. Congruent communication and high self-worth are important ingredients of this transition. Discussion of fantasies and recognition of passage into a new phase of life are accomplished by communication with spouses and others.

Functional Family Communications

Satir (1988) defined healthy families as untroubled and nurturing with the following patterns: self-worth is high: communication is direct, clear, specific, and honest; rules are flexible, human, appropriate, and subject to change; and the linking to society is open and hopeful. Healthy families have effective, functional communication (Satir, 1988; Stachowiak, 1975; Barnhill, 1979). The communication is clear and caring. Decision making in healthy families is efficient and effective. Healthy families have the ability to use metacommunication, that is, communication about communications.

Curran (1983) found that communication and listening were listed as the first trait of healthy families. Table-time conversations were listed as the thirteenth trait of healthy families. Curran noted that communication is necessary for loving relationships in families. Listening and sharing permits family members to know one another. Television has a detrimental effect on family communication (Brody & Stoneman, 1983; Curran, 1983). As the time families watch television increases, family communication reduces in quality and quantity. Curran proposed hallmarks found in healthy, communicating families. The first hallmark was that parents share the family power equally. The relationship gives the children security to become independent and risk takers.

Another hallmark for communicating families is the ability to listen. Parents sometime tend to react rather than respond. Curran (1983) suggested that reacting means responding to personal feelings and experiences rather than to those of the speaker. Empathy means responding to the feelings of the other family members. Empathy reflects the ability to listen while reacting reflects the lack of listening. Wise parents use empathetic responses to their children rather than reacting or preaching about how things were when the parents were young.

Equally important, according to Curran (1983), is the ability to recognize nonverbal messages. Communications of feelings are frequently nonverbal. Healthy families use "signs, symbols, body language, smiles, and other physical gestures to express their feelings of caring and love" (p. 47). Silences and withdrawal are accepted by healthy family members in a positive, open way. Allowing family members to have time alone is acceptable for the healthy families.

Healthy families foster independence and allow individual feelings. Family discussion contains give and take. Children are encouraged to articulate their thoughts at home, thus giving them added confidence when outside of the home.

The healthy family knows turn-off words and put-down phrases, but these families do not use them in daily communications. These families pay attention to the needs of each family member, thus reducing hurts resulting from careless remarks.

Curran (1983) explained that interruptions in family communications are common in healthy families. All family members are interrupted, but no one member is interrupted more often than any other family member. Spontaneity in family communications is also important. Communication is clear in healthy families, other family members anticipate what is about to be said by others. There is a total feeling of closeness in the family.

Curran (1983) found that healthy families "develop a pattern of reconciliation" (p. 55). Parents tend to imitate their own parents in patterns of reconciliation. If absent in the family of origin, new patterns of reconciliation are developed. Reconciliation is important in communication and in family life. Finally, Curran described healthy families as those who know they will have problems, but when they do have problems, the family handles them quickly. Negotiation is a tool the healthy family uses.

Hurley (1981) suggested healthy families have more pauses, laughter, and interruptions than unhealthy families. Mishler and Waxler (1975) found laughter was used frequently by healthy families. Riskin and Faunce (1970) found more interruptions in healthy families than in neurotic families.

Satir (1988) described a healthy family as a nurturing family. Nurturing families discuss their feeling freely with one another. Members of the family are comfortable with one another. These family members demonstrate affection toward one another. Honesty and love are found in the home. The parents work hard to create an atmosphere where each family member is valued as a unique self. High levels of self-esteem for each member are family goals.

Dysfunctional Family Communications

Dysfunctional family communications are severely troubled. Friedman (1992) defines dysfunctional communication as unclearly transmitted or received messages and/or messages with incongruent content and command aspects. Conflicts are painful for the dysfunctional family. These families avoid direct communication.

Communication patterns for dysfunctional families are characterized by long speeches, and well-functioning families have short but numerous speeches (Galvin & Brommel, 1986). Conversations are not directed to specific family members but to the family in general (Stachowiak, 1975).

Dysfunctional communication within families causes dysfunction in the family system (Miller & Janosik, 1980). A low self-esteem in the family and in individual members is a factor that generates dysfunctional communications. Self-centeredness, lack of empathy, and the need for total agreement are family values that perpetuate the low esteem in members (Friedman, 1992).

Sender Dysfunction

The communication sender is often responsible for the dysfunctional communication. The sender assumes that others think or feel the same way about events. In making this assumption, the sender may speak for others, give incomplete messages, fail to check out perceptions, or fail to express true feelings, such as express anger when really hurt (Friedman, 1992). Other common causes for dysfunctional sender communications include omitting connections between ideas; using terms as "always," "should," and "never"; lacking clarity in messages; sending double-bind messages; and showing disconfirmation and disqualification in communications.

Receiver Dysfunction

The receiver may also be the source for dysfunctional communication. Receivers may fail to listen, which results in misunderstanding or misinterpretation. In the event of an unclear message, the dysfunctional receiver fails to ask for clarification, and instead functions from assumptions. The receiver can also ignore or disqualify the message. Infrequently, the receiver assumes an attacking position by insulting or rebuffing the message. The receiver can also become involved in a double-bind situation (Friedman, 1992).

The Double Bind

The most confusing dysfunctional communication is the double bind. Bateson et al. (1956) initiated double-bind research to link family dynamics to schizophrenia. The theoretical formulation for the double bind consists of conflicting communication patterns, which were thought to be a cause of schizophrenia (Jones, 1986). Bateson et al. (1956) described the double bind as an interactional process in which one person is placed in a situation to receive two conflicting messages. The person receiving the conflicting messages cannot leave the kindred relationship.

The functional response to the double bind is the metacommunication. Individuals caught in the double bind cannot metacommunicate nor can they laugh off the situation. Nor are the individuals strong enough to withdraw from the double-bind situation.

Satir (1988) proposed that incongruent communication is a source of dysfunction. Incongruent communication means that the communicational and the metacommunicational parts of the message do not agree. According to Satir, four types of dysfunctional communication commonly occur. The four dysfunctional communication types are placating, blaming, computing, and distracting.

Each of the communication types have their own way to transmit information. Placaters talk in a disarming way; they never disagree and always want to please. They are apologizing, "yes" people. The blamers are fault finders. Problems are caused by others. Blamers are bossy and dictatorial. Computers are always correct. They do not show any feeling in their communication and distance themselves from others. They remain neutral in most situations. The distractors are attention getters who attempt to distract others from the issues and the task at hand. Distractors chatter constantly, saying very little (Satir, 1988).

EFFECTS OF COMMUNICATION ON FAMILY HEALTH STATUS

Communication is the means by which family members deal with the responsibilities of family life. There is no one correct way to communicate in a family. The way in which family members communicate with one another influences their relationships and family life. Healthy family communication is clear and effective.

Effective communication enables family members to deal with the stresses of everyday life. Cohesion, adaptability, and communication are the prime concepts in Olson's Circumplex Model of families, which was presented in Chapter 4. Communication, in that model, is the factor which facilitates movement on the two concepts of cohesion and adaptability in family behavior. Positive communication allows the families to share their feelings and to work toward family goals (Olson et al., 1983a). Negative communication prevents the sharing of needs, thereby increasing stressors found in daily life. Increased stressors affect not only family life but the health of the family and the health of each family member.

ASSESSMENT OF FAMILY COMMUNICATION

Numerous instruments are available to nurses to measure communication patterns in families. The use of these tools enables nurses to make more accurate assessments. Communication facilitates many family functions and is a subscale of FACES III (Olson et al., 1985).

Parent-adolescence communication patterns can be measured using parent and adolescent instruments constructed by Barnes and Olson (1982). Openness, freedom to exchange ideas, trust, and honesty found in both parents and the adolescents are the concepts measured. Bienvenu (1969) has also constructed the Family Communication Inventory as a tool to promote communication between parents and adolescents.

Other instruments are available to couples preparing for marriage. The instruments include the FOCCUS (Facilitating Open Couple Communication), PMI Profile (Pre-Marital Inventory), and the Prepare-ENRICH (Premarital Personal and Relationship Enrichment).

Additional instruments for measuring and assessing family communications include the Marital Communication Scale, which is part of ENRICH (Olson et al., 1982); the Marital Communication Inventory by Schumm, Anderson, and Griffen (1983); the Affective Sensitivity Scale by Danish and Kagan (1971); the Self-Disclosure Questionnaire by Jourard and Lasakow (1959); and the Interpersonal Communication Inventory by Bienvenu and McCain (1970).

Emde (1992a) suggested two ways a nurse can assess the quality of family communication. She described structured interviews and the interactional task. Two types of questions make up the structured interview. The first set of questions relate to the history of the marital relationship, while the second set focuses on the current marital relationship.

The interactional task selected by the couple must be an important one for them. The task must take about 20 minutes and fit into a nurse home visit. The task must emphasize concrete, positive behaviors. Emde (1992b) suggested parenting issues as a particularly effective task. Careful analysis of both the interview and observational data provide confirming or disconfirming communication patterns which support or deny the identity of the spouses. Careful linking of the data from both sources gives nurses strategies for effective intervention.

Although family health nurses may not be therapists, the knowledge of communication patterns and use of therapeutic approaches are useful in nursing interventions of well families. Family health nurses should make appropriate referrals when working with families whose communication problems are beyond the level of the nurse's expertise.

NURSING INTERVENTIONS TO IMPROVE FAMILY COMMUNICATION

Communication is essential to the delivery of nursing care. Nurses are responsible for the quality of the communication in the nurse-client relationship, and they facilitate communication between individuals in the family system. Nurses have several approaches available to ensure effective family communication.

Listening

One important skill for the nurse is listening. Listening includes hearing, perceiving, and interpreting sounds (Edwards and Brilhart, 1981). When listening, nurses need to listen with a purpose, to be aware of emotions, and to pay strict attention to the conversation. In addition to listening, nurses must use feedback to make certain the message has been perceived correctly by the clients (Wilson, 1970). Only then can the nurse respond to the message, seek feedback, and offer understanding and acceptance.

Nurses may include all family members in a conference at one time. Listening in such a situation demands considerable expertise and practice. Satir (1988) reported that troubled families display communication patterns that are unclear or vague, prevent growth, and reduce family harmony. In these cases, the nurse who intervenes by listening intervention can help cause changes in the family system communication patterns.

According to Kelly (1977), there are two ways to categorize listening: deliberative listening and empathetic listening. To listen deliberatively means to critically analyze what is being said, and then to understand the meaning of the words. The empathetic listener attempts to understand the speaker, and then to understand the meaning of the message. Both types of listeners have the same goal: understanding of the words spoken.

Affective and Cognitive Interventions

Wright and Leahey (1984) suggest two levels of direct interventions using communications. The first consists of doing something; the second consists of not doing something. The interventions focus on the cognitive, affective, or behavior domains of family functioning. Interventions focusing on the cognitive domain consist of giving new information on a situation. The new information gives the family a new or different perception for the situation. Change in the family system is the goal sought when the nurse introduces new information.

Interventions focusing on the affective domain are aimed at reducing or increasing emotions. For instance, a child who has forgotten to take a homework assignment to school may come home crying because the teacher was angry. The parents' response would reflect the child's feelings; "You must have been very embarrassed when the teacher fussed at you." In such a case, the child is free to explain how he or she felt in the unhappy situation. Interventions affecting the emotions often help reduce problems. With the release of emotions such as anger, hate, grieving, or depression, resolution occurs.

Interventions that focus on the behaviors are designed to assist family members to behave differently toward one another. Focusing on behavior opens the door to increased growth-producing behaviors for all members. Ericson and Rogers (1973) state that in symmetrical relationships a person acts toward another as the other acts toward him. Thus, behavior changes are encouraged as a first step to improve communications.

Nurses can teach family members to focus on the behaviors that are unacceptable to the family rather than on the individual as unacceptable. Family members should be encouraged to use the "I message" rather than to attack the other verbally. For example, when a child does not knock on a parent's closed door before entering, the parent may say "I become very angry when you forget to knock on my door. Please try to remember in the future." This "I message" is preferable to a verbal attack such as "You are bad because you never knock." The parent may also role model the appropriate behavior.

Teaching the Leveling Response

Satir (1988) emphasized the importance for parents to develop self-worth in their children. Parents who provide respect, encouragement, and unconditional positive regard to their children help to develop high levels of self-esteem in the children. She suggested the use of a communication response called leveling. This response includes voice, verbal, body language, and facial expressions which are all congruent with one another.

The leveling response is open, honest, direct, and there are not threats to the self-worth of individuals involved in the communication. Leveling remarks relate emotions felt by the speaker. The parent's "I message" to the child previously mentioned who forgot to knock on the door was a leveling response that focused on the unacceptable behavior. The behavior, not the self-worth of the child, was the focus of the remark. Observant family health nurses can teach families to focus leveling remarks, thereby preventing damage to the self-esteem.

STRATEGIES TO IMPROVE FAMILY COMMUNICATION

Children learn to express themselves as they observe their parents expressing themselves. Parents model the relationship between themselves to the children. The parental relationship sets the pattern for all family relationships and communications (Dreikus, 1964). Dreikus suggested that families meet regularly to discuss problems and to seek solutions as a group. He called the sessions family councils. Regularly scheduled family councils teach children decision-making skills and ways to solve problems.

Hendricks (1979) suggests families experiment with a variety of family meetings to enhance communication. The first is a "Family Feelings Meeting," where each member states how he or she feels using "I messages." For example, one member may say "I feel lonely when you are away." The rules for family meetings are (1) there is no criticism, (2) everyone gets to talk, (3) there is no punishment, and (4) discussion is delayed until later.

In the second type of meeting, a "Family Wants Meeting," each member shares what he or she wants in terms of material wants and interpersonal concerns. Members are allowed to clear their minds without interruption. The third type of meeting is a "What Works Meeting," which helps family members to identify behaviors that are or are not working. The purpose of the meeting is to focus on behaviors and their consequences. Explanations and problem solving are delayed until later. For example, "It works better when we share our work and meeting schedule for the week on Sunday. I feel we are better able to reduce the chaos" (pp. 44–48). Families can be encouraged to experiment with family meetings.

Nurses employed in doctor's offices, schools, hospitals, and public health agencies need to increase family education about communicating with children and adolescents. Gordon (1975) initiated an effective program called Parent Effectiveness Training (PET). These programs are held in many sections of the United States. The PET programs focus on communication techniques such as "I-messages" and "active listening method." Many families have benefited from this program.

Another approach to improved family communication is the *quid pro quo,* introduced by Lederer and Jackson (1968). Couples are encouraged to set aside an hour a week to practice bargaining with one another. Using this approach, couples learn to give and take in open communication to maintain and build self-esteem. Also, Satir (1988) provides numerous exercises for families to use for improving their communications.

Numerous other approaches are available for improving marriage and family communications. Marriage Enrichment, Marriage Encounter, and Marriage Communication Lab programs are all religion based and found in many communities. The programs all emphasize communication.

In addition, there are many self-help groups that help to improve family communications in troubled families. These groups include Alcoholics Anonymous, Al-Anon, Parents Anonymous, Parents Without Partners, Compassionate Friends, and Candlelighters.

One of the most important activities in nursing practice is research to increase understanding of family communications. Conceptual or operational schemes and methodological problems have severely hampered research. Suggested fu-

CHAPTER HIGHLIGHTS

One of the most important activities in the family is the interactional relationship known as communication.

Family communications are complex, dynamic processes that are influenced by family variables such as age, gender, power, cohesion, adaptability, rules, networks, socioeconomic status, political views, developmental stages, culture, and so on.

Healthy families and healthy marriages need the skill of effective communication.

Communication patterns, rules, and meanings are learned within families and must be negotiated each time a new family is established.

There are varied levels of communication within families that represent the willingness of members to interact.

Each family developmental stage entails new family communication dynamics and communication patterns for family members.

Effective communication facilitates a family to cope with everyday life stressors, to share feelings and work together toward family goals.

A key variable in effective nurse family interaction is effective listening.

Nursing assessment of family communication may be accomplished by observation, interview, and use of prepared assessment measures.

ture research should include measurement of the intensity of the family members' relationships. Communication patterns in families must be evaluated to define relationships (Olson, 1983b). Knowledge of family communication patterns can improve the development of specific therapeutic interventions following assessment of family communications.

REFERENCES

Barnes, H.L., & Olson, D.H. (1982). Parent-adolescent communication scale. In D.H. Olson (Ed.), *Family Inventories: Inventories Used in a National Survey of Families Across the Family Life Cycle* (pp. 33–46). St. Paul: Family Social Science, University of Minnesota.

Barnes, H.L., Schumm, W.R., Jurich, A.P., & Bollman, S.R. (1984). Marital satisfaction: Positive regard versus effective communication an explanatory variable. *The Journal of Social Psychology*. 123, 71–78.

Barnhill, L.R. (1979). Healthy family systems. *The Family Coordinator,* 28, 94–100.

Bateson, G., Jackson, D.D., Haley, J., & Weakland, K.J. (1956). Toward a theory of schizophrenia. *Behavior Science,* 1: 251–264.

Bateson, G., Jackson, D.D., Haley, J., & Weakland, K.J. (1963). A note on the double bind—1962. *Family Process,* 2: 154–161.

Bienvenu, M.J. (1969, April). Measurement of parent-adolescent communication. *The Family Coordinator,* pp. 117–121.

Bienvenu, M.J., & McCain, S. (1970). Parent-adolescent communication and self-concept. *Journal of Home Economics,* 62(5), 344–345.

Bowen, M. (1978). *Family Therapy in Clinical Practice.* New York: Aronson.

Brazelton, T.B. (1991). Our changing American values. In V.S. Flowers (Eds.), *Bill Moyers: A World of Ideas.* New York: Doubleday.

Brazelton, T.B. (1981). *On Becoming a Family.* New York: Delacorte.

Brody, G.H., & Stoneman, Z. (1983). The influence of television on family interaction. *Journal of Family Issues,* 4(2), 329–348.

Curran, D. (1983). *Traits of a Healthy Family.* New York: Ballantine Press.

Danish, S.J., & Kagan, N. (1971). Measurement of affective sensitivity. *Journal of Consulting Psychology,* 18, 51–61.

Dreikus, R. (1964). *Children: The Challenge.* New York: Hawthorn Books.

Edwards. B.J., & Brillhart, J.K. (1981). *Communication in Nursing Practice.* St. Louis: C.V. Mosby.

Emde, J.E. (1992a). Marital communication analysis: Strategies for clinicians (part 1). *NCAST National News,* 8(2), 4–6.

Emde, J.E. (1992b). Marital communication analysis: Strategies for clinicians (part 2). *NCAST National News,* 8(3), 1–4.

Ericson, P.M., & Rogers, L.E. (1973). New procedures for analyzing relational communication. *Family Process,* 12, 245–267.

Friedman, M.M. (1992). *Family Nursing: Theory and Assessment* (3rd ed.). Norwalk, CT: Appleton & Lange.

Galvin, K.M., & Brommel, B.J. (1986). *Family Communication.* Glenview, IL: Scott, Foresman.

Gordon, T. (1975). *PET: Parent effectiveness training.* New York: American Library.

Hawkins, J.L., Weisberg, C., & Ray, D.W. (1980, August). Spouse differences in communication style: preference, perception, behavior. *Journal of Marriage and the Family,* pp. 585–593.

Hendricks, G. (1979). *The Family-Centering Book.* Englewood Cliffs, NJ: Spectrum.

Hubbell, R.D., Byrne, M.C., & Stachowiak, J. (1974). Aspects of communication in families with young children. *Family Process.* 13, 215–224.

Hurley, P.M. (1981). Communication patterns and conflict in m marital dyads. *Nursing Research,* 30, 38–42.

Jones, S.L. (1986). A reformulation of the interactional approach to family therapy. In A. Whall (Ed.), *Family Therapy Theory for Nursing.* Norwalk, CT: Appleton-Century-Crofts.

Jorgensen, S.R., & Gaudy, J.C. (1980). Self-disclosure and satisfaction in marriage: The relation examined. *Family Relations,* 29, 281–287.

Jourard, S.M., & Lasakow, P. (1959). Some factors in self-disclosure. *Journal of Abnormal and Social Psychology,* 56, 91–98.

Kantor, D., & Lehr, W. (1976). *Inside the Familiy.* San Francisco: Jossey-Bass.

Kelly, C.M. (1977). Empathetic listening. In J. Stewart (Ed.), *Bridges Not Walls.* Reading; MA: Addison-Wesley.

Lederer, W., & Jackson, D.D. (1968). *The Mirages of Marriage.* New York: W.W. Norton.

Lidz, T. (1963). *The Family and Human Adaptation.* New York: International University Press.

Liss, J. (1972). *Family Talk.* New York: Ballantine Press.

McGoldrick, M., & Carter, E.A. (1980). Forming a remarried family. In E. Carter & M. McGoldrick (Eds.), *The Family Life Cycle: A Framework for Family Therapy.* New York: Gardner.

Miller, J.G. (1965). Living systems: Basic concepts. *Behavioral Science,* 10, 193–237.

Miller, J.R., & Janosik, E.H. (1980). *Family-Focused Care.* New York: McGraw Hill.

Miller, S., Wackman, D., Nunnally, E., & Miller, P. (1988). Connecting With Self and Others. Littleton, CO: Interpersonal Communication Programs.

Mishler, E.G., & Waxler, N.E. (1975). The sequential patterning of interaction in normal and schizophrenic families. *Family Process,* 14, 17–50.

Navran, L. (1967). Communication and adjustment in marriage. *Family Process,* 6, 173–184.

Neugarten, B., & Weinstein, K.K. (1964). The Changing American grandparent. *Journal of Marriage and the Family.* 26, 119–204.

Olson, D.H., Fournier, D.G., Duckman, J.M. (1982). ENRICH. Minneapolis: Prepare-ENRICH, Inc.

Olson, D.H., McCubbin, H., Barnes, H.L., Larsen, A.S., Muxen, M.L., & Wilson, M.A. (1983a). *Families: What Makes Them Work.* Beverly Hills: Sage.

Olson, D.H., Portner, J., & Lavee, Y. (1985). *FACES III.* St. Paul, MN: Family Social Sciences, University of Minnesota.

Olson, D.H., Russell, C.S., & Sprenkle, D.H. (1983b). Circumplex model of marital and family systems: VI theoretical update. *Family Process,* 22, 69–84.

Olson, D.H., Sprenkle, D.H., & Russell, C.S. (1979). Circumplex Model of marital and family systems: Cohesion and adaptability dimensions, family types, and clinical applications. *Family Process,* 18, 69–84.

Powell, J. (1977). Interpersonal encounter and the five levels of communication. In J. Stewart (Ed.), *Bridges Not Walls*. Reading, MA: Addison-Wesley.

Rausch, H.L., Greif, A.C., & Nugent, J. (1979). Communication in couples and families. In W.R. Burr, R. Hill, F.I. Nye, & I.L. Reiss (Eds.), *Contemporary Theories about Families* (Vol 1) (pp. 468–489). New York: Free Press.

Riskin, J., & Faunce, K.E. (1970, June). Family interaction scales: Part 3. Discussion of methodology and substantive findings. *Archives General Psychiatry, 22*, 527–537.

Ruesch, J. (1954). Psychiatry and the challenge of communication. *Psychiatry, 17*, 1–18.

Satir, V. (1988). *The New Peoplemaking*. Mountain View, CA: Science and Behavior Books.

Schumm, W., Anderson, S.A., & Griffen, C.L. (1983). The marital communication inventory. In E.E. Filsinge (Ed.), *Marriage and the Family Assessment*. Beverly Hills: Sage.

Stachowiak, J. (1975). Functional and dysfunctional families. In V. Satir, J. Stachowiak, & H. Tachman (Eds.), *Helping Families to Change*. New York: Aronson.

Stewart, J. (1977). *Bridges Not Walls*. Reading, MA: Addison-Wesley.

Tannen, D. (1990). *You Just Don't Understand*. New York: Ballantine Books.

Watzlawick, P., Beavin, J.H., & Jackson, D.D. (1967). *Pragmatics of Human Communication: A Study of Interaction Patterns, Pathologies and Paradoxes*. New York: Norton.

Whall, A. (1986). *Family Therapy Theory for Nursing*. Norwalk, CT: Appleton-Century-Crofts.

Wilson, L.M. (1970). Listening. In C.E. Carlson (Ed.), *Behavior Concepts and Nursing Interventions*. Philadelphia: J.B. Lippincott.

Wright, L.M., & Leahy, M. (1984). *Nurses and Families: A Guide to Family Assessment and Intervention*. Philadelphia: F.A. Davis.

Wynne, L.C., Jones, J.E., Al-Khayyal, M. (1982). Healthy family communication patterns: Observations in families "at risk" for psychopathology. In F. Walsh (Ed.), *Normal Family Processes: Implications for Clinical Practice* (pp. 142–165), New York: Guilford Press.

Zuzich, A.M., & Boyd, C. (1986). An inductively derived family therapy approach for nursing. In A. Whall (Ed.), *Family Therapy Theory for Nursing*. Norwalk, CT: Appleton-Century-Crofts.

FAMILY SOCIAL SUPPORT

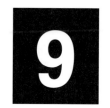

PATRICIA ROTH

A kind heart is a fountain of gladness, making everything in its vicinity freshen into smiles.

WASHINGTON IRVING

OBJECTIVES

On completion of this chapter, the reader will be able to:

1. Differentiate between the concepts of social network and social support

2. Analyze the relationship among the variables of social support, stress reduction, and well-being

3. Describe the influence of contemporary social trends on conventional and progressive family forms

4. Analyze the effectiveness of various types of networks in providing social support to families and individuals

5. Assess family needs for social support with awareness of cultural determinants

6. Evaluate the contribution of social support to the integration of health-promoting behaviors into family lifestyles

7. Develop effective strategies for implementing the concept of social support in nursing education, research, and practice

---

The advance of technology has nurtured a revolutionary age marked by rapid and dramatic change. Although the specter of an uncertain future challenges individuals and interpersonal relationships, accelerated change also presents a wealth of opportunity. These same opportunities require decisions unknown to previous generations. People seek healthier, more satisfying lifestyles and are faced with hard choices concerning the use of technology to assist fertility, improve pregnancy outcomes, deter chronic illness, and delay death, decisions that profoundly influence family life.

Changes in family life-cycle patterns have increased correspondingly during the last two decades, due to the lower birthrate, the longer life expectancy, the changing role of women, and the increasing incidence of divorce and remarriage. Previously, childrearing occupied adults for an entire life span, but it now occupies less than half of adult life prior to old age, giving new meaning to the concept of family. Since women have always been central to the functioning of the family, the changing role of women is pivotal to shifting family life-cycle patterns. Women are seeking to establish personal life goals, making career choices, establishing two-career marriages, having children later, and having fewer children or no children at all. Not surprisingly, women have difficulty establishing concurrent functions outside of the family and experience special life-cycle stresses as they are expected to bear emotional responsibility for all family relationships. Although the role of women in altering the family life cycle is significant, recognition must be given to the strain that vastly accelerated change puts on families, whether the changes themselves are enhancements or detriments (Carter & McGoldrick, 1988).

Life change, as a multidimensional concept, has been implicated in the social etiology of life stress, with the number and magnitude of life change events serving as a measure of stress. It is generally assumed that the greater life change an individual experiences, the more the individual must adapt. Although it has been hypothesized that stress is a major determinant of well-being, empirical research findings indicate that stressful events may have a limited impact on well-being, even when viewed from a longitudinal perspective (Murrell, Norris, & Grote, 1988). Thus, researchers argue that those models that explore the direct effects of stress on well-being are inadequate and that the role of social psychological resources in the stress process must be considered (Barerra, 1988). One of the most frequently examined coping resources is social support. Although the evidence is not conclusive, there is general consensus that the negative effects of life stress are reduced for persons with strong social support systems (Krause, 1990). The concept of social support has emerged as a major variable in health-related research, but there is lack of conceptual agreement on the definition of social support from study to study and how it functions to buffer the effects of stress or to protect health (Ryan & Austin, 1989). The purpose of this chapter is to explore the concept of social support as a health status variable, to consider the implications of social support for the traditional nuclear family and newer family forms, and to propose nursing interventions to improve the quality of social support for families.

THE CONCEPT OF SOCIAL SUPPORT

One of the most important distinctions to be made concerning social support is the difference between the number of relationships a person has and the person's perception of the supportive value of social interactions. The former is the social network, and the latter is perceived social support. Because the terms are frequently used interchangeably, further clarification is indicated.

A *social network* may be defined as the set of relationships of a particular individual or a set of linkages among a set of persons. Structurally, networks include size, density, accessibility, kinship-reliance, stability, and frequency of contact. (Hall & Wellman, 1985). Although the size or extent of the social network may be an indication of the degree of social support available, it is questionable to assume that benefits are directly proportional to the size of the network or that having a relationship is equivalent to getting support. These factors merit consideration when multiple social connections are used or when a single social connection, such as being married or having a confidant, is used. It is likely that a positive association exists between social network size and amount of social support. However, the prob-

lems generated from important social relationships contribute significantly to the degree of stress people experience in their lives. Therefore, consideration of the quality of the social relationship is important in addition to consideration of the availability or extent of the social network (Ryan & Austin, 1989).

Social support focuses on the nature of the interactions taking place within social relationships as these are evaluated by the individual. Perceived social support involves an evaluation of whether a pattern of interactions is helpful and to what extent. Distinguishing between social networks and social support is important because these concepts may have differing effects on the health status of the individual and considerable implications for research and clinical practice. Social support, as perceived by the individual, may be more strongly associated with health outcomes because it is a more direct indication of the support actually afforded a person, whereas the demands and constraints of network membership may dilute the beneficial effects (Schaefer et al., 1981).

Social support can have a variety of components, each serving a variety of supportive functions. Schaefer et al. (1981) identified the emotional, tangible, and informational functions separately. *Emotional* support includes intimacy, ability to confide in one another, and a sense of attachment contributing to a feeling that one is cared about or that one is a member of the group. *Tangible* support involves direct aid or services, including providing money or goods, providing a caretaking function, or performing a service. *Informational* support includes providing advice or information to assist in problem solving and giving feedback concerning an individual's progress. Thoits (1982) identified social support as the degree to which a person's basic social needs (affection, esteem, approval, belonging, identity, and security) are gratified through interaction with others. The functional aspects of social support include both socioemotional and instrumental aid. Another conceptualization of social support, based on Weiss's theory of the provisions of relationships (1974), identified five dimensions of support: intimacy, social integration, worth, nurturance, aid, and assistance (Weinert, 1987). These varying definitions are indicative of the conceptual and methodological issues that have emerged in researching the concept of social support. These issues have included inadequate conceptualization, lack of recognition of the multidimensionality of the concept, and the proliferation of measurement strategies. Ryan & Austin (1989) suggest that it is difficult to integrate the results of research on social support due to these issues. However, increased awareness of the complexity of the phenomena is apparent as researchers attempt to develop hypotheses derived from theory, and to explore both quantitative and qualitative approaches to capturing the nuances of social support.

SOCIAL SUPPORT, STRESS, AND WELL-BEING

The concept of social support has emerged as a major variable in health-related research. Much of the research has explored the concept of social support in relation to caregiving, social isolation, and stressful life events such as illness and death (Baillie, Norbeck, & Barnes, 1988; Chappell & Badger, 1989; McHaffie, 1992; Sankar, 1991). In view of the hypothesis that social support fosters better adaptation to stressful life events, some studies have explored the dimension of physical health while others have focused on psychological well-being, using both objective measures and subjective indicators.

The exact nature of the role of social support in mediating stressful life events is the subject of continuing research. Krause (1986) summarizes the buffering hypothesis in discussing social support, stress, and well-being among older adults. Proponents of this hypothesis maintain that social support reduces the impact of stress by giving greater clarity to the situation and by facilitating the development and implementation of a sensible plan of action for dealing with the problem. In addition, social support may also reinforce the individual's positive self-concept and provide assurance that although the situation is difficult, it can be tolerated, and successful outcomes may follow the plan of action.

Barrera (1988) describes stress buffering as any condition that decreases the overall positive relationship between stressful life events and psychological distress. He suggests that two distinct models might be described as illustrating stress buffering effects. In the first model, there is a positive relationship between life stress and social support that could reflect the mobilization of social support in response to life's stressors. This model further proposes that social support serves to mitigate adverse reactions to precipitating stressors. The second model portrays social support as interacting with stress, but support is not independently related to either stress or outcome variables such as physical health or psychological disorder. In the second model, there is no relationship between the occurrence of life stress and the mobilization of support hypothesized.

In attempting to determine the current status of the stress buffer model, Barrera (1988) states that there has been some evidence for the stress moderating influence of social support, but study results are contradictory. Cohen and Wills (1985) conducted an extensive literature review of stress buffering and found inconsistent support for the model. Based on their findings, Barrera (1988) suggests that there is a need to reconsider the

assumptions of the Stress Buffer Model and to specify more exactly the conditions under which it can be observed. In reappraising the model, he identifies the following issues that merit consideration: (1) buffering effects are apparent for only certain types of social support, (2) buffering effects occur when social support matches the needs presented by life event stressors, and (3) buffering effects conform to a curvilinear rather than a linear model. He proposes that there is a need to explore alternative models to explain the relationship between social support, stressful life events, and psychological distress. Further, there is a need to move beyond cross-sectional studies to more longitudinal studies to explore changes inherent in the recovery from life stress and the changing needs that emerge. Finally, Barrera (1988) notes that there is a paucity of studies that address the ways in which social support contributes to the occurrence of positive events, influences their appraisal, or is mobilized due to positive life experiences.

With these caveats in mind, clinicians must view the implications of social support realistically in planning care for clients and recognize both the value and limitations of current research efforts.

SOCIAL TRENDS AND EMERGING FAMILY FORMS

Within the past generation, family life-cycle patterns have changed dramatically, causing some to emphasize the breakdown in traditional values and behaviors and to view with alarm the decline and decay of the traditional family. Traditional families, consisting of a husband who is considered head of the household and responsible for family support and the wife who is responsible for child care and home care and their children, have had social, legal, and religious sanction. Bahr (1988) challenges the notion of family deterioration and indicates that the available evidence from this century and even from earlier times does not support a decline in family vitality, strength, solidarity, or positive influence in people's lives. He suggests that the traditional family of nostalgic memory never existed, except perhaps in a tiny segment of the population—the moneyed leisure class—and even then, historical evidence does not reveal the values, behaviors, and personal qualities associated with the traditional family. The view of the traditional family as a safe solidarity of kinship, caring, responsibility, and love is not readily supported. In reality, Bahr (1988) suggests that traditional structures were intolerant, intractable structures that produced a tragic loss of human potential—structures that stifled human creativity, opportunity, and growth. With recognition of the pain that still mars family relationships, Bahr maintains that today's families are not only viable, but stronger, more resilient, and more rewarding units in which to live than families of the past.

Nevertheless, the American family is changing and may be best characterized by horizontal movement rather than decline. There is a major shift in the proportion of families of various types, a shift of a magnitude sufficient to indicate the necessity of a thoughtful examination of the implications for the societal structure. Traditional families are a smaller proportion of American families, with families consisting of the male breadwinner and female homemaker composing a minority but still sizable component of family structures. Variant forms of family life now make a relatively large contribution to the mix of families and the increased importance of this diversity must be recognized and incorporated into the perception of American family life. These forms consist of two-earner families, single-parent families, childless families, and blended families. They may also consist of persons who live together without conventional marriage in heterosexual, gay, or lesbian relationships (Chilman, Nunnally, & Cox, 1988). Emerging family forms may include the presence of emancipated children and their offspring or elderly relatives who are unable to live independently. Thus the paradigm for middle-class American families is currently more or less mythological, relating in part to existing and emerging patterns and in part to the ideal standards of the past to which most families compare themselves.

Gender, Roles, and Family Structure

Many of the changes occurring in family forms can be viewed as adaptations to the changing images of women, their desires, and their resources. (Dornbusch & Strober, 1988). Women have always been central to the functioning of the family and their identities have been associated with the role of mother and wife, and their life-cycle phases linked to childrearing activities. A longer life expectancy means that women now have a time frame equal to that of the childrearing years to engage in other life options. Women have come to need and want a personal identity and have sought that identity through education, career, and other avenues of self-development. Technological advances have enabled women to plan their involvement in childrearing, but conflicting goals and multiple role demands continue to create considerable stress (Carter & McGoldrick, 1988).

A review of the research in gender roles and the family indicates that while more women are working outside of the home, they continue to do most of the domestic labor. Women also tend to modify their employment because of family constraints, although men usually do not. Women also engage in more kinkeeping and care of elderly relatives than do men. Not surprisingly, women face conflict between the traditional feminine roles of being nurturant, supportive, passive, and domestic as opposed to the expectation of achieving and being egalitarian (Caycedo, Wang, & Bahr, 1991). In addition to the demands of multiple roles, women continue to face occupational segregation and disparate earnings from their male counterparts, a situation that becomes increasingly complex for women who are single parents or heads of household (Strober, 1988).

Changes in family structure have also posed challenges and new life stressors for men. In discussing the role of men in families, especially fatherhood, Morgan (1990) notes that little attention has been given to the male role in family-centered research but that the situation is changing. He attributes a renewed interest in male roles to changes in patterns of employment and economic life, increasing divorce rates, and issues concerning custody of children. Changing patterns in employment have included shifts from heavy industrial work to lighter industrial, nonmanual and service occupations and the growing participation of women in the workforce. These changes affected the gender character of the workplace and further deteriorated the myth of the male breadwinner. The declining workforce participation of men due to male unemployment and, possibly, a growing disenchantment with the breadwinner role have provided another impetus. With increasing divorce rates (many petitions initiated by women), the position of men in the family has been undermined. In addition, custody of children frequently went to women, underlining the centrality of the mother's role and the marginality of the father's role. There is also some evidence to suggest that fathers suffer more from divorce, and the issue of lone fathers has begun to receive attention, although they are a minority of single-parent households. Thus attention has again shifted to the role of men in families, issues of masculinization, and sources of resistance to change.

Although men's attitudes have become more egalitarian, evidence of change in actual practice in crucial areas of child-care responsibility and domestic labor is difficult to come by. Morgan (1988) cautions that men have few motives to support change in their domestic roles and have the physical and economic power to resist such changes. Even in those situations where attitudes support change, the practical realities may limit options. While new styles of masculinity are developing in exploring the themes of tenderness, softness, and nurturing, they may lack substance and are occurring in a domestic context which has changed little. There are also factors which support change, however, including the altered work environment, the view of work as a less salient factor in identity, and the experiences and attitudes of women who are able to exert considerable influence in the family structure as well as in the social policy arena. Clearly, domestic and family life have been more resistant to change in gender relations than have some areas of employment and the public sphere.

Implications for Social Support

The continued existence of traditional family structures and the emergence of variant family forms have implications for social networks and social support for family members. In traditional families, specific roles and functions are prescribed. Therefore, the structure may be in place for developing social networks and orchestrating social support. In addition, the present social, legal, and religious structures tend to respond with a greater degree of significance to traditional families in need. Therefore, the potential may exist for eliciting social support if these social structures favor the family form and lifestyle. However, such assumptions may not always be warranted. In contrast, nontraditional families may find that some forms of social networking and sources of social support are not available to them. For example, the single parent frequently lacks the option of participating fully in school, church, or social functions due to time constraints. An elderly person lacking a spouse, children, or other significant relationships may be isolated from any significant support systems and may lack the ability to mobilize effective substitutes using existing sources. A single male, caring for aging parents, may find little support in the workplace or through existing social and health policy. A view of the continuum of family lifestyles is essential to understanding their needs, their methods for enhancing the quality of their lives and relationships, and their potential for accessing social support when confronted with life stress.

SOCIAL NETWORKS AND SOCIAL SUPPORT IN FAMILIES

The influence of the social network and of social support in mediating the effects of family stress has emerged as a major domain in family-centered research in the last decade, reflecting similar lines of inquiry and limitations as previously described concerning health-related research and social support. In addition to defining the concept and categorizing the types of social support, family-centered research has focused on what types of social networks offer support to the family in times of stress, in what ways, and for what types of stressor events.

Support Networks

The major social support networks that provide support to individuals and families include neighborhoods, family, kinship, and self-help groups. Studies of these networks indicate that they usually provide a great deal of support, which has a positive effect on stress reduction. However, the issue of accessibility is not usually addressed. In any case, there is a great deal of variability among special networks in both availability and ability to provide support. For example, Norbeck et al. (1991) found differences among the social support needs of family caregivers of psychiatric patients from the age groups. Caregivers of adult patients reported having the least support. Many support needs were expressed, but the needed support did not exist. In exploring the residential differences in the composition of helping networks of impaired elders, Coward et al. (1990) found that severely impaired elderly in nonmetropolitan communities were less apt than their urban counterparts to be receiving aid from a formal provider and are significantly more likely to be receiving assistance from informal helpers exclusively. Although these studies indicate the lack of availability of certain types of supports, Walls and Zarit (1991) substantiated the important role black churches play in enhancing the lives of elderly black individuals. Although family networks were considered more supportive than church networks, this study found that perceptions of support from the churches were associated with well-being. These and other studies indicate that there are differences in availability of networks, the kind of support they offer, and the degree to which families make use of them.

Family and Kinship Systems

In describing the characteristics of family and kinship systems when they are functioning as supportive mediators of stress, Caplan (1976) suggests that these systems act as (1) collectors and disseminators of information; (2) a feedback system; (3) sources of ideology; (4) guides and mediators in problem solving; (5) sources of practical aid and services; (6) a haven for rest and recuperation; (7) a control and reference group; (8) a source of identity; and (9) a contributor to emotional mastery. Research on the mediating effects of social support in reducing the family's vulnerability to stress has explored various facets of family life.

Stressful life events have been the subject of some studies that have explored expectations, sources, and availability of social support among family members. McHaffie (1992) found that parents with an infant in the neonatal intensive care unit expected emotional support from grandparents but there was a general feeling that they should stay in the background and become actively involved only if the parents requested. Types of support varied from visiting the baby to transport, caring for siblings, shopping, instilling a sense of hope, or simply showing that the infant and parents were a high priority.

Spousal relations have been the subject of some studies that explored social support and the spousal relationship. Living with a chronically ill spouse has a significant impact on family members, particularly those living with and caring for a homebound adult. DesRosier et al. (1992) found that women caring for husbands disabled with multiple sclerosis depended on their husband for support due to the social isolation of their caregiving responsibilities. They made personal space and time for themselves by setting apart a place in the home that was theirs or by declaring time out. These strategies help them to avoid or reduce the negative outcomes of the social support they received. In exploring the costs and benefits of social support in families, Robertson et al. (1991) found that external support can reduce the stress of individuals but it may also produce costs for the persons involved. This study substantiated that in families headed by a man with unstable work history, the wife's support from relatives and friends is associated with the husband's negativity toward the spouse.

Intergenerational support was the focus of a study conducted by Spitze and Logan (1990), who concluded that the key for older adults in receiving help is having at least one daughter, but there is no advantage to having additional children of either gender. Having daughters is most salient for phone contact, while frequency of visiting is affected by both gender and number of children. Matthews and Rosner (1988) noted that the presence of some siblings who did not help at all or helped only sporadically was associated with both the larger family size and the presence of male siblings. The effects of gender composition seem to reflect what is known about the differences in male-female helping behavior.

Attention has also been focused on working women who provide support to elderly family members. Brody and Schoonover (1986) noted that working women continued to provide various types of support to a dependent elderly relative and sought assistance only with those areas in which they were not available to provide support. Exploration of family and kinship systems in providing social support continues to be the subject of research efforts across all phases of the life span, with varying results regarding stress reduction. Results depend on the position of family members and the developed patterns or support and resources exchanged.

Mutual Self-Help Groups

Although self-help groups have existed for several decades, there has been a large expansion of both types and numbers of groups in recent years. Bumagin & Hirn (1990) identify these groups as consisting of diverse individuals who come together for a particular purpose, sometimes self-selected and other times imposed by external factors. The recent growth in self-help groups is attributed to a breakdown in traditional authority and institutions and to a need for services that may have been performed in the past by family, church, or neighborhood. Many hospitals and social service agencies often have groups that offer education and/or emotional support, while some groups have come into existence on their own, initiated by the needs of people in a given situation. Self-help groups have been formed to address multiple concerns of people, including addiction, crisis, life events, and medical conditions. Examples of such groups include Make Today Count, Parents Without Partners, Weight Watchers, Alcoholics Anonymous, Mended Hearts, Widow-to-Widow, and the Empty Candle.

Self-help groups may serve the purpose of information-sharing, emotional support, effecting behavioral change, or promoting personal growth. In addition to providing support for their members, these groups may also be action oriented and focus on changing attitudes or public opinion concerning their situation or on influencing public policy that affects their problem.

Most self-help groups function by providing information, a setting for mutual support, a reference group, and role models. The common rationale uniting professionally led groups and self-help groups is that people in similar situations can learn from and support each other (Bumagin & Hirn, 1990). Experiential knowledge is an important facet of this function, for it demonstrates that one is not alone in experiencing a problem but that others have been there and learned to cope. This approach may be used in conjunction with professional expertise, or it may be used as an alternative to standard professional care related to physical and/or mental health. George & Gwyther (1988) found that support group participation by caregivers of memory-impaired elderly had positive influences on caregivers' level of knowledge and perceptions of mutual support. They were unable to support a decrease in psychological distress.

Although self-help groups have proved beneficial for many people with various types of problems, they are not useful for everyone. For some American subcultures, discussing personal issues with a group of strangers is very difficult, creating an uncomfortable climate that is not helpful. Others find the group composition at such variance from their own background that they discontinue attendance. Additional barriers to involvement in these types of support groups may include transportation, timing of meetings, membership fees, and lack of care for dependent family members. Self-help groups are not a panacea for every type of personal or social problem, but they may be effective for those individuals who can benefit from the type of support offered and who can integrate the self-care philosophy into their personal regime for health and self-development.

APPROACHES TO ASSESSMENT OF SOCIAL SUPPORT

Prior to exploring the use of the concept of social support in clinical practice, it is essential to examine methods that would be most appropriate for assessing individual and family needs for support. The process of assessment can be facilitated through an understanding of the various components of social support, the implementation of informal techniques for gathering information, and the use of formal questionnaires.

Previous research has indicated that numerous approaches have been used to evaluate the concept of social support, indicating the diverse and multifaceted nature of the concept. One important facet of assessment of support appears to focus on its social context, the people who are actual or potential providers of support. This can be accomplished through the use of a variety of tools and techniques. For example, family members are often responsive to the use of a genogram, which is a diagram of the family's constellation that shows the structure of intergenerational relationships. A second tool that may be helpful in exploring social networks is the ecomap, which diagrams the family's contact with others outside of the immediate family and may include people, agencies, and institutions (Ross and Cobb, 1990).

Genogram

A genogram (Fig. 9–1) usually follows conventional geneologic charts and includes three generations or more if pertinent to the situation. Generational lines are indicated by horizontal rows, marital relationships by horizontal lines, and children by vertical lines. Children are rank-ordered from left to right, beginning with the eldest child. The names and the age of each individual, or the date of death if the person has died, are included in the symbol. Additional information pertinent to the health of each family member may be added as well as data concerning year of marriage, divorce, or adoption. This approach may be helpful in obtaining information about the family and its needs in a way that fosters involvement of all family members, but it may also evoke differing emotional responses from individuals as painful relationships or events are recalled. Therefore, the interviewer must be prepared to deal effectively with emotional responses that may be triggered by this process (Wright & Leahey, 1994).

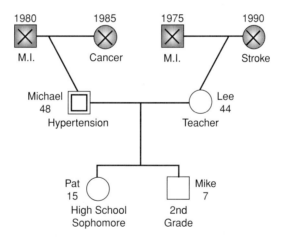

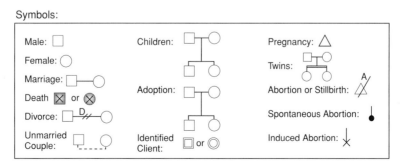

FIGURE 9–1. Family genogram.

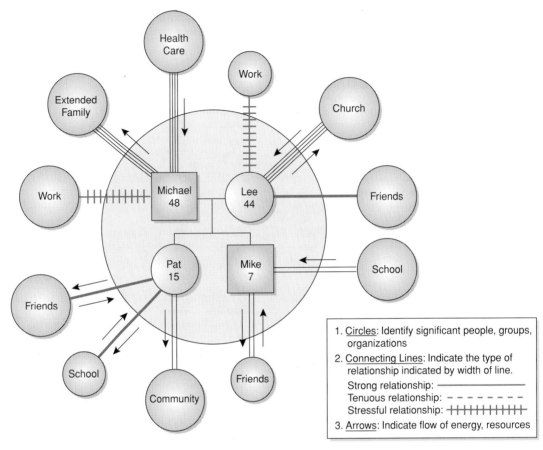

FIGURE 9–2. Family ecomap.

Ecomap

The ecomap (Fig. 9–2) provides an overview of family relationships to various persons, institutions, or agencies and pictures nurturant of stress-laden relationships. The family or household is placed in the center circle, and the outer circles represent significant relationships in the family members' lives. Lines between the inner and outer circles indicate the nature of the connection. Straight lines indicate strong connections, and dotted lines indicate tenuous connections. Slashed lines indicate stressful relationships. The strength of the relationship is indicated by the width of the line. Arrows may be added to indicate the flow of resources and energy.

Both the genogram and the ecomap are assessment tools that can be used in a variety of settings to determine how individuals are linked to significant people and how they might have opportunities to interact in ways that provide social support. As indicated earlier, the presence of potential sources of support is not necessarily an indication of support being either provided or received, nor is it an indication of accessibility (Hartman, 1978).

Indexes of Social Support

Formal methods for assessing support systems in terms of network analysis may include indexes such as the *Social Network Index* (Berkman & Syme, 1979). This tool includes information on marital status, number of close friends and relatives, frequency of contact, and membership in clubs and community organizations. The *Arizona Social Support Interview Schedule* includes measures of network size, support satisfaction, and support need (Barrera, 1981). These instruments may be useful in conducting research related to social networks or may be incorporated into family interviews or assessment guides.

In addition to network analysis, a second dimension of assessment of social support relates to the individual's subjective appraisal or relevant support dimensions. This may include happiness with key relationships, satisfaction with support, and adequency of social attachments. The *Norbeck Social Support Questionnaire* (Norbeck et al. 1983) asks respondents to identify significant persons in their lives, perceived support available, and important relationships lost. Schaefer et al.'s (1981) *Social Support Questionnaire* measures the emotional, tangible, and informational functions of social support by using a similar identification of persons involved in one's social network and a rating of each person on the identified functions. Weinert (1987) has developed a social support measure, the PRQ 85, which measures the adequacy of social support and also involves identification of the persons in the network.

A third facet of assessment of support involves specific behavioral activities that are involved in helping. This aspect involves what systems actually do, how they do it, and with what type of results. Although the tools identified above incorporate functions of social support, others such as the *Inventory of Socially Supportive Behaviors* (Barrera, 1981) address this aspect with increased attention to the type and frequency of assistance.

The assessment of social support involves an analysis of the social network to ascertain the actual and potential sources of social support available, an indication from the client regarding his or her perception of the support available from these sources, and the specific helping behaviors that would be of assistance to this family in this situation. Ryan & Austin (1989) maintain that a combination of both quantitative and qualitative approaches may best capture the nuances of social support. Several studies (Sankar, 1991; Norbeck et al., 1991, DesRosier et al., 1992) have used qualitative methods to explore the role of social support in the caregiving process with selected populations, which may further strengthen assessment strategies.

SOCIAL SUPPORT IN FAMILY HEALTH NURSING

Implementing the concept of social support in nursing care to families can be a complex and multifaceted undertaking because of the nature of the situations in which mobilization of support is indicated, the necessity of meshing formal and informal support networks, and the need for greater specificity in research concerning effective interventions and outcomes. Norbeck (1982) has identified several key assumptions to guide nurse clinicians in both assessing families and planning interventions:

1. People need supportive relationships with others throughout the life span to manage the role demands of day-to-day living, as well as to cope with life transitions and stressors that emerge.
2. Social support is given and received in the context of a network of relationships.
3. The relationships in the network have relative stability over time, especially those that compose the inner circle or primary ties for the individual.

4. Supportive relationships are basically healthy, not pathologic.
5. The type and amount of support needed is individually determined, based on individual differences and characteristics of the situation.
6. The type and amount of support that is available also is determined by characteristics of the individual and the situation.

Incorporating these assumptions into the nursing assessment is essential in order to gather relevant data regarding the actual and potential support available to the family and to develop realistic nursing interventions should the need be determined. Many interventions will relate to deficiencies in social support, and others may relate to personal or network deficiencies.

Nursing Interventions in Support Deficits

Deficits in social frequency arise from situational problems in which there is a loss of support due to death, divorce, separation, relocation, or other reasons. Although many situational problems are not health problems, they are frequently accompanied by stress-related illnesses that bring families into contact with nurses and other health care professionals in an initial attempt to organize formal sources of support. Providing direct emotional support may be an initial nursing intervention, but a more effective long-term approach may be to assist the family to assess its own needs for support and to use its own natural helping systems. Related nursing interventions include facilitating acknowledgment of the loss, recognizing the grieving process, and using appropriate timing for introduction of various types of support. Occasionally, both lay and professional persons fail to provide adequate support because they urge use of appropriate types of support at inappropriate times. For example, a newly divorced woman with a child may benefit from family emotional, financial, or child-care support initially, but she may also need to mobilize formal support services such as counseling, legal advice, and health care. She may eventually benefit from involvement in a self-help group for single parents. However, Bond & Wagner (1988) note that it is important to recognize that the needs of individuals and families may differ in regard to type of support needed depending on how far along they are in understanding and responding to the situation.

A second type of problem or deficiency occurs when the problem or event exceeds the capacity of the network to provide support. These events are usually situational in nature rather than developmental, and they are usually beyond the range of the collective experience of the network. For example, in dealing with catastrophic illness, such as a disabling stroke, it may be possible to identify a person in the network who, with professional assistance, may be able to provide support to the caregiving spouse. This may be an adult child, a sibling, or a close friend who can be assisted to provide emotional or tangible support if he or she knows what to expect during the process of rehabilitation and is aware of the adjustments that need to be made in living with chronic illness. Other options may include volunteer linking, or providing the opportunity for support from someone who has undergone a similar experience and thus can provide realistic guidance. A support group such as a stroke club may be useful to the couple at some point as well, particularly if participants share a common age, ethnic or religious affiliation, geographic location, or viewpoint about the nature and resolution of the problem (Bumagin & Hirn, 1990). If none of these avenues of support can be mobilized, it may be appropriate to continue to provide direct support or to arrange for other sources of formal or professional support.

A third type of social support deficit relates to difficulties that an individual may experience in establishing or maintaining a support network. An individual may lack the social skills necessary to maintain a social network or to increase a friendship network. Or, the individual may possess the social skills but lack the opportunity or finances due to family responsibilities or other reasons. Although social skill development or information on how to initiate contacts may be helpful in those situations where it is applicable, careful assessment of the situation is necessary to ascertain the real basis for the problem. In some cases, a support network may be available for a specific purpose that is not immediately apparent. For example, although it may appear that an older person has no immediate family and no access to transportation, closer evaluation may identify a network of neighbors who provide transportation, do daily checks, and shop for groceries. On the other hand, it may be readily apparent that an older woman who is providing care for a dependent spouse is homebound and lacks access to any type of socialization or assistance. After evaluation of the need, creative solutions can be developed through direct contact with potential sources of support. Environmental considerations may also be addressed, if and when this is possible. Some families may not have access to support because of locale, choice of neighborhood, or selection of housing. At times the decision of an older person to live with an adult child may totally isolate the older person from his or her peer group as well as other social contacts. A newly divorced individual may choose to move to a different city, eliminating all current support systems at a time when they may be badly needed, or a young couple may begin a family in a city in which they have no extended family to provide support. Sometimes these issues can be considered during the decision-making process so that benefits and negative factors can be explored. If the environmental situation cannot be changed, then alternative supports must be explored and mobilized as indicated.

Another type of deficit may relate to the network itself; relationships in the family may not always be healthy, or they may be more stressful than supportive. Examples include the existence of family violence or substance abuse in which a spouse or parent can be the source of a great deal of stress but also a source of support. Other problematic areas may include the existence of dependent relationships, overly solicitous concern, or continuous pressure to change behavior. Although some areas may require intervention by mental health professionals, other less destructive patterns may be amenable to nursing intervention. In some situations, family members can be encouraged to seek reciprocal relationships with peers outside the kin network. These friendship networks may provide the individual with needed support in order to cope with family stressors such as an aging parent, a child with behavioral problems, or an unemployed husband. In some cases, it may be necessary to decrease face-to-face contact with a family member who exerts highly negative attitudes of influence, particularly in times of high situational stress. Successful intervention is based on careful evaluation of the problem and mobilization of sources appropriate to the family and situation, using the combined efforts of family members and nurse clinicians.

Meshing Formal and Informal Supports

A major component of the professional nursing role in relation to social support concerns the mobilization of informal support systems. Because this is a frequently identified nursing intervention in many settings, it may be helpful to identify several approaches to working with informal helpers. As a professional, the nurse's philosophical orientation to practice may provide an overarching influence in relation to client care and the use of family members, friends, or volunteers to provide support. Bond & Wagner (1988) identify several factors that are useful in successful planning to prevent psychological and physical distress and to promote health. They include the importance of maintaining a multisystem, multilevel perspective; an emphasis on the promotion of competence; empowerment of individuals and groups; and sensitivity to the development process of individuals, families, and other systems. These factors can be operationalized by considering carefully the community and family context, by building on an individual's strengths, by seeing how people can help themselves or may be helped by others, by ensuring that people take responsibility for selecting the help they need, and by identifying ways for people who share problems to share solutions. Family health nurses must also recognize that informal supports can be mobilized into a partnership if recognition is given to the differences in the mode of operation between professionals and laypersons. The degree to which nurses as professionals believe that knowledge confers a superior status or authority may influence relationships with informal helpers. In some cases, such a stance may have a positive influence in the situation, and in others, it may be a serious deterrent to providing support. Taking too strong a position on any subject or alienating family members may close off access to sources of help or assistance.

Another essential component of the nursing role is to ascertain the helper's ability or readiness to take the responsibility for aiding another. For some, the role expectations may be very different from those previously encountered, and many adjustments will be necessary. In addition, family health nurses must be aware of changes in the informal helping network and be prepared to make adjustments accordingly. Changes occur in the ability of the informal helper to provide support because of life transitions, fatigue, illness, accumulated stress, and other factors. Mobilization of other sources of support may be necessary from formal and informal sources in a short period of time. Such a situation may occur when a family has been able to provide care to an elderly relative in their own home but may not be able to continue if the person begins to hallucinate, wander, or become incontinent. The ability to be knowledgeable of and combine the use of informal and formal support systems is difficult and challenging. However, due to unique relationships with families and involvement in a variety of settings, family health nurses may be in the best position to initiate successful partnerships between formal and informal support networks.

Social Support and Family Health Promotion

The family as a basic unit of health management is a critical determinant of the health status and practices of individual members. In proposing a Health Promotion Model, Pender (1987) identifies the importance of interpersonal variables on health-promoting behaviors, including the contributions of significant others, and on family patterns of health care. Significant others could be family members, confidants, or close friends who are capable of influencing another because of the close nature of their relationships. Many times these persons may share a common household, workplace, or recreational activity, which serves to strengthen the bond and provide more opportunities for interaction as well as for integration of health-promoting behaviors. Although family patterns of health care influence family members'

beliefs, values, and attitudes about health behaviors, other systems or persons influence family members to modify specific health practices or make lifestyle changes. See the Family Health Promotion Model in Chapter 2. Unit III covers content related to family nutrition, exercise, recreation, stress management, sleep, and adjustment to family transitions, which all are improved by social support.

Peer groups, teachers, counselors, and the media may also have a profound effect on the health practices of individuals, altering the influence of the family situation in a positive or a negative manner. Interaction with health professionals is another variable that may encourage diet modification, adoption of a specific exercise program, or alteration of lifestyle. Family members and significant others are important interpersonal variables in the development of health behaviors, and they are significant components of the social network. As such, they have the potential to be influential sources of social support in developing and maintaining healthful lifestyles.

Although family members and significant others may influence health behaviors and act as sources of social support, the question remains concerning what type of support under what circumstances will enhance the health and well-being of individuals and families. Research on the health protective benefits of social support has resulted in inconsistent findings and is not readily transferable to clinical practice. This is due in part to the differing conceptualizations of social support from study to study and the reliance on subjective measures of health. Anderson & Tomlinson (1992) note that the concept of health reflects differing paradigmatic influences as well as differing degrees of specificity, centrality, and reductionism. Both within and outside the discipline of nursing, the construct of family health suffers from even greater definitional confusion. Thus objective measurement is complex and elusive. Minimal research exists about understanding family process in relation to health promotion, preventing illness, or recovering from illness. However, two general strategies concerning social support and family health promotion may be helpful to consider.

The first strategy focuses on improving the supportive quality of network contacts. This strategy is based on the landmark work of Cassel (1974), who hypothesized a connection between deficiency of people's primary group ties and increased vulnerability to disease. He suggested that families and groups at risk be identified by their lack of fit with the social milieu and that the nature and form of social supports be determined and strengthened to protect these groups from disease outcomes. Family health nurses can implement this strategy in many different ways in a variety of settings. For example, developing educational programs in parenting that enhance parent-child communication and include childrearing practices that foster self-esteem can lead to enhancement of family ties, decreased stress, and a supportive atmosphere for health-promoting lifestyles. Middle-aged persons caring for aging parents can be taught methods of providing support that permit elders to maintain independence and control over their own lives as long as possible, thus decreasing the situational stress involved on both sides. Either of these approaches could be particularly helpful to persons who are distant from immediate family members or whose role demands lessen social support opportunities.

A second general preventive strategy concerns providing people with access to meaningful social ties. In order for this strategy to be successful, opportunities must be available that maximize the expression of social support. Family health nurses can implement this strategy and foster health promotion by encouraging clients to seek information and support from qualified professionals, peers, self-help groups, and educational programs appropriate to their health needs. A support group may be helpful to assist persons to stop smoking, adjust dietary habits, or participate in an exercise program. Nurses can also facilitate the formation of support groups within the context of their practice to meet the needs of particular families who may be experiencing life transitions or other stressors. Family health nurses can provide information and explore alternatives prospectively with families in life circumstances that herald the approach of certain types of life events, such as caring for a disabled member, raising a grandchild following parental separation, or coping with chronic illness. For example, based on the results of a qualitative study, Kendall (1992) notes that support groups can be very helpful for persons with HIV. She recommends such groups be focused on human connections and believes that the groups can be used to help members reformulate meaning in their lives despite the possibility of death in the future. Since many HIV-infected individuals may be isolated from family and other sources of support, such a group may be of assistance to promote wellness or quality of life.

Because the social environment is capable of radiating both support and stress and because individuals differ in their receptivity toward the skillfulness in using social support, the implementation of these strategies presupposes a comprehensive network analysis and consideration of cultural determinants. The major strategies of improving access to social support and increasing the quality of available social support may be conducive to encouraging positive health behaviors in families and promoting lifestyles that enhance their well-being both in the present and across future generations.

Implications for Nursing Research

Because family health nurses are involved in both direct and indirect clinical roles, multiple opportunities exist to define more clearly the concept of social support in relation to nursing practice. The family health system is emerging as a paradigmatic view for nursing, and Anderson & Tomlinson (1992) have proposed a classification that can be used to organize knowledge generation. The ultimate goal is the development of theory-driven interventions derived from conceptualizations about the future of family health. Kane (1988) indicates that empirical investigations of social support available to families is hampered by the lack of a theoretical basis. She proposes a conceptual model that presents family social support as a process of relationships between the family and its social environment. Both of these efforts are useful in addressing problems

CHAPTER HIGHLIGHTS

A family may have different types and qualities of social support within the family or in other social relationships; however, the family's or individuals' perceptions of the value of the beneficial effects of the social support determine the outcome.

The types of social support include emotional, tangible, and informational support.

The evidence to support relationship of social support as a buffer for stressful life events and psychological distress is inconsistently reported in the literature.

In some families the quality of interactions and network influences health status and involvement in health promotion activities.

Assessment of social support can be facilitated by a diagram of the family constellation that shows intergenerational relationships and by a diagram of the family's contact with people, agencies, and institutions outside the family.

Social support deficits occur as a result of (1) loss of support, (2) when the problem exceeds the capacity of the network to provide support, (3) difficulty in establishing or maintaining a social support network, and (4) dysfunctional relationships.

The major family health nursing role is to assess a family's social support and to assist the family to identify and mobilize informal and formal support systems within the family and the community.

related to the inadequate conceptualization of family health and social support. Barrera (1988) states that there is a necessity to explore other models beyond the Stress Buffer Model of social support to examine the effects of alternate coping resources and those variables which provide linkages between social support, stress, and distress. He also recommends further longitudinal studies to explore changes in the process of recovery from life stress and the changing needs of persons involved, as well as the relationship between positive life events and social support. Ryan & Austin (1989) note that nurse researchers are making considerable progress in developing instrumentation, hypothesis testing, and expanding theories. However, future research directions could include the exploration of problematic social ties, the timing of social support, the effectiveness of certain types of support under specifc circumstances (health, illness), and the availability and effectiveness of social support interventions. Consideration should also be given to exploring the concept with differing cultural groups and variant family forms. Although some attention has been given to family-centered research, issues of recruitment, measurement, and retention of multiple subjects provide considerable challenges (Moriarity, 1990). As family health nurses research these areas in relation to their own areas of practice, greater specificity regarding appropriate interventions and expected outcomes will be possible.

REFERENCES

Anderson, K.H., & Tomlinson, P.S. (1992). The family health system as an emerging paradigmatic view for nursing. *Image: Journal of Nursing Scholarship,* 24(1), 57–63.

Bahr, H.M. (1988). Family change and the myth of the traditional family. In L. Bond and M. Wagner (Eds.), *Families in Transition: Primary Prevention Programs That Work* (pp. 13–30). Newbury Park, CA: Sage.

Baillie, V., Norbeck, J., & Barnes, L. (1988). Stress, social support and psychological distress of family caregivers of the elderly. *Nursing Research,* 37(4), 217–222.

Barrerra, M. (1981). Social support in the adjustment of pregnant adolescents: Assessment issues. In B.H. Gottlieb (Ed.), *Social Networks and Social Support* (pp. 69–96). Beverly Hills: Sage Publications.

Barrera, M. (1988). Models of social support and life stress: Beyond the buffering hypothesis. In L. Cohen, (Ed.), *Life Events and Psychological Functioning: Theoretical and Methodological Issues* (pp. 211–236). Beverly Hills: Sage Publications.

Berkman, L.F., & Syme, S.L. (1979). Social networks, host resistance and mortality: A nine year follow-up study of Alameda County residents. *American Journal of Epidemiology,* 109, 186–204.

Bond, L.A., & Wagner, B.A. (1988). *Primary Prevention Programs That Work.* Newbury Park, CA: Sage Publications.

Brody, E., & Schoonover, C.B. (1986). Patterns of parent-care when adult daughters work and when they do not. *The Gerontologist,* 26(4), 372–381.

Bumagin, V.E., & Hirn, K.F. (1990). *Helping the Aging Family: A Guide for Professionals.* New York: Springer.

Caplan, G. (1976). The family as a support system. In G. Caplan & M. Killilea (Eds.), *Support Systems and Mutual Help: Multidisciplinary Exploration* (pp. 19–36). New York: Grune & Stratton.

Carter, B., & McGoldrick, M. (1988). *The Changing Family Life Cycle: A Framework for Family Therapy.* New York: Gardner Press.

Cassel, J. (1974). Psychosocial processes and "stress": Theoretical formulations. *International Journal of Health Services,* 4, 471–482.

Caycedo, J.C., Wang, G., & Bahr, S.J. (1991). In S.J. Bahr (Ed.), *Family Research: A Sixty-Year Review, 1930–1990.* New York: Lexington Books.

Chappell, N.L., & Badger, M. (1989). Social isolation and well-being. *Journal of Gerontology: Social Sciences,* 44(5), S169–S175.

Chilman, C.S., Nunnally, E.W., & Cox, F.M. (Eds.). (1988). *Variant Family Forms.* Beverly Hills: Sage Publications.

Cohen, S., & Wills, T.A. (1985). Stress, social support, and the buffering hypothesis. *Psychological Bulletin,* 98, 310–337.

Coward, R.T., Cutler, S.J., & Mullens, R.A. (1990). Residential differences in the composition of the helping networks of impaired elders. *Family Relations,* 39(1), 44–50.

DesRosier, M.B., Cantanzaro, M., & Piller, J. (1992). Living with chronic illness: Social support and the well spouse perspective. *Rehabilitation Nursing,* 17(2), 87–90.

Dornbusch, S.M., & Strober, M.H. (1988). *Feminism, Children and the New Families.* New York: Guilford Press.

George, L.K., & Gwyther, L.P. (1988). Support groups for caregivers of memory-impaired elderly: Easing caregiver burden. In L. Bond and B. Wagner (Eds.), *Families in Transition: Primary Prevention Programs That Work.* Newbury Park, CA: Sage.

Hall, A., & Wellman, B. (1985). Social networks and social support. In S. Cohen and S.L. Syme (Eds.), *Social Support and Health* (pp. 23–41). New York: Academic Press.

Hartman, A. (1978). Diagrammatic assessment of family relationships. *Social Casework,* 59, 465–476.

Kane, C.F. (1988). Family social support: Toward a conceptual model. *Advances in Nursing Science,* 10(2), 18–25.

Kendall, J. (1992). Promoting wellness in HIV support groups. *Journal of the Association of Nurses in AIDS Care,* 3(1), 28–38.

Krause, N. (1990). Stress, support and well-being in later life: Focusing on salient social roles. In M. Stephens, J.H. Crowther, S. Hobfoll, and D. Tennenbaum, (Eds.), *Stress and Coping in Later Life Families* (pp. 71–97). New York: Hemisphere Publishing.

Krause, N. (1986). Social support, stress and well-being among older adults. *Journal of Gerontology,* 41(4), 512–519.

Matthews, S.H., & Rosner, T.T. (1988). Shared filial responsibility: The family as the primary caregiver. *Journal of Marriage and the Family,* 50, 185–196.

McHaffie, H.E. (1992). Social support in the neonatal intensive care unit. *Journal of Advanced Nursing, 17,* 279–287.

Morgan, D.H. (1990). Issues of critical sociological theory. In J. Sprey (Ed.), *Fashioning Family Theory.* Newbury Park, CA: Sage.

Moriarity, H. (1990). Key issues in the family research process: Strategies for nurse researchers. *Advances in Nursing Science,* 12(3): 1–14.

Murrell, S., Norris, F., & Grote, C. (1988). Life events in older adults. In L. Cohen (Ed.), *Life Events and Psychological Functioning: Theoretical and Methodological Issues* (pp. 96–122). Beverly Hills: Sage Publications.

Norbeck, J.S. (1982). The clinical use of social support. *Journal of Psychosocial Nursing and Mental Health Services,* 20(12), 22–29.

Norbeck, J.L., Chaftez, L., Skodol-Wilson, H., & Weiss, S.J. (1991). Social support needs of family caregivers of psychiatric patients from three groups. *Nursing Research,* 40(4), 208–212.

Norbeck, J.L., Lindsey, A.M., & Carrieri, V.L. (1983). Further development of an instrument to measure social support: Normative data and validity testing. *Nursing Research,* 32(1), 4–9.

Pender, N. (1987). *Health Promotion in Nursing Practice.* Norwalk, CT: Appleton-Century-Crofts.

Robertson, E.B., Elder, G.H., & Skinner, M.L. (1991). The costs and benefits of social support in families. *Journal of Marriage and the Family,* 5, 403–416.

Ross, B., & Cobb, K.L. (1990). *Family Nursing: A Nursing Process Approach.* Redwood City, CA: Addison-Wesley.

Ryan, M., & Austin, A.G. (1989). Social supports and social networks in the aged. *Image: Journal of Nursing Scholarship,* 21(3), 176–180.

Sankar, A. (1991). Ritual and dying: A cultural analysis of social support for caregivers. *The Gerontologist,* 31(1), 43–50.

Schaefer, C., Coyne, J.C., & Lazurus, R.S. (1981). The health-related functions of social support. *Journal of Behavioral Medicine,* 4(4), 381–405.

Spitze, G., & Logan, J. (1990). Sons, daughters and intergenerational support. *Journal of Marriage and the Family,* 52(2), 420–430.

Strober, M.H. (1988). Two-earner families. In M. Dornbusch & M.H. Strober (Eds.), *Feminism, Children and the New Families.* New York: Guilford Press.

Thoits, P.A. (1982). Conceptual, methodological and theoretical problems in studying social support as a buffer against life stress. *Journal of Health and Behavior,* 23(6), 145–159.

Walls, C.T., & Zarit, S.H. (1991). Informal support from black churches and the well-being of elderly blacks. *The Gerontologist,* 31(4), 490–495.

Weinert, C. (1987). A social support measure: PRQ 85. *Nursing Research,* 36(5), 273–277.

Weiss, R.S. (1974). The provisions of relationships. In Z. Rubin (Ed.), *Doing Unto Others* (pp. 17–26). Englewood Cliffs, NJ: Prentice-Hall.

Wright, L., & Leahey, L. (1994). *Nurses and Families.* (2nd ed.). Philadelphia: F.A. Davis.

FAMILY STRESS

10

PERRI J. BOMAR and SHERRY COOPER

Confront the diversity of your generation, learn to live with the diversity, and ultimately come to celebrate it.

DONALD KENNEDY

Family stress—inevitable but surmountable.

DOLORES CURRAN

OBJECTIVES

On completion of this chapter, the reader will be able to:
1. Differentiate between physiological, psychological, social, and family stress
2. Describe the differences between crisis and stress
3. List the major developmental stressors of families across the life cycle
4. Identify theoretical models of family stress
5. Recognize symptoms of stress in families
6. Describe methods to assess family stress
7. Use knowledge of theoretical frameworks of family stress when intervening with families in stress

INTRODUCTION

In the 1980s and early 1990s, as the result of complex and dynamic societal, political, and cultural forces, families as a unit experienced more stress than families of previous eras. Researchers report that dynamic changes in families, such as changes in the roles of women, changing family lifestyles and forms, economic pressures, and occupational expectations, have a profound impact on quality of family life and the level of stress. It is expected that many of the family stressors of this decade will also continue well into the year 2000 (Olson & Hanson, 1990). As families are viewed from a systems perspective, it is crucial for nurses to be cognizant of family stress as they adapt to the predictable and unpredictable changes that families and family members experience across the life span (Boss, 1988; McCubbin, 1993; McCubbin & McCubbin, 1987).

This chapter will begin by defining individual stress as differentiated from family stress. Next,

the differences between crisis and stress will be discussed, followed by a review of the current theoretical models of family stress. Then the major developmental stressors of families and symptoms of family stress will be highlighted. In the last section, assessment of family stress and use of the theoretical frameworks of family stress in nursing practice will be discussed.

DEFINING STRESS

Definitions of family stress theory evolved from physiologic and psychological stress theory.

Physiologic Stress

The research of Cannon (1929) and Selye (1976) documented the physiologic impact of actual or perceived stress on the body. Selye defined *stress* as "the nonspecific response of the body to any demand, whether it is caused by or results in unpleasant conditions" (Selye, 1976, p. 51). Agents that cause the conditions of stress are called *stressors*. Stress can be differentiated in terms of negative or positive stimuli or good or bad stress. Negative or harmful stimuli are called *distress* and may result from actual or perceived threats to the body. One example might be illness or cognitive processes such as worry or fear. Pleasant or good stimuli, such as marriage or birth of a baby, are called *eustress,* or good stress (Selye, 1974, p. 74). Both distress and eustress cause nonspecific responses in the body. However, the effects of eustress cause less damage. Both eustress and distress initiate the "fight or flight" response in the body. This response includes activation of the sympathetic nervous system (vasoconstriction of blood vessels, elevated blood pressure, increased heart rate, and increased secretion of adrenaline). Prolonged stress has been shown to cause many illnesses such as ulcers, high blood pressure, and frequent infections (Selye, 1976; Brown, 1984). Selye emphasized that stress is unavoidable. However, the effects on the body can be minimized by eliminating stressors and altering one's response to stressors. Psychological stress theory explains the relationship of emotion to physiologic stress.

Psychological Stress

Lazarus (1966) explored psychological stress and stated that perceptions and cognitive processes are also stressors. The manner in which an individual copes depends on the intensity of the threat, type of personality, specific culture, locus of control, and beliefs about the stressor. Although Lazarus noted differences between physiologic, psychological, and social stress, he emphasized that the physical responses of the body are the same. Both cognitive processes and physical stress initiate the fight or flight response in the body. According to Phares (1976), the manner in which persons cope with stress depends on whether they perceive control of their environment to be within themselves (internal locus of control) or from factors beyond their control (external locus of control).

Social Stress

Social stress results from the actual or perceived threats in one's social environment, such as relationships at work, conflicts at school, or interactions within society. Examples include racism and prejudice, economic recessions, evaluations of performance at work or school, conflict with neighbors, and environmental noise (Melson, 1983). Families of different cultures may experience cultural stress from conflict with values, rituals, beliefs, customs, and lifestyle patterns (Hardy, 1993). This is particularly evident in families who anticipate migration and later immigrate to a different country or relocate to another state or neighborhood (Janosik & Green, 1992).

Family Stress

Building on Selye's (1974, 1976) physiologic model of stress and Lazarus's psychological definition, McCubbin and Patterson (1983b) defined *family stressors* as "a life event or occurrence in or impacting upon the family unit which produces change in the family social system" (p. 88). This occurrence is described as more than day-to-day changes in the family. It refers to events or transitions that require changes in family boundaries, roles, patterns, and values. Another term salient to understanding family stress is *family hardships,* which are the demands on the family unit specifically as a result of the stressor. *Family stress* "(as distinct from stressor) is defined as a state which arises from actual or perceived demand-capacity imbalance in the family's functioning and which is characterized by a nonspecific demand for adaptive behavior" (McCubbin & Patterson, 1983b, p. 88). Boss (1987) offers another definition and states that family stress is "an upset in the steady state of the family . . . anything that . . . causes uneasiness or exerts pressure on the family system" (p. 695). Like individual responses to stress, the family's responses depend on the stressor, the previous ability to handle hardships, the characteristics of the family, and the emotional and physical health of its members. Family *distress* is experienced when stress is perceived as unpleasant. An example of distress would be illness of a family member, a family argument, or unemployment of the major breadwinner. Family *eustress* is experienced when events are perceived as pleasant. A crucial element determining whether or not the event or threat is stressful is family perception. For example, a family gathering may be perceived as pleasant by one family and unpleasant by another. Family *strain* is pressure on family functioning as the result of an accumulation of stressors over time. If strains persist, the outcome is often crisis or collapse for the family (Boss, 1987).

Stress produces instability within the family system. Stressor events only have the potential of causing stress or change (Boss, 1988; McCubbin, McCubbin & Thompson, 1993). Whether stress is actually experienced depends on the meaning of the event, the family's perception, the availability of resources, and the context. Family stressors originate from multiple sources (Boss, 1988; Neuman, 1982) shown in Table 10–1. Family stress is a complex phenomenon that is influenced by numerous stressors and sources. Normative stressors that often produce family stress are events such as

TABLE 10–1. CLASSIFICATION OF FAMILY STRESSOR EVENTS

INTERNAL
Events begin within the family, such as illness of a family member or major changes in family routine.

EXTERNAL
Events that occur outside the family, such as the economy, war, or legislative policies

NORMATIVE
Developmental changes that most families experience, such as marriage, birth, holidays, graduations, aging, and death.

NONNORMATIVE
Unexpected events, such as untimely deaths, disasters of nature, war, and being laid off from a job.

AMBIGUOUS
Difficult to obtain facts about the event. One is unclear about what is happening to the family.

NONAMBIGUOUS
Clear facts obtainable about the event.

VOLITIONAL
Events that are wanted and sought out, such as a purchase of a new home, a planned pregnancy, or attending college.

NONVOLITIONAL
Events that are not sought out but just happen, such as unplanned pregnancy, or unexpected job loss.

CHRONIC
A situation of long duration such as racial discrimination, family member with Alzheimer's disease or hypertension.

ACUTE
An event that lasts a short time but is severe, such as a family member requiring major surgery or failure of a major goal.

CUMULATIVE
Events that pile up, one right after another, before the family is able to make adjustments or adaptations.

ISOLATED
An event that occurs alone when no other events seem apparent.

Data from Boss, P. (1989). *Family Stress Management* (p. 40). Newbury Park, CA: Sage.

beginning parenthood, beginning of school for children, entering adolescence, launching adult children, and facing retirement. The predictable normative transitions of individual family members affect the family as an integrated whole. Examples of normative maturational transitions are infancy to toddlerhood, school age to adolescence, graduation from high school, grandparenthood, menstruation, and the climacteric. Any maturational crisis or transition that one family member experiences affects the family as a unit. As family members progress along the life span from infancy to old age, the family as a social system may experience stress because it is an interdependent, interacting social unit. The family system as a unit simultaneously experiences stress and strains as it adapts to stressors from multiple sources.

The impact of some transitions may be minor, while others may require considerable adaptation. For example, the birth of a baby necessitates adjusting to an additional person to relate to, spending time required for child-care tasks, having time for self and as a couple, and coping with the additional financial expenditures. In addition, each parent is experiencing conflict related to clarification of spouse-parent-person roles, career development, maintenance of the home, and so on. All changes, whether normal expected life-cycle developmental changes or catastrophic events, have the potential to cause strain or hard-

ship on the family as a unit. Although many stressors may be minor and require minimal adjustments in the family, others may require considerable adaptation. For example, natural disasters, environmental changes, and nonvolitional stressors often are not within the control of the family, yet considerable family adaptation is needed.

Family stress as the result of fire (external and nonnormative stressor), serious auto accident (acute and nonnormative stressor), accidental death (nonnormative stressor), or job termination (nonvolitional stressor) requires use of multiple resources to help the family cope with the considerable changes. The decision to begin the care of an elderly parent with Alzheimer's disease in the home would require numerous adjustments and compromises in the family and marital system. Such adjustments might include less personal and couple time, more expenses resulting from another person in the home, role change conflicts, and frustrations and fear regarding progression of the disorder.

Family stress is experienced as the family attempts to adjust, reorganize, consolidate, adapt, and establish new patterns of behaviors. Transitions of individuals and families are the major cause of stress in families (Janosik & Green, 1992). As families attempt to incorporate the normative transitions of its members and the life-cycle changes of the family unit, change is often needed in role structure and relationships. In addition to adapting to changes within the family unit, the family must adapt to changes and stressors in the community and society.

Sources of stress may evolve from either within the family system or within the social system. Examples of stress that originate within the family system would be the birth of an infant, toilet training of a toddler, illness of a family member, starting a new job, and completing or beginning school. Examples of external family stressors are such events or situations as requirements of a job or school, social pressures, conflict with neighbors, and racism or prejudice.

The severity of stressors varies. Some are easy to remove and others are difficult to resolve. For example, a cold or the flu is easy to resolve and is an acute transitory stressor; whereas spousal violence, alcoholism, and chronic illnesses are chronic, difficult to resolve and are long term.

CRISIS AND STRESS

The terms "crisis" and "stress" are not interchangeable. Stress precedes crisis. When stress is unresolved or inadequate, coping strategies are used, and when there is lack of resources or inappropriate resources, stress progresses into crisis. Crisis is often abrupt and sudden. However, stress is always present at some level and progresses to crisis when the family does not have the necessary resources to adapt. Stressors such as a fire in the home or sudden death may quickly progress into crisis if the family often does not have adequate resources to cope effectively. In crisis, customary approaches to problem solving or coping are not effective. As a result, disorganization and emotional turmoil are experienced. When family can no longer cope, it exhibits the following characteristics: (1) nonperformance of roles, (2) nonmaintenance of structural boundaries, and (3) immobilization of the system (Boss, 1987, p. 700). The distinct difference between stress and crisis can be seen in Table 10–2. When the crisis is resolved, the level of family functioning will return to one of three levels: below the precrisis

level, at the precrisis level, or above the precrisis level (Boss, 1987).

THEORETICAL FRAMEWORKS OF FAMILY STRESS

There are a number of models that explain the dynamic and complex phenomenon of family stress. Most evolve from Hill's (1949) ABCX Model of family crisis (See Figure 10–1), which is as follows:

A (the stressor event)—interacting with B (the family's crisis meeting resources)—interacting with C (the definition the family makes of the event)—produces X (the crisis).

Other models are the Double ABCX Model (McCubbin & Patterson, 1983a, 1983b); the Contextual Model of Family Stress (Boss, 1987), the Typology Model of Family Adjustment and Adaptation (McCubbin & McCubbin, 1987), and The Resiliency Model of Family Stress, Adjustment, and Adaptation Model (McCubbin & McCubbin, 1993). The models are based on family research and add to the development of a theoretical framework for family stress.

The Double ABCX Model was developed by McCubbin and Patterson (1983b) from studies of families experiencing war-induced crises. The Double ABCX Model reflects the cumulative effects of stressors and builds on Hill's crisis model by including four additional post-crisis variables that seem to infect family adaptations. These post-crisis variables are as follows: (1) a pileup of additional stressors, (2) family use of existing and new resources, (3) family changes in perception of the crisis event, and (4) the results of family coping strategies influencing adaptation (McCubbin & Patterson, 1983a,b).

Further research by McCubbin and McCubbin (1987) resulted in the T-Double ABCX Model of Family Adjustment and Adaptation. Their research illuminates additional variables that determine whether the family will make the necessary adjustments to a stressor, including the variable of family type. The three family types noted were

TABLE 10–2. DIFFERENCES BETWEEN CRISIS AND STRESS

	CRISIS	STRESS
Time	Short term (limited)	Long term
	Categorical (present or not present)	Continuous (low or high levels)
	Dependent on stress	Independent of crisis
Equilibrium	Acutely disturbed	Moderately disturbed
Coping	Coping not effective	Coping maintains equilibrium
Family Functioning	Immobilized and disorganized	Continues with adjustments

Data from Boss, P. G. (1987). Family stress. In M. Sussman & S. Steinmetz (Eds.), *Handbook on Marriage and the Family* (pp. 701–702). New York: Plenum.

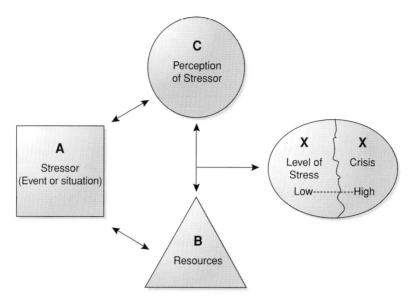

FIGURE 10–1. Hill's (1949) ABCX Model of Family Stress.

regenerative, resilient, and rhythmic. Family strengths identified include rituals, celebrations, routines, traditions, and so on.

Summarizing her Contextual Model of Family Stress, Boss (1987) stated that the meaning the family gives to an event is the most crucial factor determining whether or not the family will experience stress. She emphasized that families do not live in a vacuum. In this model, a family's stress is influenced by two contexts: internal (over which the family has control) and external (over which the family has no control). Internal contexts are the structural, sociologic, and philosophic influences. External contexts include the environmental setting (economics, politics, and culture) and the family world (heredity, culture, spirituality, and development). McCubbin, McCubbin, and Thompson (1993) substantiate Boss's claim. From their research, they noted that families tend to have a *family schema,* which appears to be the most significant factor that influences how families adjust and adapt to stressors. Family variables included in the schema are shared family values, goals, priorities, expectations, and world view. The perception is not just the group perception but a shared meaning that is influenced by individual and gender differences.

Although it is beyond the scope of this chapter to discuss each model in depth, a brief discussion of the major concepts in the models will follow. The concepts to be discussed include family adaptation and adjustment, pileup, family vulnerability, family type, family resources, family perception, family schema, and problem solving.

The Resiliency Model of Family Stress, Adjustment, and Adaptation

The Resiliency Model of Family Stress, Adjustment, and Adaptation (McCubbin & McCubbin, 1993) is the outcome of further research with families. Their findings suggest additional important variables of *family schema* and *family resilience* in conceptualizing family stress.

According to McCubbin & McCubbin (1993), families respond to life events and life transitions in two phases (Fig. 10–2). Change in families is constant, resulting from individual family member experiences or family unit changes. The adjustment phase involves the minimal transitory changes the family unit makes in its routine patterns and processes in response to an event or transition that does not pose a hardship (such as changing jobs, moving to a new residence, or minor illness of a member). The adaptation phase is a much longer phase. It begins when the family's attempts to make minimal adjustments are no longer effective and result in a crisis. Both the adjustment and adaptation phases are discussed in the following section; letters in parentheses refer to Figures 10–1 and 10–2.

Adjustment Phase

In the *adjustment phase* of the Resiliency Model (see Fig. 10–2), the family makes minor, short-term adjustments in family patterns and processes to accommodate the stressor. The family will manage the stressor with relative ease (*bonadjustment*) or poor adjustment (*maladjust-*

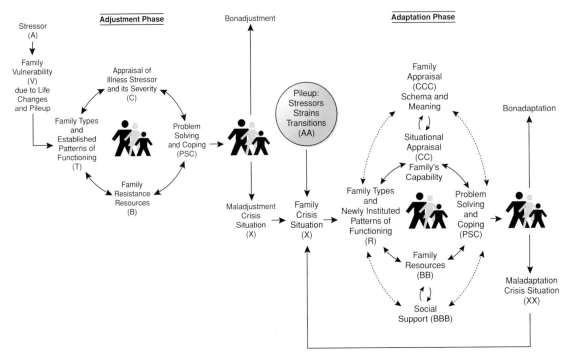

FIGURE 10–2. The Resiliency Model of Family Stress, Adjustment, and Adaptation. (From Danielson, C.B., Hamil-Bissel, B., & Winsted-Fry, P. (1983). *Family Health and Illness* (p. 23). *1993.* St. Louis: Mosby-Year Book.)

ment) to the stressor. If the stressor results in major changes in the family, such as a significant decrease in finances, they experience a crisis (maladjustment) and progress to the second stage in the model (McCubbin, 1993).

FAMILY STRESSOR (A). The family stressor (actual or perceived threat) may be from external or internal sources. External sources may be jobs, school, the neighborhood, extended family relationships, and so forth. Other stressors include family unit or member normative transitions that are common life events such as births, marriage, graduation, and retirement. Nonnormative stressors are events that are unique or rarely occur in families. The severity of the stressor interacting with ongoing family demands threatens the family equilibrium and resources.

FAMILY VULNERABILITY (V). Family "vulnerability is the fragile interpersonal and organizational conditions of the family system" (McCubbin, 1993, p. 28). This is the simultaneous accumulation or "pileup" of ongoing family demands such as finances, developmental changes of members, and family lifestyle that occur at the same time as the new event or transition. If the family has too many demands, they are more vulnerable to stress (McCubbin & McCubbin, 1987).

FAMILY TYPE (T). Family types, based on the Circumplex Model (Olson, et al., 1983b) discussed in Chapter 4, refers to a definitive set of family characteristics and patterns of family functioning in relationship with other family variables. The

suggested use of the typology is to explain and predict family responses and level of adaptation. According to McCubbin & McCubbin (1987), the typology emphasizes different aspects of family functioning in four family types that influence the adaptation process. The four family types are regenerative, resilient, rhythmic, and ritualistic.

The first is the *regenerative* family type, emphasizing family hardiness (i.e., internal strengths, control, internal meaningfulness of life, being challenged by life) and family coherence (i.e., emphasis on acceptance, loyalty, pride, trust, caring) as key factors in a family's ability to adapt to stress. The greater the family's hardiness and coherence the greater the ease with which a family will be able to adapt to crises (McCubbin, 1993). The second typology is *resilient* family patterns. The dimensions in this group are family bonding (i.e., feeling close to each family member, being open to discussing family problems, and doing things as a unit) and family flexibility (i.e., open communication and ease in changing rules, boundaries, and roles). The third family system type is the *rhythmic* model, composed of the dimensions of family time and routines and the valuing of family time and routines. The emphasis is on family togetherness and predictability in family lifestyle pattern. Rhythmic families highly value family time and routine and have a high degree of togetherness and predictability. The fourth type is the *traditionalistic* model, derived by evaluating the dimensions of family traditions and celebrations. Families who adapt more readily to stress would tend to value routines, rituals, and family bonding.

The more cohesive and adaptable the family is, the better it is able to cope with stress. In addition, good communication is a key factor in all aspects of family functioning (Curran, 1985; Galvin & Brommel, 1986).

FAMILY RESISTANCE RESOURCES (B). Family resistance resources are the collective strengths a family uses to cope. They reflect the family's abilities to address and make adjustments to meet the demands of stressors without causing a crisis in the family functioning (McCubbin & McCubbin, 1987). These resources are found within individual family members or the family unit, and include such things as family finances, personality traits, problem-solving skills, reframing, role sharing, religious beliefs, negotiation, flexibility, routines, celebrations, and communication (Curran, 1983; Olson et al. 1983a; McCubbin et al. 1987). If a family has the sufficient quality and quantity of family resources, and other variables are appropriate, a crisis can be avoided.

FAMILY APPRAISAL OF THE STRESSOR (C). Family appraisal or the meaning or perception the family gives to an event, significantly determines how the family responds to a stressor. The appraisal influences the strategies the family uses to adjust to that stressor (Boss, 1987; McCubbin & McCubbin, 1987; McCubbin & Patterson, 1983a,b; Patterson & Garwick, 1992). Some families choose to redefine or reframe the stress. For example, one family may view an acute illness as temporary and as a challenge to overcome, while another may define it as a catastrophe. Generally, when a family views a stressful situation as a "challenge" or a "growth experience," they have redefined it. Positive redefining includes (1) clarifying the issues, hardships, and tasks to render them more manageable; (2) decreasing the intensity of the emotional burdens associated with the crisis situation; and (3) encouraging the family unit to carry on with its fundamental tasks of promoting members' social and emotional development (McCubbin & Patterson, 1983b, p. 97). The unique perceptions of individual family members shape the resulting family appraisal.

FAMILY PROBLEM SOLVING AND COPING (PSC). Family problem solving and coping is the component of adjustment that includes the family's decisions and actions to relieve stress. According to McCubbin (1993), PSC is the family's efforts to organize their response into manageable steps, such as the realm of interpersonal issues and communication about how to solve the problem. Coping gears the family's cognitive, emotional, and behavioral responses toward restoring balance and relieving the family strain created by a stressor.

FAMILY BONADJUSTMENT, MALADJUSTMENT, AND CRISES (X). Stressors vary in the strain they make on a family system's balance. The extent of the hardship depends on the family type and strengths, internal and external support, perception and meaning, and coping and problem solving. When a stressor causes minor changes in the family and the adjustment to the stressor occurs with relative ease, the family experiences a positive adjustment (bonadjustment). When the family does not have adequate resources or strengths to make the needed changes, negative coping (maladjustment) and a state of crisis will occur.

The experience of family crisis requires changes in the family's established patterns of functioning (McCubbin & McCubbin, 1993). When an acute illness progresses to a chronic condition the family may be in state of crisis. For example, after the initial diagnosis of AIDS a family begins to cope with the long-term issues of a chronic disease. A family experiences maladjustment when it is unable to solve the myriad of issues related to incorporating the care of the chronically ill member into the family routine. Family crisis occurs when the family system lacks the personal and family resources, skills, and strengths to cope with the chronic illness over time. After the crisis is experienced, the family begins the adaptation process to resolve the crisis.

Adaptation Phase

The second phase in the Resiliency Model is the *adaptation phase* (see Fig. 10–2), which can be measured by the APGAR, a short questionnaire developed by Smilkstein (1978), or by the Family Maladaptation Index, created by McCubbin & Thompson (1990). The adaptation phase encompasses the family's actions during the time it takes to recover from a crisis situation (McCubbin & McCubbin, 1993). The family's goal at this time is to restore order and normalcy to family life. Adaptation "is used to describe the *outcome* of family efforts to bring about a new level of balance, harmony, coherence, and functioning to a family-crisis situation" (McCubbin & McCubbin 1993, p. 35). In this post-crisis phase, the outcome is influenced by a number of interacting components. Family pileup (the new stressor combined with existing family strains) interacts with family resiliency (determined by the family's ability to recover quickly by such activities reorganizing roles, routines, and spending). The family's resilience is supported by family and community resources, which interact with family appraisal (changes in meaning and renegotiating of goals and priorities), problem solving, and coping strategies (McCubbin & McCubbin, 1993). The end result of the adaptation is the achievement of either positive outcomes (bonadaptation) for individual members and the family unit or inadequate adaptation (maladaptation) within family unit and with the community. Maladaptation of the family unit results in disintegration of the family functioning, and the family experiences crisis again. A brief description of each aspect of the adaptation phase follows.

PILEUP (AA) OF DEMANDS. Families are seldom dealing with one simple stressor, but rather with numerous stressors that cumulate over time. Contributing to this piling up of stressors are the demand of the new stressor, combined with existing family strains and transitions (both individual family member transitions and family unit transitions), family efforts to cope, and inadequate resources. There are six categories of stresses and strains that pile up in families as they adapt to crises (McCubbin & Patterson, 1983; McCubbin & McCubbin, 1993, p. 37):

- The crisis/illness and related hardships over time
- Normative transitions in individual family members and the family as a whole
- Prior family strains accumulated over time
- Situational demands and contextual difficulties
- The consequences of family efforts to cope
- Intrafamily and social ambiguity that provides inadequate guidelines on how families should act or cope effectively with crisis and its hardships

For example, the diagnosis of an illness may be the initial stressor. Normative transitions may include such family adjustments as additional hardships to family finances; changes in family living arrangements, resulting in additional time needed for household tasks; and feelings of ambiguity about the multiple role of family members as caregivers combined with preexisting roles.

FAMILY TYPE AND PATTERNS OF FUNCTIONING (R). The family type and family patterns of functioning determines the strength of the family in adapting to stress over time (Lavec & Olson, 1991; Olson et al., 1983; McCubbin & McCubbin, 1993). The family who has a shared routine is flexible, yet bonded, and will be more resilient during periods of extreme stress. Over time, families develop new patterns of functioning to incorporate the crisis into their family life. The family's usual pattern of functioning (family type) interacts with new patterns of functioning (resiliency) and significantly influences the manner in which the family will adapt to the crisis or ongoing stressor.

FAMILY RESOURCES (BB)—STRENGTHS AND CAPABILITIES. Family resources reflect the family's potential to cope with the demands of the crisis. The strengths and capabilities are the combination of each family member's knowledge and skills, the skills of the family as a unit, and the resources of their external systems (extended family, social and medical systems). Family resources may be limitless and include such variables as communication, organization, role sharing, problem solving, affirmation of members, sense of family unity, and family hardiness. Other variables may include

family routines, rituals, and resilience. The variety, depth, and personal strengths of individual members, and the coherence, hardiness, adaptability, skills, and knowledge of the family unit, are significant factors in enhancing a family's adaptation to crises.

SOCIAL SUPPORT (BBB). Social support encompasses the external resources that the family uses to cope with the stressor. Resources may be such things as schools, churches, extended family, formal and informal support groups, employers, and social and government agencies (McCubbin, Cable & Patterson, 1992). McCubbin (1993) states that the greater the family's social support in "breadth, depth, and efficacy and the greater the quality of affirming social support the more likely the family will be able to adapt to a crisis situation" (pp. 48–49).

FAMILY APPRAISAL—SITUATIONAL (CC) AND SCHEMA AND MEANING (CCC). McCubbin and McCubbin's (1993) research has revealed that in addition to defining or giving meaning to stressors, there are two other levels of family appraisal: situational appraisal and schema and meaning. *Situational appraisal* is the family's attempt to examine family strengths and potentials in relationship to the demands caused by the crisis or pileup of stressors. This appraisal determines whether the family perceive that they have ability to manage the stressor crisis, as well as the resulting changes needed to solve the problem.

Crisis precipitates the need for the family to change the rules, organization, and patterns of family functioning. The family is impelled to explore the meaning of the illness and the resultant family changes in this stage. The *family schema* is the dynamic family's shared meaning, beliefs, values, goals, priorities, expectations, and world view McCubbin & McCubbin, 1987).

Separate from determining the meaning of an event is the consensus on family boundaries. According to Boss (1988), families may experience boundary ambiguity; that is, determining who is emotionally and physically present or absent in the family. The more cohesive, congruent, and positive the family's appraisal, the more affective they are at adapting to the crisis (McCubbin & McCubbin, 1987; McCubbin, 1993). The family's appraisal and schema are crucial variables in the outcome of their adaptation (Boss, 1988; McCubbin, 1993). The greater the congruency in family meaning of the event, the greater the ease with which they are able to adapt to the stressor (Patterson & Garwick, 1992).

FAMILY PROBLEM SOLVING AND COPING (PSC). The process that the family uses to cooperatively mobilize its resources is called problem solving. The problem-solving process interacts with the family's ability to manage a stressor. Coping is the process of securing the different resources, skills, and knowledge needed to cope with the continuing stress and its hardships. The goal of the coping process is to restore the family unit's balance while removing or reducing the stressor and its accompanying hardships through problem solving. (See Chap. 14 for a discussion of family coping.)

THE FAMILY ADAPTATION PROCESS—BONADAPTATION, MALADAPTATION, AND CRISIS (XX). The family adaptation process is on a continuum from bonadaptation to maladaptation (see Fig. 10–2). This process involves the family's unity and compromise in problem solving to manage the crisis. Interaction with external systems also enhances bonadaptation. The greater the family's strengths in coherence, flexibility, and the previously discussed variables, the greater the likelihood they will be able to adapt to the crisis. When families do not have adequate resources, family strengths, and the ability to rebound from a crisis event or situation, they will experience maladaptation. Examples of maladaptation are divorce, separation, family violence, alcoholism, or extreme family dysfunction. The outcome of maladaptation is crisis. The process of adaptation begins again with this new crisis combined with ongoing family stress.

SYMPTOMS OF FAMILY STRESS

Families as a unit often exhibit noticeable symptoms of stress and strain. Symptoms can be observed in individual family members and/or in the family as a whole. Family symptoms might be marital discord; changes in the family rules, rituals, and chores; roller-coaster–like emotional climate; changes in togetherness and cohesion; increased family communication; changes in family decision making and leadership; and increased contention (Burr et al., 1994). Negative coping behaviors and symptoms of family stress in individual family members include increased smoking; alcohol abuse; abuse of coffee, aspirin, and medications; overeating; frequent and recurring illness such as colds or sore throats; accident and injury proneness; and symptoms of anxiety and frustration. Infants and children may have recurring illnesses and be extremely irritable or exhibit acting-out behaviors. Older children may develop problems with school work, manifest behavior problems in school, and skip school. Often family processes and interactions are strained and may include marital conflict, sibling conflict, yelling, shouting, mean talk, sarcasm, swearing, moping, faultfinding, criticism, rigidity, and selfishness, and in extreme cases, family violence and divorce (Brown, 1984).

Curran (1985) noted that families who are under stress often experience the following:

- A constant sense of urgency and hurry; no time to release and relax
- A tension that underlies and causes sharp words, sibling fighting, misunderstandings

- A mania to escape—to one's room, car, or garage
- A feeling that time is passing too quickly; children are growing up too quickly
- A nagging desire for a simpler life; constant talk about times that were or will be simpler
- Little "me" or couple time
- A pervasive sense of guilt for not being or doing everything to or for all people in one's life (p. 13)

Although many families might experience a number of these symptoms at times, distress results when a family lives with all of them continuously. According to Burr et al. (1994), the experience of change and stress in families affects family functioning in five different patterns: a roller-coaster pattern, an increase in the quality and strength of functioning, no change in functioning, a decrease in functioning, and a mixture of these.

FAMILY LIFE-CYCLE STRESSORS AND STRAINS

The family's natural history or life cycle serves as a framework for observing the family experience and accompanying stressors and crises. Inevitable changes occur in families during its history. The occurrences of births, deaths, leaving the nest, and getting married may be perceived as a crisis or stress by families as they are required to make adaptation to life transitions.

In a study of 1,000 families, Olson et al. (1983a) noted that the ten most frequently reported stressors were intrafamily strains, financial strains, work-family strains, illness, marital strains, pregnancy, family transitions, and losses. The intensity of these strains varied with the family stage of development.

Factors such as chronic illness or a family member with a handicap influence family health across the life span. For example, M.A. McCubbin (1993) noted in her research of the stressors of families with handicapped children that the family experienced life-cycle strains in addition to specific strains related to the child's condition. Specific strains and stressors for single and dual parents of handicapped children included intrafamily strains due to the challenge of parenting teenage children; an increased number of tasks and chores that do not get done; financial strains from increased medical/dental care, food, clothing, energy, and housing; and illness and family care strains related to the illness of a child in the family or the death or illness of a parent or close relative.

Burr et al. (1994), in a study of 50 families from Utah experiencing family stressors, noted that nine family realms changed during the stressful period: marital satisfaction, family rituals and celebrations, quality of communication, family cohesion, functional quality of the executive sub-system, quality of the emotional atmosphere, management of daily routines and chores, contention, and normal family development versus changed or arrested development (p. 5).

Although the family life cycle is divided into stages, the progression from one stage to another is gradual rather than abrupt. The following section presents a discussion of common stressors occurring during the eight family life-cycle stages.

Stage 1

The first stage of the family life cycle is the *beginning family,* which starts when the adult leaves his or her family of origin to begin the process of forming a new family. Critical goals of family functioning during this phase is the establishing of a satisfying marriage, relating to the kin network, and family planning (Duval & Miller, 1985; Carter & McGoldrick, 1988).

Families without children experience conflict due to work-family strains, finances, and intrafamily strains. Research by Olson et al. (1983a) revealed that work-family and financial strains accounted for 70 percent of new couples' stressors and strains. An uncertain and unstable economic climate, such as that in the 1990s, results in a strong competitive factor in the labor force, which causes stress to families in this stage. According to Glick (1989), these couples experience a conflict between a desire for children and the desire for personal and material rewards from employment. Other stressors include the anticipatory strain of raising children during dynamic social and economic conditions.

Stage 2

This *early childbearing* stage begins with the birth of the first child. Stress occurs as the couple works to establish a stable family unit, reconcile conflicts, and facilitate the developmental needs of all its members. Olson et al. (1983a) reported that couples with young children experienced higher conflict in the areas of (1) work-family strains, (2) financial and business strains, (3) intrafamily strains, and (4) illness and family "care" strains (Smith & Hanrahan, 1995). Work-family strains are often related to parents changing careers or jobs, promotion or increased responsibilities, job stress, increased conflict with coworkers, and multiple role responsibilities (Kalil et al., 1993). Financial struggles included taking out loans to cover expenses, purchasing a car or other major item, medical and dental expenses, and access to and cost of safe and convenient child care (Voling & Belsky, 1993). Specific intrafamily strains reported were increased husband/father time away from the family and an increase in tasks

or chores that don't get done. An additional strain was caring for a close friend or relative who was seriously ill (Olson et al., 1983a, p. 124).

During the early childbearing stage couples often fail to nurture their marriage. According to Cowan and Hetherington (1991), the transition to parenthood may cause a strain on the marital relationship that amplifies differences between spouses and increases marital dissatisfaction.

Stage 3

Families during the *preschool stage* appear to struggle with a unique set of stressors and strains. The parents' perceptions of stress is a crucial variable in their response to the toddler's increasing autonomy and development of a sense of self. Parents are confronted with the negativism of toddlers and the need to negotiate often. During this stage, parenting hassles are a normative source of stress.

The availability and cost of child care continues to be a problem that causes role conflict between childrearing and employment for most couples with young children. According to McGovern et al. (1992), there has been a dramatic increase in the number of women with infants and toddlers who work outside the home. Women are reported to have higher levels of stress, fatigue, and assume more of the family chores and responsibilities than their mates, which creates additional family stress (Lee et al. 1994; Horschild, 1989). The complex, competing responsibilities of juggling time between work and family, incorporating new members into the family, integration of work and family life, and understanding and adjusting to the specific developmental needs and changes of early childhood are all sources of stress for the family during the preschool stage.

Stage 4

The *school-age years* represent a busy period, with families experiencing increased stress related to family unit pressures. Families with school-aged children have intrafamily strains, particularly from the increase of the children's "outside activities." Other intrafamily strains include an increase in the husband/father's time away from the family, an increase in sibling conflict, an increase in conflict with managing school-aged children, and an increase in the number of tasks and chores that do not get done. The cause of financial strain is often the same as in Stage 1 and 2 families. Last, work-family transitions and strains are experienced as the result of decreased job satisfaction and career changes (Olson et al., 1983a, pp. 125–126; Larson et al., 1994).

Since families usually reach their maximum number of members during this stage, an increase in the complexity of family roles and interrelationships can be expected. As a result, families in this stage are at risk for role strain as they attempt to meet multiple role demands. Multiple roles often cause a spillover of stress from work roles to the domain of the home. Guzelzow et al., (1991) noted that although dual-career couples experience stress related to both childrearing and career responsibilities, role strain is reduced when there is role sharing, flexibility in scheduling, and cognitive restructuring coping strategies.

Stage 5

When puberty begins the family progresses into Stage 5. During *adolescence,* perhaps more than any other stage, the family experiences biological and emotional upheaval (Janosik & Green, 1992) as the adolescent begins sexual maturation. Emotional tasks of the adolescent include identity formation and alienation, cognitive and moral development, and gradual separation from the family in preparation for leaving the family. Family emotional upheaval results as teenagers strive for independence, struggle with peer pressure, and accomplish developmental tasks needed to reach young adulthood. In some families, strain may occur due to the increased challenge of parenting teenagers, the increased amount of "outside activities" of children, higher financial expenditures, and household tasks not completed (Olsen et al. 1983). The accumulative effects of the intense developmental transitions of the adolescent combined with the family developmental tasks (i.e., maintaining family standards, nurturing the parents' marriage, developing new patterns of communication, reorganizing family power, rules, and roles) are the major sources of stress. Family life is often chaotic, requiring flexibility, while at the same time needing clearly delineated boundaries.

Stage 6

The beginning of Stage 6 of family life is distinguished by the *launching of young adults.* For middle-class families this may mean a considerable strain on the family's budget due to education costs, increasing expenses for necessities, and costs of major household items, while for poor families, the young adults may begin full-time work, but they do not make enough financially to be independent. During this stage there also tends to be an increase in the number of household tasks and chores that are not done. Another common cause of stress and strain is the transitional strain that occurs as young adults leave home for college or for work, then return for short periods of time. The serious illness of a close friend or family member may also contribute to stress and strain (Olson et al. 1983a).

The most common form of family fission takes place when a young adult leaves the parental household to establish an independent residence. A source of intrafamily conflict is the different beliefs and expectations about premarital cohabitation, which has increased over 200% in the past decade (Goldschneider & Goldschnieder, 1989).

This developmental stage may be further complicated by the need to provide for aging parents. Families are caught between the fluctuating demands of launching and rearing children and the requirements of aging parents. They may experience multiple pressures from the psychosocial problems of parental deterioration, role reversal, and the aging parents' need for emotional, financial, and physical support.

Stage 7

Families who are coping with the strain of young adults and children leaving home for college are in the *empty nest* or *middle years* stage and experience stress from a variety of sources. The critical developmental tasks of this family are to release young adults with appropriate assistance, maintain a home that is supportive when they return, and sustain kin ties with the younger and older family members. Olson et al. (1983a) noted that a major strain that parents experience is the loss of dependent children. Due to economic shifts in the 1990s, however, many young adults are returning to the "nest" or remaining longer (Glick, 1990).

Unless the marital dyad is recultivated and nourished, then accompanying the "nest-leaving" stage is the potential stressor of the disintegration of the marital relationship. Other struggles include financial strains, increased conflict with marital sexual relationships, decreased job/career satisfaction, and a serious illness or death of a close friend or family member (Olson et al., 1983a).

Stage 8

The period of *retirement and old age* (Stage 8) is accompanied by the need to adjust to the process of retirement; to cope with the aging process in oneself; and to cope with the illnesses of aging, caregiving to less healthy members, bereavement, and loneliness. The major stressors of families at this stage are finances as the result of reduced income; increased cost for health care and other necessities; and caregiving for ill and aging parents (Baum, 1991). Increased physical disabilities, combined with fewer family members in the home, result in the stress of increased responsibilities of household maintenance. Due to an increasingly mobile society and the trend to live independently, another major strain is the caregiving for ill and aging family members who live in different geographic areas. Intrafamily strains and the death of close family members or friends affect retired families significantly.

MOST FREQUENT FAMILY STRESSORS

In a survey of 450 men and women who were asked to indicate ten situations that created the most strain for their families, Curran (1985) reported the following stressors in order of priority:

1. Economic/finances/budgeting
2. Children's behavior/discipline/sibling fighting
3. Insufficient couple time
4. Lack of shared responsibility in the family
5. Communication with children
6. Insufficient "me" time
7. Guilt for not accomplishing more
8. Spousal relationship
9. Insufficient family playtime
10. Over scheduled family calendar (p. 20)

As previously discussed, all families will experience both eustress and distress. The family response to the event or situation will be significantly influenced by the variables identified in the models presented. The family nurse should be cognizant of the common stressors of families across the life span and families with variations of issues, which are discussed in the following section and in Chapter 20.

SPECIFIC STRESSORS

In addition to the stressors mentioned previously, there are the struggles that all families do not experience but that are common occurrences in the United States. Examples of circumstances that have unique and multiple stressors are divorce and remarriage (Crosbie-Burnett, 1989; Ihinger-Tallman & Pasley, 1987), dual-careers (Hochschild, 1989), co-parent families, single-parent families (Olson & Baynard, 1993), military families, clergy families, multigenerational families, and intracultural and interracial families (Olson & Hanson, 1990; Glick, 1990). Examples of family situations that cause specific stressors are racial and ethnic struggles (Dilworth-Anderson et al., 1993), migration and immigration (Janosik & Green, 1992), unemployment and poverty (Murata, 1995), homelessness, chronic illness (Danielson et al., 1993), psychiatric disorders, substance abuse, minority status, poverty in rural areas, changing economic status of farmers, and aging family members (Carter & McGoldrick, 1988; Crosbie-Burnett, 1989; Glick, 1989; & McCubbin & McCubbin, 1993). Chapter 20 includes more in-depth information about stressors in traditional and nontraditional families experiencing situational transitions.

ASSESSMENT OF FAMILY STRESS

A systematic approach to determining the presence of stress in a family is crucial. There are a number of reliable and valid assessment tools to measure family and individual stress (Table 10–3). Knowledge of the predictable, expected,

TABLE 10–3. SELECTED INDIVIDUAL AND FAMILY STRESS ASSESSMENT TOOLS

TOOL	DIMENSIONS MEASURED	SOURCE
Individual Stress Assessment Tools		
Life Change Index	Life events and changes	Holmes & Rahe (1967)
State-Trait Anxiety Inventory	General and current anxiety	Speilberger et al. (1983)
How You React to Stress	Physical and emotional symptoms of stress	McKay, Davis, & Fanning (1981)
Young Adult Family Inventory of Life Events and Changes (YA-FILES)*	Young adult life events and changes	McCubbin & Gronchowski (1987)
Adolescent Inventory of Family Life Events (A-File)*	Adolescent life events and changes	McCubbin & Patterson (1987)
Family Stress Assessment Tools		
Family Inventory of Life Events Pileup*	Family life events and changes	McCubbin & Patterson (1983) (FILE)
Family Stressors (FS)*	Family stressors	McCubbin & Patterson (1987)
Family Strains (FST)*	Family strains	McCubbin & Patterson (1987)
Family Distress Index*	Family distress	McCubbin & Patterson (1987)
Stress Kit	Pileup and coping strategies	Aid to Lutherans Association

*Most of these tools are in McCubbin, H. I., & Thompson, A. I. (Eds.). *Family Assessment Inventories for Research and Practice.* Madison, WI: The University of Wisconsin. For information write:
Family Stress Coping and Health Project
1300 Linden Drive
University of Wisconsin-Madison
Madison, WI 53706.

almost universal transitions in families can assist nurses working with families to develop coping strategies. As previously noted, family stress and strain are the result of continual dynamic changes that occur simultaneously in individuals, families, and society.

One of the most frequently used tools is the Holmes and Rahe Social Readjustment Rating Scale. This tool focuses on common stressors of individuals across the life span (Holmes & Rahe, 1967). Family scientists have noted that one family member's answers on the questionnaire are not descriptive of total family stress.

An instrument more descriptive of family stress is the Family Inventory of Life Events and Changes (FILE) that was developed by McCubbin et al. in 1987 (Fig. 10–3). It contains 71 items that reflect common normative and nonnormative life events that families often experience as a unit. It is used to record life events that a family has experienced during the last year. Both negative and positive events are included. The major concern is the amount of change that has occurred in the family during the past year. FILE can be used to determine families' stress levels and to indicate their potential risk for problems related to high levels of stress. Adult family members complete the form alone or together. The reliability is .81. The scale has nine subscales: (1) intrafamily strains and conflict, (2) marital strains, (3) pregnancy or childbearing strains, (4) finance and business strains, (5) work-family transitions and strains, (6) illness and family "care" strains, (7) losses, (8) transitions "in and out," and (9) family legal violations.

The family score for the FILE is determined as follows:

1. Adult family members complete one form together or two separate forms.
2. The respondents check yes or no if their family has experienced the strain or stressor listed on the questionnaire in the past year.
3. Total the number of yes answers assigned for each item on the questionnaire. If both adult family members complete a form, scoring is calculated by totaling the yes responses item by item. If either or both of the couple check yes for an item, the family-couple score would be considered as one yes and added to the total score.
4. If the family-couple completes one form, the family-score is calculated by totaling the number indicated for each item marked yes.

For information on scoring subscale scores, consult *Family Assessment Inventories for Research and Practice* by McCubbin and Thompson (1987, 1991). Families with high scores (over 750) and moderate scores (501–749) should be informed of the significance of their stress score and assisted to establish positive coping strategies such as those discussed in Chapter 14. In addition, it is crucial to assist them in recognizing support systems and resources. Scores of 0–100 are low and indicate minimal pileup.

Also, McCubbin and Thompson's (1987, 1991) manual contains a compilation of tools developed by family stress researchers. For example, the YA-FILES is an inventory created for the measurement of stressors in families with young adults (Grochowski & McCubbin, 1987). The family assessment measures are based on the T-Double ABCX Model of Family Adjustment and Adaptation. They measure family demands, vulnerability, family typologies, family resources, coping and problem solving, social and community support, schema and coherence, adjustment and adaptation, and stress, strain, and distress (McCubbin & Thompson, 1987, 1991). These measures are useful in assisting family nurses in determining family pileup, specific stressors, family strengths, bonding, flexibility, social support, and so forth.

Another useful tool to determine family stress is the *Stress Kit* produced by the Aid Association for Lutherans (1989), which is based on the Double ABCX Model. It contains an excellent card game called "PileUp," which is an innovative approach to assist a family to determine their stressors and strains. It can be used either by the family alone or by a family health nurse along with the entire family or with a group.

Family scientists continue research on family stress across the life span as it relates to the lifestyles of families as they strive toward higher levels of wellness. Family nurses are encouraged to contribute to the body of knowledge by identifying family stressors in their realm of nursing practice.

NURSING IMPLICATIONS

It is crucial for nurses to be cognizant of the profound impact of stress on the family system. Families often are not aware of the repercussions of stress on the family unit. Piling up of stressors affects family functioning and the quality of family life. Nurses often have opportunities to observe families and to anticipate or note signs of stress and strain in individual family members and within the family as a unit.

Major roles of the family nurse are to (1) recognize situations that predispose families to stress; (2) recognize symptoms of stress in the family and individual members; (3) assess individuals and family members for vulnerability, strengths, and levels of stress; (4) assist families to recognize the stressors and symptoms of stress in individual members and in the family as a unit; and (5) teach health-promoting and health protecting behaviors to enhance family adjustment and adaptation to stress.

FAMILY STRESS COPING AND HEALTH PROJECT
1300 Linden Drive
University of Wisconsin-Madison
Madison, WI 53706

Family Health Program
FORM C
1983
© H. McCubbin

ID 7 ☐ ☐ ☐ ☐
GID ☐ ☐ ☐
FID ☐ ☐ ☐ ☐

FILE

Family Inventory of Life Events and Changes

Hamilton I. McCubbin   Joan M. Patterson   Lance R. Wilson

PURPOSE

Over their life cycle, all families experience many changes as a result of normal growth and development of members and due to external circumstances. The following list of family life changes can happen in a family at any time. Because family members are connected to each other in some way, a life change for any one member affects all the other persons in the family to some degree.

> "FAMILY" means a group of two or more persons living together who are related by blood, marriage or adoption. This includes persons who live with you *and* to whom you have a long term commitment.

DIRECTIONS

"DID THE CHANGE HAPPEN IN YOUR FAMILY?"
Please read each family life change and decide whether it happened to any member of your family—**including you.**

- DURING THE LAST YEAR
  First, decide if it happened any time **during** the last 12 months and check
  YES or NO.

During Last 12 Months
Yes   No
☐   ☐

FAMILY LIFE CHANGES	DID THE CHANGE HAPPEN IN YOUR FAMILY?			FAMILY LIFE CHANGES	DID THE CHANGE HAPPEN IN YOUR FAMILY?		
	During Last 12 Months Yes	No	Score		**During** Last 12 Months Yes	No	Score
I. INTRA-FAMILY STRAINS				12. Increased difficulty in managing infant(s) (0-1 yr.) 35	☐	☐	
1. Increase of husband/father's time away from family 46	☐	☐ 12		13. Increase in the amount of "outside activities" which the child(ren) are involved in 25	☐	☐	
2. Increase of wife/mother's time away from family 51	☐	☐		14. Increased disagreement about a member's friends or activities 35	☐	☐	
3. A member appears to have emotional problems 58	☐	☐		15. Increase in the number of problems or issues which don't get resolved 45	☐	☐	
4. A member appears to depend on alcohol or drugs 66	☐	☐		16. Increase in the number of tasks or chores which don't get done 35	☐	☐	
5. Increase in conflict between husband and wife 53	☐	☐		17. Increased conflict with in-laws or relatives 40	☐	☐ 32	
6. Increase in arguments between parent(s) and child(ren) 45	☐	☐		**II. MARITAL STRAINS**			
7. Increase in conflict among children in the family 48	☐	☐		18. Spouse/parent was separated or divorced 79	☐	☐	
8. Increased difficulty in managing teenage child(ren) 55	☐	☐		19. Spouse/parent has an "affair" 68	☐	☐	
9. Increased difficulty in managing school age child(ren) (6-12 yrs.) 39	☐	☐		20. Increased difficulty in resolving issues with a "former" or separated spouse 47	☐	☐	
10. Increased difficulty in managing preschool age child(ren) (2½-6 yrs.) 36	☐	☐		21. Increased difficulty with sexual relationship between husband and wife 58	☐	☐ 34	
11. Increased difficulty in managing toddler(s) (1-2½ yrs.) 36	☐	☐					

Subtotal 1 _____

Please turn over and complete ◆
Subtotal 2 _____

Figure 10–3. Family inventory of life events and changes. (From McCubbin, H.I., & Thompson, A.K. (Eds.), (1987). *Family Assessment Inventories* (pp. 97–98) Madison, WI: University of Wisconsin. Reprinted with permission.)

FAMILY LIFE CHANGES	During Last 12 Months Yes	No	Score
III. PREGNANCY AND CHILDBEARING STRAINS			
22. Spouse had unwanted or difficult pregnancy 45	☐	☐	
23. An unmarried member became pregnant 65	☐	☐	
24. A member had an abortion 50	☐	☐	
25. A member gave birth to or adopted a child 50	☐	☐ 45	
IV. FINANCE AND BUSINESS STRAINS			
26. Took out a loan or refinanced a loan to cover increased expenses 29	☐	☐	
27. Went on welfare 55	☐	☐	
28. Change in conditions (economic, political, weather) which hurts the family business 41	☐	☐	
29. Change in Agriculture Market, Stock Market, or Land Values which hurts family investments and/or income 43	☐	☐	
30. A member started a new business 50	☐	☐	
31. Purchased or built a home 41	☐	☐	
32. A member purchased a car or other major item 19	☐	☐	
33. Increasing financial debts due to over-use of credit cards 31	☐	☐	
34. Increased strain on family "money" for medical/dental expenses 23	☐	☐	
35. Increased strain on family "money" for food, clothing, energy, home care 21	☐	☐	
36. Increased strain on family "money" for child(ren)'s education 22	☐	☐	
37. Delay in receiving child support or alimony payments 41	☐	☐ 63	
V. WORK-FAMILY TRANSITIONS AND STRAINS			
38. A member changed to a new job/career 40	☐	☐	
39. A member lost or quit a job 55	☐	☐	
40. A member retired from work 48	☐	☐	
41. A member started or returned to work 41	☐	☐	
42. A member stopped working for extended period (e.g., laid off, leave of absence, strike) 51	☐	☐	
43. Decrease in satisfaction with job/career 45	☐	☐	
44. A member had increased difficulty with people at work 32	☐	☐	
45. A member was promoted at work or given more responsibilities 40	☐	☐	
46. Family moved to a new home/apartment 43	☐	☐	
47. A child/adolescent member changed to a new school 24	☐	☐ 77 / 78-01	

Subtotal 3 _____

FAMILY LIFE CHANGES	During Last 12 Months Yes	No	Score
VI. ILLNESS AND FAMILY "CARE" STRAINS			
48. Parent/spouse became seriously ill or injured 44	☐	☐ 12	
49. Child became seriously ill or injured 35	☐	☐	
50. Close relative or friend of the family became seriously ill 44	☐	☐	
51. A member became physically disabled or chronically ill 73	☐	☐	
52. Increased difficulty in managing a chronically ill or disabled member 58	☐	☐	
53. Member or close relative was committed to an institution or nursing home 44	☐	☐	
54. Increased responsibility to provide direct care or financial help to husband's and/or wife's parent(s) 47	☐	☐	
55. Experienced difficulty in arranging for satisfactory child care 40	☐	☐ 26	
VII. LOSSES			
56. A parent/spouse died 98	☐	☐	
57. A child member died 99	☐	☐	
58. Death of husband's or wife's parent or close relative 48	☐	☐	
59. Close friend of the family died 47	☐	☐	
60. Married son or daughter was separated or divorced 58	☐	☐	
61. A member "broke up" a relationship with a close friend 35	☐	☐ 26	
VIII. TRANSITIONS "IN AND OUT"			
62. A member was married 42	☐	☐	
63. Young adult member left home 43	☐	☐	
64. A young adult member began college (or post high school training) 28	☐	☐	
65. A member moved back home or a new person moved into the household 42	☐	☐	
66. A parent/spouse started school (or training program) after being away from school for a long time 38	☐	☐ 41	
IX. FAMILY LEGAL VIOLATIONS			
67. A member went to jail or juvenile detention 68	☐	☐	
68. A member was picked up by police or arrested 57	☐	☐	
69. Physical or sexual abuse or violence in the home 75	☐	☐	
70. A member ran away from home 61	☐	☐	
71. A member dropped out of school or was suspended from school 38	☐	☐ 50 / 78-02	

Subtotal 4 _____
Grand Total ____

FIGURE 10-3. *Continued.*

Although many family nurses are not taught family therapy techniques, family nursing practice can include teaching families to anticipate stress, collaborating with them to develop strategies that promote family resiliency and a healthy family lifestyle, encouraging the development of family rituals and routines to relieve and cope with stress, and facilitating family problem solving. Vulnerable and high-risk families should be referred to programs that provide family preservation, family life education, and support (Hawkins, Roberts, Christiansen & Marshall, 1994).

Unit 3 and particularly Chapter 14 in this text include a variety of interventions to strengthen a family's ability to cope with the myriad of stressors that result from internal and external environments. It is crucial for family nurses to be aware of health policies, family policies, and the economic, political and other environmental factors that influence the quality of family life. It is also imperative that family nurses conduct family research to determine the affects of stressors and strains resulting from the normative and nonnormative individual and family transitions of varied family types on the quality of family health.

CHAPTER HIGHLIGHTS

Family stressors can be positive (eustress) or negative (distress).

Families seldom experience a single stressor at one time.

Transitions of family members and the family unit can be the major source of family stress.

Stress is a normal phenomenon in families that results from the accumulation of stressors that occur during the developmental transitions of individual family members, during family transitions across the life cycle, and in interaction with multiple external family environments.

Family resiliency and appraisal are major factors in determining whether an event or situation is a stressor and in determining the family's ability to manage it effectively.

Families experience stress from sources that are internal, external, normative, nonnormative, ambiguous, nonambiguous, volitional, nonvolitional, chronic, acute, cumulative, or isolated.

The primary implications for the family nurse are to understand family stress, assess the family level of stress, collaborate with families to manage the stress, to be familiar with community resources for families, and to teach families ways to reduce their vulnerability and anticipate potential stressors.

REFERENCES

Aid Association for Lutherans (1989). *Stress Kit.* Duluth, MN: Whole Person Press.

Baum, C.M. (1991). Addressing the needs of the cognitively impaired elderly from a family policy perspective. *American Journal of Occupational Therapy,* 45(7), 594–606.

Boss, P.G. (1980). Normative family stress: Family boundary changes across the life-span. *Family Relations,* 29, 445–150.

Boss, P.G. (1987). Family stress. In M. Sussman & S. Steinmetz (Eds.), *Handbook on Marriage and the Family* (pp. 695–723). New York: Plenum.

Boss, P.G. (1988). *Family Stress Management.* Newbury Park, CA: Sage.

Brown, B. (1984). *Between Health and Illness: New Notions on Stress and the Nature of Well-being.* Boston: Houghton Mifflin.

Burr, W.R., Klein, S.R., et al. (1994). *Reexamining Family Stress.* Thousand Oaks: Sage.

Cannon, W.B. (1929). *Bodily Changes in Pain, Hunger, Fear and Rage.* New York: Appleton.

Carter, E.A., & McGoldrick, M. (Eds.). (1988). *The Changing Family Life Cycle.* New York: Gardner.

Cooke, R.A., & Rousseau, D.M. (1984). Stress and strain from family role and work related expectations. *Journal of Applied Psychology,* 69, 252–260.

Cowan, P.A., & Hetherington, M. (Eds.). (1991). *Family Transitions.* Hillsdale, New Jersey: Erlbaum.

Crosbie-Burnett, M. (1989). Application of family stress theory to remarriage: A model for assessing and helping step families. *Family Relations,* 38, 323–331.

Curran, D. (1983). *Traits of the Healthy Family.* Minneapolis, MN: Winston.

Curran, D. (1985). *Stress and the Healthy Family.* Minneapolis, MN: Winston.

Danielson, C.B., Hamel-Bissell, B., Winstead-Fry, P. (1993). *Families, Health, and Illness: Perspectives on Coping and Intervention.* St. Louis: Mosby Year Book.

Dillworth-Anderson, P., Burton, L.M., & Johnson, L.B. (1993). Reframing theories for understanding race, ethnicigy and families. In P.G. Boss, W.J. Doherty, R. LaRossa, W.R. Schumm, & S.K. Steinmetz (Eds.), *Source Book of Family Theories and Methods* (pp. 627–645). New York: Plenum.

Duval, E.M. (1977). *Marriage and Family Development* (5th ed.). Philadelphia: Lippincott.

Duval, E.M., & Miller, B.C. (1985). *Marriage and Family Development* (6th ed.). New York: Harper & Row.

Galvin, K.M., & Brommel, J.B. (1986). *Family Communication: Cohesion and Change* (2nd ed.). Glenview, IL: Scott Foresman.

Girando, D.A., & Everly, G.S. (1979). *Controlling Stress and Tension: A Holistic Approach.* Bowie, MD: Brady.

Glick, P.C. (1989). The family life cycle and social change. *Family Relations,* 38, 127–134.

Goldschnieder, F.K., & Goldschnieder, C. (1989). Family structure and conflict: Nest-leaving expectations of young adults and their parents. *Journal of Marriage and the Family, 51,* 87–97.

Grochowski, J., & McCubbin, H.I. (1987). YA-FILES young adult family inventory of life events and changes. In H.I. McCubbin & A.I. Thompson (Eds.), *Family assessment inventories for research and practice* (pp. 113–124). Madison, WI: University of Wisconsin.

Guzelzow, M., Bird, G., & KoBall, E.H. (1991). An exploratory path analysis of the stress process for dual-career men and women. *Journal of Marriage and the Family*, 51, 151–164.

Hardy, K. (1993). Implications for practice with ethnic minority families. In P.G. Boss, W.J. Doherty, R. LaRossa, W.R. Schumm, & S.K. Steinmetz (Eds.), *Source Book of Family Theories and Methods* (pp. 645–650). New York: Plenum.

Hawkins, A.J., Roberts, T., Christiansen, S., & Marshall, C.M. (1994). An evaluation of a program to help dual-earner couples share the second shift. *Family Relations*, 43, 213–220.

Hill, R. (1949). *Families under stress: Adjustment to Crisis of Separation and Reunion*. New York: Harper & Row.

Holmes, T.H., & Rahe, R.H. (1967). The social readjustment scale. *Journal of Psychosomatic Research*, 11, 213–218.

Hochschild, A. (1989). *The Second Shift: Working Parents and the Revolution at Home*. New York: Harper & Row.

Ihinger-Tallman, M., & Pasley, L. (1987). *Remarriage*. Newbury Park, CA: Sage.

Janosik, E., & Green, E. (1992). *Family Life: Process and Practice*. Boston: Jones & Bartlett.

Kalil, K.M., Gruber, J.E., Conley, J., & Michael, S. (1993). Social and family pressures on anxiety and stress during pregnancy. *Pre- and Peri-Natal Psychology Journal*, 18(2), 113–118.

Larson, J.H., Wilson, M.S., and Beley, R. (1994). The impact of job insecurity on marital and family relationships. *Family Relations*, 43, 138–143.

Lavee, Y., & Olson, D.H. (1991). Family types and response to stress. *Journal of Marriage and the Family*, 53, 786–798.

Lazarus, R.S. (1966). *Psychological Stress and the Coping Process*. New York: McGraw-Hill.

Lee, K.A., Lentz, M.J., Taylor, D.L., Mitchell, E.S., & Woods, F. (1994). Fatigue as a response to environmental demands in women's lives. *Image*, 26(2), 149–154.

McCubbin, H.I., Cauble, E., & Patterson, J. (Eds.). (1982). *Family Stress and Social Support*. Springfield, IL: Springer.

McCubbin, H.I., & Patterson, J. (1983a). Family transitions: Adaptation to stress. In H.I. McCubbin & C.R. Figley (Eds.), *Stress and the Family: Vol. 1. Coping with Normative Transitions* (pp. 5–25). New York: Brunner/Mazel.

McCubbin, H.I., & Patterson, J. (1983b). Family stress adaptation to crises: A double ABCX model of family behavior. In D.H. Olson & B.C. Miller (Eds.), *Family Studies Review Year Book* (Vol. 1). (pp. 87–106). Beverly Hills: Sage.

McCubbin, H.I., Thompson, A.I., (Eds.). (1987, 1991). *Family Assessment Inventories for Research and Practice*. Madison, WI: University of Wisconsin.

McCubbin, M.A., & McCubbin, H.I. (1987). Family stress theory and assessment: The t-double ABCX model of family adjustment and adaptation. In H.I. McCubbin & A.I. Thompson (Eds.), *Family Assessment Inventories for Research and Practice* (pp. 3–32). Madison, WI: University of Wisconsin.

McCubbin, M.A., & McCubbin, H.I. (1993). Families coping with illness: The resiliency model of family stress, adjustment and adaptation. In C.B. Danielson, B. Hamel-Bissell, & P. Winstead-Fry (Eds.), *Families, Health, and Illness: Perspectives on Coping and Intervention* (pp. 21–63). St. Louis: Mosby Year Book.

McCubbin, M.A., McCubbin, H.I., & Thompson, A.I. (1987). The family hardiness index. In H.I. McCubbin & A.I. Thompson (Eds.), *Family Assessment Inventories for Research and Practice* (pp. 125–130). Madison, WI: University of Wisconsin.

McCubbin, H.I., McCubbin, M.A., & Thompson, A.I. (1993). Resiliency in families. In T.H. Brubaker (Ed.), *Family Relations: Challenges for the Future. Vol. 1. Current Issues in Families* (pp. 153–177). Newbury Park, CA: Sage.

McCubbin, M.A. (1993). Family stress theory and the development of nursing knowledge about family adaptation. In S.L. Feetham, S.B. Meister, M.J. Bell, & C. Gillis (Eds.), *The Nursing of Families: Theory, Research, Education and Practice.* (pp. 46–57). Newbury Park, CA: Sage.

McCubbin, H.I., & Thompson, A.I. (1990). The family maladaptation index. Madison, WI: University of Wisconsin.

McKay, M., Davis, M., & Fanning, P. (1981). *The Art of Cognitive Stress Intervention*. Richmond, CA: New Harbinger.

McGovern, P.M., Gjerdingen, D.K., & Frogerg, D.G. (1992). The parental leave debate: Implications for policy-relevant research. *Women & Health*, 18, 97–118.

Melson, G.F. (1983). Family adaptation to environmental demands. In H.I. McCubbin & C.R. Figley (Eds.), *Stress and the Family: Vol. 1. Coping with Normative Transitions* (pp. 149–162). New York: Brunner/Mazel.

Murata, J.M. (1995). Family stress, mother's social support, depression and son's behavior problems: Modeling nursing interventions for low-income inner-city families. *Journal of Family Nursing*, 1(1), 41–62.

Neuman, B. (1982). The Neuman systems model. Norwalk, CT: Appleton-Century-Crofts.

Olson, D.H., McCubbin, H.I., Bames, H.L., Larsen, A.S., Muxen, M.J., & Wilson, M.A. (1983a). *Families: What Makes Them Work*. Beverly Hills: Sage.

Olson, D.H., Russell, L.S., & Sprenkle, D.H. (1983b). Circumplex Model VI: Theoretical update. *Family Process*, 27, 69–83.

Olson, D.H., & Hanson, M.K. (1990). *2001: Preparing Families for the Future*. Minneapolis, MN: National Council on Family Relations.

Olson, S.L., & Banyard, V. (1993). "Stop the world I want to get off for a while": Sources of daily stress in the lives of low-income single mothers of young children. *Family Relations*, 42, 50–56.

Patterson, J.M., & Garwick, A.W. (1992). Family meanings in family stress theory: The "C" factor. Paper presented at the Theory Construction and Research Methodology Workshop, Annual Meeting of National Council of Family Relations, Orlando, FL.

Phares, E.J. (1976). *Locus of Control and Personality*. Morristown, NJ: General Learning Press.

Selye, H. (1974). *Stress Without Distress*. New York: The New American Library.

Selye, H. (1976). *The Stress of Life* (rev. ed.). New York: McGraw-Hill.

Smilkstein, G. (1978). The family APGAR: A proposal for a family function test and its use by physicians. *Journal of Family Practice,* 6, 416–436.

Smith-Hanrahan, C. (1995). Postpartum early discharge: Impact on maternal fatigue and funtional ability. *Clinical Nursing Research,* 4(1), 50–56.

Speilberger, C.D., Gorsach, R.L., Lushene, R., Vagg, P.R., & Jacobs, G.A. (1983). *Manual for the State Trait and Anxiety Inventory.* Palo Alto, CA: Consulting Psychologists.

Voling, B.L., & Belsky, J. (1993). Parent, infant, and contextual characteristics related to maternal employment decisions in the first year of infancy. *Family Relations,* 42, 4–12.

ADDITIONAL READINGS

Barnfather, J.S., & Lyon, B.L. (Eds.). (1994). *Stress and Coping: State of the Science and Implications for Nursing Theory, Research and Practice.* Indianapolis: Sigma Theta Tau International, Inc.

Conger, R.D., Eler, G.H., Lorenz, F. O., Simmons, R.L., & Whitbeck, L.B. (1994). *Families in Troubled Times: Adapting to Change in Rural America. Social Institutions and Change.* New York: Gruyther.

Menagan, E.G. (1994). The daily grind: Work stress, family patterns, and intergenerational outcomes. In W.R. Avison & I.H. Gotlib (Eds.), *Stress and Mental Health: Contemporary Issues and Prospects for the Future* (pp. 115–147). New York: Plenum.

FAMILY SPIRITUALITY

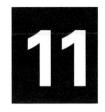

CARMEN GERMAINE WARNER

The faith . . . that is in you . . . dwelt first in your grandmother Lois and your mother Eunice.

2 TIMOTHY 1:5

OBJECTIVES

On completion of this chapter, the reader will be able to:

1. Distinguish between religion and spirituality
2. Explore differences in the major religions
3. Discuss the role of religion in family life across the life span
4. Explain the influence of religion on family health across the family life span
5. Examine the role of religion in selected family crises and transitions
6. Discuss the role of the nurse in assisting families in spiritual distress and in the promotion of spiritual health

Families in the 1990s are facing considerable stresses, problems, and challenges unlike those of previous decades. The economy is dealing with the harshest attack since the Great Depression; the incidence of divorce and family breakup has soared to an unbelievable level; and reports of violence, abuse, and addiction are at an all time high (Bronson-Gray, 1992).

Unemployment, abandonment, impending death, and total loss and destruction—these are the faces of discouragement and despair that are confronting families every day. As family nurse clinicians, we must deal with situations like the following case examples on a regular basis.

CASE EXAMPLES

1. For the past nineteen years, Tom, father of five, held a position as parts mechanic at a local aircraft plant. Now, at the age of 49, Tom has been laid off, with no alternate positions in sight. After frantically searching for a job, Tom develops severe abdominal pain, for which the doctor sees no medical cause. "What do I do?" Tom asks as he discusses the future of his family with his wife, now six months pregnant. "Where do I turn? Who can help us?"

2. Glen, at the age of 15, has suddenly become quiet, withdrawn, and isolated from his mother and younger sister. Although Glen had once led an active life of sports and model car racing with his father, he is now alone, without a father. Glen's father left the home over three years ago. Even his close childhood friends do not come around the house anymore. When Glen's mother inquires about what has happened, he shouts, "Leave me alone! I don't want anything from anybody—I can take care of myself."

3. Cindy is 29 years old. She looks back at her life and smiles. She has a wonderful husband and two young children. Even her job offers her more income and professional gratification than she had known before. Now that her twin daughters are in school full time, Cindy is exploring outside activities and has enrolled in graduate school. During a recent medical examination, Cindy was discovered to have a lump in her right breast. Upon surgical exploration, cancer was diagnosed, with metastasis to her liver and kidney. Having been active in church all her life, Cindy turns away from her church family and displays her anger toward God. "Why me? What did I do wrong in my life? I hate you, God, for ruining my life and my family's lives."

4. It was 3:00 A.M., Monday, August 24th. The winds had built up over the past several hours, but protective boards had been placed on the windows, and the family was huddled together in their basement. "We'll make it," Joe said in a comforting voice to his wife and three

children. "We've suffered these tropical storms before." At 6:00 A.M. after the brunt of Hurricane Andrew had passed, Joe and his family began to emerge from the pile of debris and rubble. Their house was completely destroyed—everything was gone. "Oh, my God, my God! What has happened? What do we do now? Where, oh where, do we begin?"

These are examples for which nursing intervention, listening skills, and resource counseling may not be adequate in addressing the core of a client's pain, pressure, or problem. As families struggle with real life, textbook references, client care plans, and case study situations may not provide the depth of healing and hope that is crucial and of paramount importance.

The healthy personality is reflected in people who take alert and responsive care of themselves, and who find life, with some satisfaction and some accepted suffering, meaningful (Jourard, 1968). As mentioned, there are times when situations place considerable pressure on all people. It is not uncommon for family health nurses to see families turn to God while facing desperate needs. When everything else fails, prayer, worship, and focus on God become the only foundation on which they can stand. Strength, hope, and a sense of survival grow out of people's religious belief as they turn toward God.

RELIGION AND SPIRITUALITY: DISTINGUISHING CHARACTERISTICS

For clarity and uniformity of meaning in this text, the following definitions are introduced.

Religion The term "religion" relates to the inward and outward expression of belief, not the content of that belief. It is an aspect of the spiritual dimension of life. It is the belief in the reverence for God or some supernatural power that is recognized as the creator and ruler of the universe (Lockyer, 1986). Religion also is defined as a belief in a supernatural or divine force that has power over the universe and commands worship and obedience (Guralnik, 1972). A personal definition may be expressed as an individual and communal commitment to a diety involving a belief system, a value/ethical system, and a worship system.

There is a hesitancy today to use the word *religion* either in the context of the Christian faith or of its expression in worship and service. This is because Christianity reflects an outward expression by believers—not as an attempt to secure salvation, but as a thanks offering for it.

Religiosity Although it is different, often religiosity is used interchangeably with spirituality. There are a number of definitions in the literature. According to Meager, O'Brien and Aherne (1979) religiosity is one's relationship with their God and things or persons that are sacred. It also may refer to a continual human striving for spiritual growth in a community of spiritual people. Religiosity, noted as intensive excessive or affected religiousness, was proposed by Batson and Ventis (1982) to demonstrate psychodynamically different ways of being religious. The extrinsic religious orientation is one in which religion is used to justify self-centered ends in a strictly utilitarian way for one's safety, social standing, and solace, and for endorsing one's chosen way of life. By contrast, the intrinsic religious orientation is one in which religious commitments are carefully thought out and taken seriously as a major goal in life. "The extrinsically motivated individual uses his religion, whereas the intrinsically motivated lives his" (Batson & Ventis, 1982).

Spirituality Spirituality is a component of health related to the essence of life. It is the vital principle in human beings that gives life to the physical organism in contrast to its purely material aspects, and relates to the soul as opposed to the body (Hill & Smith, 1990). It also is clarified as a sensitivity or commitment to religious values and sacred matters (Douglas, 1980). Spirituality is associated with specific things of the spirit, as distinguished from that which is material.

Shafranske and Maloney (1990) note that there is a difference between religion and spirituality. Religion can be noted as ". . .adherence to the beliefs and practices of an organized church or religious institution," and spirituality as ". . . those more personal practices of a religious nature which may or may not emanate from a particular religious institution" (Douglas, 1980, p. 74).

Family Spirituality The family as a unit is held together by interwoven threads. These threads represent the various paths and patterns of family life, including areas of security and protection, food and shelter, education and growth, and spiritual cohesiveness and purpose. It is this important area of spiritual bonding that affords the basis for family strength, endurance, and growth.

Family spirituality is the means by which a God-centered focus provides the basis for the harmony, communication, and wholeness among and between family members from which all other family activities, ties, and beliefs are influenced, guided, and directed.

It is this grounding and foundation building that allow the opportunity for individual and family growth, the ability to challenge and test one another and remain mutually respectful, and the beauty of granting freedom to one another, yet accepting the responsibility for both individual and family spiritually focused roles.

COMMON CHARACTERISTICS OF MAJOR RELIGIONS

The health and well-being of each family may involve a variety of religions and practices that may not be familiar or comfortable to the family nurse. Depending on the religious preference of the patient, one may be either relatively comfortable or uneasy. Despite any existing differences, the ability of practitioners to guide, direct, and work with each religious preference will establish a trusting relationship and an open means of communication.

To facilitate optimum interaction with clients, nurses should have a basic understanding of the common characteristics of religion, which are as follows:

- Basis of authority or source(s) of power
- Portion of scripture or sacred word
- Ethical code that defines right and wrong
- Psychology and identity that fits its adherents into a group, and that define the world
- Aspirations or expectations
- Ideas about what follows death

The major world religions are divided into three groups (Okamoto, 1976). The first group includes Christianity, Judaism, and Islam. Taoism, Confucianism and Shintoism are assembled in the second group. The third group includes Buddhism and Hinduism. Table 11–1 depicts various religions and their beliefs, practices, and specific relationships to family needs.

ROLE OF RELIGION IN FAMILY LIFE

The Puritans were the first Anglo-Americans to establish viable families, and this proved crucial to the survival of subsequent revitalization of their religious system (Perry, 1990). Religion, family, and society intersect, especially at times of developmental life transitions, including birth, puberty, marriage, and death. These vital moments in the life cycle were given meaning and significance in the religious ideologies and rituals that social groups employed and enacted to interpret them. Even in ancient societies, there was the belief that religion and its influence ruled human destiny (Hill & Smith, 1990). Treatment was administered by tribal shaman or medicine men, with later treatment being administered in temples by priests.

Over the course of many years, religion and spiritual influence have changed. Today, physicians and nurses have become increasingly more specialized, and sophisticated machinery has been deemed essential. As modern health care has evolved, the importance of the religious dimension has decreased to the extent that it has been deemed least important and caused the client to become increasingly dehumanized. It was only as a result of the dehumanization process that an eventual upsurge in religion and spiritual well-being evolved (Hill & Smith, 1990).

In the course of the elevation of religion in family living, people have turned away from organized religion and the notion of one true God. In a misguided attempt to find God inside themselves, people have turned to so-called new age religions. These religions claim to be the new and improved spirituality that can be practiced "individually" through some mixture of metaphysical concepts, workshops and awareness training programs, star charts, crystals, channels, and out-of-body experiences (Pearsall, 1990). "Religion can also be harmful to individuals and families" (Abbot, et al., 1990, p. 143). Examples of harmful activities include excessive corporal punishment of children, promotion of sexism and racism, sexual abuse, rigid doctorines, delay of health care, and disapproval of the use of family planning methods. Regardless of the type of religion practiced, its value and its role in the family is important to family health nurses, because even though religion is seen as a personal belief, it is truly a group (family) involvement, as well.

FAMILY SPIRITUAL HEALTH MODEL

The family spiritual health model is important to understand and apply with respect to both personal and family beliefs. The family spiritual health model (Fig. 11–1) depicts an inward flow of communication, beginning with the all-encompassing existence of God (Supreme Being). The presence of God flows through each dimension of life, including community, family, child and parent. The effects of God's presence culminates in the inner focus of family existence, noted as the core of spirituality.

The model reflects the dynamics of a constant flow of God's presence back and forth, encompassing the totality of family dynamics. As each circle of communication expands, beginning with the core of spirituality, the network broadens, moving from parent to child to family and finally to the community. These concentric circles relate to the expanded communication evident in the ongoing expansive level of family spiritual health.

Between each circle of expanding communication, there is a perforated ring representing the focus and ongoing movement toward God, beginning with one's basic spiritual grounding in a relationship with God and expanding to include others. The base line of the model indicates that this flow is throughout time in an unceasing, ever constant manner over the family's life course.

Each ring reflects the characteristics and notations of family values that are nurtured and

TABLE 11–1. BELIEFS, PRACTICES AND FAMILY NEEDS OF VARIOUS RELIGIOUS GROUPS

RELIGION	BELIEF	PRACTICE	RELATION TO FAMILY NEEDS
Adventist	Dead are asleep; to be resurrected when Christ returns Divine healing Literal interpretation of Bible	Anoint with oil in prayer Adult baptism by immersion Children dedicated No alcohol, tobacco, narcotics, or stimulants No special practice regarding death Prohibit eating meat, primarily pork Oppose hypnosis Sabbath is Saturday No immunizations or blood transfusions	Healing through prayer Bible provides support Importance of nutrition in religious beliefs
American Indian	300 different tribal groups; each has its own nature-oriented religion Disease has two forms—the presence of a material object in the body, and the absence of the soul from the body Super-human powers are used for protection against disease	Practice elements of magic, disease treatment, and herbal medicine Medicine men and shamans perform symbolic rites against disease	Super-human powers used to protect from disease Use herbs as treatment Medicine men to be contacted during illness
Armenian	No conflict between church and medicine	Infants baptized by immersion 8 days after birth Confirmation (called chrismation) follows immediately Communion is performed as last rites and also may be given earlier, in infancy and throughout life Laying on of hands Fasting during Lent and before Communion	Child baptized as infant Communion near death Prayer with and for one another
Baptist (over 27 different groups in the U.S.)	Bible is supreme authority God works through the physician	Baptize only believer by immersion No infant baptism No alcoholic beverages Laying on of hands Prayer with clergy if near death	Have Bible by bedside If death is imminent, call clergy Prayer very important May delay seeking medical care
Buddhist	No conflict between church and medicine Illness is a trial to aid development of soul	Discourage use of alcohol, tobacco, or drugs Last-rite chanting practice at bedside after death Body cremated	Celebrated holy days: Jan. 1, 16; Feb. 15; March 21; April 8; May 21; July 15; September 9, 23; December 8, 31
Christian Scientist	Denies reality of illness Sickness and sin are errors of human mind, eliminated by spiritual truth, not drugs	Have own practitioners to offer care No infant baptism No alcohol, coffee, tea, tobacco, or drugs No blood transfusions, biopsies, and autopsies—only by law Cremation and burial acceptable No physical medicine	Secure physicians and nurses of like faith Restrictions to be closely adhered to
Church of Christ	No conflict between church and medicine Recognize human limitations of medicine	Communion Anoint with oil Laying on of hands for healing No alcohol or last rites Baptism by immersion after 8 years of age	Pray with others for healing If child is older than 8 and critically ill, see clergy

TABLE 11–1. BELIEFS, PRACTICES AND FAMILY NEEDS OF VARIOUS RELIGIOUS GROUPS *Continued*

RELIGION	BELIEF	PRACTICE	RELATION TO FAMILY NEEDS
Church of God	Divine healing through prayer	No alcohol or tobacco No baptism or last rites of cremation Speak in tongues	Pray with others for healing
Church of Jesus Christ of Latter-Day Saints (Mormons)	Believe in revelations through prophecies Blessing of the ill by anointing and laying on of hands by elders	Baptism by immersion after age 8 Baptism by proxy for the dead No alcohol, coffee, tea or caffeine of any kind, or tobacco Use meat sparingly	Observe diet Be aware of dress code Buried with temple garments on
Disciples of Christ (Christian Church)	No conflict between church and medicine	No infant baptism—only a dedication service Adult baptism by immersion Communion important in worship and in hospital	Spiritual support by clergy and elders May desire communion in hospital
Eastern Orthodox	No conflict between church and medicine	Baptism within 40 days after birth Baptism by immersion, followed by immediate confirmation (chrismation) and communion in infancy Last rites obligatory Cremation discouraged Anointing of sick by healing through prayer	Christmas is on Jan. 7 and New Year's on Jan. 14 Observe baptism requirements Prayer very important
Episcopal (Anglican)	No conflict between church and medicine	Infant baptism Baptism urgent if newborn is likely to die Last rites not mandatory Spiritual healing in some cases Some fast before Communion and reserve eating meat	Baptism if child's life is in danger May desire prayer for spiritual healing
Grace Brethren	No conflict between church and medicine	No infant baptism Dedication for children Baptism only for those old enough to profess faith Anointing of sick for physical and spiritual healing No last rites Clergy needed at time of death Abstinence from alcohol, tobacco, and illicit drugs Cremation permitted Stillborns to be buried	Clergy called for anointing of sick and at time of death Stillborns to be buried
Greek Orthodox	No conflict between church and medicine Oppose euthanasia; try to preserve life	Chrismation and communion within 40 days of birth Communion as last rites Autopsies and cremations discouraged Selective fasting on Wednesday and Friday and during Lent Holy communion provided by priest on request	Call priest for communion when patient near death Fasting is important and may need to be coordinated with diet Christmas and Easter observed according to different calendar format
Hindu	Most accept modern medical practices	Prescribed rites follow death Priest ties a thread around the neck or wrist signifying a blessing Priest pours water into mouth of corpse; family washes the body Bodies cremated Many dietary restrictions; do not eat beef	Be aware of special rituals concerning death Dietary requirements are important to follow

Table continued on following page

TABLE 11–1. BELIEFS, PRACTICES AND FAMILY NEEDS OF VARIOUS RELIGIOUS GROUPS *Continued*

RELIGION	BELIEF	PRACTICE	RELATION TO FAMILY NEEDS
Jehovah's Witnesses	Oppose false teachings of other religions Attempt to convert others	No infant baptism No last rites Alcohol discouraged Cremation acceptable Autopsy by personal decision No abortion or blood transfusions	Be aware of infant and death rites Will not accept blood or abortions
Judaism	No conflict between church and medicine Someone to be with person when soul leaves the body	Male circumcision on 8th day after birth Fetus, organs, and body parts must be buried Abortion only to save life of mother Many special dietary requirements Opposed to euthanasia, autopsy, and cremation Observe Sabbath through rest and worship Burial within 24 hours (not on Sabbath)	In case of impending death, read Psalm 23, 103, or 139 Special dietary needs are important Family present during circumcision
Lutheran (10 different branches)	No conflict between church and medicine	Baptism 6–8 weeks after birth by immersion or sprinkling Anointing may be requested	Baptism important Clergy valuable during illness
Mennonite	No conflict between church and medicine Self-determination is important	No infant baptism; but baptism in teens No last rites, communion, or other sacraments No alcohol Prayer very important Women may wear head coverings during hospitalization	No religious rites or sacraments Prayers crucial in time of illness or personal need
Methodist (over 20 different groups)	Belief in divine judgment (good rewarded and evil punished) Clergy counsels but does not hear confession	Baptism for child and adults Communion, prayer, and scripture important Donation of organs encouraged	Seek prayer, scripture, and communion at time of need
Moravian	Disease is not a form of divine punishment, although breaking from God can lead to physical problems	Infant baptism No last rites Patient to be comfortable, but not to extend life at all costs Communion and laying on of hands are important	Physical touch and prayer are most important Communion desired
Muslim (Islam)	Conservative groups can have fatalistic view which can effect compliance with therapy	No baptism Fetus aborted after 130 days must be buried according to custom Abortion forbidden Women can't sign consent forms One must confess sins before death to preserve family Family washes and prepares body after death No autopsies unless required by law Bury as soon as possible after death No cremation No alcohol or pork Koran has many holy requirements to be kept Jewelry may have special meaning	Multiple religious rules and regulations must be observed Diet and death have many special requirements

TABLE 11–1. BELIEFS, PRACTICES AND FAMILY NEEDS OF VARIOUS RELIGIOUS GROUPS *Continued*

RELIGION	BELIEF	PRACTICE	RELATION TO FAMILY NEEDS
Nazarene	No conflict between church and medicine Belief in divine healing but not exclusive to medical treatment	Baptism optional No last rites Cremation permitted Stillborns are buried Communion and laying on of hands by pastor No alcohol or tobacco	Special attention to stillborns Prayer and communion important
Pentecostal (Assembly of God; Foursquare)	Illness seen as an intrusion of Satan Deliverance from illness is provided in atonement	Baptism by immersion after age of accountability No last rites Divine healing through anointing, prayer, and laying on of hands No alcohol, tobacco, or illicit drugs No eating of strangled animals or anything to which blood has been added No pork products	Prayer, anointing and laying on of hands for healing
Presbyterian (10 different groups)	Science used for relief of suffering and recognized gift from God Full forgiveness through repentance for any illness connected with a sin	Infant baptism Last rites not a sacrament; involves prayer and scripture Communion may be required	Communion beneficial to patient Prayer valuable
Quaker (Friends)	No creed, thus a diversity of personal beliefs Pacifists God is in every man and may be approached directly Individual choice and decision making very important	No baptism at birth No rituals related to death Decisions left up to individual Avoid alcohol and drugs	Discuss desires and needs with individual for their choice
Roman Catholic	No conflict between church and medicine except for abortion upon demand May donate or transplant organs if no harm to donor	Infant baptism mandatory Emergency baptism for neonates with poor prognosis, stillborns, and fetuses (if not clinically dead) Anointing of the sick is mandatory Fasting and abstinence from meat on Ash Wednesday and Good Friday (exceptions okay in hospital)	Baptism mandatory Priest to be called if death is eminent Communion important to patient
Russian Orthodox	No conflict between church and medicine	Baptism by priest only Chrismation and communion in infancy No autopsies, embalming, or cremation After death, arms crossed with fingers in a cross formation Clothing to be of natural fiber to decompose faster Crosses worn and important; to be left in place No meat or dairy products on Ash Wednesday and during Lent	

Table continued on following page

TABLE 11–1. BELIEFS, PRACTICES AND FAMILY NEEDS OF VARIOUS RELIGIOUS GROUPS *Continued*

RELIGION	BELIEF	PRACTICE	RELATION TO FAMILY NEEDS
Salvation Army	No conflict between church and medicine, except for abortion on demand Bible is the only rule for one's faith	Infant dedication No particular baptism, communion, or death practices	Abortion on demand not accepted Bible is important to one's daily life
Unitarian (Universalist)	Reason and practicality are most important Each person has right to approach values individually Clergy are not always needed if patient is assuming responsibility for self	Baptism by choice, but without formula of the Trinity Dedication of children No sacraments officially Agree to organ donation Prefer cremation Belief in immortality differs	One's own choice and decision is important regarding religious matters

From A. Schroeder (1993). Emotional and spiritual support. In T.C. Kravis, C.G. Warner, & L. Jacobs (Eds.), *Emergency Medicine Review* (3d ed.). New York: Raven Press.

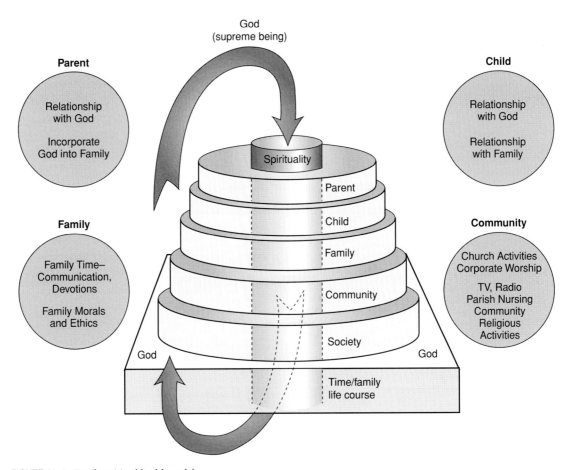

FIGURE 11–1. Family spiritual health model.

expanded through this model. The model also clarifies the means by which religion and spiritual growth can support the total well-being of the family unit.

Religion provides the ultimate way by which one may worship in fellowship with others. It has been noted that over 40% of the population seeking guidance in an emotional problem will turn to a religious leader first before any other professional leadership (Beitman, 1992). Thus, through this contact, families are becoming closer to one another and to God, and are developing and experiencing valuable family strengths. Research supports the belief that values and religiosity are specific qualities related to family strengths (Olson et al., 1983; Stinnett, 1981; Schumm et al., 1990). Researchers found religiosity to be the most reliable predictor of family strengths. Religion contributed to family strengths in the following five ways: (1) beliefs or values; (2) beneficial practices or behaviors; (3) social benefits related to organizations with a religious affiliation; (4) family recreation and activities; and (5) assistance in seeking divine intervention with individual and family religious counseling and spiritual direction (Abbot, 1990, Bringman & Keating, 1991).

FAMILY STRENGTH THROUGH RELIGION

Family health clinicians can look for growth-producing elements in each family's life and value system that will encourage them to demonstrate flexibility, forgiveness, patience, love, tolerance, cooperation, communication, and develop a purposeful meaning for the family way of life. As these family strengths grow and mature, the following specific family characteristics evolve.

- *Faith:* Allows families to discover meaning and purpose in life and enter into fundamental commitment, as well as identifying how one perceived life
- *Hope:* Provides a sense of optimism in times of stress and difficulty
- *Love:* A means of promoting an opportunity for support and nurturing
- *Parenthood of God:* Individuals may be strengthened by enhancing ego strength
- *Forgiveness and grace:* Allows the family the ability to resolve conflicting situations
- *Reverence and commitment:* Fosters commitment to one's family and reverence to the concept and purpose of family (Brigman, 1992).

According to Pearsall (1990), if religion is truly to be a source of strength to the family, it must be a religion of closeness and unity with others. Associated with this unity is the opportunity provided through church attendance. Pearsall says that it is primarily through ongoing church attendance that family members learn to nurture, care for, and support one another. This caring association knits families together and provides strength and hope in times of need.

INFLUENCES IN THE LIFE CYCLE

The importance of a religious influence in the family is a life-long process—from the cradle to the grave.

CHILDHOOD. Ideally, an infant's first involvement with feelings and emotions is the development of a sense of trust and the belief in a secure environment. The child feels loved and comforted, which is the initial step in the development of self-esteem and self-love. Spiritual and religious values are conveyed to the infant in a nonverbal manner throughout these early years, which establishes a basis for future beliefs (Hill & Smith, 1990).

Parents who want to influence the health of their children by providing a religious foundation, can do the following:

1. Teach children the value of kindness, goodness, patience, faithfulness, gentleness, and self-control.
2. Read books to children, and encourage them to read books, demonstrating the incorporation of these qualities in one's life and in the lives of notable individuals.
3. Read and study selections from the writings of one's faith (scripture) as part of a daily family devotional, discussing personal application to one's situation.
4. Discuss and point out examples of how religious beliefs and principles can be applied.
5. Celebrate religious holidays as a family unit, and establish family rituals and practices associated with these holidays.
6. Plan family outings and activities in connection with religious holidays.
7. Discuss the value and importance of daily prayer as individuals and as a family.
8. Stress that prayer need not be fancy nor formal, but an open, natural communication with God (or one's higher power).
9. Pray for one another as a family (for example, before meals, at the beginning and end of each day, and throughout the day) for such things as preparation for school work, guidance at work or in meetings, and strength during times of illness or discouragement.
10. In some traditions, families will establish a prayer partner (another parent or church/synagogue member) who will commit to pray for the family and be present for love and support.

11. Commit to having each child baptized or dedicated in accordance with one's church, synagogue, or other religious institution.
12. Prepare children for their commitment to God through the celebration of the sacraments or the rite of passage such as confirmation, first communion, bar mitzvah, and bat mitzvah, or ritual as prescribed by one's faith.
13. Attend religious services, classes, and fellowship as a family unit.
14. Teach the importance of giving of the family's money, talent, prayers, and service to one's place of worship.

ADOLESCENCE. Adolescence is a crucial time in the development and formation of an individual's identity (Maslow, 1968). The primary risk during this particular stage is to resolve identity versus role diffusion. A significant part of an adolescent's personal identity relates to how he or she views himself or herself with respect to the opposite sex. To be part of the group is very important; and frequently, group pressure might lead to early sexual activity.

An important factor in helping the adolescent deal with the issue of sexuality is the spiritual health and well-being of the family unit. A strong family spiritual foundation, grounded in solid moral beliefs, will afford an adolescent the desire, words, and actions to reject sexual activities and to stand firm on personal beliefs, resisting peer pressure and influence. One way to secure this is through the recognition that sex education and the pertinent values must be broached long before adolescence if the child is to develop psychosexually (Cavanagh, 1983).

Adolescents need to openly and honestly address the question of who they are and what their place is in the world. Adolescents are adjusting to a new, dramatic awareness of self, causing them to debate, and question everything presented to them. They are attempting to determine values, roles, and responsibilities in a world where there is confusion, doubt, and emphasis on personal gain. Individual feelings and emotions are real, but frequently unexplainable. Parents can incorporate religion into their communication with adolescents in the following ways:

- Discuss sexual values and religious beliefs.
- Pray with your child concerning specific needs, desires, and wants.
- Join with other parents from your church, synagogues, or school and pray for your children and other classmates. "Moms-in-Touch" (MIT) is a group of mothers from schools throughout the country who meet weekly for this very purpose.
- Involve children in various youth groups and activities to provide spiritual, social, and peer support during these challenging times.

- Encourage the involvement of family church activities, especially focusing on recreation, sport, and eating activities.
- Initiate a time when an open forum of communication and sharing is possible—a time when a particular event or activity can be related to scripture.

It is the critical stage of adolescence that Carson (1989) identifies as a time of conflict and rebellion leading to one's search for self-identity and purpose. During this process, the adolescent seeks faith and purpose from group contact and interaction. Such contact, for example from a church or synagogue, will support, influence, and affirm the adolescent and encourage a commitment to his or her religious belief. This affirmation affords a stepping stone to the next stage of young adulthood.

YOUNG ADULT. Only when adolescents have explored and come to terms with who they are can they commit to an intimate relationship as a young adult (Carson, 1989). The personal sacrifices of such a commitment may produce a challenge. Fowler (1974) notes that during this time, individuals make a conscious decision concerning their commitment to religious symbols, religious beliefs, and a supreme being. It is now that the young adult begins the searching part of his or her faith. During this process, a personal conversion experience may occur, usually in a very soft and subtle manner.

Parents can draw on their religion to assist the young adult in the following ways:

- Encourage the young adult to openly share feelings, struggles, and questions.
- Facilitate an opportunity for the young adult to discuss ideas and to ask questions of the family pastor, rabbi, priest, or other religious leaders.
- Support and encourage the value of open prayer and communication between young adults and their God.
- Seek printed materials that will support the testing, learning, and decision-making process of the young adult's religious commitment.
- Be in daily prayer for guidance, direction and peace.

ADULTHOOD. Life's challenges do not end with young adulthood. In fact, the pressures of this time often extend that difficult period of transition into the years of adulthood. Adulthood is a time of planning for the future, reexamining one's focus and purpose for life, and integrating one's religious beliefs into a format for life. Adults must examine and confirm their values, morals, and religious foundations. There is a need to understand and communicate with one's inner self, thus providing solid guidelines on which to reflect and make concrete decisions. It has been stated that during adulthood "there is nowhere you have to go to work on yourself other than where you are at this moment. Everything that is happening to you is part of your work on yourself" (Dass, 1976, p. 12).

Adults can maintain the importance of religion in the family in the following ways:

- Participate in a support group that will provide a forum for shared concerns, challenges, and choices.
- Become involved in learning/growth groups that deal with such issues as finance, parenting struggles, and personal support groups.
- Join a sacred writings study group or prayer support group for fellowship, spiritual growth, direction, and prayer in one's chosen way.
- Secure a prayer partner for daily prayer, even if not in person. (One person commits to initiating a mutual prayer time. This person, at a previously agreed upon time, calls the prayer partner, lets the telephone ring once, and then hangs up. This one ring calls both parties to prayer.)

SENIOR ADULT. At the end of the life cycle, when the pressures of work and raising children have ceased, older adults frequently have more time for, investing in, and devotion to religion and its role in their lives. This trend is consistent with the belief that the first quarter of life relates to growth, the second quarter relates to work, the third quarter to play, and the fourth quarter to spirituality (Hill & Smith, 1990).

Adults may rely on spirituality, especially during this fourth quarter, to help them deal with issues of chronic illness, pain, suffering, and even death. For example, individuals facing old age might have come to grips with an illness that has no cure, but might be seeking emotional and spiritual comfort (Taylor & Ferszt, 1990). For many people, the strength, support, and inner peace they can receive from their religion not only assists them in dealing with physical pain, but provides them with the coping skills needed to relate to the future and the family. During this time, older adults are spending part of their lives preparing for death. Acceptance of death comes with a sense of fulfilled potential.

Fear, resentment, and despair may occur when an individual has not become all that he or she thought was possible (Kavanaugh, 1972). Individuals may need the reassurance of faith, a sense of purpose, and a feeling of well-being about life after death. Such feelings will help the individual develop a positive attitude toward death, a feeling of peace about where one is in his or her life cycle, and the humility to love, accept, and forgive oneself and others. Wisdom is the gift and virtue to see one's life as a whole and accept past failures and successes with balance. Personal integrity seems to be the foundation of growth in advanced years.

Senior adults can incorporate religion into their family life in the following ways:

- Join a support group of mutual interests related to hobbies, recreation, or social gatherings.
- Participate in a grief and loss support group if one person has lost his or her mate.
- Establish a means by which people check on each other at a prearranged time.
- Seek church activities that encourage and develop personal gifts and talents.
- Welcome church or community groups that incorporate programs such as "adopt-a-grandparent."

INFLUENCE OF RELIGION ON FAMILY HEALTH

Family health clinicians are confronted with a responsibility to mobilize, encourage, and reaffirm the internal strengths, goals, and resources of their families. Throughout this process, nurses are able to assist individuals in finding the meaning in health, illness, and suffering (Stoll, 1979). The true meaning of life and living unfolds as family members are able to focus on and openly share a religious base or core in their lives. Curran (1983) comments that the issues of faith, strength, and responsibility are instrumental as building blocks for a shared family religious core. Faith in God provides the basic foundation on which all activities, beliefs, and conversation within a family unit are grounded. The strength of the family support system as a whole, building upon the existing foundation, evolves from the religious core within the family. Finally, the responsibility for passing on and integrating one's faith provides the means by which families bond together in a positive and meaningful manner.

In reviewing the model of family spiritual health, eight benefits can be identified that will influence and support the value of religion in the total health and well-being of the family: goodness, kindness, joy, love, patience, self-control, faithfulness, and peace. These benefits are defined as follows:

- Goodness bridges together the community at large and the structured church.
- Kindness is shared between and among those who worship in the corporate church or synagogue setting.
- Joy becomes evident when the family-based spiritual values extend and radiate into the community.
- Love knits together each member of the family unit.
- Patience encourages interaction between child and parent.

- Self-control establishes a personal awareness between one's self and God.
- Faithfulness encourages and directs a parent to integrate God into the family structure.
- Peace is experienced as one seeks a closeness with God.

There are several enablers of one's spiritual perspective that can be identified, encouraged, and developed through the direction and guidance of others. These enablers include love and affirmation, understanding or wisdom, and pivotal life events. Specifically, love and understanding evolve though the involvement and association of significant others, teachers, and role models like family health nurses. It is precisely the pivotal life events one faces that provide situations that develop a spiritual perspective (Newman, 1989).

Love and Affirmation

A basic human need, in addition to one of the primary ingredients of life, is the gift of love. Integrated throughout religious teachings is the principle and call to "love one another" (John 15:12), for it is indeed through the gift of love that people are healed, families are held together, disagreements are resolved, futures are built, and lives are restored.

These examples of love in action become evident in family life through the examples and teachings one secures in a religious environment. In and through a religious community, families experience the fruits of love, including support, affirmation, remembrance, dedication, and fellowship.

Support is important in the face of adversity, as well as the building up and maintenance of one's concept of self. In a religious community, one will experience the shared joys and celebrations, along with the tears and tribulations. Daily life often requires the loving support of a comforting arm, a listening ear, and the quiet presence of one who is just there for you. The availability of this support is a primary foundation in one's religious surrounding, as evidenced through small groups, prayer, worship, and pastoral care.

The need for and value of personal affirmation builds self-esteem and strengthens personal worth amidst the difficulties, challenges, and trials often experienced in a family. A strong foothold and grounding in one's faith is facilitated by application of the spiritual readings to personal affairs.

As one is affirmed regarding his or her value and worth in God, so, too, is the importance of experiencing the value of the affirmation through being remembered and recognized as valuable, worthwhile, and wanted. All family members grow and thrive on the knowledge that they are accepted and remembered as unique, special human beings. Even though one may face joys and sorrows, strengths and weaknesses, health and

illness, sin and forgiveness, past heritage and future destiny (Belgum, 1992), there is the assurance that one can seek and receive a sense of personal identity in his or her own creation.

Special activities and events within the life of a church are encouraged so that family members of all ages will be received, recognized, and remembered at important times and occasions in their life.

Understanding

From the time that a small child begins his or her grounding of truths, there is an understanding of the basic concept of right and wrong and sound moral teachings. These truths are taught and reinforced through learning in class, reading the scripture, and listening to sermons. Not only is one informed of the difference between right and wrong, but one is taught how to apply these truths and where to seek help and strength when the application may be difficult.

Pivotal Life Events

Pivotal events may develop as a result of peak experiences along life's journey. Some of those experiences, as identified by Olson, et al. (1982), are as follows:

- Transitions relating to the role or status of family members, the addition of family members, or the relocation of an individual or the family as a unit
- Sexuality focusing on pregnancy, childbearing, and the onset of sexual activity
- Personal losses, such as the loss of a family member, relative, or friend, as well as the loss of property or income
- Responsibilities and strains relating to interpersonal tensions, or stressors in relation to health care and finances
- Substance use, referring to the use of drugs or alcohol, and the disagreement over the use of a substance
- Legal conflict addressing the arrest or assault of a family member

During such pivotal life events, nurses frequently co-experience with their clients both wellness and suffering. It is believed that during these interactions, both nurse and client "become more in accordance with their human potential" (Paterson & Zderad, 1976). Health can be associated with the ability to transcend ordinary living situations in order to enhance and develop all aspects of self.

A union can develop between client and nurse through such experiences. In addition, religious rituals have proven to be very stabilizing forces. Kneeling, fasting, Bible study, praying, meditating, and chanting are outward and visible expressions of faith.

Family health clinicians should be observant for family life course transitions such as birth, baptism, first communion, confirmation, graduation, marriage, and funerals. These transitions unite and connect both the spiritual and the social cultural realms. After experiencing these transitions that are strengthened by their spirituality, families become more resilient for future life course events (Pearsall, 1990; Olson et al, 1983).

SEEKING DIRECTION FOR FAMILIES

One discovers and applies his or her source of energy in the family unit. As the energy from each member emanates, it joins together to unify the force of the family as a whole. This is evident when families simply sit down together and share that which is physical, emotional, or spiritual. Family ties are the closest when they are not separated by television, video games or conflicting outside experiences. In fact, the greatest harmony evolves from talking, sharing, and reflecting on one another's ideas.

An excellent example of this principle in action comes from the practice of making scripture come alive. This can be accomplished at mealtime. A scripture verse is chosen, read aloud, and applied to the activities of everyday life. The situational sharing can be both challenging and rewarding, as each member can communicate not only their activities but their feelings as well. Such building of family reverence that can knit members together so that during times of stress, trial, and tribulation, family unity is the stronghold and not the weakest link.

Pearsall suggests three distinct paths to be taken in establishing a grounding in family reverence (Pearsall, 1990). These paths are family time-saving, finding space for the family, and self as a cell.

Family Time Saving

We often feel that time is flying by, but really our lives are flying. With each passing day, there is less time available to spend with your loved ones. You can never make up for lost time once you discover someone has a fatal illness. The days in your past are gone forever, yet families can be guided and directed by sitting down with one another, sharing with each other, praying for one another, and just being in the presence of each other. It is this precious time together that reflects the blessing of love as noted in the personal family time (see Fig. 11–1). This family savings time is the best investment one can make in total family health and well being.

Finding Space for the Family

One may feel that in order to accomplish anything, you must always be "doing." The idea of life being worthwhile only if it is filled with constant activity is a falsehood. There is greater value and worth in just being with your family than all the aimless, frantic doings we perceive to be so meaningful. When family members take the time and effort to meditate on what they have created as a family, they bring the joy of reverence for humanness to each day of their lives. If families practice the art of creating space in their families by gearing down to "slow" and "stay" speeds, the reward will be enormous.

The Self as a Cell

Self really means the "us" of our family. In many ways, this can be portrayed in the phrase, "we are us" (Pearsall, 1990). This is a valuable point to be adhered to daily. We need to think each day of what we are actually doing to keep our family close together. Simulations, prearranged quiet times of prayer and reflection (wherever one might be), family pictures carried by each member, and a concerted effort to join hands together in the morning for prayer and scripture will keep the tie that binds ever meaningful and ever close. This closeness is especially important to implement with children during their infancy and toddler periods. Brief moments of family time together can become a way of life if initiated when children are young.

The focus and direction of the family unit is a top priority, especially concerning spiritual health and wholeness. The following three elements closely knit the family into a pattern of harmony and purpose:

- The investment of love spent through quality time together
- The gift of joy displayed by just being with each other
- The treasure of patience portrayed in knowing the closeness of one another

ROLE OF RELIGION IN CRISES AND TRANSITION

Life is a journey of day-to-day uncertainties. Despite all the advances in technology, communication, health care, and research, no human being can predict the future. However, a religion or faith can often help individuals deal with the future.

Benefits of Religion

For those who are grounded in a sound religion, the fear for tomorrow and the events of the future are minimized. Support, comfort, and direction in times of need and crises are provided through religious belief, a spiritual leader, and the love and support of other faith members, such as those in the local church.

Religion, in fact, helps individuals to make sense of life (Gilbert, 1992). People, through religion, are able to bridge life on this earth to life in the hereafter. Through this belief, hope and strength are provided as a guide during difficult times. There are seasons in a person's life, however, when family members are weak, ill, or in pain and unable to deal with life's crises on their own. It is during these times of doubt, confusion, and grief that fellow church members can provide valuable and necessary support, by listening, praying, and giving of their time. (Taylor & Ferszt, 1990).

Religion and Barriers to Health

Althouth religion has many positive factors, there is evidence that some individuals use their belief in a supreme being in a way that may be detrimental to their health. For example, in a qualitative report of rural African American women with hypertension, Bomar reports some participants believe that "God is in control. If I take pills, I don't have faith" (Bomar, 1995). Others may believe that their time of death is predestined and they should not interfere. For example, Powe (1995) noted significant fatalism about the outcome of cancer in her study of elderly African Americans. In addition to offering alternative options to delaying or omitting treatment based on religious beliefs, health professionals may assist individuals and families to make informed decisions about their self-care and to continue the practice of their religion.

When Religion is Absent from Family Life

Family health nurses at times may be intervening with families who either do not have a religion or who have expressed feelings of anger and resentment against God.

During contact with families, one should never attempt to force religious beliefs on a family or attempt to talk them out of their feelings toward their God. Instead, it is important to assess the family's spirituality, to focus on the values of religion, and to remain sensitive to the variability in the meaning of God and religion. Rather than confronting any feelings of denial or anger, thus creating possible alienation, one must be patient and allow the individuals an opportunity to explore their emotions, to speak their feelings, and to receive openness and honesty from others.

It is essential to inquire of the family what *they* want and what *their* needs might be. Families, if allowed to be themselves, will more likely be open for an honest response to feelings, thus enabling an opportunity for appropriate nurturing and compassionate care.

Stages of Crisis and Transition

Throughout one's life cycle, there are multiple occasions for celebrating, rejoicing, grieving, adjusting, and refocusing. In each stage, one will experience many events and opportunities for religious support. Some of these events are identified in Table 11–2.

As families deal with issues of stress, trauma, and disruption, it is valuable for members to be laced together in a common bond of unity. It is through the strength of an agreed-upon commitment that families are held together in a steadfast and solid manner that will support them during periods of transition and crisis. An idea this author has developed for the integration of such a bond is noted in Figure 11–2.

As a family faces crises together, they are supported through their faith and prayer. Individual members feel supported by the prayers of family members (Curran, 1983). During these times, it is essential for the family (one) to respond to their crisis being led, focused and strengthened by their God rather than by their emotions.

TABLE 11–2. RELIGION IN FAMILY TRANSITIONS AND CRISIS

EVENT	CEREMONY OR RITUAL	RELIGIOUS SUPPORT
Marriage	Wedding	Rejoicing; celebrating; unifying of family
Birth of child	Baptism	Commitment to God in presence of other believers
Childhood (entering adulthood)	Confirmation (at times)* or Bar mitzvah or Bat mitzvah	Learn laws of the church; assume personal responsibility for religious direction of one's life
Death	Funeral	Celebration of one's life; public affirmation of life after death
Loss, grief, financial concerns, moves	Support groups	Support and/or prayer groups; educational groups; establish connectional networks

*In the Roman Catholic church, first communion is given before confirmation or during the same ceremony. Theologically, confirmation is *not* perceived as a puberty rite even though it may be misunderstood as such.

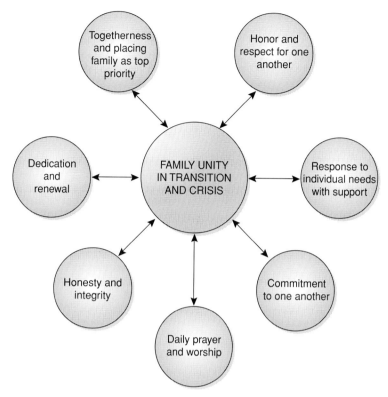

FIGURE 11–2. Seven integrating beliefs in the family structure.

Family health nurses can encourage family members to share these ideas noted in figure 2 with one another, focus on that which is most valuable, and pray about the specifics of what is important. The value and importance of prayer should be addressed in an open, nonthreatening way so family members can feel comfortable in the practice of prayer.

Belief in the Power of Prayer

The power of prayer not only has deeply touched the lives of those believing in its worth and applying it to their daily lives, but its outcomes have become evident through scientific studies.

Dr. Randy Byrd (1986), a cardiologist formally from the University of California, conducted a ten-month study of 393 patients admitted to the coronary care unit at San Francisco General Hospital. A computer randomly assigned these patients to two separate groups. One group of 192 patients were prayed for by prayer groups in their homes, while a second group of 201 patients did not have people praying for them.

Strict scientific, double-blind controls were placed on this study. Groups from across the country representing Protestant, Catholic, and Jewish faiths were asked to pray for between five and seven patients. The prayer groups were provided with the names and the condition of each patient. However, guidelines on how to pray were not provided.

The results of Byrd's (1986) study were impressive. Those who were prayed for by prayer groups in homes were five times less likely than the unremembered group to require antibiotics (three patients compared to sixteen patients). Those receiving prayer were three times less likely to develop pulmonary edema, (six patients compared to eighteen patients). None of the prayed-for group required endotracheal intubation, while twelve in the unremembered group required mechanical ventilatory support). Fewer patients in the prayed-for group died (although this difference was not statistically significant).

In his book *Mind Beyond Body*, Dr. Dossey (1989) discusses the importance of prayer by professionals in such places as a hospital setting. Dossey emphasizes the fact that there is no energy nor signal producing power from the mind during prayer. In fact, he states that the effectiveness of prayer is not influenced by distance.

Keeping this in mind, as caregivers, our prayers can and will provide visible healing results without our ever needing to touch or speak with the person for whom we are praying. Our caring can be felt if we fully live the ultimate of this caring.

NURSING PROCESS AND FAMILY SPIRITUAL HEALTH

Unlike applying the nursing process to physical needs, Carson (1989) relates that spiritual needs must be inferred from client behavior, where nurses apply the tool of themselves and their gifts of compassion, listening, and kindness.

Although the emphasis on holistic care has been encouraged and advocated throughout nursing practice, the emphasis and comfort relative to the spiritual portion has not been openly and willingly dealt with (Labun, 1988). Equally so, schools of nursing stress biopsychosocial needs and minimally, if at all, relate to the spiritual aspect of the individual (Brunner, 1984).

This void in the sensitivity and appreciation of the value of spirituality in nursing stems from several areas of focus. Initially, nurses are more comfortable dealing with facts rather than feelings. Throughout the nursing process, it is easier to relate to that which one can see, hear, or touch—that of the physical. The issue of spirituality is often awkward and uncomfortable, almost as if the nurses feel it is none of their business. Second, nurses may not wish to "get involved." If one can relate solely to a disease, a symptom, or a causative factor, the process is easier. However, when one touches the issues that are of a spiritual nature, the nurse's own spiritual dimensions and issues may come into focus.

Lastly, the issue of role definition also contributes to the lack of sensitivity and true appreciation of the spiritual health of the family. There are others, such as pastors, priests, rabbis, and chaplains, who are available to assist families with the issue of spiritual matters. However, the crucial factor is the recognition of spiritual distress and the collaborative involvement of the family health practitioner in the initial referral.

Assessment of Family Religious Orientation

Much of this chapter has dealt with the importance of family unity, focus, and direction. In order for the nurse to relate and intervene with families, the family as a unit and each member must be first assessed regarding his or her individual spiritual development and growth. For example, prayer, although it is basically talking with God, may mean something different to each family member. Some members may feel comfortable with sharing their prayers openly, others may prefer to read prayers that are already written, and others may be uncomfortable with even the idea of prayer. However, the primary focus should be on how the family as a unit relates to and incorporates prayer.

The spiritual health of the family, however, is more commonly assessed by basically inquiring of the family's involvement or membership in a particular religion. This surface assessment does not reveal the important feelings and spiritual benefits identified in Table 11-3.

However, the Family Spiritual Health Assessment tool presented in Table 11–4 may be helpful in assisting the nurse with assessing the spiritual health of family units.

Recognizing that a spiritual assessment is not easy to discuss, one may consider the following points:

- Inquiries may be made in response to comments or statements made by family members.
- Questions may be asked based on observations made in the home (obvious religious pictures or literature).
- Dialogue may be stimulated through nonverbal communication, or in response to the ease or discomfort of responses.
- Every question does not need to be asked and additional questions relative to a particular topic may be added.
- A clear explanation should be provided by the nurse concerning the assessment process.

Throughout the assessment process, it is important to emphasize family members' strengths and not their weaknesses. Preaching or directing their lives is not of value at this time.

For some families, religion may serve as a source of strength, calm, inner peace, and guided direction. Others may be cool toward God, even

TABLE 11–3. FAMILY SPIRITUAL HEALTH

BENEFITS	FAMILY SPIRITUAL HEALTH RELATIONSHIPS
Goodness	Expands knowledge and enlightenment and bridges to church
Kindness	Integrates spiritual and social activities into corporate spiritual growth
Joy	Extends family values into the community
Love	Encourages personal/family time
Patience	Facilitates interaction between child and parent
Self-Control	Stimulates relationship of child with God
Faithfulness	Integrates spirituality into family process
Peace	Facilitates oneness with God

TABLE 11–4. FAMILY SPIRITUAL HEALTH ASSESSMENT

1. Is religion or a Supreme Being important to your family? What do you call your Supreme Being?
2. Do all your family members believe in the same Supreme Being?
3. Describe the relationship of each family member to God (Supreme Being).
4. What is your God like?
5. How do you communicate with your God?
6. How does God (Supreme Being) relate to your family and to each member?
7. What does faith mean to your family life and to each member?
8. How has your faith influenced your life?
9. Is there anything that has happened in your life or that of your family that has either separated you from or brought you close to God (Supreme Being)? Explain.
10. Where is the source of your hope?
11. To whom do you talk when in need of spiritual direction?
12. Are there any religious beliefs, practices, or rituals that are important to your family today?
13. Do you read scriptures or religious literature as a family or individually? If so, what do you read? Who reads the most?
14. Do you pray as a family? How often? Do you pray in silence or aloud? Do you pray for each other?
15. What happens when you pray? Does prayer benefit your family?
16. Are there any religious medals, jewelry, or statues that are important to your family?
17. Do you worship as a family or individually? How often do you attend?
18. What are your beliefs about death and life after death?
19. Do you worship as a family? How often do you attend?
20. Describe the value of worship to your family and to each member.
21. What relationship have you established at your place of worship?

Data from Carson, V.B. (1989). Spirituality and the nursing process. In V.B. Carson (Ed.), *Spiritual Dimensions of Nursing Practice* (pp. 150–179). Philadelphia: Saunders.

angry, questioning the nature of suffering, apparent abandonment, and death. No matter what the situation may be, family health practitioners are not to judge, condemn, or criticize a person's religious influence. Instead, the nurse's role is to provide an open ear and affirming support to assist family members.

Nursing Diagnosis

All the data and information the nurse is able to obtain—whether it be verbal, nonverbal, visible, situational, or through family relationships—will provide the necessary basis for accurate interpretation. It remains crucial that the nurse continually validate the information to prevent any false assessments, interpretations, or judgments. An open, reflective dialogue will facilitate this opportunity.

A common nursing diagnosis in the realm of family spiritual health is *spiritual distress* (Carpentino, 1991). This is a "state where an individual or group experiences or is at risk of experiencing a disturbance in the belief or value system that provides strength, hope and meaning to one's life" (pg. 264–265). The distress may be major or minor and related to pathophysiology, recommended treatment regimens, personal factors, or environmental factors.

The North American Nursing Diagnosis Association (Nanda) taxonomy has addressed the following three spiritual needs of an individual: (1) love and relatedness, (2) forgiveness, and (3) meaning and purpose. These identified needs, plus observations made from behavior responses, actions or reactions, and direct responses to questions, lead the nurses in making an appropriate nursing diagnosis.

Intervention

Just as intervention is necessary when a family is confronted with a physical or emotional situation, it is also valuable during times of spiritual distress, conflict, or when a spiritual leader is needed. The following are examples of situations where spiritual intervention is frequently needed:

- Baptism, confirmation, communion, or marriage of a family member
- Times of illness, loss, impending death or death
- Times of separation, divorce, parent/child problems, financial distress, and other distressing events
- Times of celebration, joy, and reunion when special religious events are in order

In the case studies at the beginning of the chapter, each case demonstrates the strength, guidance, calm, and peace that are stabilizing factors during times of turmoil, and spiritual intervention.

Intervention may begin through the process of caring and opening up lines of communication. In fact, when family members begin to acknowledge and verbalize their concerns, all they may need is permission to follow through in the manner in which they already believe to be correct. Each family is a unique unit, comprised of persons with individual beliefs, spiritual commitments, and ideas for the place of religion in their lives. There are multiple contributing factors that constitute the spiritual wholeness of each person. Some factors include personal relationships with others, cultural and ethic background, life experiences, influence by written materials or worship services, and personal prayer. Consequently, the spiritual profile of each family is quite detailed and unique as is their personal level and practice of faith.

In fact, this level and practice of faith, although different for each family member, may contribute to the perceived spiritual intervention for the family as a unit. Aden (1976) has identified the spiritual development of a family across the life span in relationship to faith. The author's applied definition of faith progresses from trust, courage, obedience, assent, and identity through adolescence to surrender, unconditional surrender, and unconditional acceptance, concluding in maturity (Aden, 1976).

Concomitant with the assessment process is the means by which family members can set priorities. In essence, establishing priorities is a matter of making choices regarding the importance of one's religion in daily activities, the commitment to prayer, the practice of worship, the pattern of daily scripture reading, the refocusing of one's lifestyle and example as set forth in religious teachings, and the commitment to live one's religious belief through action and not mere words.

As nurses begin to work with priority identification within the family, a process of goal setting might prove valuable. Personal goals can be designed by each family member in order to address his or her religious belief and its integration in each aspect of daily living.

Whether or not a nurse clinician is committed to a particular faith, he or she should be aware of the religious community resources available, including the availability of religious leaders, worship services, support services, and reading materials (Steiger & Lipson, 1985). Resources to consider with the family's or client's permission might include:

- Contacting chaplains within particular health facilities
- Intervening with the family's pastor, priest, or rabbi
- If a parish connection has not been established, locating houses of worship in the neighborhood
- Identifying available radio and television religious programming
- Informing family members of local religious bookstores

- Providing information concerning various churches and synagogues, related activities, support groups, or visitation services
- Inquiring about the availability of a parish nurse within a nearby congregation (where a nurse functions as a referral and resource service within a parish community)

Information provided in Table 11—1 can serve as a working tool for referral and reference purposes. It is helpful throughout the implementation process for the family health practitioner to recognize the meaning and value of each religion's sacraments, specific prayers, ceremonies, and specific printed resources. Each religion has its own book of scripture readings and resources relative to specific family needs and issues.

Frequently, a clinician can read from religious works as a means of offering guidance, support, understanding, and peace. Inquiring of an individual's favorite scripture or story might afford an opportunity for reading aloud. Some of the most valuable reading comes from the texts such as the book of *Psalms,* the *Bible,* the *Torah,* the *Koran,* and the *Book of Mormon.*

Ideas that might benefit the growth and intervention within a family structure, initiated by a parent might include the following:

- Selected scriptures or passages from such books as the *Bible,* the *Torah,* or the *Koran.*
- Inquire about verses or readings that might have a pertinent family value.
- Encourage family members to join in the religious readings.
- Read specific prayers from a prayer book, relevant to individual or family needs.
- Pray with or for the family or an individual related to particular requests or needs.
- Teach young children right and wrong based on religious tenets.
- Carry specific tapes of either musical or voice inspiration.
- Identify one's prayer requests to be shared with a prayer support group, prayer chain, a church, or a personal prayer group.
- Encourage families to become involved in scripture studies, home support, or fellowship groups and other spiritually fulfilling relationships.
- Introduce people to the purpose and value of prayer and spiritual journaling.
- Discuss moral and ethical issues with children.

Beckmann-Murray and Proctor-Zentner (1985) have identified specific practices or ideas that proved helpful for individuals from the Catholic, Protestant, and Jewish religions. The results of their questionnaire noted that for all three relig-

TABLE 11–5. SAMPLE LIST OF PRAYER AND MEDITATION BOOKS

Pastoral Care of the Sick and Dying (1984)
Office of Publishing Services
U.S. Catholic Conference
1312 Mass. Ave N.W.
Washington, D.C. 20005

Praying in the Catholic Tradition (1990)
Author: P. Schineller
Publisher: Liquori Publishing

Prayer Book for Young Catholics
Author: Fox
Publisher: Our Sunday Visitor

Prayer Handbook for Today's Catholic
Author: E. Tobin
Publisher: Liquori

Prayers That Avail Much
Publisher: Harrison House

Prayers for Children
Author: J. Hormen
Publisher: Viking Press

Prayers for the Very Young
Author: D. Roberts
Publisher: Concordia Press

Prayers of Jesus for Children
Author: I. Savary
Publisher: Regina Press

Miracle Hour: A Method of Prayer That Will Change Your Life
Author: Linda Schubert
Publisher: Linda Schubert
P.O. Box 4034
Santa Clara, CA 95056

Jewish Spiritual and Torah Meditations
Author: Rabbi Bernard Raskas
Publisher: Ktav Publishers

The Prayers of Islam
Author: Elijah Mohammod
Publisher: The Nation of Islam

Prayer*
Author: Spencer W. Kimball et. al.
Publisher: Deseret Book Co.

Hope*
Author: Ezra T. Benson et .al.
Publisher: Deseret Book Co.

*The Church of the Latter-Day Saints has only a few written prayers. These are primarily read with the sacraments. These two books by Mormon authors are for prayer and meditation.

ious, reading from the Bible, religious writings, and religious books and magazines were valuable in their spiritual growth, and praying using one's own words, praying with a religious leader, or praying aloud with a group was meaningful.

The sample list of prayer books provided in Table 11–5 might be helpful for family use.

Evaluation

It might be helpful to encourage individual and personal journaling as a reflective means by which the family health practitioner could evaluate the effectiveness and value of the spiritual intervention. Much of this awareness will be reflective of one's comfort in sharing and identifying personal feelings. It might also be helpful for an individual or family member to respond openly to questions, such as the following:

- How are we doing as a family?
- Are we openly and honestly addressing spiritual needs and challenges?
- Are we practicing what we have been taught and have read?
- How can we improve in love, reverence, forgiveness, and in our relationship with God (or a Supreme Being)?
- Have we been open and honest in our dialogue with our family health nurse?

These questions can be used reflectively as the nurse and the family or individual compare personal questions with previously established goals.

IMPLICATIONS FOR FAMILY NURSING PRACTICE

The family health nurse fulfills several roles. Each role is a valuable component in the relationship between nurse and family. Fostering a family's religiosity requires playing the role of a supporter and encourager, as well as incorporating listening, empathy, vulnerability, humility, and commitment (Fish & Shelly, 1985).

The Role of the Supporter and Encourager

One of the most valuable tools in a nurse's ability to meet spiritual needs simply is his or her presence. Personal contact has a physical, emotional, and spiritual effect. The relationship between nurse and client evolves over a period of time as each family member begins to develop a sense of trust and confidence in his or her nurse. As this relationship of trust matures, there is a shared opportunity for both nurse and family to be open and supportive, allowing the uniqueness of the family to be revealed. During this process the nurse can demonstrate support and encouragement while learning about the family's needs, desires, hopes, aspirations, wants, dreams, hurts, joys, and ambitions. At this time, the nurse is able to communicate personal spiritual strength and a sincere willingness to care, to listen, and to just be present with the family. The nurse's unspoken message of acceptance of a client as a unique spiritual being provides a wonderful opportunity for spiritual healing and wholeness.

Travelbee (1966, p. 17) expands on this belief:

The nurse possesses a profound understanding of the human condition. The nurse realizes that personal spiritual values, or philosophical beliefs about human beings, illness, and suffering will determine the extent to which he or she will be able to help others find meaning (or no meaning) in these situations.

Travelbee's approach and response calls nurses to continually self-examine their personal strength, limitations, motivations, and needs. It is through this development of self-knowledge that a nurse's presence is most able to be effective, and his or her ability to support and comfort others becomes a living reality.

The art and skill of fostering a family's religiosity requires the following essential elements: listening, empathy, vulnerability, humility, and commitment (Fish & Shelly, 1985).

The Role of the Listener

Good listeners know that it is both an art and a skill—that is, the learned response. The family nurse must be attentive with his or her eyes, ears, mind, and heart. Listening is an active skill, requiring both concentration and commitment.

Frequently, family members may hide their true feelings and may not speak openly regarding either fact or their personal feelings. In this way, they do not have to risk the embarrassment of dealing with their own pain or fears. Neither do they have to risk the chance of dealing with a negative or questioning response from the listener.

Frequently, lack of communication may be a result of existing barriers that prohibit the nurse from actively listening. Some barriers might include:

- Outside distractions that prevent the nurse from concentrating completely
- An inability to assess the individual's exact meaning of a word, comment, or body gesture
- The interjection of personal feelings or responses into the patient's conversation, thus preventing open, honest dialogue
- The formulation of specific responses or solutions while the other person is speaking, which interrupts the level of concentration required to hear exactly what is being said

It is important for the nurse to focus on his or her ability to be rather than to do, to listen rather than speak, to be open rather than judge. These qualities are valuable not only for the nurse, but for each member of the family.

The Role of the Empathizer

A nurse who has the gift of empathy has the ability to experience vicariously the feelings of another individual. It is crucial for a nurse to have the capability of putting specific feelings into

words and, at the same time, be able to remain objective during the process of seeking alternatives.

It is important to be able to distinguish between empathy and sympathy. Carson (1989) clarifies that with sympathy the listener is allowed to share in the feelings of another person, but in the process of sharing, the listener loses objectivity and is unable to differentiate between his or her feelings and those of the speaker. Empathy, on the other hand, allows the nurse to be present with his or her patients, to be supportive in an attempt to understand the patients' feelings, and to encourage the patient while they begin to examine their own alternatives. Thus, the nurse would not make the decision or process alternatives, but would work with and stay with the patient throughout this process.

If a nurse should find this process difficult, it might be of value to pray, in a manner consistent with your own beliefs, prior to visiting the patient. This may provide peace and wisdom.

The Role of Being Vulnerable

As part of the art of caring and the gift of empathy, the ability to be vulnerable allows the nurse to experience the feelings of the family (Watson, 1988). The nurse encourages each family member to deal realistically with his or her inner feelings. A nurse's vulnerability prevents him or her from remaining uninvolved, aloof, or judgmental. This affords the family additional strength, knowing they are not alone in making decisions and choosing alternatives that will facilitate them to move forward. The nurse can share in the patient's feelings of pain and abandonment, as well as their feelings of joy and anticipation.

Just as the nurse has received guidance, direction, and strength through prayer, he or she can make a personal reserve of strength, faith, and hope available to each individual member and the family unit as a whole.

The Role of Being Humble

It is through a knowledge and experience of humility that a nurse will come face-to-face with his or her own limitations. In fact, it is through one's limitations and weaknesses that God can most effectively work through an individual to assist others. In essence, an individual's pride is removed and the door is open for God's strength to prevail. It takes great humility and inner strength for someone to admit that he or she does not have all the answers, but that the necessary answers will be sought.

The gift of humility increases the level of faith and trust between nurse and client. Each accepts the other for who they are, not what they desire to become.

The Role of Commitment

Commitment is based on the availability of the nurse throughout the time the family needs support. To be committed to a nurse/client relationship requires that the nurse will be present through all stages of emotional and spiritual growth, and not abandon his or her client when the relationship becomes challenging or uncomfortable. This is especially true during the time of a terminal illness or even death. To be truly committed indicates a nurse's inner spiritual strength, which is passed on to the family.

A family health nurse who is involved in the spiritual well-being of each family may benefit from areas of individual spiritual renewal and freshment. Some of these opportunities might include:

- Joining a nurses' spiritual growth and support group, such as Nurses Christian Fellowship.
- Organizing or participating in a nurses' prayer support group.
- Subscribing to a journal (such as *Journal of Christian Nursing, Journal Transcultural Nursing* and *Journal of Multicultural Nursing and Health*).
- Participating in or organizing a "spiritual grand rounds" at your facility.
- Inquiring about the role and function of a parish nurse (a health minister for the congregation).

IMPLICATIONS FOR NURSING EDUCATION AND RESEARCH

The caring and spiritual dimension of nursing continues to pose areas of resistance and reluctance for many nurses, largely due to a lack of awareness, knowledge, assessment, and integration skills and support concepts (Leininger & Watson, 1990). In order for nursing to be more supportive in this area, some of the following ideas might be considered.

For education:

- Include spiritual assessment and its relationship to family healing and wholeness in the curriculum design.
- Establish student discussion and integration forums relating to spirituality in the family.
- Introduce case studies—both written and oral—in lab settings where the challenges and the opportunities are presented.
- Provide courses or specialist education in parish nursing.

For research:

- Develop and evaluate instruments to be used to measure spiritual concepts.

- Examine the relationship of nursing diagnosis indicators to physical health.
- Identify factors related to the development of spirituality throughout the life span.
- Identify factors that would encourage the nurse to provide spiritual care to families.
- Assess the effectiveness of nursing intervention on spiritual outcomes for patients.
- Identify the influence of religiosity on health care and outcomes.
- Evaluate both the negative and positive influence of religiosity on the health of families and individual members.

CHAPTER HIGHLIGHTS

The terms *religion* and *spirituality* are often used interchangeably, yet their meanings are not the same. Religion is the belief in a supernatural or divine force that has power over everything. Spirituality is a philosophical orientation regarding to relationships that produces behaviors and feelings of hope, love, trust, and faith which provide a meaning for existence.

The major religions are divided into three groups: group one (Christianity, Judaism and Islam), group two (Taoism Confucianism, Shintoism) and group three (Buddhist and Hinduism).

Religiosity may enhance family strengths by contributing to the formation of family beliefs and values, encouraging healthy behaviors and practices, providing social interactions with others, providing recreational interaction, and enhancing family coping during crises and transitions across the life span.

The effects of religion on the total health and well-being of the family unit include goodness, kindness, joy, love, patience, self-control, faithfulness, peace, affirmation, forgiveness, reverence for family life, support, and understanding.

The family health nurse should assess family religion and spirituality and help families to strengthen this trait.

The nurse's role in family spiritual health includes being humble, vulnerable, a supporter, an encourager, a listener, an empathizer, and committed to holistic family health promotion.

SUMMARY

For a family nurse practitioner to provide and be sensitive to the spiritual strength of families is a demonstration of the nurse's spiritual life. A nurse will demonstrate his or her gifts of kindness, love, gentleness, compassion, understanding, honesty, and patience throughout the assessment, intervention, and evaluation process. As nurses share these gifts with others, their qualities are strengthened within their own selves.

When nurses share themselves, they are fostering spirituality and serving as a bridge between the family and their perception of a higher strength and power.

REFERENCES

Abbott, D.A., Berry, M., & Meredith, W.H. (1990). Religious beliefs and practice. A potential asset in helping families. *Family Relations,* 39; 443–448.

Aden, L. (1976). Faith and the development cycle. *Pastoral Psychology,* 24(2), 215–230.

Batson, C., & Ventis, W. (1982). *The Religious Experience: A Social-Psychological Perspective.* New York: Oxford University Press.

Beitman, B.D. (1982). Pastoral counseling centers: A challenge to community mental health centers. *Hospital Community Psychiatry,* 33(3), 486.

Belgum, D. (Spring 1992). Guilt and/or self-esteem as consequences of religion. *Journal of Religion and Health,* 31(1), 84.

Bomar, P. (1995, October). A comparison of rural and urban African-American women: Factors influencing adherence to health promoting lifestyle. Paper presented at North American Congress on Women's Health Issues. Galveston, TX.

Brigman, K.M. (1992). Religion and family strengths: Implications for mental health professionals. *Topics in Family Psychology and Counseling,* 1(1), 39–52.

Brigman, K.M., & Keating, B.R. (1989). Religious attitudes and family strengths: Examining the relationship. Unpublished paper.

Bronson-Gray, B. (1992). Kids in crisis. *Nurse Week,* 5(16), 8–13.

Brunner, L. (1984). The spiritual dimension of holistic care. *Imprint,* 4, 44–45.

Byrd, R. (1986). Cardiologist studies: Effect of prayer on patients. *Brain/Mind Bulletin,* 11(7), 1.

Carpentino, L. J. (1991). *Handbook of Nursing Diagnosis.* (4th ed.). Philadelphia: Lippincott.

Carson, V. (1989). *Spiritual dimensions of nursing practice.* Philadelphia: Saunders.

Cavanagh, M. (1983). the impact of psychosexual growth on marriage and religious life. *Human Development* 4,(3), 16–24.

Curran, D. (1976). *Grist for the Mill* (p. 12). Santa Cruz, CA: Unity Press.

Dass, R. W. (1976). *Grist for the Mill.* Santa Cruz, CA: Unity Press.

Dossey, L. (1989). *Mind beyond Body.* New York: Bantam Press.

Douglas, J.D., et al. (1982). *New Bible Dictionary* (2nd ed). Wheaton, IL: Tyndale House Publishers.

Fish, S., & Shelly, J. (1985). *Spiritual Care: The Nurse's Role.* Downers Grove, IL: Inter-Varsity Press.

Fowler, J.W. (1974). Toward a developmental perspective on faith. *Religious Education* 69(2), 207–219.

Gilbert K. (1992). Religion as a resource for bereaved parents. *Journal of Religion and Health,* 31(1), 20.

Guralnik, D. (Ed.) (1972). *Webster's New Word Dictionary of the American Language* (2nd college ed). New York: World Publishing.

Hill, L., & Smith, N. (1990). *Self-Care Cursing: Promotion of Health.* Norwalk, CT: Appleton & Lange.

Jourard, S.M. (1968). *Disclosing Man to Himself.* Princeton, NJ: Van Nostrand, 1968.

Kavanaugh, R. (1972). *Facing Death* (p. 12). New York: Penguin,

Labum, E. (1988). Spiritual Care: An element in nursing care planning. *Journal of Advanced Nursing,* 13, 314–320.

Leininger, N. & Watson, J. (1990). *The caring imperative in education.* New York: National League for Nursing.

Lockyer, H. (1986). *Nelson's Illustrated Bible Dictionary* (p. 907). New York: Thomas Nelson Publishers.

Maslow, A. (1968). *Toward a Psychology of Being.* (p. 112). New York: Van Nostrand Reinhold.

Meagher, P.K., O'Brien, T., Aherne, C.A. (1979). *Encyclopedic Dictionary of Religion.* Washington, DC: Corpus.

Murray, R.B. & Zentner, J.P. (1985). Religious influences on the person. In R. B. Murray & J.P. Zentner *Nursing Concepts for Health Promotion* (3d ed). (p. 475). Englewood Cliffs, Nj: Prentice Hall.

Newman, M. (1989). The spirit of nursing. *Holistic Nursing Practice,* 3, 1–6.

Okamoto, A. (1976). Religious barriers to world peace. *Journal of Religion and Health,* 15(1), 26–33.

Olson, D.H., McCubbin, H.I., Barnes, H.L., Larsen, A.S., Muxen, M.J., & Wilson, M.C. (1983). *Families: What Makes Them Work.* Beverly Hills: Sage.

Olson, D.H., McCubbin, H.I., Barnes, H.L., Larsen, A.S., Muxen, M.J., & Wilson, M.C. (1982). *Family Interventions.* St. Paul, MN: University of Minnesota.

Paterson, J.G., & Zderad, L.T. (1976). *Humanistic Nursing* (p. 7). New York: John Wiley & Sons.

Pearsall, P. (1990). *Power of the Family* (p. 185). New York: Bantam.

Perry, J.P. (1990). The formation of a society on Virginia's Eastern shore. In G.F. Moran (Ed.), *Religion, Family, and Life Course* (pp. 1615–1655). Ann Arbor, MI: Michigan University Press.

Powe, B. D. (1995). Cancer fatalism: A predictor of colorectal cancer screening among elderly African Americans. In J. E. Wang (Ed.). *Proceedings of the Second International Interdisciplinary Health Research Symposium.* (pp. 71–78). Morgantown: University of West Virginia, School of Nursing.

Schroeder, A. (1993). Emotional and spiritual support. In. T.C. Kravis, C.G. Warner, & L. Jacobs (Eds.), *Emergency Medicine: A Comprehensive Review* (3rd ed.). New York: Raven Press.

Schumm, W.R., Hatch, R.C., & Schumm, K.R. (1990). Family strengths project: Preliminary data report. Paper presented at Family Strengths Conference, Washington, DC.

Shafranske, E.P., & Maloney, H.N. (1990). Clinical psychologists religious and spiritual orientations and their practice of psychotherapy. *Psychotherapy,* 27(1), 72–78.

Steiger, N.J., & Lipson, J.C. (1985). Psychological and spiritual well-being. In N.J. Steiger & J.C. Lipson (Eds.), *Self-Care Nursing:Theory and Practice* (pp. 208–235). Bowie, Md: Brady Communications.

Stinnett, N. (1981). In search of strong families. In N. Stinnett, B. Chesser, & J. DeFrain (Eds.), *Building Family Strengths: Blueprints for Action*. Lincoln, NE: University of Nebraska Press.

Stoll, R. (1979). Guidelines for spiritual assessment. *American Journal of Nursing,* 79 1574–1577.

Taylor, P.B., & Ferszt, G.G. (1990). Spiritual healing, *Holistic Nursing Practice,* 4(4), 32–38.

Travelbee, J. (1966). *Interpersonal Aspects of Nursing.* Philadelphia: F.A. Davis.

Watson, J. (1988). *Nursing science and human care: A theory of nursing.* New York: National League for Nursing.

Westerhoff, J. (1976). *Will Our Children Have Faith?* New York: Seabury Press.

ADDITIONAL READINGS

Caine, R. (1991). Incorporating CARE into caring for families in crisis. *AACN Clinical Issues in Critical Care Nursing,* 2, 236–241. the word CARE is an acronym for four basic behaviors identified by the author as a foundation for humanistic concern. These are communication, advocacy, reciprocity, and empathy.

Fitchett, G. (1993). *Assessing Spiritual Needs: A Guide For Caregivers.* Minneapolis, MN: Augsburg.

Mayer, J. (1992). Wholly Responsible for a Part, or Partly Responsible for a Whole. *Second Opinion,* 17(3), 26–55.

Mentgen, J., & Trapp-Bulbrook, M.J. *Healing Touch.* (1994). Carrboro, NC: North Caroline Center for Healing Touch.

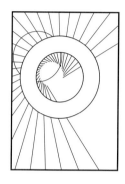

UNIT III

Family Health
Nursing Process

FAMILY HEALTH ASSESSMENT AND INTERVENTION

12

SHIRLEY M.H. HANSON
and KAREN B. MISCHKE

Every family, in its own way, is an unexplored mystery.

HENRYK J. SOLALSKI

OBJECTIVES

On completion of this chapter, the reader will be able to:

1. Explain the family nursing process and the family as client
2. Discuss the steps of the family nursing process (nursing diagnosis, nursing goals, and nursing outcomes)
3. Identify the components of contracting with families for family health care
4. Discuss the Neuman Systems Model
5. Describe the Family Systems Stressor-Strength Inventory (FS^{3}I)
6. Suggest clinical situations where the model and assessment/measurement instrument can be applied

INTRODUCTION

There are many ways to conceptualize families that serve as a basis for family nursing assessment and intervention (Clemen-Stone et al., 1991; Helvie, 1991; Bullough & Bullough, 1990; Hanson & Boyd, 1996). Three traditional approaches (Nye & Berardo, 1981) that have been used by family social scientists are developmental (Duvall, 1977), structural-functional (Bales, 1950; Parsons, 1951), and symbolic interaction (Burgess, 1926; Mead, 1934). Three approaches used by nursing include viewing the family as a system, as the context for individual development, as a component of society, and as a client (Hanson & Boyd, 1996).

The family as a system is the conceptual framework used by Friedman (1992), Ross and Cobb (1990), and Neuman (1980, 1982, 1989). They view the family as a living social system and support the notion that an adequate understanding of its members can only be gained when individuals are viewed within the context of their families. Therefore, family nursing assessment and intervention are directed both toward the family as

client and toward the family as context. Miller and Janosik (1980), building on systems theory, view the family as a social system composed of a structural complex of elements. These elements are related in such a way that patterns are formed between the elements. "The family is characterized by wholeness, nonsummativity and equifinality" (p. 14). Using this family conceptualization, nurses address the dimensions of family structure and family function.

Wright and Leahey (1994) also build on general systems theory and expand the conceptualization of the family to include categories of family structure and family process, together with individual and family development. Nursing assessment and intervention strategies are built on the application of systems theory, communication theory, and developmental theory to family structure and process.

A comparison of the Family Assessment and Intervention Model and the Family Systems Stressor Strength Inventory discussed in detail in this chapter and the Friedman's Family Assessment Model and Form and the Calgary Family Assessment Model (CFAM) have been presented elsewhere. Readers are referred to Hanson & Kaakinen (1996) and Hanson & Boyd (1996).

The family assessment process described in this chapter provides an opportunity for families and caregivers to acquire relevant information from which to develop individually tailored plans for promotive and protective health care. The family as the primary social structure within society provides the context in which family members learn and practice health-promoting behaviors (Pender, 1987; Pender et al., 1992). Families have the primary responsibility for (1) developing self-care competencies in individual members; (2) providing sufficient social and physical resources for each member; (3) facilitating autonomy and individuality of family members; and (4) promoting family behaviors that are undertaken to increase the family's well-being and quality of life. The responsibility for maintaining and enhancing health should be an integral part of the family lifestyle (Pender et al., 1992; Houldin et al., 1987; Clemen-Stone, et al., 1991; Mauksch, 1974; Anderson & Tomlinson, 1992).

ASSESSMENT IN FAMILY NURSING PRACTICE

Nurses are taught to recognize that each individual is a unified whole: People exist as individuals and as members of a family within the larger context of the community. Most nurses embrace the notion that nursing is family centered, even though the family as the unit of service for client assessment and intervention is a relatively new concept to the nursing profession (Berkey & Hanson, 1991; Wright & Leahey, 1994). Little documentation exists relative to the family-centered nature of actual family nursing practice or what is included in family nursing practice (Speer & Sachs, 1985). For example, until the past decade, there has been a limited focus on family health promotion and prevention as specific family needs (Anderson & Tomlinson, 1992; Pender, 1987).

In the past, numerous deterrents prohibited nurses from instituting family-centered health promotion and prevention activities. The lack of time, organizational support, economic incentives, and knowledge about family assessment were but a few of the obstacles to implementing family health approaches (Speer & Sachs, 1985). However, as insurmountable as these obstacles appear to be, it is vitally important to conduct family assessments since the information obtained greatly influences family nursing practice. As the nursing profession progresses into the 21st century, it must continue to broaden its scope of practice and include the entire family in the assessment, diagnosis, intervention, and evaluation process (Hanson & Boyd, 1996; Hanson & Kaakinen, 1996; Hanson et al., 1992; Hanson & Heims, 1992; Gilliss, 1991; Whall & Fawcett, 1991; Gilliss et al., 1989; Murphy, 1986; Bell et al., 1990).

FAMILY ASSESSMENT INSTRUMENTATION

Webster defines "assess" in the following way: to determine the amount of, importance of, or value of an outcome. In this context, assessment is neither instantaneous nor static but is a continuous, evolving process. "In theory and practice, assessment is a means by which the assessor, by drawing on the past and the present, is able to predict or plan for the future" (Braden & Herban, 1976, p. 63).

There are a number of sophisticated family assessment/measurement instruments described in the literature (Hanson & Boyd, 1996; Hanson & Kaakinen 1996; Berkey & Hanson, 1991; Filsinger, 1983; Forman & Hagan, 1984; Humenick, 1982; McCubbin & Thompson, 1987; Olson et al., 1983; Strauss & Brown, 1978). These instruments have been developed and used by psychologists, sociologists, social workers, family life professionals, and marriage and family practitioners and applied to clients in their respective fields. Each of these helping professionals use the measurement instruments with specific foci and purposes in mind (Speer & Sachs, 1985). For example, the primary concern of sociologists has been marital satisfaction, decision making, and role delineation. Psychologists have focused on the interactional patterns of parents and children (Patterson, 1971). Social workers have emphasized parental coping abilities (Hurwitz et al., 1965), and marriage and family clinicians have focused on marital/family dysfunction (Speer & Sachs, 1985). Most of these instruments applicable to the therapeutic domain are nonnursing in nature, and although they may be valid and reliable, they do not always demonstrate a clear relevance to nursing. The primary reasons are that the family assessment perspective has been closely aligned with individual disciplines (Speer & Sachs, 1985) and the measurement implementation has been used to quantify a particular aspect of family health for research purposes.

Several nurse academicians have developed instruments and/or assessment tools that can be used with families (Berkey & Hanson, 1989; Clemen-Stone et al., 1991; Feetham, 1983; Freidman, 1992; Hanson, 1985, 1986, 1996; Pender, 1987; Pender et al., 1992; Stanhope & Lancaster, 1992; Wright & Leahey, 1994). These assessment tools, like those developed in the social and behavioral sciences, have strengths and weaknesses. One limitation attributed particularly to the nursing tools is that of psychometric validation. Nursing family assessment instruments for the most part are not psychometrically sound nor have they as yet been thoroughly field tested. As a consequence, nurses have looked outside of their discipline for valid and reliable family assessment instruments. Table 12–1 summarizes selected nursing and nonnursing assessment instruments. The reader is referred also to the References for more detail. Criteria for the selection of instruments are contained in Table 12–2. The Family Assessment/Intervention instrument discussed in this chapter is another effort to design a tool for assessing and measuring family health.

DEFINITION OF FAMILY

Numerous definitions for the family unit are found in the literature (Helvie, 1991; Neuman, 1989; Spradley, 1990; Duvall, 1977; Hill & Han-sen, 1960). The definition of family adopted for this chapter is from the Neuman Systems Model. It addresses the membership of the system, the relationship of the members to each other, and the factors of commitment and caring that make relationships meaningful. Neuman states (1982), "The family as a system . . . is composed of individual family members harmonious in their relationships—a cluster of related meanings and values that govern the family and keep it viable in a constantly changing environment" (p. 241). It consists of a "group of two or more persons who create and maintain a common culture; its most central goal is one of continuance" (Neuman, 1982, p. 241).

When placed in the context of a systems framework, this definition appears to develop a life of its own—one that is rich in meanings, values, movement, and identifiable relationship patterns (Berkey & Hanson, 1991).

TABLE 12–1. SELECTED FAMILY ASSESSMENT AND MEASUREMENT INSTRUMENTS*

DEVELOPED BY NONNURSES

Name: A-FILE
Purpose: Adolescent-family inventory of life events and changes
Source: Olson, Sprenkle, & Russell (1979)
            Olson, Bell, & Portner (1980)
            Olson, Russell, & Sprenkle (1980)
            Olson, et al. (1982, 1983)
            Olson & Portner (1983)

Name: DYADIC ADJUSTMENT SCALE
Purpose: Measure marital adjustment
Source: Spanier & Filsinger (1983)

Name: ENRICH
Purpose: Enriching and nurturing family relationship; communication and happiness
Source: Olson, Sprenkle, & Russell (1979)
            Olson, Bell, & Portner (1980)
            Olson, Russell, & Sprenkle (1980)
            Mountain (1982)
            Olsen et al. (1982, 1983)
            Olson & Portner (1983)

Name: FAMILY ADAPTABILITY AND COHESION EVALUATION SCALE (FACES I)
Purpose: Family interactions as a system of behavior; cohesion and adaptability
Source: Olson, Sprenkle, & Russell (1979)
            Olson, Bell, & Portner (1980)
            Olson, Russell, & Sprenkle (1980)
            Olsen et al. (1982, 1983)
            Olson & Portner (1983)
            Speer & Sachs (1985)

Name: FAMILY ADAPTABILITY AND COHESION EVALUATION SCALE (FACES III)
Purpose: Shortened version of FACES I and II: Family satisfaction; parent-adolescent communication
Source: Olson, Portner, & Lavee (1985)
            Olson, Sprenkle, & Russell (1979)
            Olson, Bell, & Portner (1980)
            Olson, Russell, & Sprenkle (1980)
            Olsen et al. (1982, 1983)
            Olson & Portner (1983)
            Speer & Sachs (1985)

Table continued on following page

TABLE 12.1 SELECTED FAMILY ASSESSMENT AND MEASUREMENT INSTRUMENTS (continued)

Name:	FAMILY APGAR
Purpose:	Family functioning: adaptability, partnership, growth; affection, and resolve
Source:	Smilkstein (1978)
	Good et al. (1979)
	Smilkstein, Ashworth, & Montano (1982)
	Speer & Sachs (1985)
Name:	(MCMASTER) FAMILY ASSESSMENT DEVICE (FAD)
Purpose:	Family health: problem solving, communication, roles, affective responsiveness, affective involvement, behavior control, and general functioning
Source:	Epstein, Baldwin, & Bishop (1983)
	Speer & Sachs (1985)
Name:	FAMILY ENVIRONMENT SCALE (FES)
Purpose:	Family environment: relationships, personal growth, system maintenance and change
Source:	Moos (1974)
	Moos & Moos (1983)
	Speer & Sachs (1985)
Name:	FAMILY FUNCTIONING INDEX (FFI)
Purpose:	Multidimensional complexities of family functioning: communication, togetherness, closeness, decision making, child orientation
Source:	Pless & Satterwhite (1973)
	Speer & Sachs (1985)
Name:	FAMILY INVENTORY OF LIFE EVENTS (FILE)[*]
Purpose:	Normative and nonnormative family stress over one year
Source:	McCubbin & Patterson (1983)
	McCubbin & Thompson (1987)
Name:	FAMILY STRENGTHS
Purpose:	Family strengths
Source:	Olson et al. (1983)
Name:	F-COPES
Purpose:	Family coping strategies
Source:	Olson, Sprenkle, & Russell (1979)
	Olson, Bell, & Portner (1980)
	Olson, Russell, & Sprenkle (1980)
	Olson et al. (1982, 1983)
Name:	HOME OBSERVATION FOR MEASUREMENT OF THE ENVIRONMENT
Purpose:	Parameters within the home that nurture development of infants and children
Source:	Caldwell & Bradley (1970)
	Bradley (1982)
	Calloway (1982)
Name:	INVENTORY OF FAMILY FEELINGS (IFF)
Purpose:	Family's affective structure; delineates patterns of conflict, relationships, and alliances; positive/negative feelings toward each member
Source:	Margolin & Fernandez (1983)
	Lowman (1980)
	Speer & Sachs (1985)
Name:	QUALITY OF LIFE
Purpose:	Quality of life
Source:	Olson et al. (1983)
Name:	STRUCTURAL FAMILY INTERACTION SCALE (SFIS)
Purpose:	Minuchin's theory of family functioning; enmeshment; disengagement; neglect/overprotection; rigidity/flexibility; conflict/avoidance; patient management; triangulation of parent/child coalition; detouring
Source:	Perosa, Hansen, & Perosa (1981)
	Speer & Sachs (1985)

DEVELOPED BY NURSES

Name:	CALGARY FAMILY ASSESSMENT MODEL (CFAM)
Purpose:	Assess families using family structure, family development, functional assessment
Source:	Wright & Leahey (1994)

TABLE 12.1 SELECTED FAMILY ASSESSMENT AND MEASUREMENT INSTRUMENTS (continued)

Name:	CHRONICITY IMPACT AND COPING INSTRUMENT; PARENT QUESTIONNAIRE (CICI:PQ)
Purpose:	Parental perceptions of stressors; problematic situations or resources; parent's coping strategies for managing stressors
Source:	Hymovich (1983)
	Speer & Sachs (1985)
Name:	FAMILY ASSESSMENT GUIDE
Purpose:	Assess families in the community
Source:	Clemen-Stone, Eigsti, & McGuire (1991)
Name:	(The) FAMILY ASSESSMENT TOOL
Purpose:	Assessment guide for school nurses; family perception, health interview, family history
Source:	Holt & Robinson (1979)
Name:	FAMILY ASSESSMENT TOOL: FAMILY HEALTH CARE PLAN
Purpose:	Assess families for purpose of planning health care: family health care plan, family-community health nurse contract, health assessment guide, family problem-solving guide
Source:	Stanhope & Lancaster (1992)
Name:	FAMILY COPING INDEX
Purpose:	Assess nursing needs of family and determine level of coping; physical independence, therapeutic independence, knowledge of condition, principles of personal hygiene, attitude toward health care, emotional competence, family living patterns, physical environment, use of community resources
Source:	Freeman & Heinrich (1981)
Name:	FAMILY HEALTH INVENTORY
Purpose:	Measure physical and mental health of individuals in families
Source:	Hanson (1985)
	Hanson (1986)
Name:	FAMILY HEALTH PROMOTION-PROTECTION PLAN
Purpose:	Assessment of family health status and the development of a plan to improve health behavior
Source:	Pender (1987)
	Pender, Barkauskas, Hayman, Rice, & Anderson (1992)
Name:	FAMILY SYSTEMS STRESSOR STRENGTH INVENTORY (FS^3I)
Purpose:	Assessment and measurement of family stressors and strengths. Includes a family care plan schematic
Source:	Berkey & Hanson (1991)
Name:	FEETHAM FAMILY FUNCTIONING SURVEY (FFFS)
Purpose:	Measures parent's perception of relationships among family members and their abilities to function in the outside world
Source:	Roberts & Feetham (1982)
	Feetham & Humenick (1982)
	Speer & Sachs (1985)
Name:	FRIEDMAN FAMILY ASSESSMENT MODEL
Purpose:	Assess families suing structural-function framework: developmental stage, family history, family structure, family functions, family coping, family health
Source:	Friedman (1992)

*See references related to family nursing measurement, particularly Berkey & Hanson (1991).

GENERAL SYSTEMS THEORY AND THE NEUMAN SYSTEMS MODEL

Neuman (1980, 1982, 1989) and others (Feetham, 1983, 1990; Wright & Leahey, 1994; Ross & Cobb, 1990) believe that general systems theory provides a framework that is useful in assessing the large number of variables, relationships, and developments that occur within family units. Systems theory helps nurses conceptualize appropriate nursing actions that are applicable to family health and assists them with the identifica-

tion of parameters that contribute to and detract from healthy family functioning.

The Neuman Systems Model contains concepts that can be applied to the family, the health care provider, and the health care system (Neuman, 1989). These concepts help to identify actual and potential family health problems as well as problems surrounding the delivery of needed family services. The concepts adopted from the Neuman Systems Model, which was originally designed for individuals and modified for use with the family system, are client; basic structure; flexible line of

TABLE 12–2. CRITERIA FOR SELECTING FAMILY ASSESSMENT INSTRUMENTS

In selecting family assessment instruments, nurses need to be cognizant of parameters that contribute to the instruments' effectiveness. These parameters are (1) understandability, (2) administration and scoring, (3) reliability and validity, (4) client appropriateness, and (5) clinical relevance (Speer & Sachs, 1985).

The instruments selected for assessment of family health must be clear, uncomplicated, and easily understood. The questions need to be worded at a grade level that family members with poor reading skills and/or limited vocabularies can comprehend. Speer & Sachs (1985) suggest the reading level be set at a sixth grade level.

Families are more likely to complete assessment instruments, and nurses are more apt to use them if they can be administered in a short time period. To be useful in busy clinics, 15 or 20 minutes is probably the maximum amount of time that nurses and families can devote to this process. Another factor worth considering is the *ease of scoring* and the length of time involved in interpreting results.

Reliability and validity, the third area for consideration when selecting a family assessment tool, involves judgment about the instrument's consistency and whether or not the results honestly reflect what the tool is attempting to measure. It is important that the tool be both valid and reliable.

In order for an assessment instrument to be effective, it needs to be constructed in such a way that the questions are *appropriate* for the majority of families. The composition of words, phrases, and concepts should not be geared to a particular social class, age group, or ethnic background. The questions need to be universal in scope. They must also address topics the family deems reasonable and appropriate, or the family may hesitate to participate.

The last area to consider is the clinical relevance of the instrument. Nurses need assessment tools that assist them with gathering relevant clinical material. If the tool is easy to understand, administer, and score but is not relevant, it is ineffectual. Speer and Sachs (1985), Berkey & Hanson (1991), and Neuman (1989) supported the notion that family health measurement tools must focus on those areas of need for which nursing interventions may be planned.

defense; normal line of defense; lines of resistance; stressors; degree of reaction; primary, secondary, and tertiary prevention; reconstitution; and intrapersonal, interfamily, and extrafamily factors. Each of these concepts is defined by Neuman (1989) and elaborated on the authors (Table 12–3).

Concepts from the model related to the nurse or health care providers include primary prevention, secondary prevention, tertiary prevention, nursing diagnosis, and the profession of nursing. Additional concepts applicable to the family but not specifically defined by Neuman are health, health promotion, wellness, and illness.

Neuman Systems Model Basic Assumptions

The basic assumptions inherent within the Neuman Systems Model relate to an individual client as a system, or to a group of any size as client (Neuman, 1989, pp. 17, 21–22). For purposes of clarity and focus the authors have designated the concept family as the *client*. The following assumptions, termed *propositions* by Fawcett (1989), define, describe, and link the concepts of the model.

- Though each family as a family system is unique, each system is a composite of common, known factors or innate characteristics within a normal, given range of response contained within a basic structure.
- Many known, unknown, and universal environmental stressors exist. Each differs in its potential for disturbing a family's usual stability level, or normal line of defense. The particular interrelationships of family variables—physiologic, psychological, sociocultural, developmental, and spiritual—at any time can affect the degree to which a family is protected by the flexible line of defense against possible reaction to one or more stressors.

- Over time, each family/family system has evolved a normal range of response to the environment, referred to as a normal line of defense, or usual wellness/stability state.

- When the cushioning, accordion-like effect of the flexible line of defense is no longer capable of protecting the family/family system against an environmental stressor, the stressor breaks through the normal line of defense. The interrelationships of variables—physiologic, psychological, sociocultural, developmental, and spiritual—determine the nature and degree of the system reaction or possible reaction to the stressor.

- The family, whether in a state of wellness or illness, is a dynamic composite of the interrelationships of variables—physiologic, psychological, sociocultural, developmental, and spiritual. Wellness is on a continuum of available energy to support the family in its optimal state.

- Implicit within each family system is a set of internal resistance factors, known as lines of resistance, which function to stabilize and return the family to the usual wellness state

TABLE 12–3. CONCEPTS AND DEFINITIONS

CONCEPTS OF HEALTH CARE SYSTEM MODEL	CONCEPTS DEFINED BY NEUMAN	CONCEPTS ADOPTED BY MISCHKE-BERKEY, WARNER, HANSON
1. Client		System: Individual, family, group, or community units of society. Each unit functions as a whole and contains the elements of basic structure, normal line of defense, and lines of resistance (Johnson et al., 1982; Neuman, 1989).
a. Individual		a. Individual: Smallest living member or unit of society.
b. Family	A group of two or more persons who create and maintain a common culture; its most central goal is one of continuance (Neuman, 1983, pp. 241).	b. Family: A group of two or more individuals who create and maintain a common culture harmonious in their relationship and possess meanings and values that govern the family and keep it viable in a constantly changing environment. A group of individuals closely related by blood, marriage or friendship ties (nuclear family, cohabitating couple, single parent, blended families, etc.). May be characterized by commitment, mutual decision making, and shared goals.
c. Community		A collection of people organized as a social system that develops and uses in common some agencies and institutions and that shares a physical environment (Moe, 1977).
2. Basic Structure	Basic physiologic, psychological, sociocultural, developmental and spiritual factors that are common to all human beings (Neuman, 1989, p. 29).	Characteristics, functions, energy resources, and interactive patterns common to the family system that are influenced by physiologic, psychologic, sociocultural, and spiritual characteristics of the family members. Family's state of wellness designated by health care activities initiated by the individual and family that seek to promote and expand positive potential for health behaviors (Pender, 1987).
3. Flexible Line of Defense	Dynamic state of wellness; individual's current state, which is particularly vulnerable to situational or maturational crises. Can be viewed as a protective buffer for preventing stressors or tensions from breaking through normal line of defense. Factors such as loss of sleep, undernutrition, developmental state (Neuman, 1982, p. 15).	It encompasses the dynamic level of family health attained following a temporary response to problems, perceived situational and maturational crises impinging on the system (Johnson et al., 1989).
4. Normal Line of Defense	State of wellness; what the "individual has become over time or his so-called 'normal' range of responses which maintains his stability, e.g., lifestyle, coping patterns" (Neuman, 1982, p. 12).	Family's state of wellness over time and the process of adaptations members consider "normal" for family unit.
5. Lines of Resistance	Resistant factors or forces that attempt to stabilize individual and return him or her to normal line of defense should a stressor break through it (Neuman, 1982, p. 12.)	Factors or forces within the family system that are activated to protect/preserve the stability of its basic structure subsequent to the stress impactor penetrating the family's normal line of defense (Johnson et al., 1982; Neuman, 1989).

Table continued on following page

TABLE 12–3. CONCEPTS AND DEFINITIONS (continued)

6. Stressor	Any problem, condition, etc., capable of causing instability of the system by penetration of the normal line of defense; can be viewed as intra,,- inter-, or extrapersonal in nature (Neuman, 1982, p. 14). "Stressors are neutral until the outcome effects determine their real nature as positive or negative" (Neuman, 1987).	Any problem, condition, or situation capable of causing family system instability by penetrating any of the family's lines of defense. The problem, condition, or situation as an impactor can be intra-, inter-, or extrafamily in nature. Outcome effects determine whether or not condition or situation is positive or negative (Neuman, 1987).
7. Degree of Reaction	Amount of system instability caused by a stressor penetrating through the normal line of defense (Neuman, 1982, p. 15).	Amount of family system instability caused by stress impactor penetration through any of the family lines of defense. It is demonstrated in amounts of tension.
8. Reconstitution	The system attempts to resolve impact of a stressor. Moves from the deepest degree of reaction back toward the normal line of defense; may reconstitute to a level higher or lower than penetration (Neuman, 1982, p. 13).	Restoring family functions that have been impaired as a result of the family's response to the problem or situation penetrating the lines of defense (Johnson et al., 1982; Neuman, 1989).
9. Factors/Forces	Factors considered related to stressors, reactions, and reconstitution.	Factors/forces that designate the level of penetration by stress/problem on the family system, the degree of reaction, and the family's adaptation to it.
10. Health	"Health or wellness is the condition in which all parts and subparts (variables) are in harmony with the whole of man" (Neuman, 1982, p. 9).	Health is the actualization of inherent and acquired human potential through satisfying relationships with self, family, and others; it is goal-directed behavior that includes competent personal and family care while adjustments are made as needed to maintain system stability and structural integrity (Fishbein & Ajzen, 1975).
11. Health Promotion	"A goal inherent within primary prevention concept; primarily nursing action is one of education with a specific goal outcome and support mechanisms to continue the health promoted" (Neuman, 1987).	Consists of specific health care activities directed toward increasing the level of well-being and actualizing the health potential of individuals, families, and communities (Pender, 1987).
12. Illness	"A state of insufficiency—disrupting needs are yet to be satisfied" (Neuman, 1982, p. 10).	Illness for the family and its subsystems is defined in terms of its variance from wellness. There has been a decrease in the systems ability to function at a high level of wellness because of stressors penetrating its basic structure and normal line of offense and defense.
13. Wellness Activities	"Wellness is a state of saturation—one of inertness free of disrupting needs." Nursing acts to move organism toward wellness (Neuman, 1982, p. 10).	Family or nurse actions instituted to promote and expand family's positive potential for health.
14. Interventions	Prevention as intervention format is conceptualized as modes for facilitating integrative processes necessary to attain/maintain stability and integrity of the client/client system (Neuman, 1982, p. 19).	Interventions: Family or nurse actions institute to modify and/or regulate the family system's potential for health-promoting activities and/or actual response to stress impactors (Johnson et al., 1982; Neuman, 1982).
a. Primary prevention	"Relates to general knowledge that is applied to individual patient assessment in an attempt to identify and allay the possible risk factors associated with stressors" (Neuman, 1982, p. 12).	Relates to general knowledge applied to family assessment in an attempt to identify and allay the possible risk factors associated with the stress impactors' penetration of the family's flexible line of defense.
b. Secondary prevention	"Relates to the symptomatology, appropriate ranking of interventions, priorities, and treatment" (Neuman, 1982, p. 14).	Relates to treating family system responses subsequent to the stress impactor penetrating the family's normal line of defense (Johnson et al., 1982; Neuman, 1989).

TABLE 12–3. CONCEPTS AND DEFINITIONS (continued)

c. Tertiary prevention	"Relates to the adaptive process as reconstitution begins, and moves back in a circular manner toward primary prevention" (Neuman, 1982, p. 14).	Relates to the healing restoration of those functions that have been impaired as a result of the family system's response to the stressor penetrating the normal line of defense (Johnson et al., 1982; Neuman, 1989).
15. Nursing Diagnosis	Acquiring an appropriate database in order to objectively determine variances from wellness. From this determination, relevant nursing goals can be established . . . analytic outcomes can be accomplished through purposeful interventions using one or more of these prevention modes (Neuman, 1982, p. 19).	Conceptual definition: The family system's potential to initiate health-promoting activities or stabilize family's actual response to identified potential and actual stress impactors (Johnson et al., 1982; Neuman, 1989). Operational definition: Nursing diagnostic statement contains three parameters: (1) family system's health-promoting behaviors, (2) family system's response to potential or actual tension-producing stress impactor, and (3) family system's identification of tension-producing stress impactor (Johnson et al., 1982; Neuman, 1989).
16. Nurse	The nurse assists individuals, families, and groups to attain and maintain a total wellness by purposeful interventions aimed at reduction of stress factors and adverse conditions that affect optimal functioning in a given patient situation (Neuman, 1982, p. 19).	The nurse assists individuals, families, and groups to attain and maintain a total wellness by purposeful interventions aimed at encouraging health promotion behavior and reducing stress factors and adverse conditions that affect optimal functioning in a given patient situation.
17. Nursing	Nursing can be viewed as a unique profession that considers all variables affecting an individual's response to internal and external stressors (Neuman, 1980). Nursing consists of knowledge of relationships among humans, the environment, and reaction to stress and the maintenance of stability and integrity of the system through reconstitution (Neuman, 1982, p. 19).	Nursing is seen as a unique profession because it concerns all variables affecting the family's health-promoting actions and their response to stressors. Nursing consists of knowledge of relations between humans and environment and human reaction to stress and reconstitution.
18. Nursing Intervention	Nursing intervention reduces possibility of stress and strengthens the individual's flexible line of defense (Neuman, 1982, p. 19).	Nursing intervention encourages health-promoting self-care activities, reduces possibility of stress, and strengthens the family's flexible lines of offense and defense. Nursing involves knowledge of all factors that influence the family's perceptual field.
	The nurse validates meaning of stressor that patient has with the nurse's own perceptual field that influences his or her assessment of patient's situation (Neuman, 1982, p. 19).	The nurse validates the meaning a family holds toward a stress impactor with his or her own perceptions, which influence the assessment of the family situation.

Data from Neuman, B. (1980). The Betty Neuman health-care systems model: A total person approach to patient problems. In J. Riehl & C. Roy (Eds.), *Conceptual Models for Nursing Practice* (pp. 119–134). New York: Appleton-Century-Crofts, and Venable, J. (1982). The Neuman health-care systems model: An analysis. In J. Riehl & C. Roy (Eds.), *Conceptual Models for Nursing Practice* (pp. 135–141). New York: Appleton-Century-Crofts.

(normal line of defense), or possibly to a higher level of stability, following an environmental stressor reaction.

- *Primary prevention* relates to general knowledge that is applied to family assessment and intervention in identification and mitigation of risk factors associated with environmental stressors to prevent possible reaction.

- *Secondary prevention* relates to symptomatology following reaction to stressors, appropriate ranking of intervention priorities, and treatment to reduce their noxious effects.

- *Tertiary prevention* relates to the adjustive processes taking place as reconstitution begins and maintenance factors move the client back in a circular manner toward primary prevention.

- The family is in dynamic, constant energy exchange with the environment.

Operationalization of the Neuman Systems Model

The family intervention model developed by Neuman (1989) can be operationalized for family health assessment and intervention (Fig. 12–1). Congruous with earlier definitions, "the family as client" is viewed as an open and dynamic system in interaction with its environment. This system is subject to the resultant tension and stress that is produced when stressors impinge on or penetrate through the family's defense system. The reaction of the family system is dependent on the penetration depth of the stressor. For example,

did the stressor impinge on the flexible line of defense and/or penetrate through the normal line of defense to the lines of resistance which protect the family's basic structure? Included in this basic structure are the characteristics, functions, and energy resources of the family unit. It also contains the patterns of family interaction. The basic structure must be protected at all costs, otherwise the demise of the family system will occur.

Reconstitution or adaptation is the work a family undertakes to preserve or restore impaired family unit functions. These family unit functions have been altered by stressors penetrating the family lines of defense.

Nursing interventions are defined as actions instituted to assist, modify, and/or regulate the family system's ability to generate its own health-

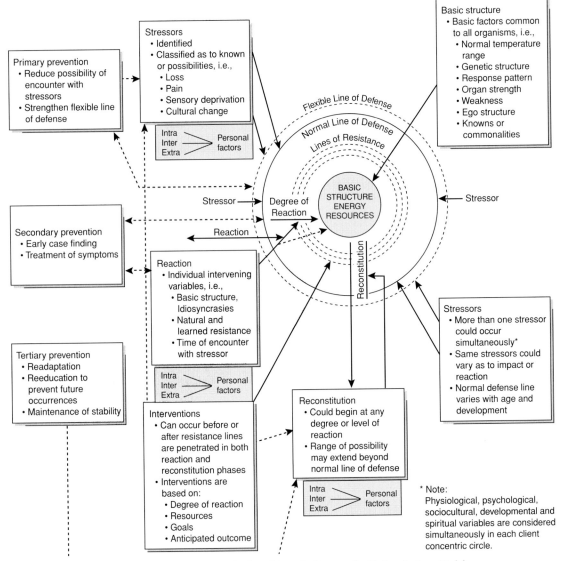

FIGURE 12–1. Family Assessment/Intervention Model, adapted from the Neuman Health-Care Systems Model.

promoting care or to respond to potential or actual stressful situations. This is accomplished by implementing health-promoting actions in concert with primary, secondary, or tertiary interventions that restore and stabilize the family system.

The Neuman Systems Model and Health Promotion

The family assessment process needs to include family wellness that is proactive as well as reactive in nature. Families must take responsibility for their own wellness and initiate self-care behaviors prior to the occurrence of stressful situations. The Neuman Systems Model includes selected health care behaviors and activities that families can institute at the flexible line of defense. These activities are implemented to prevent possible reactions to single stressors or a combination of stressors, thereby maintaining homeostasis (Neuman, 1989). In terms of intervention, the flexible line of defense becomes the primary level for intervention.

Much of the preventive health literature subsumes health-promoting behaviors and health-protecting activities under primary preventions (Leavell & Clark, 1965; Murray & Zentner, 1985; Shamansky & Clausen, 1980). From a narrow perspective, prevention simply means inhibiting the development of a disease and/or dysfunction before it occurs (Mausner & Kramer, 1985). In current usage, however, prevention has been extended to include measures that interrupt or slow the progression of disease (Mausner & Kramer, 1985). Several levels of prevention are said to exist. Included in the first level, primary prevention, are general health promotion behaviors and specific protective measures (Leavell & Clark, 1965).

Health care providers make philosophic and ethical decisions about whether or not they view health promotion from a proactive/wellness stance or from a reactive/illness stance. The reactive posture becomes a reaction to a potential disease or stressor threat. For example, does the caregiver view the family as instituting health-promoting behaviors to enhance its level of self-actualization, well-being, and fulfillment, or is it instituting such measures to prevent disease and dysfunction? Measures to prevent disease and instability include actions directed toward decreasing the probability of encountering illness or stressors by actively protecting the body against unnecessary stressors or detecting illness at an early stage (Pender, 1987).

The Neuman Systems Model (1989), being a wellness-oriented model, encourages health promotion from both a proactive wellness position and a reactive position. Health promotion should always be a goal in prevention and intervention. For example, if a family is threatened by a stressor, they might strengthen the flexible line

of defense by using one health-promoting behavior, thus assuming a reactive stance (Neuman, 1987). However, the outcome effect of this reactive posture may be generalized to the normal line of defense and lines of resistance, thereby strengthening them as well. This outcome is achieved via a proactive wellness position (Neuman, 1987). In another instance, a family might plan to institute several specific health-promoting behaviors based on one stressor threat (Neuman, 1987), thereby strengthening all lines of defense.

The authors view health promotion from a high-level wellness perspective and consider it to be a major focus of primary prevention. Selected concepts from the Neuman Systems Model focusing on wellness include basic physiologic structure and condition; system stability; socioeconomic background, developmental state, cognitive skills, age, and sex. The authors have added the following concepts: importance of health, perceived control, desire for competence, self-awareness, self-esteem, perceived health status, and perceived benefits of health-promoting behaviors. Added to these selected individual perceptions are family conditions that occur at home, work, and school and conditions that promote healthy living. These are good nutrition, adequate clothing, shelter, rest, recreation, productive interpersonal family relating styles, and strategies for managing family stress (Berkey & Hanson, 1991). This wellness focus also encompasses the broad area of health education, including instruction in hygiene, sex education, anticipatory guidance for children and parents, regular exercise patterns, and counseling in preparation for retirement (Berkey & Hanson, 1991).

The Neuman Systems Model and the Family Nursing Process

The Neuman Systems Model (1989) supports a unique approach to the nursing process. The traditional stages of the nursing process include nursing assessment, diagnosis, planning, intervention, and evaluation. Neuman reduces these five stages to three: *nursing diagnosis, goals,* and *outcomes* (Neuman, 1989). The authors modified Neuman's assumptions to encompass a family focus, as well as an individual focus. The modified assumptions include the following: (1) good assessment requires knowledge of all factors that influence the family's perceptual field; (2) most nursing care delivered to families occurs during transition periods, such as transitions to parenthood or development transitions of children; (3) the well family demonstrates a spectrum of abilities, insights, and strengths; (4) family members of the dynamic unit are engaged in tasks aimed at personal development and continuation of the family system; (5) the family, as well as the caregiver, validates the meaning a stressor holds for the family; and (6) factors in the nurse's perceptual field that influence assessment of the family situation will become apparent.

Nursing Diagnosis

Nursing diagnosis includes the synthesis of Neuman's systems theory with the family assessment data. One purpose of this synthesizing effort is to determine the wellness level of family systems, based on selected relevant client data and theory. Wellness is defined as a state of well-being that individuals and families strive to achieve (Brubaker, 1983). It is the goal of health-promoting behaviors. Additional purposes for the synthesizing efforts include identification of family stability needs and availability of resources to accomplish desired outcomes. Nursing diagnosis consists of a database regulated by the family's and the clinician's identification and evaluation of health-promoting behaviors and the actual or potential stressors that pose a threat to family stability. This is determined by analyzing the following: the family's basic structure and energy resources; the family's lines of defense, lines of resistance, and potential reaction; the family's possibilities for reconstitution; and the identification of potential/actual stressors that influence the family's interactive patterns. Nurses also need to identify past, present, and potential coping strategies that contribute to family stability; identify and evaluate internal and external resources that contribute to family health; and clarify perceptual differences that occur between the family's interpretation of the problem and the caregiver's impressions. If differences exist, a plan needs to be developed relative to resolving the perceptual differences.

Nursing diagnoses that have a family focus and include health care promotion can best be understood by looking at the following example:

Mr. and Mrs. Anderson took their one-month-old daughter Tamara to their family physician's office for a well-baby checkup. They were seen by a certified family nurse practitioner. The infant's physical examination was within the normal range of development. The assessment revealed that Tamara's nutritional and elimination patterns were appropriate, as were her sleeping activities.

Both Mr. and Mrs. Anderson have adjusted well to the addition of Tamara into their family structure. Parental roles are shared. However, Mr. Anderson often assumes additional parenting responsibilities so that his wife can have additional rest. The marital couple has a satisfying sexual relationship and express some questions about the best birth control methods that would fit their needs.

Nursing Diagnoses #1: "Effective family coping associated with attention to emotional needs of each family member as evidenced by: successful adjustment to meet family addition; and flexibility of roles; spouses' expressed satisfaction with their relationship" (Houldin et al., 1987, p. 180).

Nursing Diagnoses #2: "Adequate sexual function associated with adaptation to changes associated with childbearing, as evidences by: Report of satisfying sexual relationship. Over the next six months, spouses will continue to experience a satisfying sexual relationship" (Houldin et al., 1987, p. 184).

Nursing Goals

When working with families, the goals of intervention are to attain/maintain the maximum level of wellness and family stability. Therefore, all nursing intervention strategies are designed with these goals in mind. How the goals are accomplished is a negotiable process. The nurse and family negotiate with each other and decide what prescriptive changes are necessary, based on the family's strengths, problems, needs, and resources identified in the nursing diagnosis.

After these changes are identified, a clinician-client contract is established with the family. Loveland-Cherry (1992) defines a family contract as any working agreement continuously renegotiable between the family and the nurse (clinician). These parties share an understanding of the desired prescriptive changes and how these changes might be accomplished. Contracts can be formal (written) or informal (verbal) depending on the family's needs. They identify the responsibilities of both family and caregiver. The process of contracting encourages families to act for themselves in health promotion or self-care rather than become passive recipients of health care. Contracting also encourages collaborative participation between the family and the caregiver in the development, implementation, and evaluation of the process (Loveland-Cherry, 1992). Chapter 7 discusses the types of family self-care contracts.

The example of the Anderson family (Table 12–4) and the nursing diagnoses identified for them can be elaborated on to illustrate nursing goals and nursing interventions (Houldin et al., 1987, pp. 180–185). These goals and interventions are delineated in the nursing contract either formally or informally and are evaluated in the nursing outcomes.

Nursing Outcomes

Nursing outcomes are determined by instituting a health promotion mode within one of the three prevention/intervention modes. The *primary prevention/intervention* mode focuses on the movement of the individual and family toward a positively balanced state of increased health (Pender, 1987) and on the family actions necessary to retain system stability (Neuman, 1989). The *secondary prevention/intervention* mode addresses actions that are necessary to attain system stability, and the *tertiary prevention/intervention* mode encompasses those actions instituted to maintain system stability (Neuman, 1989). Evaluation of the outcome goals, subsequent to intervention, con-

TABLE 12–4. FAMILY NURSING PROCESS CASE EXAMPLE

NURSING DIAGNOSIS #1: FAMILY COPING: POTENTIAL FOR GROWTH

Nursing Goals	Nursing Interventions	Nursing Outcomes
1. Family will make adequate lifestyle changes over the next six months as they respond to the addition of a child into their family structure.	Encourage marital dyad to continue communicating their feelings regarding changes in their lifestyle.	At the six-month interval, parents will: 1. Discuss adaptations made to accommodate lifestyle changes; 2. Continue to cope effectively with each member's needs; 3. Continue to problem solve effectively; 4. Understand normal growth and development needs of infant; and 5. Know health needs and recognize minor health problems of infants.
2. Family's emotional needs will be adequately met over the next six months.	Assist with identification of family's coping and problem-solving ability. Praise, support, and encourage their efforts.	
3. Effective problem-solving techniques will be used over the next six months.	Teach parents principles of normal growth and development and parenting to enhance infant's development.	
4. Parents will continue to provide for the physical, emotional, and developmental needs of their infant over the next six months.	Assist parents to recognize and prepare for minor problems infant may encounter by teaching parents about common health needs and problems.	

NURSING DIAGNOSIS #2: ADEQUATE SEXUAL FUNCTIONING

Nursing Goals	Nursing Interventions	Nursing Outcomes
1. Marital dyad will successfully adapt to emerging parenting roles and family changes over the next six months.	Discuss sexual functioning with marital dyad and ask them to identify areas in which the nurse can provide information.	At the six-month interval, spouses will: 1. Continue satisfying sexual relationship; 2. Successfully adapt to child-rearing demands and schedule; 3. Continue to express affection; and 4. Use of appropriate family-planning measure.
2. Marital dyad will continue to demonstrate expressions of intimacy and affection over the next six months.	Discuss the energy demands and adaptations appropriate in the childrearing period.	
3. Marital dyad will mutually choose family planning method that will be used over the next six months.	Provide information about selected birth control measures including advantages and disadvantages.	

firms whether or not the goals were accomplished, and/or documents the need for goal reformation. Nurses wanting to consider intermediate and long-range goals for the family system need to structure their actions in relation to having short-term goals and outcome.

Using the Anderson family as an example, the goals delineated covered a six-month time frame. These are considered to be short-term goals by both the nurse and the family. Houldin et al. (1987) identified the following evaluative outcomes for the two nursing diagnoses presented, recognizing that the family outcome validates the nursing process (Neuman, 1989).

The Neuman Systems Model gives structure and substance to nursing actions (Neuman, 1982). In concert with health promotion models and family theory, the Neuman Systems Model gives nurses a blueprint for systematic family assessment and intervention (see Fig. 12–1). This model addresses activities related to health promotion and wellness and prevention/intervention.

HEALTH PROMOTION ACTIVITIES

Health promotion, as defined by Pender et al. (1992), refers to activities that are directed toward developing resources of clients for the purpose of maintaining or enhancing well-being. Prevention, on the other hand, refers to activities that attempt to protect clients from potential or actual health threats that might result in system instability (Neuman, 1989). Although the literature uses these terms synonymously, they are conceptually distinct (Pender, 1987).

In developing this family assessment and intervention instrument, the authors grouped health promotion activities and preventive health activities together. This approach was based on the recommendations of Neuman (1987) and an extensive literature review (Bullough & Bullough, 1990; Leavell & Clark, 1965; Spradley, 1990). Both aspects involve raising the family's level of wellness. When families are engaged in health-promoting activities, clinicians direct their efforts toward increasing the family's understanding of health and assisting families in developing more positive health practices (Spradley, 1990).

PREVENTION/INTERVENTION ACTIVITIES

In considering prevention/intervention activities, credence is given to the fact that families are confronted with potential and actual problem situations each day. These situations could jeopardize the stability of the family unit. When faced with these situations, families develop and use coping strategies to prevent any decrease in family function. This action is directed toward protection of the basic family structure and its energy resources. The basic structure encompasses family characteristics, family functions, and patterns of interaction that are influenced by the physiologic, psychologic, sociocultural, developmental, and spiritual characteristics of the individual members. If the integrity of the basic structure is not preserved, the viability of the system ceases.

Stability of the family system is the common goal of both families and clinicians. Frequently they work together in therapeutic partnerships to preserve the family system. This alliance occurs when families, faced with potential or actual situations that could lead to or contribute to family instability, are unable to resolve their issues without outside assistance. Depending on the stressful situation, families may have the resources to take their problems in stride and adapt easily; as a consequence, family functioning is only temporarily impaired. However, there are situations that families perceive as overwhelming, and they are unable to summon sufficient internal or external resources to deal with the situations. When that occurs, family system stability is in jeopardy.

Families facing potential or actual stressful circumstances experience varying amounts of stress and react with varying degrees of restorative or adaptive ability. The amount of stress experienced is dependent on the family's perception of the situation. The degree of reconstitution/adaptation is based on the family's ability to restore impaired family functions (Neuman, 1989). Some families have difficulty mobilizing their energy resources to focus on system reconstitution. The reasons for this are as varied as the families. Some families lack information; others have attempted to use their usual coping strategies, which fail to work in this situation; and some families perceive the problem as unsolvable.

Neuman (1989) provides a systematic method of identifying appropriate interventions that can be used to assist families with restoration of family functions. Nursing interventions can be implemented at any level of family functioning and with any degree of family instability. As nurses assist families in maintaining their stability and normal family functions, they focus on different areas of the assessment and intervention process. However, family nurses are alert to the fact that the assessment and intervention process moves back and forth from one area to another.

There are three broad areas of concentration: (1) wellness/health promotion and classification of the problems with identification of family member/stressors at the lines of defense; (2) family reactions and the degree of instability at the lines of defense (the family experiences tension as it reacts to the stressful situation); and (3) restoration of family stability and family function at levels of prevention (see Fig. 12–1).

Wellness/Family Strengths and Problem Identification/Stressors at Lines of Defense

Wellness/Health Promotion Activities

The initial focus of the clinician and family is on wellness and the identification of behaviors the family uses to increase their health-promoting activities. The increase in these activities results in the family's movement toward higher levels of health. The family is acting on its environment rather than reacting to potential threats imposed by the environment (Pender, 1987). The wellness activities include family values, beliefs, and actions that influence, facilitate, or sustain health-promoting activities. These values, beliefs, and actions include (1) the importance and valuing of health; (2) perceived control of individual and family health; (3) desire for competence in the family's ability to interact or transact effectively with the environment; (4) individual and family awareness of health-promoting behaviors; (5) self-esteem of family members; (6) definition of health to which the family subscribes; (7) perceived health status, which contributes to frequency and intensity of health-promoting behaviors; and (8) perceived benefits of instituting health-promoting behaviors (Pender, 1987).

Health-promoting activities based on the family's values and belief system are energized by the strengths operating within the unit itself. Family strengths are those caring, nurturing, and growth-facilitating qualities held by individual family members that are blended together in a chorus of supportive interactive relationships. Nurses and family members alike need to be able to identify these nurturing qualities in order to promote the continuation of healthy relationship patterns.

Wellness/Family Systems Strengths

Family nurses recognize that most families are able to identify the problems or stressors occurring in the family unit but they may not be able to identify their inherent family system strengths. Therefore, it is imperative for nurses to assist families with the identification of their strengths and then to acknowledge and reinforce them. The family strengths serve as a catalyst for healthy family functioning. Emphasizing family strengths encourages family members to feel better about themselves (Stinnett & DeFrain, 1985) by fostering a positive self-image, promoting self-confidence, and decreasing the family's feeling of hopelessness (Berkey & Hanson, 1991). Focusing on family strengths also vitalizes the family's efforts and unleashes their potential for developing their system's capacities (Spradley, 1990). The knowledge gained from incorporating strengths into a family care plan can contribute significantly to the family's ability to resolve problem issues (Stinnett & DeFrain, 1985).

A number of family-focused researchers have attempted to delineate characteristics and behaviors of healthy families (McCubbin & Patterson, 1983; Moos & Moos, 1983; Otto, 1973; Peters, 1982; Pratt, 1976; Satir, 1972; Stinnett & DeFrain, 1985). Their research findings contributed to the family-focused research of Curran (1983), who focused on identifying overall family strengths and the identifiable hallmarks of success that contribute to the attainment of family system goals. Fifteen of the family system strengths delineated by

Curran (1983) were incorporated into the family assessment instrument. Each of these strengths have a great influence on family system stability.

Problem Identification

The secondary focus for both nurses and families is threefold: (1) the identification of any problem, situation, or stressor capable of causing family instability; (2) the intensity of the stressor; and (3) the family members involved in the problems situation. For example, is the family involvement (factor) intrapersonal, interfamily, or extrafamily in nature? *Intrapersonal involvement* designates the event as having an impact within the individual family member, and *interfamily involvement* implies the problem is occurring between family members. *Extrafamily involvement* implies that the family is experiencing some degree of instability between itself and society.

The term *line of defense* refers to the protective strategies families institute to guard their basic structural unit from the stressful situation or problem (Hoffman, 1982; Neuman, 1989). The *flexible line of defense* refers to the dynamic level of health families attain following a temporary response to a stressful situation impinging on the system (Johnson et al., 1982; Neuman, 1989). Examples of problems or situations that may impinge on the flexible line of defense are career changes, marriage, and children entering the family (Reed, 1989).

Inside the flexible line of defense is the normal line of defense. The *normal line of defense* refers to the family's state of wellness over time (Neuman, 1989). It includes the family's process of adaptation and/or reconstitution. Families respond to situations in ways they consider to be "normal" for their individual unit, and over time develop patterns they consider appropriate or "normal" for certain situations. Examples of stressful situations/problems that may affect ways of coping and behaving considered "normal" for the family unit are marital difficulty, unemployment, and death of a family member (Reed, 1989).

The *lines of resistance* are found within the circle of the normal line of defense, and they protect the family's basic structure (Neuman, 1989). These lines of resistance are forces within the family system that can be activated to protect and preserve the stability and energy resources of the basic unit. These forces are brought into play when problems or stressful situations penetrate the family's normal line of defense. Examples of problems that cross the normal line of defense and threaten the viability of the family structure are substance abuse by a family member, family violence and abuse, chronic physical or mental illness, or loss of a family member's physical abilities.

The *basic family structure and energy resources* refers to the characteristics, functions, and survival skills common to the family system (Neuman, 1989). These characteristics and functions are influenced by the physiologic, sociocultural, and spiritual components of the individual family members. This basic core of the family must be diligently protected if the family unit is to remain healthy and functional.

Identifying tension producing situations/stressors was the focus of investigation of family researcher Curran (1985). Her research revealed similarities among healthy well-functioning families and similarities among dysfunctional families. All family systems experience somewhat similar stressors as they grow and develop over the life cycle, but some families are more successful in stressor management than others. Twenty-five common stressors identified by Curran (1985) as influencing family health and stability have been incorporated into the family assessment instruments.

Problem Identification/Stressors

Families that are able to transform stresses into positive forces are able to maintain and retain system stability and health. Other families facing similar growth and developmental demands tend to lose control and react in ways that jeopardize family system function.

Family units living with distress and instability as a way of life exhibit symptoms that nurses can recognize while performing family assessments (Curran, 1985, p. 13). These include the following:

- A constant sense of urgency and hurry; no time to release and relax
- Tension that underlies and causes sharp words, sibling fighting, and misunderstandings
- A mania to escape—to one's room, car, garage, away
- Feelings of frustration over not getting things done
- A feeling that time is passing too quickly, children are growing up too fast
- A nagging desire for a simpler life; constant talk about times that were or will be simpler
- Little "me" or couple time
- A pervasive sense of guilt for not being and doing everything to and for all of the people in one's life

Most families experience these symptoms at one time or another, but for some the symptoms become the family's modus operandi. The family members learn to live with negativity, distress, and instability. How families react to stressors is evident at the lines of defense and resistance.

Family Reactions and Instability at Lines of Defense and Resistance

The assessment focus here is on the amount of stress produced when families react to a problem or stressful condition. Various amounts of stress or tension can occur within a family member, between family members, or between the family and society. This stress is demonstrated by the amount of instability that occurs at any of the lines of defense and/or resistance. Instability at the flexible line of defense can be assessed by being alert to the dynamic state of the family as it manages the ongoing encounter with a stressful situation. The dynamic state of the family includes such elements as conflict-resolution mechanisms, decision making, task allocation, family bonding patterns, institution of family roles, and family rules (Miller & Janosik, 1980).

Instability or stress occurring at the normal line of defense can be assessed by being cognizant of the manner in which families normally respond to stressful situations. "This line of defense acts as a wellness standard against which to determine health variance from a more immediate or situational condition" (Neuman, 1989). Nurses need to keep in mind that the term "normal" is defined by the families involved. However, the nurse can determine the amount of family instability by assessing the following elements: communication patterns, problem-solving mechanisms, actions instituted to meet family member needs for intimacy and affection, and ways of dealing with loss and change (Reed, 1989).

Problem situations creating instability for the family that are controlled by the flexible and normal lines of defense are conceptualized as "normal" stressors (Neuman, 1989). These include events surrounding the family's activities of daily living or the "nitty gritty" daily business of family life (Reed, 1989).

The elements found within both the flexible and the normal lines of defense also compose the family's normal coping mechanisms. When the problem or stressful situation is of such an intensity that prescribed coping mechanisms from the two lines of defense prove ineffective, the tension level builds, and family lines of resistance are called into operation.

The lines of resistance are composed of internal factors that can be mobilized to control or defend the basic family structure against the stressor(s) (Neuman, 1989). These lines are arranged in such a way that stressors must break through the normal coping mechanisms employed by the family at the lines of defense in order to penetrate the basic energy resources of the family. Assessment of the amount of stress and tension at the lines of resistance includes evaluation of internal factors found in the family's basic structure. They are interrelatedness, interdependence, values, and beliefs (Reed, 1989). These internal factors may be viewed differently by each family member, and the intensity of the member reaction is related to how the problem is perceived. Perception of problems and their subsequent resolution is often based on the characteristics the couple dyad initially brought to the beginning family structure. Each member of the couple brings certain beliefs, values, and ways of relating that were learned in their family of origin. As the new family structure (family of procreation) begins to develop, the couple dyad has to mesh their different belief systems, value judgements, and patterns of relating and dependence. This results in the creation of new family characteristics. How the young family grows and matures is in part based on the interrelatedness of these internal elements. As families mature, all family members may not continue to support the original couple beliefs, and the way problems are perceived may vary. Stress may become excessive.

Restoration of Family Stability and Family Functions at Levels of Prevention/Intervention

In an effort to restore family stability, the clinician must assess the family's ability to restore stability and function subsequent to a potential or actual problem situation. All families attempt to cope with stressful situations at some level, and each family reacts in its own way. Each stressor is different in its potential to disturb the family's equilibrium (Neuman, 1989). Moreover, the relationship of physiologic, psychological, sociocultural, developmental, and spiritual characteristics of individual members can affect the degree to which the family is able to mobilize its flexible line of defense to defend against problems.

There is a close link between assessment at the lines of defense and prevention/intervention levels. Intervention goals for families always include the results of the assessment focus: optimal family functioning, family stability, and family's reaction to the instability.

The prevention and intervention mode is conceptualized as a way of facilitating the integrative processes of the family. This integration is necessary for the family to retain, attain, or maintain its health and integrity as a unit (Neuman, 1989).

The intervention strategies are instituted at the designated defense lines. Supportive and coping strategies are designed for the family members involved. For example, if stressors occur within a family member, intrapersonal intervention strategies are designed by the clinician and family member at the designated intervention level. If problem situations are between family members, interfamily intervention strategies are developed at the appropriate line of defense. If the stressful conditions are between the family unit and society, extrafamily intervention strategies are developed.

Primary Prevention Level

Intervention coping strategies at the primary prevention level include actions initiated by families, family members, or nurses before or after encountering a problem or stressful situation (Neuman, 1989). These strategies encompass actions families undertake to decrease the possibility of encountering potential or actual problems as well as those actions that strengthen the flexible line of defense in the presence of stressors (Neuman, 1980). Neuman (1989) cites additional intervention strategies nurses can use: (1) provide the family with information related to existing family strengths; (2) support the family's coping abilities and functioning capabilities; (3) desensitize existing or potential harmful stressors in the family; (4) encourage the family's attempts toward wellness; and (5) educate and/or reeducate family members. Examples of intervention measures at this level are classes on growth and development of children and adults, premarital counseling, parenting classes, and marriage enrichment groups.

Secondary Prevention Level

Intervention strategies designed for the secondary prevention level include actions initiated after the family encounters stressors. This encompasses early case findings by the health care provider and treatment of family instability following its reaction to problem situations. Additional strategies include (1) protecting the family's basic structure; (2) mobilizing and maximizing both the internal and the external family resources toward family stability and energy conservation; (3) facilitating the family's purposeful manipulation of problems or stressful conditions and their reaction to them; (4) educating families and assisting them with the development of their own health care goals; (5) assisting families to use appropriate treatment and intervention measures; (6) supporting the family's positive reaction toward illness; (7) advocating for families by assisting them with health care service coordination; and (8) providing primary prevention/intervention to families as needed (Neuman, 1989). Examples of intervention measures at this level include family crisis intervention, treatment of family member illness, marital counseling, employment counseling, and grief work (Reed, 1989).

Tertiary Prevention Level

Intervention strategies at the tertiary prevention level are initiated after treatment has been completed. Health care providers and families focus on reconstitution, rehabilitation, and reeducation of the family unit and/or its individual members. Nursing actions are directed toward (1) maintaining maximum level of family wellness and stability; (2) educating, reeducating, and/or reorienting of the family as appropriate; (3) supporting the family unit in its effort to set appropriate health goals and institute needed changes; (4) coordinating health service resources for families; and (5) providing families with primary and/or secondary prevention/intervention as needed (Neuman, 1989). Examples of tertiary preventive measures are family counseling, support groups of all types, and rehabilitation groups (Reed, 1989).

FAMILY SYSTEMS STRESSOR-STRENGTH INVENTORY (FS³I)

The Family Systems Stressor-Strength Inventory (FS³I) is a family health assessment/measurement instrument intended for use with families. The instrument itself is located in Appendix A and the scoring summary in Appendix B. It focuses on identifying stressful situations occurring in families and the strengths families use to maintain healthy functioning. Selected demographic data are requested: name, age, sex, marital status, education, occupation, religious preference, referral source, ethnic group, and member relationship.

The FS³I is divided into two sections: Section I, Family Perception Scores and Section 2, Clinician Perception Scores. These two sections are further divided into three parts: (1) Family Systems Stressors: General; (2) Family Stressors: Specific; and (3) Family System Strengths. Each part has quantitative and qualitative aspects. Family members are asked to complete an individual form prior to an interview with the clinician. Questions can be read aloud to any members who are unable to read.

The interview with the clinician focuses on clarifying the perceived general stressors, specific stressors, and family strengths as identified by the individual family members. The interview process also gives the clinician an opportunity to evaluate family functioning and stability. The clinician evaluates family members on their stressors and strengths, using the same format as those of family members, and notes these findings in a designated section on the family form.

The clinician records the individual family member's score and the clinician perception score on the Quantitative Summary. A different color code is used for each family member. The clinician also completes the Qualitative Summary synthesizing the information gleaned from all participants. Clinicians can use the Family Care Plan to prioritize diagnoses, set goals, develop prevention/intervention activities, and evaluate outcomes (Appendix B, p. 0).

Family Systems Stressor (General): Family and Clinician Perceptions

Part 1 of the instrument is based on the family research of Curran (1985) and the systems work of Neuman (1989). Curran (1985) identified 45 areas of concern and/or stressor situations that influence family health. Twenty-five stressors dealing with some aspect of normal family life were used to develop the items for the assessment/measurement instrument. Each question requires the respondent to answer in a five-point Likert scale format. Family members are requested to circle the amount of stress they experience. The answers can range from little stress to high stress. A nonapply option is available to each item. Additional stressors can be identified and family remarks made at the end of each question. Stress levels are viewed in terms of the family's actions or reactions to situations penetrating the lines of defense.

Clinician perceptions are identified in an interview with family members. The clinician asks the individual members about the various stressors occurring in their family and then ranks the stressors according to how he or she perceives their family effects. The clinician can add additional stressors when identified and make descriptive remarks subsequent to each question. The scoring format for Part 1 is described in Appendix B.

The numerical scores designate the intensity of stressor effect, the degree of stressor penetration, and family reaction. The qualitative scores are matched with the appropriate lines of defense and resistance. The identified lines of defense and resistance determine the prevention/interventions level: primary, secondary, and tertiary intervention. Clinicians check the appropriate intervention level where therapeutic actions are to be initiated. All qualitative information is recorded on a Qualitative Summary.

Family Systems Stressor (Specific): Family and Clinician Perceptions

Part 2 of the instrument is based on the systems work of Neuman (1989). It begins with family members identifying a specific stress-producing situation/problem affecting the health and stability of their family unit. Following problem/stressor identification, family members are asked to answer seven questions directly related to this problem (Neuman, 1989). Four additional questions focus on overall family/family member functioning. All closed-ended questions are answered on a five-point Likert scale format and followed by space for descriptive remarks. The answers range from little stress to high stress. Stress levels are viewed in terms of the family's actions or reactions to a particular situation penetrating the lines of defense.

Clinician perceptions are identified in an interview with family members. The clinician asks each individual member about the various problem/situation occurring in the family and then ranks this stressor according to how he or she perceives its family effects. The clinician makes descriptive remarks subsequent to each question. The scoring format for Part 2 is described in Appendix B.

The numerical scores designate the intensity of stressor effect, the degree of stressor penetration, and family reaction. The quantitative scores are matched with the appropriate lines of defense and resistance. The identified lines of defense and resistance determine the prevention/intervention level: primary, secondary, and tertiary intervention. Clinicians check the appropriate intervention level where therapeutic actions are to be initiated. All qualitative information is recorded on a Qualitative Summary.

Family System Strengths: Family and Clinician Perceptions

Part 3 of the instrument is based on the family research of Curran (1983). Family members are asked to identify the extent to which fifteen family traits/strengths are operationalized in their family system. The closed-ended questions are answered on a five-point Likert scales form at: 1 designates seldom; 5 designates always. A non-apply column is also an option. A space for family remarks follows each question. The numerical response and general remarks pinpoint the extent to which family members perceive their family strengths.

Clinician perceptions are identified in an interview with family members. The clinician asks the individual members about the various family strengths occurring in their family and then ranks these according to their presence and consistency. The clinician makes descriptive remarks subsequent to each question when appropriate. The scoring format for Part 3 is described in Appendix B.

The numerical scores designate the presence and consistency of family strengths. The family member quantitative scores are matched with the appropriate lines of defense and resistance. The identified lines of defense and resistance determine the prevention/intervention level: primary, secondary, and tertiary intervention. Clinicians check the appropriate intervention level where therapeutic actions are to be initiated. All qualitative information is recorded on a Qualitative Summary (Appendix B).

The investigators believe that awareness of family strengths facilitates and gives direction to the prevention/intervention process. Families and nurses work together to identify stressful family situations and the family strengths available to support prevention and intervention activities. Family strengths can prevent family instability and wellness variances by enhancing the family's problem-solving and reconstitution ability.

Family Systems Stressor-Strength Inventory: Family Care Plan

The family care plan was formulated using the Neuman Systems Model (1989). The broad areas of nursing diagnosis, nursing goals, and nursing outcomes are divided into five sections: (1) nursing diagnosis, (2) family strengths, (3) prioritized family goals, (4) prevention/intervention mode, and (5) outcomes including evaluation and replanning (Appendix B).

NURSING DIAGNOSIS. Formulating nursing diagnoses requires the nurse to carry out several functions: (1) analyze all data collected from the quantitative and qualitative summaries, (2) identify the actual and potential family stressors and prioritize them, (3) state the nursing diagnosis based on the causative stressor(s) in the family system, and (4) incorporate the family's reaction to stressor(s) using subjective and objective data which support the nursing diagnosis. Following synthesis of this data, nurses are able to make comprehensive nursing diagnostic statements based on the family's system variance from wellness.

FAMILY STRENGTHS. The nurse records the strengths and/or the supportive resources available to the family from both inner and external sources.

GOALS. Establishing wellness and stability is the end point of goal setting by the nurse and family members. Goal consideration includes stressor identification, family strengths, and the internal and external environment resources available to family unit. The nurse negotiates with the family to formulate appropriate prevention/intervention strategies.

PREVENTION/INTERVENTION MODE. The quantitative and qualitative data designates the most appropriate preventive/intervention mode. Once identified the selection and development of prevention/intervention activities can be accomplished. Intervention modes include (1) primary prevention activities, focusing on actions to *retain* family system stability; (2) secondary prevention activities, focusing on actions to *attain* family system stability; and (3) tertiary prevention activities, focusing on actions that *maintain* family unit stability.

OUTCOMES, EVALUATION AND REPLANNING. Evaluating outcomes for the family care plan requires that both nurse and family members re-examine the prioritized goals previously set and determine whether they were achieved. This evaluation process centers on analyzing the effectiveness of the nurse prevention/intervention activities supporting goal attainment. If the goals were not achieved a new plan needs to be made.

Replanning of family goals is considered when outcome goals have not been achieved. New plans are designed when any of the following conditions exist: (1) changes in the nature of the family stressors, (2) changes in the family member variables and/or changes in the family system variable; and (3) changes in priorities of goals in relation to the primary, secondary, and tertiary prevention modes. The nurse needs to add a statement of replanning actions to the Family Care Plan, for example: "change intervention to . . ."; "continue present intervention"; "discontinue, goal met"; "redefine nursing diagnosis"; and so on (Neuman, 1987).

ACKNOWLEDGEMENTS

The authors of this chapter would like to recognize the following people:

Dr. Mischke wishes to thank the mentors who have consistently supported her professional and personal growth: Shirley Hanson, Leitte Brostoff, and Doris Julian. She also wishes to acknowledge the nurturing support of her three children: Tamara, Mark, and Todd.

Dr. Hanson wishes to acknowledge some professional colleagues who have contributed to her scholarly career:

CHAPTER HIGHLIGHTS

The focus of concern in the family nursing process is the family as context (the interactions and health of the family system as a unit).

The purpose of family assessment is to provide an opportunity for families and health professionals to determine relevant data from which a unique plan can be developed for a family's health promotion and health protection.

The components of the family nursing process using the Betty Neuman Model are nursing diagnosis, goals, and outcomes.

The broad categories of foci of family nursing assessment and intervention include classification of family health promotion needs and family stressors; determination of family stability during family transitions; and restoration of family stability and function after transitions or crises.

The three levels of family intervention include primary prevention, secondary prevention, and tertiary prevention.

Family health may be assessed using nursing and nonnursing family assessment measures such as the Family Systems Stressor-Strength Inventory (FS^{3}I).

Perri Bomar, Marilyn Friedman, Vivian Gedaly-Duff, Catherine Gillis, Marsha Heims, Doris Julian, Maureen Leahey, Karen Mischke, and Lorraine Wright. Children Derek, Gwen, and Joseph, as well as sisters Marjorie, Peggy, and Kathleen all deserve special thanks for their patient understanding of time spent away from home activities.

REFERENCES

Anderson, K., & Tomlinson, P. (1992). The family health system as an emerging paradigmatic view for nursing. *Image* 24(1), 57–63.

Bales, R. (1950). *Interaction Process Analysis.* Reading, MA: Addison-Wesley.

Bell, J.M., Watson, W.L., & Wright, J.M. (Eds.). (1990). *The Cutting Edge of Family Nursing.* Calgary: Family Nursing Unit Publications.

Berkey, K.M., & Hanson, S.M. (1991). *Pocket Guide to Family Assessment and Intervention.* St. Louis: Mosby.

Braden, C., & Herban, N. (1976). *Community Health: A Systems Approach.* New York: Appleton-Century-Crofts.

Bradley, R.H. (1982). The home inventory: A review of the first fifteen years. In N.J. Anastasiow & A. Fandal (Eds.), *Identifying the Developmentally Delayed Child* (pp. 87–100). Baltimore: University Park Press.

Brubaker, B. (1983). Health promotion: A linguistic analysis. *Advances in Nursing Science,* 5(3), 1–14.

Bullough, B., & Bullough, V. (1990). *Nursing in the Community.* St. Louis: C.V. Mosby.

Burgess, E. (1926). The family as a unity of interacting personalities. *The Family,* 7, 3–9.

Caldwell, B.M., & Bradley, R.H. (1970). *Home Observation for Measurement of the Environment.* Little Rock, AR: University of Arkansas.

Calloway, S.J. (1982). Home observation for measurement of the environment. In S.M. Humenick (Ed.), *Analysis of Current Assessment Strategies in the Health Care of Young Children and Childbearing Families* (pp. 252–258). Norwalk, CT: Appleton-Century-Crofts.

Clemen-Stone, S., Eigsti, D., & McGuire, S. (1991). *Comprehensive Family and Community Health Nursing* (3rd ed.). St. Louis: McGraw-Hill.

Clemen-Stone, S., Eigsti, D., & McGuire, S. (1987). *Comprehensive family community health nursing* (2nd ed.). St. Louis: McGraw-Hill.

Curran, D. (1983). *Traits of a Healthy Family.* Minneapolis, MN: Winston Press.

Curran, D. (1985). *Stress and the Healthy Family.* Minneapolis, MN: Winston Press.

Daniel, L. (1986). Family assessment. In B. Logan & C. Dawkins (Eds.), *Family-Centered Nursing in the Community* (pp. 184–208). Reading, MA: Addison-Wesley.

Danielson, C.B., Hamel-Bissell, B., & Winstead-Fry, P. (1993). *Families, Health and Illness: Perspectives on Coping and Intervention.* St. Louis: C.V. Mosby.

Duvall, E. (1977). *Family Development.* Philadelphia: J.B. Lippincott.

Epstein, N., Baldwin, L., & Bishop, D. (1983). The McMaster family assessment device. *Journal of Marital and Family Therapy,* 9, 171–180.

Fawcett, J. (1989). *Analysis and Evaluation of Conceptual Models of Nursing* (2nd ed.). Philadelphia: F.A. Davis.

Feetham, S. (1983). *Feetham Family Functioning Survey.* (Available from Children's Hospital National Medical Center, 111 Michigan Avenue NW, Washington, D.C.)

Feetham, S.L. (1990). Conceptual and methodological issues in research in families. In J. Bell, W. Watson, & L. Wright (Eds.), *The Cutting Edge of Family Nursing* (pp. 35–49). Calgary: Family Nursing Unit Publications.

Feetham, S.L., & Humenick, S.S. (1982). The Feetham family functioning survey. In S.S. Humenick (Ed.), *Analysis of Current Assessment Strategies in the Health Care of Young Children and Childbearing Families* (pp. 259–268). Norwalk, CT: Appleton-Century-Crofts.

Filsinger, E. (Ed.). (1983). *Marriage and Family Assessment: A Sourcebook for Family Therapy.* Beverly Hills: Sage.

Fishbein, M., & Ajzen, I. (1975). *Belief, Attitude, Intention, and Behavior: An Introduction to Theory and Research.* Reading, MA: Addison-Wesley.

Forman, B.D., & Hagan, B.J. (1984). Measures for Evaluating Total Family Functioning. *Family Therapy,* 11(1), 1–36.

Freeman, R.B., & Heinrich, J. (1981). *Community Health Nursing Practice* (2nd ed.). Philadelphia: W.B. Saunders.

Friedman, M.M. (1992). *Family Nursing: Theory and Assessment* (3rd ed.). Norwalk, CT: Appleton-Lange.

Gilliss, C.L. (1991). Family nursing research, theory and practice. *Image: Journal of Nursing Scholarship,* 22, 19–22.

Gilliss, C.L., Highley, B.L., Roberts, B.M., & Martinson, I.M. (Eds.). (1989). *Toward a Science of Family Nursing.* Reading, MA: Addison-Wesley.

Good, M.D., Smilkstein, G., Good, B.J., Shaffer, T., & Arons, T. (1979). The family APGAR index: A study of construct validity. *Journal of Family Practice,* 8, 577–582.

Hanson, S.M.H. (1996). Family nursing assessment and intervention. In S.M.H Hanson & S.T. Boyd. *Family Health Care Nursing: Theory, Practice and Research.* Philadelphia: Davis.

Hanson, S.M.H., & Boyd, S.T. *Family Health Care Nursing: Theory, Practice and Research.* Philadelphia: Davis.

Hanson, S.M.H., & Kaakinen, J. (1996). Family assessment. In M. Stanhope & J. Lancaster (Eds.) *Community Health Nursing: Process and Practice for Promoting Health* (4th ed.). St. Louis: Mosby.

Hanson, S.M.H. (1985). Family health inventory: A measurement. Paper presented at the National Council of Family Relations, Dallas, TX.

Hanson, S.M.H. (1986). Healthy single parent families. *Family Relations,* 35(1), 125–132.

Hanson, S.M.H., & Heims, M.L. (1992). Family nursing curricula in U.S. schools of nursing. *Journal of Nursing Education,* 31(7), 303–308.

Hanson, S., Heims, M., & Julian, D. (1992). Education for family health care professionals. *Family Relations,* 41, 49–53.

Helvie, C. (1991). *Community Health Nursing: Theory and Practice.* New York: Springer.

Hill, R., & Hansen, D. (1960). The identification of conceptual frameworks utilized in family study. *Marriage and Family Living,* 22, 299–311.

Hoffman, M. (1982). From model to theory construction: An analysis of the Neuman health-care systems model. In B. Neuman (Ed.), *The Neuman Systems Model: Application to Nursing Education and Practice* (pp. 44–54). Norwalk, CT: Appleton-Century-Crofts.

Holt, S., & Robinson, T. (1979). The school nurses assessment tool. *American Journal of Nursing,* 79(5), 950–953.

Houldin, A., Saltstein, S., & Ganley, K. (1987). *Nursing Diagnosis for Wellness: Supporting Strengths.* Philadelphia: J.B. Lippincott.

Humenick, S.S. (1982). *Analysis of Current Assessment Strategies in the Health Care of Young Children and Childbearing Families.* Norwalk, CT: Appleton-Century-Crofts.

Hurwitz, J., Kaplan, D., & Kaiser, E. (1965). Designing an instrument to assess parental coping mechanisms. In H. Parad (Ed.), *Crisis Interventions: Selected Readings* (pp. 339–348). New York: Family Service Association of America.

Hymovich, D. (1983). The chronicity impact and coping instrument: Parent questionnaire. *Nursing Research,* 32, 275–281.

Johnson, M.N., Vaughn-Wrobel, B., Ziegler, S.M., Hough, L., Bush, H.A., & Kurtz, P. (1982). Use of the Neuman health-care systems model in the master's curriculum: Texas Women's University. In B. Neuman (Ed.), *The Neuman Systems Model: Application to Nursing Education and Practice* (pp. 130–152). Norwalk, CT: Appleton-Century-Crofts.

Leavell, H., & Clark, E. (1965). *Preventive Medicine for the Doctor in His Community: An Epidemiologic Approach* (3rd ed.). New York: McGraw-Hill.

Loveland-Cherry, C. (1992). Issues in family health promotion. In M. Stanhope and J. Lancaster (Eds.), *Community Health Nursing: Process and Practice for Promoting Health* (pp. 470–483). St. Louis: C.V. Mosby.

Lowman, J. (1980). Measurement of family affective structures. *Journal of Personality Assessment,* 44(2), 130–141.

Margolin, G., & Fernandez, V. (1983). Other marriage and family questionnaires. In E.E. Filsinger (Ed.), *Marriage and Family Assessment: A Sourcebook for Family Therapy* (pp. 317–338). Beverly Hills: Sage.

Mauksch, H. (1974). A social service basis for conceptualizing family health. *Social Science and Medicine,* 8, 521–523.

Mausner, J., & Kramer, S. (1985). *Epidemiology—An Introductory Text.* Philadelphia: W.B. Saunders.

McCubbin, H.I., & Patterson, J.M. (1983). Stress: The family inventory of life events. In E.E. Filsinger (Ed.), *Marriage and Family Assessment: A Sourcebook for Family Therapy* (pp. 275–298). Beverly Hills: Sage.

McCubbin, H.I., & Thompson, A.I. (1987). *Family Assessment Inventories for Research and Practice.* Madison, WI: University of Wisconsin.

Mead, G. (1934). *Mind, Self, and Society.* Chicago: University of Chicago Press.

Miller, J.R., & Janosik, E. (1980). *Family-Focused Care.* San Francisco: McGraw-Hill.

Mischke-Berkey, K., Warner, P., & Hanson, S.M.H. (1989). Family health assessment and intervention. In P. Bomar (Ed.), *Nurses & Family Health Promotion: Concepts, Assessment and Intervention* (pp. 115–151). Baltimore, MD: Williams & Wilkins.

Moe, E.O. (1977). Nature of today's community. In A.M. Reinhardt & M.D. Quinn (Eds.), *Current Practice in*

Family-Centered Community Nursing (Vol. 1) (pp. 99–112). St. Louis: C.V. Mosby.

Moos, R. (1974). *Family Environment Scales.* Palo Alto, CA: Consulting Psychologists Press.

Moos, R.H., & Moos, B.S. (1976). A typology of family social environments. *Family Process, 15,* 357–371.

Moos, R.H., & Moos, B.S. (1983). Clinical applications of the family environment scale. In E.E. Filsinger (Ed.), *Marriage and Family Assessment: A Sourcebook for Family Therapy* (pp. 253–274). Beverly Hills: Sage.

Mountain, K.L. (1982). Faces: A family dynamics assessment based on cohesion and adaptability. In S.S. Humenick (Ed.), *Analysis of Current Assessment Strategies in the Health Care of Young Children and Childbearing Families* (pp. 269–277). Norwalk, CT: Appleton-Century-Crofts.

Murphy, S. (1986). Family study and nursing research. *Image, 18*(4), 170–174.

Murray, R., & Zentner, J. (1985). *Nursing Assessment and Health Promotion Through the Life Span.* Englewood Cliffs, NJ: Prentice-Hall.

Neuman, B. (1980). The Betty Neuman health-care systems model: A total person approach to patient problems. In J.P. Riehl & C. Roy (Eds.), *Conceptual Models for Nursing Practice* (2nd ed.). (pp. 119–134). New York: Appleton-Century-Crofts.

Neuman, B. (1982). *The Neuman Systems Model.* Norwalk, CT: Appleton-Century-Crofts.

Neuman, B. (1983). Family intervention using the Betty Neuman health care systems model. In I. Clements & F. Roberts (Eds.) *Family Health: A Theoretical Approach to Nursing Care* (pp. 239–254). New York: Wiley.

Neuman, B. (1987, 1992, July). Personal correspondence with Betty Neuman, author of *The Neuman Systems Model.* Norwalk, CT: Appleton-Century-Crofts.

Neuman, B. (1989). The Neuman Systems Model. In B. Neuman (Ed.). *The Neuman Systems Model* (pp. 1–64). Norwalk, CT: Appleton & Lange.

Nye, F.I., & Berardo, F.M. (1981). *Emerging Conceptual Frameworks in Family Analysis.* New York: Praeger Scientific.

Olson, D.H., Bell, R., & Portner, J. (1980). *Family Adaptability and Cohesion Evaluation Scales.* St. Paul, MN: University of Minnesota Press.

Olson, D., McCubbin, H.I., Barnes, H., Larsen, A., Muxen, M., & Wilson, D. (1982). *Family Inventories.* St. Paul, MN: University of Minnesota.

Olson, D.H., McCubbin, H.I., Barnes, H.L., Larsen, A.S., Muxen, M.J., & Wilson, M.A. (1983). *Families: What Makes Them Work.* Beverly Hills: Sage.

Olson, D.H., & Portner, J. (1983). Family adaptability and cohesion evaluation scales. In E.E. Filsinger (Ed.), *Marriage and Family Assessment: A Sourcebook for Family Therapy* (pp. 299–316). Beverly Hills: Sage.

Olson, D.H., Portner, J., Lavee, Y. (1985). *FACES III.* St. Paul, MN: Family Social Sciences, University of Minnesota.

Olson, D., Russell, C., & Sprenkle, D. (1980). Circumplex model of marital and family systems II: Empirical studies and clinical intervention. In J.P. Vincent (Ed.), *Advances in Family Intervention, Assessment, and Theory* (pp. 88–97). Greenwich, CT: JAI Press.

Olson, D.H., Sprenkle, D.H., & Russell, C.S. (1979). Circumplex model of marital and family systems I: Cohesion and adaptability dimensions, family types, and clinical applications. *Family Process, 18,* 3–28.

Otto, H.A. (1973). A framework for assessing family strength. In A. Reinhardt & M. Quinn (Eds.) *Family-centered community nursing: A sociocultural framework* (pp. 87–94). St. Louis: Mosby.

Parsons, T. (1951). *The Social System.* Glencoe: Free Press.

Patterson, G.R. (1971). *Families: Application of Social Learning Theory to Family Life.* Champaign, IL: Research Press.

Pender, N. (1987). *Health Promotion in Nursing Practice* (2nd ed.). Los Altos, CA: Third Party.

Pender, N., Barkauskas, V., Hayman, L., Rice, V., & Anderson, E. (1992). Health promotion and disease prevention: Toward excellence in nursing practice and education. *Nursing Outlook, 40*(5), 106–109.

Perosa, L., Hansen, J., & Perosa, S. (1981). Development of the structural family interaction scale. *Family Therapy, 8*(2), 77–90.

Peters, M. (1981). Making it black family style: Building on the strength of black families. In N. Stinnet, T. Derain, K. King, D. Knaab, & Rowe, G. (Eds.) *Family strengths 3: Roots of well-being* (73–91). Lincoln: University of Nebraska Press.

Pless, I.B., & Satterwhite, B. (1973). A measure of family functioning and its application. *Social Science and Medicine, 7,* 613–621.

Pratt, L. (1976). *Family Structure and Effective Health Behavior.* Boston: Houghton-Mifflin.

Reed, K. (1989). Family theory related to the Neuman Systems Model. In B. Neuman (Ed.) *The Neuman Systems Model* (pp. 385–395). Norwalk, CT: Appleton & Lange.

Roberts, C.S., & Feetham, S.L. (1982). Assessing family functioning across three areas of relationships. *Nursing Research, 31*(4), 321–335.

Ross, B., & Cobb, K.L. (1990). *Family Nursing: A Nursing Process Approach.* Redwood City, CA: Addison-Wesley.

Satir, V. (1972). *Peoplemaking.* Palo Alto, CA: Science and Behavior Books.

Shamansky, S., & Clausen, C. (1980). Levels of prevention: Examination of the concept. *Nursing Outlook, 28*(2), 104–108.

Smilkstein, G. (1980). The cycle of family functioning: A conceptual model for family medicine. *The Journal of Family Practice, 11*(2), 223–232.

Smilkstein, G. (1978). The family APGAR: A proposal for a family function test and its use by physicians. *Journal of Family Practice, 6, 1231—1239.*

Smilkstein, G., Ashworth, C., & Montano, D. (1982). Validity and reliability of the family APGAR as a test of family function. *Journal of Family Practice, 15,* 303–311.

Spanier, G.B., & Filsinger, E.E. (1983). The dyadic adjustment scale. In E.E. Filsinger (Ed.), *Marriage and Family Assessment: A Sourcebook for Family Therapy* (pp. 155–168). Beverly Hills: Sage.

Speer, J.J., & Sachs, B. (1985). Selecting the appropriate family assessment tool. *Pediatric Nursing, 11,* 349–355.

Spradley, B. (1990). *Community Health Nursing: Concept and Practice.* Boston: Little, Brown.

Stanhope, M., & Lancaster, J. (1992). *Community Health Nursing: Process and Practice for Promoting Health.* St. Louis: C.V. Mosby.

Stinnett, N., & DeFrain, J. (1985). *Secrets of Strong Families.* Boston: Little, Brown.

Strauss, M.A., & Brown, B.W. (1978). *Family Measurement Techniques: Abstracts of Published Instruments, 1935–1974.* Minneapolis: University of Minnesota Press.

Webster's New Collegiate Dictionary (9th ed.). (1986). Springfield, MA: Merriam-Webster.

Whall, A., & Fawcett, J. (Eds.). (1991). *Family Theory Development in Nursing: State of the Science and Art.* Philadelphia: F.A. Davis.

Wright, L.M., & Leahey, M. (1994). *Nurses and Families: A Guide to Family Assessment and Intervention.* Philadelphia: F.A. Davis.

ADDITIONAL READINGS

Clements, I.W., & Roberts, F.B. (Eds.). (1983). *Family Health: A Theoretical Approach to Nursing Care.* New York: Wiley.

Feetham, S.L., Meister, S.B., Bell, J.M., & Gillis, C.L. (Eds.). (1993). *The Nursing of Families: Theory/Research/Education/Practice.* Newbury Park, CA: Sage Publications.

Grotevant, H.D., & Carlson, C.I. (1989). *Family Assessment: A Guide to Methods and Measures.* New York: Guiford Press.

Holman, A.M. (1983). *Family Assessment: Tools for Understanding and Intervention.* Beverly Hills: Sage.

Reed, K.S. (1993). *The Neuman Systems Model.* Thousand Oaks, CA: Sage.

Reed, K. (1982). The Neuman systems model: A basis for family psychosocial assessment and intervention. In B. Neuman (Ed.), *The Neuman Systems Model: Application to Nursing Education and Practice* (pp. 188–195). Norwalk, CT: Appleton-Century-Crofts.

Touliatos, J., Perlmutter, B.F., & Straus, M.A. (Eds.). (1990). *Handbook of Family Measurement Techniques.* Newbury Park, CA: Sage.

Wegner, G.D., & Alexander, R.J. (Eds.). (1993). *Readings in Family Nursing.* Philadelphia: J.B. Lippincott.

APPENDIX A

FAMILY SYSTEMS STRESSOR-STRENGTH INVENTORY (FS^{3}I)

Karen B. Mischke, RN, OGNP/WHCNP, PhD, CFLE
Hillsboro Womens Clinic
620 SE Oak Street
Hillsboro, Oregon 97123

Shirley M. H. Hanson, RN, PMHNP, PhD, FAAN, CFLE, LMFT
Professor, School of Nursing, Department of Family Nursing
Oregon Health Sciences University, Portland, Oregon 97201
Telephone: 503-494-8382/3869, Fax 503-494-3878,
E-Mail: hanson@ohsu.edu

Instructions for Administration

The Family Systems Stressor-Strength Inventory (FS^{3}I) Scoring Summary is divided into two sections: Section 1, Family Perception Scores and Section 2, Clinician Perception Scores. These two sections are further divided into three parts: Part I, Family Systems Stressors: General; Part II, Family Systems Stressors: Specific; and, Part III, Family Systems Strengths. Each part contains a Quantitative Summary and a Qualitative Summary.

Quantifiable family and clinician perception scores are both graphed on the Quantitative Summary. Each family member has a designated color code. Family and clinician remarks are both recorded on the Qualitative Summary. Quantitative summary scores, when graphed, suggest a level for initiation of prevention/intervention modes: Primary, Secondary, and Tertiary. Qualitative summary information, when synthesized, contributes to the development and channeling of the Family Care Plan.

Family Name _____ Date _____

Family Member(s) Completing Assessment _____

Ethnic Background(s) _____

Religious Background(s) _____

Referral Source _____

Interviewer _____

	Family Members	Relationship in Family	Age	Marital Status	Education (highest degree)	Occupation
1.						
2.						
3.						
4.						
5.						
6.						

Family's current reasons for seeking assistance?

_____

_____

Source: Variations of this form appear in the following:
Mischke-Berkey, K. & Hanson, S. M. H. (1991). *Pocket guide to family assessment and intervention.* St Louis: Mosby Year Book.
Hanson, S. M. H. (1996). Family nursing assessment and intervention. In S. M. H. Hanson and S. T. Boyd's, *Family Health Care Nursing: Theory, Practice, and Research.* Hanson, S. M. H. & Mischke, K. (1996). Family Health Assessment and Intervention. In P. J. Bomar. *Nurses and Family Health Promotion: Concepts, Assessments, and Interventions.* Philadelphia: W. B. Saunders.

FAMILY SYSTEMS STRESSOR-STRENGTH INVENTORY (FS³I)

Part I: Family Systems Stressors (General)

Directions: Each of the 25 situations/stressors listed here deals with some aspect of normal family life. They have the potential for creating stress within families or between families and the world in which they live. We are interested in your overall impression of how these situations affect your family life. Please circle a number (0 through 5) that best describes the amount of stress or tension they create for you.

Stressors	Family Perception Score						Clinician Perception
	Not Apply	Little Stress	Medium Stress		High Stress		Score
1. Family member(s) feel unappreciated	0	1	2	3	4	5	_____
2. Guilt for not accomplishing more	0	1	2	3	4	5	_____
3. Insufficient "me" time	0	1	2	3	4	5	_____
4. Self-image/self-esteem/feelings of unattractiveness	0	1	2	3	4	5	_____
5. Perfectionism	0	1	2	3	4	5	_____
6. Dieting	0	1	2	3	4	5	_____
7. Health/Illness	0	1	2	3	4	5	_____
8. Communication with children	0	1	2	3	4	5	_____
9. Housekeeping standards	0	1	2	3	4	5	_____
10. Insufficient couple time	0	1	2	3	4	5	_____
11. Insufficient family playtime	0	1	2	3	4	5	_____
12. Children's behavior/discipline/sibling fighting	0	1	2	3	4	5	_____
13. Television	0	1	2	3	4	5	_____
14. Over scheduled family calendar	0	1	2	3	4	5	_____
15. Lack of shared responsibility in the family	0	1	2	3	4	5	_____
16. Moving	0	1	2	3	4	5	_____
17. Spousal relationship (communication, friendship, sex)	0	1	2	3	4	5	_____
18. Holidays	0	1	2	3	4	5	_____
19. In-laws	0	1	2	3	4	5	_____
20. Teen behaviors (communication, music, friends, school)	0	1	2	3	4	5	_____
21. New baby	0	1	2	3	4	5	_____
22. Economics/finances/budgets	0	1	2	3	4	5	_____
23. Unhappiness with work situation	0	1	2	3	4	5	_____
24. Overvolunteerism	0	1	2	3	4	5	_____
25. Neighbors	0	1	2	3	4	5	_____

Additional Stressors:_____

_____

Family Remarks: _____

_____

Clinician: Clarification of stressful situations/concerns with family members.
Prioritize in order of importance to family members:_____

_____

FAMILY SYSTEMS STRESSOR-STRENGTH INVENTORY (FS³I)

Part II: Family Systems Stressors (Specific)

Directions: The following 12 questions are designed to provide information about your specific stress-producing situation/problem, or area of concern influencing your family's health. Please circle a number (1 through 5) that best describes the influence this situation has on your family's life and how well you perceive your family's overall functioning.

The specific stress-producing situation/problem or area of concern at this time is: _____

_____

_____

Stressors:	Family Perception Score					Clinician Perception Score
	Little		**Medium**		**High**	
1. To what extent is your family bothered by this problem or stressful situation? (e.g. effects on family interactions, communication among members, emotional & social relationships)	1	2	3	4	5	_____
Family Remarks: _____						
Clinician Remarks: _____						
2. How much of an effect does this stressful situation have on your family's usual pattern of living? (e.g. effects on lifestyle patterns and family developmental tasks)	1	2	3	4	5	_____
Family Remarks: _____						
Clinician Remarks: _____						
3. How much has this situation affected your family's ability to work together as a family unit? (e.g. alteration in family roles, completion of family tasks, following through with responsibilities)	1	2	3	4	5	_____
Family Remarks: _____						
Clinician Remarks _____						

Has your family ever experienced a similar concern in the past?

    1. YES   If YES, complete question 4

    2. NO   If NO, complete question 5

Stressors:	Family Perception Score					Clinician Perception
	Little		Medium		High	Score
4. How successful was your family in dealing with this situation/problem/ concern in the past? (e.g. workable coping strategies developed, adaptive measures useful, situation improved)	1	2	3	4	5	_____
Family Remarks: _____						
Clinician Remarks: _____						
5. How strongly do you feel this current situation/problem/concern will affect your family's future? (e.g. anticipated consequences)	1	2	3	4	5	_____
Family Remarks: _____						
Clinician Remarks: _____						
6. To what extent are family members able to help themselves in this present situation/problem/ concern? (e.g. self-assistance efforts, family expectations, spiritual influence, and family resources)	1	2	3	4	5	_____
Family Remarks: _____						
Clinician Remarks _____						
7. To what extent do you expect others to help your family with this situation/ problem/concern? (e.g. what roles would helpers play; how available are extra-family resources)	1	2	3	4	5	_____
Family Remarks: _____						
Clinician Remarks _____						

Stressors:	Family Perception Score					Clinician Perception
	Poor	Satisfactory			Excellent	Score

8. How would you rate the way your family functions overall? (e.g. how your family members relate to each other and to larger family and community)

1 2 3 4 5   _____

    Family Remarks: _____

    _____

    Clinician Remarks: _____

    _____

9. How would you rate the overall physical health status of each family member by name? (Include yourself as a family member; record additional names on back.)

1 2 3 4 5   _____

    a. _____   _____

    b. _____   _____

    c. _____   _____

    d. _____   _____

    e. _____   _____

10. How would you rate the overall physical health status of your family as a whole?

1 2 3 4 5   _____

    Family Remarks: _____

    _____

    Clinician Perceptions _____

    _____

11. How would you rate the overall mental health status of each family member by name? (Include yourself as a family member; record additional names on the back.)

1 2 3 4 5   _____

    a. _____   _____

    b. _____   _____

    c. _____   _____

    d. _____   _____

    e. _____   _____

Stressors:	Family Perception Score						Clinician Perception
	Poor		Satisfactory			Excellent	Score
12. How would you rate the overall mental health status of your family as a whole?	1	2	3		4	5	

Family Remarks: _____

_____

Clinician Perceptions _____

_____

Part III: Family Systems Strengths

Directions: Each of the 16 traits/attributes listed below deal with some aspect of family life and its overall functioning. Each one contributes to the health and well-being of family members as individuals and to the family as a whole. Please circle a number (0 through 5) that best describes the extent that the trait applies to your family.

My Family	Family Perception Score						Clinician Perception
	Not Apply	Seldom		Usually		Always	Score
1. Communicates and listens to one another	0	1	2	3	4	5	

Family Remarks: _____

_____

Clinician Remarks _____

_____

2. Affirms and supports one another	0	1	2	3	4	5	

Family Remarks: _____

_____

Clinician Remarks _____

_____

3. Teaches respect for others	0	1	2	3	4	5	

Family Remarks: _____

_____

Clinician Remarks _____

_____

4. Develops a sense of trust in members	0	1	2	3	4	5	

Family Remarks: _____

_____

Clinician Remarks _____

_____

My Family	Family Perception Score						Clinician Perception
	Not Apply	Seldom		Usually		Always	Score
5. Displays a sense of play and humor	0	1	2	3	4	5	_____
Family Remarks: _____							
_____							
Clinician Remarks _____							
_____							
6. Exhibits a sense of shared responsibility	0	1	2	3	4	5	_____
Family Remarks: _____							
_____							
Clinician Remarks _____							
_____							
7. Teaches a sense of right and wrong	0	1	2	3	4	5	_____
Family Remarks: _____							
_____							
Clinician Remarks _____							
_____							
8. Has a strong sense of family in which rituals and traditions abound	0	1	2	3	4	5	_____
Family Remarks: _____							
_____							
Clinician Remarks _____							
_____							
9. Has a balance of interaction among family members	0	1	2	3	4	5	_____
Family Remarks: _____							
_____							
Clinician Remarks _____							
_____							
10. Has a shared religious core	0	1	2	3	4	5	_____
Family Remarks: _____							
_____							
Clinician Remarks _____							
_____							

My Family	Family Perception Score					Clinician Perception
	Not Apply	Seldom	Usually		Always	Score
11. Respects the privacy of one another	0	1	2	3	4 5	_____
Family Remarks: _____						
Clinician Remarks _____						
12. Values service to others	0	1	2	3	4 5	_____
Family Remarks: _____						
Clinician Remarks _____						
13. Fosters family table time and conversation	0	1	2	3	4 5	_____
Family Remarks: _____						
Clinician Remarks _____						
14. Shares leisure time	0	1	2	3	4 5	_____
Family Remarks: _____						
Clinician Remarks _____						
15. Admits to and seeks help with problems	0	1	2	3	4 5	_____
Family Remarks: _____						
Clinician Remarks _____						
16a. How would you rate the overall strengths that exist in your family?	0	1	2	3	4 5	_____
Family Remarks: _____						
Clinician Remarks _____						

16b. Additional Family Strengths: _____

_____

_____

_____

16c. Clarification of family strengths with individual members: _____

_____

_____

_____

APPENDIX B

FAMILY SYSTEMS STRESSOR-STRENGTH INVENTORY (FS³I) SCORING SUMMARY

Karen B. Mischke, RN, OGNP/WHCNP, PhD, CFLE
Hillsboro Womens Clinic
620 SE Oak Street
Hillsboro, Oregon 97123

Shirley M. H. Hanson, RN, PMHNP, PhD, FAAN, CFLE, LMFT
Professor, School of Nursing, Department of Family Nursing
Oregon Health Sciences University, Portland, Oregon 97201
Telephone: 503-494-8382/3869, Fax 503-494-3878,
E-Mail: hanson@ohsu.edu

The Family Systems Stressor-Strength Inventory (FS³I) Scoring Summary is divided into two sections: Section 1, Family Perception Scores and Section 2, Clinician Perception Scores. These two sections are further divided into three parts: Part I, Family Systems Stressors: General; Part II, Family Systems Stressors: Specific; and, Part III, Family Systems Strengths. Each part contains a Quantitative Summary and a Qualitative Summary.

Quantifiable family and clinician perception scores are both graphed on the Quantitative Summary. Each family member has a designated color code. Family and clinician remarks are both recorded on the Qualitative Summary. Quantitative summary scores, when graphed, suggest a level for initiation of prevention/intervention modes: Primary, Secondary and Tertiary. Qualitative summary information, when synthesized, contributes to the development and channeling of the Family Care Plan.

Source: Variations of this form appear in the following:
Mischke-Berkey, K. & Hanson, S. M. H. (1991). *Pocket guide to family assessment and intervention*. St Louis: Mosby Year Book.
Hanson, S. M. H. (1996). Family nursing assessment and intervention. In S. M. H. Hanson and S. T. Boyd's, *Family Health Care Nursing: Theory, Practice and Research*. Hanson, S. M. H. & Mischke, K. (1996). Family Health Assessment and Intervention. In P. J. Bomar. *Nurses and family Health Promotion: Concepts, Assessments, and Interventions*. Philadelphia: W. B. Saunders.

FAMILY SYSTEMS STRESSOR-STRENGTH INVENTORY (FS^{3}I) SCORING SUMMARY

Section 1: Clinician Perception Scores

Part I Family Systems Stressors (General)

Add scores from questions 1 to 25 and calculate an overall numerical score for Family System Stressors (General). Ratings are from 1 (most positive) to 5 (most negative). The Not Apply (0) responses are omitted from the calculations. Total scores range from 25 to 125.

Family Systems Stressor Score: General

$$\frac{(\quad)}{25} \times 1 = \underline{\hspace{2cm}}$$

Graph score on Quantitative Summary, Family Systems Stressors: General (Clincian Perception).

Record Clinicinas' clarification of general stressors in Part I, Qualitative Summary: Family and Clinician Remarks.

Part II. Family Systems Stresors: Specific

Add scores from questions 1–8, 10, and 12 and calculate a numerical score for Family Systems Stressors: Specific. Ratings are from 1 (most positive) to 5 (most negative). Questions 4, 6, 7, 8, 10, and 12 are reverse scored.* Total scores range from 10–50.

Family Systems Stressor Score: Specific

$$\frac{(\quad)}{10} \times 1 = \underline{\hspace{2cm}}$$

Graph score on Quantitative Summary : Family Systems Stressor: Specific. (Clinician Perception).

Summarize data from questions 9 and 11 (reverse scored) and record Clinician Remarks in Part II, Qualitative Summary: Family and Clinician Remarks.

Part III Family Systems Strengths

Add scores from questions 1 to 16 and calculate a numerical score for Family Systems Strengths. Ratings are from 1 (seldom) to 5 (always). The Not Apply (0) responses are omitted from the calculations. Total scores range from 16 to 80.

$$\frac{(\quad)}{16} \times 1 = \underline{\hspace{2cm}}$$

Graph score on Quantitative Summary: Family Systems Strengths (Family Member Perception).

Record Clinicians' clarification of family strengths in Part III, Qualitative Summary: Family and Clinician Remarks.

---

*Reverse Scoring:
  Question answered as (1) is scored 5 points
  Question answered as (2) is scored 4 points
  Question answered as (3) is scored 3 points
  Question answered as (4) is scored 2 points
  Question answered as (5) is scored 1 point

FAMILY SYSTEMS STRESSOR-STRENGTH INVENTORY (FS^{3}I) SCORING SUMMARY

Quantitative Summary
Family Systems Stressors: General & Specific
Family & Clinician Perception Scores

Directions: Graph the scores from each family member inventory by placing an "X" at the appropriate location. (Use first name initial for each different entry and different color code for each family member.)

Scores for Wellness and Stability	Family Systems Stressors: General		Scores for Wellness and Stability	Family Systems Stressors: Specific	
	Family Member Perception Score	Clinician Perception Score		Family Member Perception Score	Clinician Perception Score
5.0			5.0		
4.8			4.8		
4.6			4.6		
4.4			4.4		
4.2			4.2		
4.0			4.0		
3.8			3.8		
3.6			3.6		
3.4			3.4		
3.2			3.2		
3.0			3.0		
2.8			2.8		
2.6			2.6		
2.4			2.4		
2.2			2.2		
2.0			2.0		
1.8			1.8		
1.6			1.6		
1.4			1.4		
1.2			1.2		
1.0			1.0		

PRIMARY Prevention/Intervention Mode: Flexible   Line 1.0–2.3
SECONDARY Prevention/Intervention Mode: Normal   Line 2.4–3.6
TERTIARY Prevention/Intervention Mode: Resistance   Lines 3.7–5.0
Breakdown of numerical scores for stressor penetration are suggested values

FAMILY SYSTEMS STRESSOR-STRENGTH INVENTORY (FS³I) SCORING SUMMARY

Quantitative Summary
Family Systems Strengths
Family & Clinician Perception Scores

Directions: Graph the scores from each family member inventory by placing an "X" at the appropriate location. (Use first name initial for each different entry and different color code for each family member.)

Sum of strengths available for prevention/ intervention mode	Family Systems Strengths	
	Family Member Perception Score	Clinician Perception Score
5.0		
4.8		
4.6		
4.4		
4.2		
4.0		
3.8		
3.6		
3.4		
3.2		
3.0		
2.8		
2.6		
2.4		
2.2		
2.0		
1.8		
1.6		
1.4		
1.2		
1.0		

PRIMARY Prevention/Intervention Mode: Flexible   Line 1.0–2.3
SECONDARY Prevention/Intervention Mode: Normal   Line 2.4–3.6
TERTIARY Prevention/Intervention Mode: Resistance   Lines 3.7–5.0
Breakdown of numerical scores for stressor penetration are suggested values

FAMILY SYSTEMS STRESSOR-STRENGTH INVENTORY (FS³I) SCORING SUMMARY

Qualitative Summary: Family and Clinician Remarks

Part I: Family Systems Stressors: General
Summarize general stressors and remarks of family and clinician. Prioritize stressors according to importance to family members.

_____

_____

_____

Part II: Family Systems Stressors: Specific
A. Summarize specific stressor and remarks of family and clinician.

_____

_____

_____

B. Summarize differences (if discrepancies exist) between how family members and clinician view effects of stressful situation on family.

_____

_____

_____

C. Summarize overall family functioning.

_____

_____

_____

D. Summarize overall significant physical health status for family members.

_____

_____

_____

E. Summarize overall significant mental health status for family members.

_____

_____

_____

Part III: Family Systems Strengths
Summarize family systems strengths and family and clinician remarks that facilitate family health and stability.

_____

_____

_____

FAMILY SYSTEMS STRESSOR-STRENGTH INVENTORY (FS³I) SCORING SUMMARY

FAMILY CARE PLAN*

| Diagnosis General and Specific Family System Stressors | Family Systems Strengths Supporting Family Care Plan | Goals Family and Clinician | Prevention/Intervention Mode | | Outcomes Evaluation and Replanning |
			Primary, Secondary or Tertiary	Prevention/ Intervention Activities	

*Prioritize the three most significant diagnoses.

FAMILY NUTRITION AND WEIGHT CONTROL

13

KATHY SHADLE JAMES

The ritual of a family dinner to end the day, a time to eat in peace and quiet and the comforting support of the family, is the one best thing anyone can do for their own health.

PAUL PEARSALL (p. 54)

OBJECTIVES

On completion of this chapter, the reader will be able to:

1. Describe changing dietary patterns in the United States and the effect on a family's nutritional status
2. Explain the relationship between diet and health
3. Identify one nutritional concern associated with each growth and development stage
4. Identify sociocultural and other factors that affect a family's nutritional behaviors
5. Assess a family's application of the U.S. dietary guidelines
6. Discriminate "healthful diets" from "fad diets"
7. Explain the relationship between lifestyle and weight control
8. Formulate nursing diagnoses related to a family's nutritional status
9. Identify nursing approaches to improve a family's nutritional health
10. Establish guidelines for a family to evaluate its nutritional and/or weight control plan

This chapter will discuss dietary issues as well as weight control and will provide guidelines for the professional whose goal is to guide families in the attainment of optimal weight and nutritional status throughout their life cycle. The nurse's goal is to instill that the key for nutritional wellness comes from within the family. The family becomes the provider of health care by teaching healthful behaviors. The family's learning of health-promoting behaviors begins at birth, with the family providing the stimulus to incorporate health into its member's value system. The degree of family support often determines the extent to which new behaviors will be adopted (McCarthy, 1990). In addition, the more knowledge people have, the more likely they are to choose and maintain healthy lifestyles (Herron, 1991).

Many families feel overwhelmed at the deluge of nutrition information. This chapter presents nutritional information pertaining to the needs of family members of all ages. The guidelines are relative to anyone choosing to alter their diet for optimal health and weight control.

The family health nurse will be provided with the knowledge and tools to assist families by teaching, guiding, and supporting decision making regarding health-promoting lifestyle changes.

CHANGING DIETARY PATTERNS IN THE UNITED STATES

A vast body of evidence from the *Surgeon General's Report on Nutrition and Health* (U.S.

Department of Health and Human Services [U.S. DHHS], 1988) indicates that the current American diet contains too much fat, sugar, and protein and not enough whole grain foods and cereals, vegetables, and fruits. A common American habit is to eat from the refrigerator at all times of the day as well as at desks, in cars, and in front of the television.

The U.S. Human Nutrition Information Service published results of a survey of individuals' food intakes during 1985 and compared the results to an earlier study in 1977. The findings indicated that dietary intake was lower in fat and higher in carbohydrate in 1985 than in 1977. Food energy intakes for women and children were higher in 1985 than in 1977 (National Nutrition Monitoring System, 1986).

On a national level, few large-scale surveys have been reported since 1989 on U.S. dietary changes. However, as a result of the past surveys, extensive reports have been published such as *Diet and Health* (National Research Council [NRC], 1989) and *Healthy People 2000* (U.S. DHHS, 1990a).

Although reports indicate that populations are consuming less fat, the U.S. population as a whole has relatively high intakes of fat, saturated fatty acids, and cholesterol. The once prevalent nutrient deficiencies have been replaced by excesses and imbalances of some food components as the principal concern. The proportion of calories from fat averages 41%. This is too high when compared to the recommendations by groups such as the American Heart Association and the National Research Council (1989), Food and Nutrition Board. They recommend limiting total fat intake to 30% of total calories.

Fat and sugar constitute 60% of daily calories. It appears that caloric intakes have either increased or physical activity has decreased, since the National Institutes of Health (NIH) consensus report (1985) indicates that 34 million Americans between the ages of 20 and 75 are overweight. Overweight affects about 26% of the population. It is a particular problem for the poor and minority populations, affecting 44% of black women below poverty levels (Stern, 1992).

Dietary patterns have been affected by many factors. Mealtimes are no longer regular. Family members eat at different times and consume different foods. Three out of four have improper breakfasts or skip breakfast altogether. Lunch is often skipped or includes junk food or cafeteria food. Dinner is often the largest meal, consisting of easy-to-prepare foods or fast foods, which constitute 25% of all meals.

A report by the National Nutrition Monitoring System (1986) concluded the following:

- In the U.S. today, food supply is safe, adequate, and abundant.
- The principal nutrition problem is the overconsumption of certain food components—

fat, saturated fat, fatty acids, cholesterol, and sodium.
- Overall, Americans maintain low levels of physical activity.
- Dietary and biochemical data indicate that intakes of iron and vitamin C are low in certain subgroups.
- Iron deficiency exists in young children and females of childbearing age, in 11- to 14-year-old boys, and in black children and women.
- Vitamin C depletion is seen most among low-income groups, especially in adult males who smoke cigarettes.

The low intake of calcium among women is a concern because calcium deficiency is implicated as a contributor to osteoporosis among postmenopausal women. From the population as a whole, intakes of calcium from food averaged below the recommended dietary allowances (RDA) 87%, with 68% of the population not meeting the RDA.

The prevalence of health conditions related to nutrition are highest among low-income populations. The food components warranting public health monitoring were based on the findings from three-day dietary intakes. High dietary consumption included food energy (calories), total fat, saturated fat, cholesterol, sodium, and alcohol. Low dietary consumption included vitamin C, calcium, iron, and fluoride. The health data showed that low levels of serum albumin (indicator of protein status) and of serum vitamin A were rarely found and were not associated with race or poverty status. The same nutritional concerns continue to exist and are reflected in the government's health status objectives found in the report *Healthy People 2000* (U.S. DHHS, 1990a).

U.S. DIETARY RECOMMENDATIONS

The main conclusion from the first Surgeon General's report in 1979 on nutrition and health (U.S. DHHS) indicated that overconsumption of certain dietary components was a major concern for Americans. With the focus on the relationship between diet and chronic diseases increasing, the U.S. Department of Agriculture, along with the U.S. DHHS, published a third edition of *Dietary Guidelines for Americans* (1990b). These guidelines are easy to follow and are available to the public.

Dietary factors are associated with five of the ten leading causes of death in the United States: coronary heart disease, cancer, stroke, non-insulin–dependent diabetes mellitus, and atherosclerosis. According to government reports, for two out of three Americans who neither drink or smoke, eating patterns may shape their long-term health status more than any other personal choice.

The public has been confused with the plethora of nutrition information in recent years with little guidance on how to separate fact from fiction. Based on an in-depth analysis of the overall relationship between diet and major chronic disease, the National Research Council (NRC, 1989) committee on Diet and Health presented dietary recommendations (Table 13–1). The recommendations are to be used in combination with the RDAs to achieve a highly desirable pattern for the maintenance of good health.

ROLE OF NUTRITION AND FAMILY HEALTH

Although it is customary to think of nutrition as an individual activity, a systems framework illustrates how food consumption depends on many factors (Table 13–2). The issue of family nutrition and food consumption involves complex interactions of social, family, and individual systems. Social, cultural, economic, cognitive, and physiologic characteristics influence the family and its members (Melson, 1980; Mellin, 1991). Family health nurses who are aware of these factors will be able to direct families to stay well, to work, to feel good about themselves, to meet their nutrition goals, and to live longer. By identifying potential barriers and setting realistic goals, the family will be successful in making desired changes.

Diet and Health Consequences

Making good food choices has important health implications. Adequate nutrition and caloric intake are essential for growth and development, physical activity, reproduction, lactation, recovery from illness and injury, and maintenance of health throughout the life cycle. The role of nutrients in diseases such as heart disease, adult-onset diabetes, high blood pressure, dental caries, and some types of cancer (especially cancers of the esophagus, stomach, large bowel, breast, lung, and prostate) is becoming clearer as epidemiologic studies offer important insights of possible relationships between diet and health consequences.

Choosing health foods begins with understanding the composition and use of food in the body. Although people vary in size, age, race, appearance, and activity, all need varying amounts of the same nutrients: protein, carbohydrate, fat, vitamins, minerals, and water. Family health nurses work to increase families awareness of nutrition and of potential risks associated with dietary choices.

Protein Requirements and Use

Because the body cannot store protein, it needs a new supply daily. Protein plays a crucial role in the growth and maintenance of body tissue and is composed of 22 different amino acids. Of the 22, 8 must be provided by the diet, and the other 14

TABLE 13–1. DIETARY GUIDELINES FOR AMERICANS

To reduce risk of diet related chronic diseases:
1. *Reduce total fat intake to 30%* or less of total calories. Reduce saturated fatty acid intake to less than 10% of calories, and the intake of cholesterol to less than 300mg daily. The intake of fat and cholesterol can be reduced by substituting fish, poultry without skin, lean meats, and low or non-fat dairy products; by choosing more vegetables, fruits, cereals, and legumes; and by limiting oils, fats, egg yolks, and fried and other fatty foods.
2. *Every day eat five or more servings of a combination of vegetables and fruits,* especially green and yellow vegetables and citrus fruits.
3. *Increase intake of starches and other complex carbohydrates* by eating six or more daily servings of a combination of breads, cereals, and legumes.
4. *Maintain protein intake at moderate levels.* The committee recommends maintaining total protein intake at levels lower than twice the RDA for all age groups (e.g., less than 1.6g/kg body weight for all adults.
5. *Balance food intake and physical activity* to maintain appropriate body weight. A steady loss of $\frac{1}{2}$ pound to 1 pound a week is generally safe. Avoid extreme measures to lose weight. Refer to Chapter 16 for estimating basal metabolic rate and caloric expenditure of activities.
6. *Alcohol consumption is not recommended.* For those who drink alcoholic beverages, limit consumption to the equivalent of less than 1 ounce of pure alcohol in a single day. This is the equivalent of two cans of beer, two small glasses of wine, or two average cocktails. Pregnant women should avoid alcoholic beverages.
7. *Use salt and sodium only in moderation.* Salt enters the diet in three ways: one-third is present naturally, including dairy, meats and seafood; one-third comes from salt added at home or in restaurants during cooking and at the table; and one-third is introduced during food processing.
8. *Maintain adequate calcium intake.* Include low- or non-fat dairy products and dark-green vegetables, which are rich sources of calcium.
9. *Avoid taking dietary supplements in excess* of the RDA in any one day.
10. *Maintain an optimal intake of fluoride,* particularly during the years of primary and secondary tooth formation and growth.

Data from National Research Council (1989). *Recommended Dietary Allowances* (9th ed). Washington, D.C.: National Academy of Sciences.

TABLE 13–2. FACTORS INFLUENCING NUTRITIONAL HEALTH

SOCIETY
Technology
Media
Status
Foods
Fast-Food
Availability of Food
Ecology

FAMILY SYSTEM
Rituals
Meal-Time
Environment
Culture
Values
Religion
Communications
Finances
Family
Structure

INDIVIDUAL SYSTEM
Self-Concept
Exercise
Nutrients
Eating Habits
Knowledge
Age
Sex
Physical Requirements

Data from Melson, G.F. (1980). *Family and Environment: An Ecological Perspective* (pp. 145–165). Minneapolis, MN: Burgess.

TABLE 13–3. PROTEIN REQUIREMENTS

GROUP	PROTEIN G/DAY[*]
Infants	
0 to 1 yr	13
Children	
1 to 3 yrs	16
4 to 6 yrs	24
7 to 10 yrs	28
Boys	
11 to 14 yrs	46
15 to 18 yrs	59
19 to 24 yrs	58
Girls	
11 to 14 yrs	46
15 to 18 yrs	44
19 to 24 yrs	46
Women (63 kg)	50
Pregnancy	60
Lactation	65
Men (79 kg)	63

*All requirements listed are approximate.

can, with the necessary materials, be made by the body. The Food and Nutrition Board of the National Academy of Sciences has established a daily recommended dietary allowance (RDA) of protein, based on age, weight, and general physical state (see Table 13–3).

Special periods of rapid growth, such as the growth of a fetus and maternal tissue during pregnancy, also require added protein, as does any illness and disease. Traumatic injury, post-surgical states, or extensive tissue destruction (as in burns) requires a considerable increase in protein intake for the healing process.

The RDA protein standard for adults is 0.8 g/kg of body weight. This amounts to about 63 grams of protein per day for a man weighing 174 pounds (79 kg) and 50 grams per day for a woman weighing 138 pounds (63 kg) (Williams, 1990). It is possible to get the recommended amount of protein without eating meat. Other sources of protein include milk and cheese, beans and peas, tofu, rice, and nuts (Dudek, 1993). The position of the American Dietetic Association (Havala & Dwyer, 1988) is that vegetarian diets are healthful and nutritionally adequate when appropriately planned.

In contrast, too much protein may have negative effects on the body. High-protein diets have been shown to increase the loss of calcium from bones and to increase the production of uric acid in the blood, which may lead to gout. In people with kidney disease, excess protein can further impair kidney functioning as the kidneys work hard to remove the nitrogen part of the protein molecule that is not needed for building or rebuilding tissues. After the body disposes of the unneeded nitrogen supply, the remainder becomes a source of calories. You can get just as fat by eating too much steak as you can by eating too much chicken or too many doughnuts (Clark, 1990).

Fat Requirements and Use

In the United States fat intake contributes about 40% of daily total calories, although dietary guidelines from the American Heart Association and the National Cholesterol Education Program (NCEP) recommend reducing total fat intake to not more than 30% of one's total calories or less, and reducing saturated fat to 10%. If you know how many calories you need, you can determine the 30% into fat grams. For example, someone who eats 1500 calories per day would have a desired fat intake of about 50 grams of fat per day.

Fat is an essential nutrient which, in addition to supplying the highest density of energy (9 calories per gram) among the energy nutrients, protects vital organs from damage and insulates the body against low temperatures. It also aides in the formation of cell membrane structure, the transport of molecules such as protein and certain fat-soluble vitamins to the cells, the transmission of nerve impulses, and the production of metabolic precursors (Williams, 1990).

Fats are composed of glycerol and attached fatty acids of varying degrees of saturation and length. Essential fatty acids cannot be manufactured by the body. The major one is linoleic, a polyunsaturated fat found primarily in vegetable oils. It's functions include prolonging clotting time, lowering serum cholesterol levels, improving skin integrity, and developing prostaglandins, which are involved in tissue activities including platelet aggregations and maintaining smooth muscle tone of blood vessels (Williams, 1990). If fat intake makes up only 10% or less of a diet's daily calories, the body cannot obtain adequate amounts of the essential fatty acids.

Dietary factors in individuals and in entire populations have important effects on blood cholesterol levels. High blood cholesterol levels clearly play a role in coronary heart disease (CHD). This disease continues to kill more than 500,000 Americans annually. About 1,250,000 Americans suffer myocardial infarctions each year. In addition to its impact on the nation's health, CHD costs the U.S. economy over $50 billion annually, according to the NIH report *Population Strategies for Blood Cholesterol Reduction* (1990). Implementations of recommendations to reduce dietary fat and cholesterol will help most Americans lower their levels of blood cholesterol.

Carbohydrate Requirements and Use

Carbohydrates were thought of as "the bad guys" in weight management. Today, carbohydrates are back in favor—especially complex carbohydrates. Complex carbohydrates, which are large chains of glucose molecules, consist mainly in all plant foods. The storage form of carbohydrates in humans is glycogen. Carbohydrates are transformed to glucose—the main sugar in the blood and the body's basic fuel.

The primary function of carbohydrates is to provide energy, since carbohydrates are digested and absorbed more rapidly than protein or fat. Under normal conditions, glucose is the only energy source for the central nervous system. Carbohydrates maintain liver, heart, brain, and nerve tissue function. They also prevent the breakdown of fats and protein for energy which results in toxic metabolic byproducts (Williams, 1990).

There are two basic types of carbohydrates: simple or complex. Simple carbohydrates are easily digested and provide quick energy. Ordinary table sugar is an example of a simple carbohydrate. Complex carbohydrates are promoted over simple carbohydrates because a high concentration of sugar in large amounts, such as in a piece of cake, is more than the body can use at one time. The excess will be stored as fat. Complex carbohydrates promote energy release more slowly and prevent large fluctuations in blood glucose levels. U.S. dietary guidelines recommend that about 50% to 60% of total calorie value of the diet come

from carbohydrates, with a greater portion of that allowance coming from complex carbohydrates and including foods such as whole wheat grains, beans and peas, potatoes, and fruits.

OVERVIEW OF NUTRITION CONCERNS AND RESEARCH

There have been numerous research reports on the effects of polyunsaturated fatty acids, monosaturated fatty acids, dietary cholesterol, fiber, food additives, and calcium on health. The following will offer an overview of conclusions from scientific reports by the NRC (1989).

Polyunsaturated Fatty Acids

Human diets do not naturally have high levels of polyunsaturated fatty acids, and there is a dearth of information about the long-term consequences of high polyunsaturated fatty acid intakes. There has been evidence from clinical and animal studies that omega-6 polyunsaturated fatty acids found in safflower, corn, and other oils result in a lowering of serum cholesterol and low-density-lipoprotein (LDL) cholesterol, and usually some lowering of high-density-lipoprotein (HDL) when substituted for saturated fatty acids. The requirement for omega-6 polyunsaturated fatty acids can be met by 1% to 2% of calories as linoleic acid.

Monosaturated Fatty Acids

Some research studies show that substitution of monosaturated for saturated fatty acids can lower total cholesterol and LDL cholesterol without a reduction in HDL cholesterol. Examples of oils that contain predominantly fatty acids are olive oil and canola oil (Applegate, 1991).

Dietary Cholesterol

Dietary cholesterol raises serum total cholesterol and LDL cholesterol levels and increases the risk of CHD and atherosclerosis. There is individual variability in this response. The American Heart Association recommends a cholesterol intake of 300 mg with additional recommendations to limit consumption to 100 mg per 1000 calories (NRC, 1989).

The National Cholesterol Education Program states that all children, whatever their family history, can benefit from a heart-healthy diet. After the age of two, children should switch to low-fat dairy products and should keep fat intake to about 30% of their daily caloric intake. Only children who have a family history of very high cholesterol levels and/or heart disease—and particularly those with a parent who suffered a heart attack before the age of 50—should have their cholesterol levels measured. That includes as many as one-quarter of this nation's children (NIH, 1990).

In cross-sectional studies, strong correlations have been found between the mean serum cholesterol of a population and the incidence of coronary heart disease. In a seven-country study (Belmaker & Cohen, 1985), countries with high mean cholesterol levels (United States and Finland) had death rates from coronary heart disease three to four times higher than countries with low mean cholesterol levels (Japan, Greece, Yugoslavia) (Belmaker & Cohen, 1985). People vary in their response to altering dietary cholesterol. For most individuals, following a low-fat diet will keep cholesterol within recommended levels. Research shows that a high consumption of saturated fats increases the amount of cholesterol in the general circulation. Fats from animal foods (lard, butterfat, chicken fat, etc.) tend to be highly saturated. Fats from fish are less saturated than other animal fats, and in fact, fish oil seems to protect against heart disease.

Typically, doctors take no measures to lower a patient's cholesterol level until it exceeds 250 mg/dl, at which point dietary modification is recommended. A desirable blood cholesterol is less than 200 mg/dl for adults; a desirable LDL cholesterol level is considered to be less than 130 mg/dl. Table 13–4 lists moderate and high-risk values of blood cholesterol.

Total serum cholesterol may not be the best predictor for coronary heart disease risk, although the risk of developing a premature coronary attack rises as serum cholesterol is elevated. Other risk factors include sex (male), family history of premature coronary heart disease, cigarette smoking, hypertension, low LDL cholesterol concentration, diabetes mellitus, history of definite cerebrovascular or occlusive peripheral vascular disease, and severe obesity (greater than 30% overweight).

To date, HDL cholesterol level is claimed to be the strongest predictor of coronary heart disease (CHD). HDLs appear to retard the atherosclerotic process by removing early cholesterol deposits and transporting them back to the liver for processing. (In diabetics, however, low density lipoproteins appear to be better correlated with risk of CHD than high-density lipoproteins.)

Factors that appear to influence the HDL level are race, sex, body weight, smoking, alcohol in-

take, physical activity, hormones, and drugs. Blacks have higher HDL levels than whites; females have higher HDL levels than males; obesity is associated with lower HDL levels; cigarette smoking lowers HDL levels; moderate use of alcohol increases HDL levels; exercise increases HDL levels; estrogens increase HDL levels and androgens lower them; and clofibrate, nicotinic acid, and heparin increase HDL levels, while zinc supplements lower them.

Low-density lipoproteins (LDL) are cholesterol-rich particles that transport cholesterol to peripheral tissues and possibly promote entrance of cholesterol into cells. An elevated LDL level (also called hypercholesterolemia) is believed to accelerate the atherosclerotic process and to increase risk of CHD (NRC, 1989).

The ratio of HDL to LDL, indicating the balance between the cholesterol delivery and removal systems, may be more important than serum levels. An ideal ratio is under 3.5. A ratio lower than about 4.5 suggests that the risk for CHD is below average; with a ratio higher than that, one has a higher than average risk. A high HDL:LDL ratio is desirable.

Fiber and Health

In the early 1970s, several researchers, notably British epidemiologist Dr. Dennis Burkett, linked a high-fiber intake among rural Africans with the low incidence of diseases common in the Western industrialized countries. The various types of fiber may help to prevent or improve disorders such as constipation, irritable bowel syndrome, and diverticulosis, although people with these disorders should consult their physicians before starting a high-fiber diet. Colon cancer is rare among people with a diet low in meat and rich in high-fiber foods. Fiber may reduce bacteria that interact with fat and bile acids to create carcinogens as stools move quickly through the digestive track. A high-fiber diet may also benefit obese persons because fibrous foods take longer to chew and provide a full feeling. Diabetics may also benefit because of the effect of fiber on blood sugar levels. There is no conclusive evidence that it is dietary fiber, rather than the other components of vegetables, fruits, and cereal products, that reduces the risk of those diseases (NRC, 1989).

The source of fiber is plants. Fiber is the plant material that doesn't get digested when eaten. There are two basic types of fiber. Type I, insoluble fibers, include cellulose, hemicellulose, and lignin. Type I fiber is like a sponge: It absorbs many times its weight in water swelling up within the intestine. Cellulose, hemicellulose, and lignin are found primarily in whole grains and beans and other plant products, especially bran. Because insoluble fibers are nondigestible by humans, they are not useful as fuel (Applegate, 1991).

TABLE 13–4. RISK VALUES OF CHOLESTEROL

AGES	MODERATE (MG/DL) RISK	HIGH RISK
2–19	170	185
20–29	200	220
30–39	200	240
40 and above	240	260

Type II, soluble fibers, include pectin, gums, and mucilages, which are found in fruits, certain vegetables and legumes, oat bran, and most plant foods. Type II fiber does appear to have some hypercholesterolemic effect of hyperlipidemics. Guar supplements tend to lower LDL cholesterol, whereas oat bran has been shown in some studies to reduce triglycerides. The gums also help manage blood sugar. Although not conclusive, epidemiologic studies are consistent in showing that a high-fiber diet containing vegetables and a relatively low level of meat and fat products is beneficial with respect to cancer of the colon and possibly atherogenesis. According to the National Research Council it is reasonable to recommend a diet containing a high level of fiber-rich foods. There is little evidence to support direct supplementation of the diet with fiber products.

Fiber is available in a variety of foods, and the recommended amount is 20 to 30 grams per day, which is twice what the average American usually eats. Clients should not be coerced into thinking that fiber is some type of medicine that ought to be added to an otherwise unrefined diet. Instead, they should be encouraged to eat a variety of foods while incorporating high-fiber foods.

Food Additives

Foods in their natural state are mixtures of chemicals. Some of these are nutrients (carbohydrate, protein, fat, minerals, vitamins, and water). Others are nonnutritive substances, such as colors, flavors, emulsifiers, antioxidants, and chelating agents.

Intentional additives are designed to perform a specific function, such as to prevent spoilage or oxidation or to improve nutritional value. Incidental additives serve no functional purpose in the final food product. Examples include pesticides, fertilizers, adjuvants to animal feed, and packaging materials, such as polyvinyl chloride, that migrate from the wrapping to the food. There are safe and unsafe doses of all chemicals, both natural and synthetic. For example, solanine (a toxic alkaloid) is present in potatoes. Common table salt is toxic in doses three to five times the normal usage. More is known about the relative safety of food additives than about naturally occurring toxicants.

The Food and Drug Administration regulates the use of additives in food by defining criteria and tolerance levels for additives and by continually monitoring their use. In recent years, cyclamates and the colorants red dye #2 and #4 and carbon black were removed from use because of hazardous effects in animals, even though there have been no observable effects in humans.

There are benefits and risks of additives. Without their use, the scope of the food supply would be limited, and many aesthetic and convenience qualities would be lost. For example, baked goods would go stale overnight, canned fruits and vegetables would be mushy and discolored, and table salt would harden. Three fifths of food additives are artificial flavors and colors, emulsifiers, stabilizers, and thickeners, whose main purpose is to make food more attractive. Other additives are used as preservatives or as leavening, anti-staling, or mold-retarding agents.

Practically any varied well-selected diet that excludes excessive amounts of highly processed foods can be nutritionally adequate. Clients should be informed that natural, organic, and health foods are neither more nor less nutritious than similar foods available at supermarkets (Lewis, 1986).

Of the well-known additives, nitrates and nitrites are probably carcinogenic when converted in the body to nitrosamines. Although nitrites are present in human saliva and the body is capable of producing nitrites on its own, it is wise to limit food sources such as smoked, salt-cured, and nitrite-cured meats because they may increase the risk of breast, colon, and prostate cancers. According to the NRC (1989) report, nitrates appear to be neither carcinogenic nor mutagenic. Nitrites are probably not direct carcinogens, but they are mutagenic in microbial systems. There is some evidence that nitrites and N-nitroso compounds play a role in the development of gastric and esophageal cancer. In addition, various mutagens and carcinogens are formed when broiling, charring, and grilling meat and fish, and browning of foods. The amounts formed may be too small to pose a serious risk for the development of cancer in humans. More epidemiologic studies are needed to assess the carcinogenity of such mutagens.

Additional diet recommendations related to cancer prevention include (1) limit alcohol consumption that may lead to cancer of the mouth, larynx, esophagus, and liver; and (2) increase dietary sources of vitamins A, E, and C. Following these recommendations does not guarantee against cancer, but they are prudent and reasonable precautions.

Sodium Intake and Hypertension

Studies show that population groups who consume a lot of sodium tend to have a higher incidence of hypertension. In northern Japan, salt consumption is enormous—20 to 25 grams per day, and prevalence is also high. In Kenya, preliminary findings indicate that the Luo tribe, who live in a countryside where the diet is low in sodium, tend to have a lower incidence of hypertension. When members migrate to other areas, incidence goes up. Many are reluctant to draw conclusions from such studies because some rural diets include large amounts of fresh vegetables that are rich in potassium, a mineral that may protect against hypertension. A high-sodium environment may favor the expression of acquired hypertension variables that may be more common in blacks or those predisposed to hypertension (Kumanyika & Adams-Campbell, 1991). According to reports from *Diet and Health,* potassium may modulate the blood-pressure–raising effects of sodium and provide some protection against death from stroke, even when blood pressure is not reduced.

The body's daily requirement for sodium varies with each individual but is quite small. The minimal requirement is about 100 to 200 mg per day, the amount in one-tenth of a teaspoon. The NRC (1989) recommends that intake of salt (sodium chloride) be less than 6 grams a day and that less than 4.5 grams is even more desirable. The estimated minimum requirement is even less—500 mg per day (National Academy of Sciences, 1989).

Estimates indicate that 90% to 95% of the population is sodium resistant, that is, their blood pressure does not show a significant increase with increased sodium in the diet. The prudent approach recommended in Dietary Guidelines for Americans (U.S. DHHS, 1990b) is to use salt sparingly, if at all, in cooking and at the table and to check labels for the amount of sodium in foods.

Calcium and Osteoporosis

Osteoporosis is a major public health problem affecting 20 million women—or one in four over 65 years of age. "Porous bones" are associated with increased risk of fractures of the hip, wrist, and spine (Riggs & Melton, 1986). Approximately 20% of women in the United States suffer one or more osteoporotic fractures by age 65, and as many as 40% sustain fractures after age 65.

A low intake of calcium and dietary factors that negatively influence its absorption include alcohol, aluminum-containing antacids, foods high in phosphorus, foods high in oxalic acids, and/or overconsumption of protein. Those at highest risk for osteoporosis are Caucasian females (usually fair-skinned and of northern European descent). Risk factors include a small body, early menopause, sedentary lifestyle, calcium deficiency, family history of osteoporosis, smoking, and consuming more than five cups of coffee or tea per day.

Prevention should begin early, preferably by the early 30s, but it is important throughout life. Nutrition scientists are recommending 1000 mg daily for most adults and 1500 mg for pregnant women, postmenopausal women, and female adolescents (Dudek, 1993; Riggs & Melton, 1986; Roe, 1986). Evidence also suggests that intakes of calcium up to 2000 mg/day are safe for teenagers and adults.

Although milk and cheese are the best dietary sources of calcium, many people do not eat these foods because of personal preferences, lactose intolerance, or acquired allergies. These people should be encouraged to use other good sources of calcium since daily calcium intake is essential (Clark, 1990). Foods high in calcium include milk, yogurt, cottage cheese, ice cream, canned red salmon, sardines with bones, kale, collards, turnip greens, mustard greens, dandelion greens, okra, broccoli, and soybeans (cooked).

Immunity and Nutritional Status

The study of nutrition and immunity is still new, but Sherman (1986) describes ways in which nutrients play a role. Nutrients are important in the anatomic development of lymphoid tissue, skin health, cell proliferation, intracellular killing, synthesis of immunicologically active proteins, cellular activity and movement, and modulation and regulation of the immune process. Because the immune response is a rapidly acting system, nutrient functions have dramatic effects on the system's responsiveness.

NUTRITIONAL NEEDS THROUGHOUT THE LIFE CYCLE

It is well recognized that nutritional needs change. When assessing the family, the nurse should be alert to specific needs related to development level.

Pregnancy and Lactation

For hundreds of years, advice given to pregnant women regarding weight gain and nutrition was based on hearsay rather than on scientific research. The Health Professionals' Committee for Nutrition Education (1986), which monitors developing, testing, and distributing patient education materials, published a historical perspective on past and current information on weight gain and recommendations for achieving optimal nutritional status during pregnancy.

Table 13–5 is a food plan that may be used as a guideline for counseling pregnant adults regarding their nutritional needs. It has been estimated that an additional 30 grams of protein and 300 calories is needed during pregnancy to meet the increased energy demands for tissue building. This amounts to about 2500 calories a day. Active, large, or nutritionally deficient women may require more. Appropriate weight gain during pregnancy will indicate whether sufficient calories are being consumed. Adding two glasses or servings of milk or milk products to the diet to total four servings will contribute to the protein requirements and meet the additional 400 mg of calcium needed daily during pregnancy. This is a total of 1200 mg per day of calcium (Williams, 1990).

By including a variety of foods, it is possible to meet the RDA for vitamins and minerals, with the possible exception of iron and folic acid. These are traditionally supplemented (Abrams & Laros, 1986; Lewis, 1986).

TABLE 13–5. DAILY FOOD PLAN FOR PREGNANCY AND LACTATION (ADULTS)

FOOD	NONPREGNANT WOMEN	PREGNANCY	LACTATION
Milk and cheese Includes whole, nonfat, evaporated, reliquified dry, buttermilk, yogurt, cheese, and foods made with milk or cheese	2c	3 or more c	4 or more c
Meat-poultry-fish-beans Lean meat, fish, poultry, eggs, legumes, nuts, peanut butter, seeds	2 servings (4–6 oz)	2½ servings (5–7 oz) Encourage use of liver	3 servings (6–9 oz)
Vegetables and fruit Some raw daily Dark green or deep yellow Vitamin-C rich food Good sources Citrus fruit or juice, green peppers, cantaloupes, fresh strawberries, broccoli Fair sources Other melons, tomatoes, cabbage, potatoes cooked in skins, other green vegetables	1 serving 1 good source or 2 fair sources	1 serving 1 good source 1 good source and 1 fair or 2 good sources	1–2 servings Same
Other vegetables and fruits	1–2 servings	2 servings	Same
Bread and cereal Enriched or whole grain	3–4 servings	4–5 servings	5 servings
Butter or fortified margarine	Amount as kcal level permits	Same	Same
Additional foods	More of these listed or other foods with amounts adjusted to rate of weight gain		Additional foods as needed to maintain weight
Iron and vitamin supplements	Use according to physician's instructions		

From C. M. Lewis (1986). *Nutrition and Nutritional Therapy* (p. 159). Norwalk, CT: Appleton & Lange. Copyright 1986 by Appleton-Century-Crofts. Reprinted by permission.

Data suggest a relationship between maternal weight gain and infant birthweight. Low birthweight infants, under 5.5 pounds, have an increased rate of infant mortality and health complications (Kline, 1986).

Pregnant adolescents have additional nutritional requirements because of their dual growth demand: that of the fetus and that of the teenager (Lewis, 1986). Table 13–6 describes a daily food plan for the pregnant adolescent.

The recommended weight gain during pregnancy is approximately 22 to 27 pounds. With twins, an additional 10 pounds is added. The cumulative gain (lb) at the end of each trimester includes approximately 1.6 pounds during the first trimester, nine pounds after the second trimester, and 20.5 pounds during the third trimester (Kline, 1986). Although a relatively wide range of weight gains can support healthy pregnancies and healthy babies, some approximate ranges based on prepregnant weight may serve as general guidelines (Williams, 1990):

- Normal weight women: 24–32 pounds
- Underweight women: 28–36 pounds
- Overweight women: 16–24 pounds

Special concerns during pregnancy related to diet include pregnancy-induced hypertension, gestational diabetes, and nausea. Hypertension is often identified by edema and proteinuria after the 20th week. A balanced diet without salt restriction or diuretics is used for management, along with bed rest and decreased activity.

Gestational diabetes is common during pregnancy when body cells are more resistant to insulin. Ninety percent of all pregnant diabetics have this form of diabetes. After delivery, the gestational diabetes usually disappears when the cells are no longer insulin resistant (Kline, 1986).

Nausea is often diminished by avoiding an empty stomach, eating small meals often, separating meals and fluids, and eating before getting out of bed. Nausea is sometimes a symptom of folacin deficiency (Williams, 1990).

Nutritional Needs in Early Years

The first year of life is an important time for good nutrition. The rapid growth and metabolism demand ample nutrition. The tremendous growth is a composite of the various growth patterns of internal organs. Birthweight usually doubles

TABLE 13–6. DAILY FOOD PLAN FOR THE PREGNANT ADOLESCENT

FOOD	AMOUNT
Milk and cheese Includes whole, nonfat, evaporated, reliquefied dry, buttermilk, yogurt, cheese, and foods made with milk or cheese	4 c milk (or 4 servings cheese—1$\frac{1}{3}$ oz/serving)

Meat-poultry-fish-beans
    Lean meat, fish, poultry, organ meats, and eggs
    Legumes, nuts, peanut butter, and seeds
	Equivalent of 4 (2–3 oz) servings meat plus 1–2 eggs

Vegetables and fruit
    Some raw daily
    Dark green leafy or yellow-orange vegetable/fruit at least every other day
2 good sources (or 1 good source and 1 fair source) vitamin C food daily. Good sources of vitamin C are citrus fruit or juice, peppers, cantaloupe, strawberries, broccoli. Fair sources are tomatoes, cabbage, collard greens, mustard greens, peas
	3–4 servings fruit
	2–3 servings vegetable
	
	($\frac{1}{2}$ c servings fruit and vegetable or $\frac{1}{4}$ c serving dried fruit)

Bread and cereal Whole grain or enriched	7 servings
Butter, fortified margarine, and other fats	Amount as caloric level permits
Additional foods Includes desserts or additional amounts of the above listed foods	As needed to maintain desired rate of weight gain; select nutritious dessert, i.e., pudding, fruit pie, peanut butter or oatmeal cookie

during the first four months from 7 to 14 pounds, and in the next eight months, another 7 pounds is added (Lewis, 1986). By the end of the first year, the growth rate has slowed, with a resultant gain of approximately 5 pounds between one and two years of age. At about one year of age children need approximately 1000 calories, and only 1300 to 1500 calories by age 3. Parents who are reminded of this normal decreased need for calories will avoid conflict with the child's refusal of food (Williams, 1990). A sample meal plan for toddlers and preschool children is suggested in Table 13–7.

Babies spend an average of 2$\frac{1}{2}$ hours per day eating, which equals about 1000 hours a year—as much time as a college student spends in classes in two years of full-time study. While obtaining nutrients for growth, babies are also learning about their world—about food, about themselves, and about behaviors that win approval and those that do not. Eating can make a great contribution to a child's future well-being physically and psychologically.

Nutritional cautions for mothers include avoiding giving babies honey because of the risk of botulism, and avoiding milk anemia by adding other foods after the child has had 2 to 3$\frac{1}{2}$ cups of milk per day. To prevent excess weight gain, allow the child to stop when the stomach is full.

Family health nurses should encourage parents to give the child food according to the developmental readiness and to encourage self-feeding skills. Hand-eye coordination may be developed by offering finger foods and spoons or a cup as the child is ready.

Nutritional Needs for School-Age Children and Adolescents

Except for during pregnancy, nutrient requirements are higher in adolescence than at any other time. The adolescent growth spurt begins at 10 or 11 years of age in girls, reaches its peak at 12 years of age, and is completed by about 15 years of age. In boys, the growth spurt usually begins at 12 or 13 years of age, peaks around 14 years of age, and ends by about 19 years of age (Lifshitz et al., 1991).

Because there are wide variations of growth and development at any age period, parents should understand that these variations do not necessarily indicate abnormal growth. Normally, a child approximately doubles body weight from 8 to 12 years of age but rarely at a constant rate. Body fat measurements increase temporarily for boys in early puberty. A persistent increase is seen in girls throughout adolescence. The increase in fatness usually occurs directly after the peak in growth. Thus, it is important to differentiate a temporary tendency toward fatness from a permanent acquisition (Peck & Ullrich, 1985).

Because of the rapid growth, energy and protein needs are high. Boys tend to gain more weight at a more rapid rate, which accounts for their higher energy and protein needs. They are laying down more muscle and less body fat than girls. Boys end up with about 8% body fat, whereas girls average 20%. The higher percentage of body fat and the lower level of physical activity means that girls need fewer calories than boys, even if they both weigh the same. Individual caloric needs vary. Girls consume fewer calories than boys—from

TABLE 13–7. DAILY FOOD PLAN FOR TODDLERS AND PRESCHOOL CHILDREN

FOOD	NUMBER OF SERVINGS	SIZE OF SERVINGS TODDLER 1–2 YEARS	PRESCHOOL 3–5 YEARS
Milk and cheese Milk (whole, skim, low-fat, reliquefied evaporated, soy), yogurt, ice cream, ice milk, cheese. Calcium equivalent of 1 c milk: 1 c plain yogurt, 1⅓ oz Swiss or cheddar cheese, 1½ c ice cream or ice milk, 2 c cottage cheese	2 servings	1 serving = 1 c milk	
Meat-fish-poultry-beans Lean cooked meat, poultry, fish; dry beans, soybeans, lentils, peanut butter, seeds. Protein equivalent of 1 oz meat: 1 egg, ½–¾ c legumes; 2 tbsp peanut butter, ¼–½ c nuts or seeds	2 servings	½–1 oz or 1–2 tbsp	1½–2½ oz or 3–5 tbsp
Vegetables and fruit Dark green or deep yellow fruit or vegetables rich in vitamin A content (e.g., carrots, sweet potatoes, green leafy vegetables, green peppers, cantaloupe, apricots, peaches)	4 servings daily to include 1 serving at least every other day of a food rich in vitamin A	⅓–½ c orange juice or other high vitamin C food: Size of serving for other foods: 1–2 tbsp or ⅛ c	⅓–½ c orange juice or other food high in vitamin C; Size of serving for other foods: 3–5 tbsp or ¼ c
Vitamin C-containing foods Good sources: citrus fruit or juice, peppers, cantaloupe, fresh strawberries, broccoli, brussel sprouts	1 serving of a good source or 2 servings of a fair source daily		
Vitamin C-containing foods Fair sources: other melons, tomatoes, cabbage, potatoes cooked in skins, green leafy vegetables, tangerine and lemon, asparagus tips, cauliflower, rutabagas			
Other vegetables and fruit	1–3 servings One serving of raw fruit or vegetable should be selected daily		
Bread and cereal Whole grain or enriched	4 servings (If no cereal is eaten, an additional serving of bread or baked goods should be selected)	½ slice bread or ¼–½ oz dry cereal or 1–2 tbsp (⅛ c) cooked cereal	1 slice bread or ½–1 oz dry cereal or 3–5 tbsp (¼ c) cooked cereal
Additional foods Butter, margarine, and other fats; desserts and additional amounts of foods from the four food groups	Amount as needed to meet kcal needs	Some vegetable oil should be included daily. Foods that provide only kcal (e.g., candy, sweets) should be used sparingly. Select nutritious desserts such as pudding, fruit, and cookies made with oatmeal or peanut butter.	

Data from C. M. Lewis, (1986). *Nutrition and Nutritional Therapy* (p. 195). Norwalk, CT: Appleton & Lange. Copyright 1986 by Appleton-Century-Crofts. Reprinted with permission.

1800 to 2500 calories per day; boys need 2500 to 3500 calories per day. Many girls eat less than this to have the thin bodies that society emphasizes. The pressure to restrict food intake for weight control may inhibit their ability to acquire the nutritional reserves for later reproduction (Lifshitz et al., 1991). Table 13–8 translates the nutri-

ent requirements of school-age children and teenagers into a daily food plan that may be used as a guideline for families.

There is little evidence of insufficient protein intake in the United States. Caloric needs might fall below the recommended amount in young people because of economic reasons or because of

TABLE 13–8. SUGGESTED DIETARY GUIDELINES FOR SCHOOL CHILDREN AND TEENAGERS

FOOD	7–10 YEARS	10–TEEN YEARS

Milk and cheese (whole, dry, skim, reliquefied evaporated, soy milk, buttermilk, and other daily products)
Calcium equivalent of 1 c milk:
  1 c plain yogurt
  2 c cottage cheese
  $1\frac{1}{2}$ c ice cream
  $1\frac{1}{3}$ oz cheddar cheese or
  Swiss cheese
	6–9 years: 2–3 c
	9–10 years: 3 or more c
		10–12 years: 3–4c 12–16 years: 4 c Pregnant teens: 5–6 c

Meat-fish-poultry-beans
  Substitutes for protein for 1 oz meat:
  1 egg
  $\frac{1}{2}$–$\frac{3}{4}$ c cooked dry beans, dry peas, soybeans, lentils
  $\frac{1}{4}$–$\frac{1}{2}$ c nuts or seeds
  2 tbsp peanut butter
	2 servings ($1\frac{1}{2}$–2 oz/serving)	2 servings (2–3 oz/serving)

Vegetables and fruit
  Eat one vitamin C source daily (e.g., citrus fruit, melon, strawberries, broccoli, tomatoes, raw cabbage)
  Eat one vitamin A source at least every other day (e.g., deep yellow-orange or very dark green vegetable or fruit)
  Use unpeeled fruits and vegetables and those with edible seeds frequently
	4 or more servings ($\frac{1}{3}$ c each)	4 or more servings ($\frac{1}{2}$ c each)

Bread and cereal (whole grain or enriched bread, cereal, rice, or pasta). One serving is:
  1 slice bread
  1 roll, muffin, or biscuit
  $\frac{1}{2}$–$\frac{3}{4}$ c cooked cereal, rice or pasta
  1 oz dry cereal
	4 servings or more (very active children need more for energy)	4 servings or more
		Teenage boys: 6 or more servings (very active teens and athletes need more)

Additional foods Fats and oils, such as butter, margarine, mayonnaise, and vegetable oils; sweets and desserts; a source of vitamin D	As needed to meet kilocaloric needs; sweets should be consumed in moderation; a source of vitamin D is recommended throughout the growth period (such as vitamin D-fortified milk)	

Kilocaloric needs	2400 (7–10 years)	Girls:
		  11–14 years: 2200
		  15–22 years: 2100
		Boys:
		  11–14 years: 2700
		  15–18 years: 2800
		  19–22 years: 2900

From C. M. Lewis (1986). *Nutrition and Nutritional Therapy* (p. 207). Norwalk, CT: Appleton & Lange. Copyright 1986 by Appleton-Century-Crofts. Reprinted by permission.

attempts to lose weight. When energy is limited, dietary protein will not be available for synthesis of new tissue. The result is a reduction in growth rate, even though protein intake appears to be adequate.

American adolescents tend to be low in their optimal intake of folacin, calcium, iron, and zinc. It is estimated that 5% to 15% of American adolescents are anemic. Because of the increased muscle mass and blood volume, the body's need for iron is especially high. After menstruation, girls need to replace the iron lost in the menstrual flow. Symptoms of iron-deficiency anemia in-

clude lack of energy, fatigue, pale complexion, and increase susceptibility to infection.

Because of the adolescent's precarious balance between striving for independence and needing to depend on the family for basic physical and emotional needs, the family's role in nutrition is variable. Peers should be involved in any plan for change (Mellin, 1991). They may be involved directly if the client is willing by inviting them to a counseling session so that specific problems and strategies can be worked out. Indirectly, friends are involved as the counselor includes information in the assessment about what friends do and think to determine if they will be an obstacle to reaching a goal.

Factors influencing adolescents' dietary patterns include:

- Lack of time because of involvement in many activities
- Priority of peer activities over eating
- Lack of guidance in the selection of foods away from home
- Fear of underweight or lack of muscle
- Desire to excel in athletics
- Concern of certain foods aggravating acne
- Lack of knowledge regarding nutritional needs
- Fear of obesity (Mellin, 1991)

Because about one-fourth of a teen's calories come from snacks, parents should provide snack foods that contain some essential nutrients, such as milk, fruit juice, yogurt, whole grain breads, fresh vegetables, crackers, cheese, nuts, and popcorn.

Parents need reassurance that feeding and eating patterns stabilize after the adolescent phase and persist into adult life (Lifshitz et al., 1991) Young adults who are well nourished feel better, have more energy, and are better able to withstand psychological and physiologic stress than those with inadequate intakes. If appropriate eating patterns have been established during the adolescent years, there is no need to change the type or quality of food in adulthood.

A common concern of parents and teens is obesity. Twenty to 25% of today's teens are obese, an increase of approximately 40% in the last 15 years. Fifty to 95% of obese adolescents will become obese adults. Often, they are caught in a downward spiral of overeating, depression, inactivity, lowered self-esteem, social isolation, and weight gain (Epstein, 1986; Jonides, 1990; Mellin, 1991).

For children, age-specific growth charts facilitate a more accurate evaluation of a child's weight since they are based on age, sex, and channels of growth of many children across the United States. Generally, children who are greater than 20% to 25% above the ideal weight for height on these graphs are considered obese (Mellin, 1991). Triceps-skin-fold measurements may also be used to determine obesity. Use of these measurements is based on evidence that approximately 50% of body fat is located subcutaneously. A triceps-skin-fold measurement above the 85th percentile is indicative of obesity.

Family health nurses who work in pediatric clinics or schools may identify adolescents who are at risk for future weight problems and refer them to programs or work with the family and teen to establish goals and a weight-reduction plan.

Anorexia and Bulimia

Society's preference for plumpness or thinness tends to set the standard for what is considered to be the ideal body shape or image. Often it also sets the stage for eating disorders.

Eating serves different functions physiologically and symbolically. Apart from the person's desire for thinness, eating disorders can have physiologic origins or be a part of family dynamics.

Anorexia is a refusal to maintain body weight over a minimal normal weight for age and height. Anorexics usually have a weight loss of 15% of their usual body weight and have an intense fear of becoming obese even when underweight (Lifshitz et al., 1991). Anorexia nervosa is characterized by a relentless pursuit of thinness that results in life-threatening emaciation and an almost delusional preoccupation with food and body image accompanied by withdrawal from family and friends. It is frequently reported to be an outcome of persistent attempts to lose weight and occurs most frequently among adolescents and young women from the upper and middle socioeconomic classes. Anorexia occurs 10 times more frequently in females than in males.

The term *anorexia* is actually a misnomer since the appetite is not lost—the client simply refuses to eat. Hyperactivity, exercising to the point of exhaustion with a denial of fatigue, and a drive for intellectual excellence are also typical of the anorexic. Pursuing a thin body becomes an isolated area of control in a world in which the individual feels ineffective; the dieting provides an artificial sense of mastery and control. In any child who does not gain weight or who ceases to grow, an eating disorder and/or an inappropriate health belief that distorts their dietary intake must be considered (Health and Public Policy Committee, 1986).

The goal of treatment is to assist the client with developing a positive and secure self-image and a change in attitude about food. For clients who have a mild form of the disorder, counseling may be provided on adolescent growth, normal nutrition, and the serious consequences of malnutrition. If the disorder is complicated by stresses such as family problems or depression, the nurse can shift the focus to deal with the particular stress.

The American Psychiatric Association (1994) defines *bulimia nervosa* as eating binges occurring at least twice a week followed by purging, either by self-induced vomiting, strict dieting or fasting, vigorous exercise to prevent weight gain, or use of diuretics or laxative. Bulimia is a disorder affecting young women usually 18 years of age or older; there is a much lower incidence with males. The majority of bulimics are in their 20s, and about one-fourth are married. Most come from upper socioeconomic groups and are college students, actresses, or models. Over half of bulimics are of normal weight, but they have an exaggerated fear of becoming fat. Symptoms of bulimia sometimes begin at the conclusion of weight-reduction diets. Other causes of chronic bulimia may include unresolved grief, traumatic neurosis, history of sexual abuse leading to guilt, and repetitive attempts at self-purification.

Bulimia is characterized by the sudden ingestion of large amounts of food in short periods of time. As much as 4000 to 5000 kcal may be consumed, followed by fasting, vomiting, or purging, particularly with laxatives or enemas. Foods eaten are usually those clients are attempting to exclude from their diet.

Sometimes the binging is precipitated by feelings of depression, anxiety, boredom, or loneliness. Frequently, the binging is done secretly and is planned. Afterward, there is often a period of drowsiness and a feeling of depression, guilt, and self-disgust.

The initial stages of the bulimic episode are not necessarily unpleasant as there is a temporary release from the rigors of strict dieting, a distraction from current problems, and a temporary decline in any feeling of depression or anxiety (Brownell & Wadden, 1986).

Nurses should be aware that binges can lead to obesity and that binges followed by fasting, vomiting, or purging may lead to severe electrolyte imbalance, dehydration, and malnutrition. Esophageal irritation and extensive dental erosion and decay are also common.

Dietary counseling of the bulimic may focus on appropriate quantities of food needed for weight maintenance. The nurse can help the client to structure the daily eating schedule and provide guidelines. This will give the client a feeling of control and assurance of adequate nutrition. Assistance with time management and stress management may help the client to avoid the extremes in overactivity and boredom. The nurse should identify stress relievers and strategies that enable the client to cope with emotions without the use of food. Other goals of treatment involve exploring body image, early dieting behaviors, and issues related to separating from the family to establish intimacy and authentic peer relationships. Individual, group, and family therapies are used in treatment.

Eating disorders require attention and should not be ignored with the hope that the adolescent will grow out of it. The psychological and physiologic health hazards warrant professional assistance. Optimal management involves combined approaches including nutritional rehabilitation, psychotherapy, behavior modification, family therapy, and at times, psychotropic medications. Hopefully, by teaching children and young persons the importance of good nutrition and by setting examples of an appropriate way to achieve and maintain a normal body weight, the incidence of eating disorders will decrease.

Adulthood

The adulthood years span approximately 40 years (from ages 21 to 60) and represent a heterogeneous group. Resting metabolic rates decrease approximately 2% each decade after age 30, thus decreasing energy requirements. Due to decreased production of estrogen and lowered metabolism, many menopausal and postmenopausal women are reported to have increased weight gain (Brzezinski & Wurtman, 1993). Family nurses may assist women and their families to understand the changes that occur during this stage and provide health teaching about modification of dietary patterns and understanding of the relationship of exercise, food intake and weight maintenance (Stoppard, 1994).

Exercise and reduced food intake provide a means by which weight gain can be prevented. Energy and nutrition needs differ for younger versus older adults. Nutrient needs for exercising versus less-active adults remain virtually the same with the possible exception of riboflavin and vitamin B6.

Nutrition needs of the exercising adult can be met by some basic guidelines:

- Eat a variety of foods to get nutrients without relying on supplements.
- Use vitamin and mineral supplements with caution.
- Choose foods high in calcium to prevent osteoporosis and possibly to control high blood pressure.
- Choose iron-rich meats such as red meat, fish, and poultry.
- Eat vitamin C–rich foods, such as oranges, with nonmeat sources of iron such as nuts, beans, and fortified cereal to help prevent iron-deficiency anemia (particularly a concern of menstruating women).
- Practice moderation in exercise and eating.
- Read about nutrition research with discretion.

Nutrition and the Elderly

The elderly population has not been studied to any great extent. Major gaps still exist in our knowledge of energy and nutrients of elderly adults. The present number of elderly people is expected to double by the year 2030, thus nurses

TABLE 13–9. SUGGESTED DAILY DIET PLAN FOR THE ELDERLY

FOOD	AMOUNT	SIZE OF SERVINGS AND SUBSTITUTIONS
Milk and cheese (Includes whole, nonfat reliquefied evaporated, and reliquefied dry milk, buttermilk, yogurt, fortified soy milk, cheese, and foods made with milk))	2 c	Calcium equivalent of 1 c milk: $1\frac{1}{2}$ c ice cream 2 c cottage cheese $1\frac{1}{3}$ oz American cheese 1 c plain yogurt
Meat-poultry-fish-beans	2 servings	1 serving = 2–3 oz cooked lean meat, fish, poultry Protein equivalent of 1 oz meat: 1 egg $\frac{1}{2}$–$\frac{3}{4}$ c cooked legumes $\frac{1}{4}$–$\frac{1}{2}$ c nuts or seeds
Vegetables and fruit Dark green or deep yellow fruits or vegetables for vitamin A (carrots, sweet potatoes, green leafy vegetables, green peppers, yellow or orange fruit)	4 servings daily to include 1 serving at least every other day	1 serving = 1 c raw leafy vegetable $\frac{1}{2}$ c cooked vegetable or fruit 1 medium-sized fruit, such as an apple or peach
Vitamin C-containing foods Good sources: citrus fruit or juice, peppers (green and red sweet), cantaloupe, fresh strawberries, broccoli, brussel sprouts Fair sources: other melons, tomatoes, cabbage, potatoes cooked in skins, green leafy vegetables, tangerines, and lemons, asparagus tips, cauliflower, rutabagas	1 good source or 2 fair sources	
Other vegetables and fruits, use peeled vegetables and fruits and those with edible seeds frequently	1–3 servings	
Bread and cereal (whole grain or enriched)	4 servings (If no cereal eaten, eat an additional serving of bread or baked goods)	1 serving = 1 slice of bread $\frac{3}{4}$ c cold cereal $\frac{1}{2}$ c cooked cereal, macaroni, spaghetti 5 saltines 1 small biscuit or muffin 2 graham crackers
Butter-fortified margarine, other fats	Amount as kcal level permits	Select foods from this group carefully because of their high kcal content; many fats have little nutritional value
Additional foods (Desserts, alcohol, additional amounts of above listed foods)	Amount as kcal level permits	Select nutritious desserts such as fruit and pudding, and cut down on calorie-containing foods, such as sugar and alcohol

From C.M. Lewis (1986). *Nutrition and Nutritional Therapy* (p. 228). Norwalk, CT: Appleton & Lange. Copyright 1986 by Appleton & Lange. Reprinted by permission.

need to be cognizant of their nutritional concerns. Table 13–9 provides a guideline for planning a diet for the elderly.

The nutritional status of the older adult is affected by physiologic and psychological parameters. The effects of physiologic parameters, such as chronic disease, often coexist with psychosocial factors such as inadequate income or social isolation.

Today's elderly population is a heterogeneous group that varies widely in age (65 to 115 years), income level, educational level, lifestyle, dietary habits, and health status. The only commonality is chronological age, which is a poor indicator of biologic age or health status.

The family health nurse should assess the individual concerns of the older adult and plan a diet with, not for, the adult. Difficulty with food ingestion, such as decreased ability to bite, chew, or swallow, decreased taste and smell acuity, and other physical limitations, such as vision or mobility limitations, may affect nutritional status (Lewis, 1986).

Digestive and absorptive functioning may decrease with age and lead to vitamin B_{12} deficiency, decreased calcium absorption, and gastrointestinal distress. Symptoms such as heartburn, gas, and abdominal distention are common and may be related to poor eating and bowel habits, a preoccupation with food, and emotional tension (Lewis, 1986).

The older adult may be concerned with an increase in weight, which often occurs with dropping basal metabolism. As muscle cells disappear, they are replaced by fat and fibrous connective tissue. Encouraging as much activity as tolerated may decrease the physiologic changes that come with aging. In spite of the large number of changes that occur with aging, most functions are affected to only a moderate degree.

According to Erickson (1956), the psychosocial development of the adult is integrity versus despair. Older adults who can look back and feel satisfied with their lives will feel a sense of integrity. In contrast, a feeling of despair may result if life is seen as a succession of wrong turns, futile efforts, and missed opportunities. Achievement of this developmental task may have a bearing on the client's nutritional status.

Psychosocial deterrents to good nutritional status include limited income, substandard housing, inadequate transportation, social isolation, and long-established food habits. Nurses should assess for the effects of these factors on the availability of food (Lewis, 1986).

WEIGHT CONTROL

Being obese, or at a level of 20% or more above desirable body weight, is a health risk. As many as 40 million Americans may have weight problems, and the numbers are rising, making obesity one of the most common health problems. Excessive weight increases the risk for gout, gallbladder disease, elevated blood pressure, coronary heart disease, and some types of cancer, and has been associated with the development of osteoarthritis. The prevalence of obesity is high in many populations, especially women, the poor, and members of some ethnic groups (NIH, 1992).

A measure of fatness that correlates highly with direct measures of body fat is the Body Mass Index. Calculate the body mass index to define and determine a healthy weight that is reasonably independent of height. The panel of obesity experts at the National Institute of Health recommends that professionals adopt this index for evaluation. Table 13–10 demonstrates how to determine body mass.

Over 65 million people are on a diet at any given time. They go on then off—losing then regaining. There are three factors working against the dieter:

1. When calories are restricted by lowering food intake, the body adapts by lowering its metabolic rate and thus resists burning the fat stores. Then, when the person becomes tired of the restricted diet and increases food intake, the body treats the intake as excess and weight is regained, even though food intake is less than before the diet.
2. Weight lost in the early part of a strict diet is mostly water, not fat. The initial rapid loss is a result of a loss of body sodium and water, which is felt to be secondary to the usual carbohydrate restriction.
3. When dieters consume fewer than 1200 calories a day, they lose muscle tissue as well as fat. The dieter actually becomes fatter than before the diet because the percentage of muscle has gone down and fat percentage increases ("First Understand," 1986).

TABLE 13–10. BODY MASS INDEX

Body mass index (BMI) is the figure obtained by dividing body weight in kilograms by the square of the body height in meters.
1. To convert weight to kilograms, divide pounds without clothes by 2.2 _____ .
2. Convert to meters, divide the height in inches (without shoes) by 39.4 (   ), then square it: _____ .
3. Divide numbers obtained in step (1) by step (2). Body mass index = _____ .

	BMI MALES	BMI FEMALES
Desirable	22–24	21–23
Overweight	above 28.5	above 27.7
Seriously overweight	above 33	above 31.5

TABLE 13–11. PRACTICAL SUGGESTIONS FOR WEIGHT CONTROL

1. Identify what contributes to weight gain.
2. Set realistic goals. A healthy weight loss is 1 pound per week. Focus on changing habits by working on one habit change each week.
3. Reduce caloric intake. Find out how many calories are eaten daily. Reduce the *intake by* 500 to 1000 calories. Do not go below 1000 calories without professional supervision. If necessary, increase the exercise level instead of reducing the intake any further.
4. Limit fat intake to 30% or less of your total calories. Pay attention to how much fat is eaten daily.
5. Exercise aerobically regularly for optimal changes in body fat and lean body mass. An ideal time range is to work up to 45 minutes 4 to 5 times per week.
6. Find substitutions for "problem foods" or high-fat, high-sugar foods. If there is none, decide on a desirable serving size.
7. Listen to the hunger level. Eat when hungry and stop when just satisfied.
8. Establish a regular eating pattern. Eating 3 to 5 times a day provides the body with small amounts of energy throughout the day.
9. Plan ahead for special occasions. If you are going out for dinner, plan to eat lighter during the day (without skipping a meal).
10. Use "smart talk." Try to avoid labeling food and yourself as good or bad. You are not a good or bad person based on what you ate that day.
11. Accept sole responsibility for your dietary choices and health practices. Eating healthy and maintaining weight involves making personal choices and values that only you can make.
12. Separate food and emotions by asking yourself what you are feeling when you want to eat. If it isn't hunger, take care of the feeling (boredom, anger, frustration, sadness, etc.).
13. Be patient and keep practicing until your new habits become a part of you. Weight management takes daily practice.

When counseling the overweight family member, the nurse should encourage a combination of reduced caloric intake and exercise. Because exercise builds muscle tissue and burns more calories, an improved muscle-fat ratio is ensured. Table 13–11 includes some key factors in learning to control weight.

A walking program of one hour per day three times a week will burn about 324 calories per session, 972 per week, 3888 per month, and 46,656 per year. This is equivalent to 13 pounds of body fat. If exercise is accompanied with a 100-calorie per day decrease, the individual will lose a total of 23 pounds without dieting! Chapter 16 presents additional guidelines for exercise.

Guidelines for Selecting a Diet Program

Nurses should ask the following questions when recommending a weight reduction program for families:

- Does the program provide a comprehensive approach, combining diet, behavior modification, and exercise?
- Is the program individualized or based on a standard program that is given to everyone?
- Is the program medically supervised?
- Will the frequency of the program meet the client's needs?

- Will the meetings be on a one-to-one basis or will there be a group format?
- What is the program's success record?
- Is there a maintenance program?
- Are special meals or products required?
- Are family members included in any meetings?
- What are the credentials of the staff?
- Are several diet options offered and will they interfere with any medications?
- Is there a contract?

Additional features may include training in stress reduction techniques, cognitive therapy (learning to change self-talk), and assertiveness. Family members may be referred to the American Society of Bariatric Physicians, which is a group composed of physicians and nurses who practice prevention, treatment, and study of overweight and related conditions (see References).

Steps to Weight Loss and Control

A safe diet that promotes long-term weight loss will also meet the following guidelines:

- Satisfy all nutrient needs except energy
- Minimize hunger
- Can be adapted to suit the tastes and habits of the individual

- Include easily obtained foods
- Encourage the establishment of life-long eating habits

If the minimum recommended number of servings for adults are consumed from the four food groups, the protein, carbohydrate, and fat supply will be less than 1100 calories a day. Diets of less than 1000 calories are not recommended because they restrict the sources of essential nutrients. Diets above 1600 calories a day may result in very slow weight loss for women. Men, however, may lose weight rapidly at this level.

Between-meal hunger is often a problem for many weight watchers. Snacks high in simple sugars or small meals are rapidly digested and absorbed into the bloodstream, causing a sharp rise in blood glucose, which stimulates insulin production. Insulin removes the glucose from the blood to the cells. If it removes too much, the blood glucose level can drop rapidly to a level even lower than before the meal or snack, leaving the person feeling tired, dizzy, and hungry. If between-meal hunger is a problem, the nurse can suggest small servings of cheese, crackers, or fruit for snacking (Wurtman, 1986).

Another common barrier to successful weight loss is irregular consumption of meals. A study conducted on 12 moderately obese men compared the same 1800 calorie diet when eaten as one, three, and six meals a day. The one-meal-a-day regimen caused more dramatic rises and falls in blood glucose levels than the other two patterns. Feelings of hunger are associated with low glucose levels, thus making it difficult to abstain from eating.

Past studies help to explain why low-carbohydrate dieters often feel tired and listless and often have trouble sleeping. Wurtman's (1986) research at Massachusetts Institute of Technology has indicated that carbohydrate deprivation depletes the brain of serotonin, an important neurotransmitter of nerve messages, which acts as a sleep inducer and a calmer. It may be that when brain levels drop too low, cravings are likely to occur. Low-carbohydrate dieters crumble at the sight of a cookie or a piece of bread.

The rule of thumb for any weight loss scheme should be "Don't go on anything that you are not willing (or able) to stay on forever." Going on a diet implies that one will someday go off of it. When clients are told that certain foods are forbidden, those foods become "special" and are often used as rewards or treats. By allowing "heavy" or "junk" foods in small quantities, the weight watcher never has to go off the diet. In the author's work with overweight persons, clients are encouraged to eat "heavy" foods, as they would if they were at their ideal weight now. For example, to maintain a slim 120 pounds, af-

ter deciding to eat pie clients are encouraged to imagine eating a sliver of pie instead of one fourth of the pie. This principle may be applied to the management of difficult or high-risk situations. The author asks the client to imagine successful behavior adaptations in previously disastrous occasions.

A final consideration is that the diet should accommodate the personal tastes of people. The nurse should consider the client's age, sex, and ethnic group.

The Impact of Obesity on the Family

The obese condition of a family member affects the family system, and the family situation affects the obesity through family structure and interaction. Bruch and Touraine's (1940) categories of family characteristics are still used today to predict how a family will respond to dietary modification of a family member. Bruch's descriptions of family characteristics are still pertinent for understanding the family system. The three classifications include (1) consistent, but not rigid, cooperation within the family, (2) rigid and over-perfectionistic family dynamics, and (3) severe family discord.

In the *consistent* classification, the family reaction is characterized as consistent but not rigid in cooperating with the family member making dietary changes. The entire family would probably act as a team in adjusting eating habits to help the obese member. Food is not used as a reward nor as a form of discipline. No great hardships or feelings of deprivation are suffered. The dieter in this situation has good chances of being successful.

Families who are *rigid* in their eating and lifestyle patterns will often respond with excessive cooperation but without real communication about the problem. Emotional reactions are often not shared; thus outwardly, communications appear smooth and normal but in reality are often lacking, and family members are inwardly tense.

A child may be treated as a possession and may be given food or material objects instead of love and opportunity to develop effective coping skills. Children with perfectionistic parents often have a difficult time reacting to stressful situations that require independent and adaptive behavior. They often have not learned to interpret their needs or to define their goals. They often grow up to be dependent and insecure and are unable to express aggression. They may feel as though they have no control over their lives.

Family histories of families with obese children suggest discrepancies in parental status, with imbalances in who has power, who makes decisions, or who is recognized as important.

The child needs help to develop self-awareness, gain insight into food habits and behavior, and develop skills to resolve conflicts. Encouragement from friends may help the child outgrow obesity. Strict adherence to a diet can result in despair and a return to overeating. Intimidating and disciplinary measures are often detrimental and unsatisfactory (Bruch & Touranine, 1940; Mellin, 1991).

An extension of the rigid, perfectionistic family is the family with *severe family discord.* The family usually demonstrates aggression, antagonism, dissatisfaction, marital disharmony, or mutual contempt. As a result, the child learns to respond to all kinds of feelings as hunger and cannot discriminate between fear, anger, anxiety, or hunger. Food has often been used as a substitute for love, security, and satisfaction. In this type of family, common interests, communication, and participation in social life are absent. Parents of these children often experienced a childhood of loneliness and unfulfilled hopes. They were deprived of affection or family support and lacked a parental figure.

Still accepted is the idea that obese child in the discordant family often lose weight but break their diets and have difficulty accepting a reducing diet. The underlying social problem increases the child's feeling of guilt and frustration. Without the chance to develop independence, the child feels ineffective, out of control, depressed, defiant, un-able to cope, and rejected. The child may also feel shame, self-hatred, or disgust.

Family living skills and positive self-image for a child may be needed before a formal program is offered. Living skills include learning to share thoughts, feelings, and concerns; to be supportive in trying times; to seek outside resources or alternatives; and to develop decision-making skills (Hertzler & Vaughan, 1979; Mellin, 1991). The nurse who focuses on family dimensions and personal development will enhance program success for families with or without problem behaviors.

Guidelines for Counseling the Family in Weight Loss or Control

The nurse should first identify the individual's and family's level of motivation and reasons for desiring to make nutritional changes. The author frequently asks clients to identify the "costs" and "benefits" of losing weight. Fear of failure is often combined with motivation. The nurse can build confidence by helping the client to set realistic, attainable goals. The nurse and client together write long- and short-term goals. The nurse may also teach the use of positive self-statements and nonfood rewards.

Provisions for psychological and social support are critical for clients with a significant

TABLE 13–12. FAMILY NUTRITION ASSESSMENT TOOL

FAMILY MEMBERS	AGE	EDUCATIONAL LEVEL	DEVELOPMENTAL LEVEL
1.			
2.			
3.			
4.			
5.			
6.			

Family's perception of health status (describe)

Nutritional practices

Who decides on the menu?
Who does the grocery shopping?
Who prepares the meals?
Number of meals consumed per day?
Describe mealtime (Who is present, when, where, and atmosphere)
Does mealtime serve a particular function? (For example, are the day's activities planned? Are problems discussed?)
Snacks consumed and frequency
Knows food sources from the food pyramid
24-hour food recall

Dietary fat

Use of red meat, fish, and poultry (once a week, three times, etc.)
How often do you eat cheese? What kinds do you purchase?

TABLE 13-12. FAMILY NUTRITION ASSESSMENT TOOL (continued)

FAMILY MEMBERS	AGE	EDUCATIONAL LEVEL	DEVELOPMENTAL LEVEL

How often do you use cold cuts?
How often do you use fish/chicken? (Describe preparation)
How often do you use processed foods such as bakery products, frozen dinners?
How much milk or other dairy products do you consume? What types?

Cholesterol and saturated fat

How many eggs does the family eat per week?
What kind of fat do you use in cooking?
What kind of vegetable oil do you use?

Complex carbohydrates and fiber

How often do you eat fruit? How do you eat it (juices, fresh, canned)?
What kind of vegetables do you eat (canned, frozen, fresh)?
What kind of bread do you eat (whole grain, white)?

Sugar consumption

Do you use sugar in cooking? Do you buy candy, pastries, sweetened cereals?

Sodium

How often do you use processed foods (canned or packaged such as macaroni and cheese)?
Do you add salt to food?

Alcohol consumption

How often do you use alcohol?

Caffeine

How much coffee and tea do you drink per day?

Supplements

Do you take vitamins or mineral supplements? What and how much? Reason.

Cultural influences

"Special" foods
Eating habits unique to culture
Family food preferences or restrictions

Economics

Do you receive any supplementary income to purchase food items?

Eating problems

Do you have problems with indigestion, vomiting, nausea, sore mouth?

Do you have any difficulty swallowing liquids or solids or chewing and feeding yourselves?Medications

Are you on any medications? Do they affect your appetite or weight?

Weight

Has weight changed in the last six months? How much? Describe events associated with the change.

Elimination pattern

Describe bowel and urinary patterns

Activity and exercise patterns

Usual daily/weekly activities of family members

Source of nutrition information

(magazines, family member, schools, health food store)

Family work patterns

Do family members work outside of the home? Type of work and hours

Physical assessment

Describe appearance of the family
Height
Weight
Blood Pressure

TABLE 13-12. FAMILY NUTRITION ASSESSMENT TOOL (continued)

FAMILY MEMBERS	AGE	EDUCATIONAL LEVEL	DEVELOPMENTAL LEVEL

Pulse/Respirations
Percent Body Fat (or Body Mass Index)

Relative Weight $\frac{\text{actual weight} \times 100}{\text{ideal weight}}$

Example:
160 (actual weight) × 100 = 16000
(16000 divided by ideal weight of 140 = 114%)
The closer relative weight is to 100%, the better.
120–139 mild obesity
140–159 moderate obesity
160 + severe obesity
Family strengths/weaknesses
(Identify nutritional concerns of the family)
Barriers to change? Are there reasons why the family cannot change the problem area?

Assessment Summary

Check Problem Area or Potential Problems
1. Dietary fat
2. Cholesterol and saturated fat
3. Complex carbohydrates and fiber
4. Sugar
5. Sodium
6. Alcohol
7. Caffeine
8. Supplements
9. Cultural influences
10. Economics
11. Eating problems
12. Medications
13. Weight changes
14. Elimination pattern
15. Activity and exercise
16. Nutrition resources
17. Work patterns
18. Notes of concern

Nursing diagnosis

Plan and interventionEvaluation

Supplementary assessment for obesity problems

Physical assessment (Height, weight, body fat composition, blood pressure, pulse, respirations)
Highest and lowest weight
Why do you want to lose?
What are the contributing factors to weight gain?
Family weight history
   Maternal   Paternal
Eating patterns
Diets attempted
Medical problems associated with obesity
Activity level
Developmental stage, stresses, significant life events
Nursing diagnosis:
Goal:
Plan:
Evaluation:

amount of weight to lose. The nurse should suggest professional, commercial, or self-help groups after the initial assessment and program plan has been made and encourage continued follow-up for at least two years after the weight has been lost.

A comprehensive weight management program includes behavioral modification, exercise, cognitive change, social support, and nutrition (NIH, 1992). Recommendations include:

- Longer treatment programs (at least 16 to 20 weeks)
- Increased use of in vivo techniques
- Assessment of rate and amount of food eaten (in the clinic instead of working with "reports")
- Examination of thoughts and emotional factors that disrupt weight control efforts
- Differentiation of tasks involved in weight loss and weight maintenance
- Examination of social support and relationships between obese person and spouses, coworkers, and friends
- Evaluation of exercise and activity patterns to design an appropriate program

APPLYING THE NURSING PROCESS TO FAMILY NUTRITION

The family health nurse should begin the family assessment by discussing nutritional practices. An assessment tool is offered in Table 13–12. It is intended as a guideline for data collection and to help the nurse assist the family in reviewing their dietary habits and their thoughts and feelings related to food.

Through use of a comprehensive nutrition tool, important data become available that increase the family's awareness of behaviors supportive of health. The information also facilitates nursing intervention and serves as a basis for decisions concerning desired nutritional practices.

After the data collection, the nurse and family identify their concerns, and a nursing diagnosis is made. Individual assessments are not specifically dealt with because of the desired focus on the family as a unit. Individual problems or needs are often a concern of the entire family and should be discussed.

With the input of the family members, the nursing plan and interventions are determined. Suggestions have been described in earlier sections for guiding the family in planning for dietary and

TABLE 13–13. RESOURCES FOR NUTRITION AND WEIGHT LOSS

American Diabetes Association 1 West 48th Street (600 Fifth Avenue) New York, NY 212-683-7444	Health Professional Committee for Nutrition Education Distribution Center 7700 Edgewater Drive, Suite 215 Oakland, CA 94621
American Dietetic Association (ADA) Journal of the American Dietetic Association 216 West Jackson Suite 800 Chicago, IL 60606-6995 312-899-4853	Human Nutrition Information Service USDA 6505 Belcrest Road Room 325-A Hyattsville, MD 20782
American Public Health Association (APHA) American Journal of Public Health 1015 15th St. N.W. Washington, DC 20005 202-789-5600	The Learn Education Center The Weight Control Digest 1555 W. Mockingbird Lane, Suite 203 Dallas, TX 75235 800-736-7323
American Society of Bariatric Physicians 5600 S. Quebec St., Suite 160D Englewood, CO 80111 303-779-4833	National Dairy Council Ohare National Center 10255 W. Higgins Rd., Suite 900 Rosemont, IL 60018-4233 708-803-2000
Center for Adolescent Obesity Balboa Publishing Corporation 11 Library Place San Anselmo, CA 94960 415-453-8886	Nutrition Foundation, Inc. Nutrition Reviews 1126 16 St. N.W. Suite 100 Washington, DC 20250 202-872-0778
Consumer Information Center Pueblo, CO 81009 303-544-5277, ext. 370	Office of Consumer Communications (HFG-10) Food and Drug Administration Room 15 B-32 Parklawn Building 5600 Fishers Lane Rockville, MD 20857
The Food and Nutrition Information Center National Agriculture Library, Room 304 10301 Baltimore Blvd. Beltsville, MD 20705 301-344-3719	Society for Nutrition Education Journal of Nutrition Education 2001 Killebrew Dr. Suite 340 Minneapolis, MN 55425-1882 612-854-0035

lifestyle changes that affect their health. Table 13–13 presents a selected list of nutritional resources for families and individuals.

The nurse's role is not finished until a follow-up evaluation has been made of the family's progress and/or attainment of goals. At that time, goals are adjusted and plans may include additional follow-up meetings with the family health nurse, or care may be discontinued if the nurse and family believe that the goals have been accomplished.

CHAPTER HIGHLIGHTS

Although it is customary to think of nutrition as an individual activity, it is best understood from a systems perspective because social, cultural, cognitive, and biological variables influence family and individual nutrition.

The average family diet can be described as imbalanced in nutrients and excessive in fat, sugar, and protein.

Key tasks of families with children is assuring adequate nutrient intake, teaching children the importance of good nutrition to achieve a normal body weight and growth, and to role model eating a variety of foods that provide adequate nutrients.

Nursing assessment of family nutrition should include determination of family and individual developmental levels, family nutritional practices and patterns, dietary intake, beliefs, values, culture, economics, preparation, and exercise.

The family nurse's role includes assisting the family by anticipatory guidance, teaching, and supporting nutritional lifestyle changes.

REFERENCES

Abrams, B., & Laros, R. (1986). Prepregnancy weight, weight gain, and birth weight. *American Journal of Obstetrical Gynecologists,* 154(3), 503.

Applegate, L. (1991). *Power Foods.* Emmaus, PA: Rodale Press.

American Psychiatric Association. (1994). *Diagnostic and Statistical Manual of Mental Disorders* (4th ed.). Washington, DC: American Psychiatric Association.

Belmaker, E., & Cohen, J. (1985). The advisability of the prudent diet in adolescence. *Journal of Adolescent Health Care,* 6, 224–232.

Brownell, K., & Wadden, T. (1986). Behavior therapy for obesity: Modern approaches and better results. In

K. Brownell & J. Foreyt (Eds.), *Handbook of Eating Disorders: Physiology, Psychology, and Treatment of Obesity, Anorexia, and Bulimia* (pp. 180–197). New York: Basic Books.

Bruch, H., & Touraine, A. (1940). Obesity in childhood: The family frame of obese children. *Psychosomatic Medicine,* 2, 141.

Brzezinski, A., & Wurtman, J. (1993). Managing weight through the transition years. *Menopause Management* 11(10), 18–23.

Clark, N. (1990). *Nancy Clark's Sports Nutrition Guidebook.* Champaign, IL: Leisure Press.

Dudek, S. (1993). *Nutrition Handbook for Nursing Practice* (2nd ed.). Philadelphia: Lippincott.

Epstein, L. (1986). Treatment of childhood obesity. In K. Brownell & J. Foreyt (Eds.), *Handbook of Eating Disorders: Physiology, Psychology, and Treatment of Obesity, Anorexia, and Bulimia* (pp. 159–177). New York: Basic Books.

Erickson, E.H. (1956). The problem of ego identity. *Journal of the American Psychoanalytic Association,* 4, 6–121.

First, understand what causes weight gain. (1986, January). *Tufts University Diet and Nutrition Letter,* pp. 3–6.

Havala, S., & Dwyer, J. (1988). *Position of the American Dietetic Association: Vegetarian Diets—Technical Support Paper,* 88(3), 352.

Health Professionals' Committee for Nutrition Education. (1986). *Weight Gain and Diet During Pregnancy.*

Health and Public Policy Committee. (1986). American College of Physicians. Position paper. Eating Disorders: Anorexia Nervosa and Bulimia. *Annals of Internal Medicine,* 105, 790–794.

Herron, D. (1991). Strategies for promoting a healthy dietary intake. *Nursing Clinics of North American,* 26(4), 875–884.

Hertzler, A., & Vaughan, C. (1979). The relationship of family structure and interaction to nutrition. *Journal of the American Dietetic Association,* 74, 23–26.

Jonides, I. (1990). Childhood obesity: An update. *Journal of Pediatric Care,* 4 244–251.

Kline, D. (1986). *Nutrition and Pregnancy: Diet and Disease Prevention.* San Diego: Nutrition Dimension.

Kumanyika, S., & Adams-Campbell, L. (1991). Obesity, diet, and psychosocial factors contributing to cardiovascular disease in blacks. In E. Saunders & A. Brest, (Eds.), *Cardiovascular Diseases in Blacks. Cardiovascular Clinics* 21(3). Philadelphia: F.A. Davis.

Lewis, C. (1986). *Nutrition and Nutritional Therapy.* Norwalk, CT: Appleton-Century-Crofts.

Lifshitz, F., Finch, N.M., & Lifshitz, J.Z., (1991). Obesity. In F. Lifshitz, N.M. Finch, & J.Z. Lifshitz (Eds.), *Children's Nutrition* (pp. 295–322). Boston: Jones and Bartlett.

McCarthy, N. (1990). Health promotion and the family. In C. Edelman & C. Mandle (Eds.), *Health Promotion Throughout the Life span* (pp. 111–132). St. Louis: C.V. Mosby.

Mellin, L. (1991). *Shapedown* (4th ed.). San Anselmo, CA: Balboa Publishing.

Melson, G.F. (1980). *Family and Environment: An Ecological Perspective.* Minneapolis, MN: Burgess.

National Academy of Sciences. (1989). *Recommended Dietary Allowances.* Washington, DC: National Academy Press.

National Institutes of Health. (1992). *Methods for Voluntary Weight Loss and Control.* Technology Assessment

Conference Statement. Bethesda, MD: Office of Medical Applications of Research.

National Institutes of Health. (1990). *Facts about Blood Cholesterol.* (Publication No. 90-2696). Washington, DC: National Academy Press.

National Nutrition Monitoring System. (1986). Nationwide food consumption survey: Continuing survey of food intakes of individuals. *Nutrition Today,* May/June, 18–22.

National Research Council. (1989). *Recommended Dietary Allowances* (9th ed.). Washington, DC: National Academy of Sciences.

Peck, E., & Ullrich, M. (1985). *Children and Weight: A Changing Perspective.* An ad hoc committee on children and weight. Berkeley: Nutrition Communications.

Riggs, B., & Melton, L. (1986). Involutional osteoporosis. *New England Journal of Medicine,* 314, 1676–1684.

Roe, D. (1986). Nutritional needs and concerns of American women. *Nutrition News,* 49(3), 9–11.

Sherman, A. (1986). Alterations in immunity related to nutritional status. *Nutrition Today,* 7–12.

Simonson, M., & Heilman, J. (1983). *The Complete University Medical Diet.* New York: Rawson.

Stern, J. (1992). Obesity prevention, research needed in high-risk minorities. *Obesity,* March/April, (5).

Stoppard, M. (1994). *Menopause.* New York: Dorling Kindersley.

Updated advice for a healthier heart. (1986, October). *Tufts University Diet and Newsletter,* p. 1.

U.S. Department of Health, Education and Welfare. (1979). *Healthy People. The Surgeon General's Report on Health Promotion and Disease Prevention.* (DHEW Publication No. 79-55071). Washington, DC: U.S. Government Printing Office.

U.S. Department of Health and Human Services. (1988). *The Surgeon General's Report on Nutrition and Health.* (DHHS-PHS Publication No. 88-50210). Washington, DC: U.S. Government Printing Office.

U.S. Department of Health and Human Services. (1990a). *Healthy People 2000: National Health Promotion and Disease Prevention Objectives.* (Publication No. (PHS) 91-50213). Washington, DC: U.S. Government Printing Office.

U.S. Department of Health and Human Services (1990b). *Nutrition and Your Health. Dietary Guidelines for Americans* (3rd ed.). Home and Garden Bulletin No. 232.

Williams, S. (1990). *Essentials of Nutrition and Diet Therapy* (5th ed.). Boston: Times Mirror/Mosby College Publishing.

Wurtman, J. (1986). *Managing Your Mind and Mood Through Food.* New York: Rawson.

FAMILY STRESS MANAGEMENT

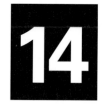

ANNE ROE MEALEY
HAROLDYNE RICHARDSON
and GRETCHEN DIMICO

Family stress-inevitable but surmountable.

DOLORES CURRAN

OBJECTIVES

On completion of this chapter, the reader will be able to:

1. Define family stress adaptation and coping
2. Discuss the role of the professional nurse in family coping
3. Assess how well the family copes with stress
4. Use the nursing process in the development of a nursing diagnosis related to family stress/coping
5. Discuss specific strategies for adaptation and coping with family stress

All human beings are born into a primary group, known as the family, and all members of the family experience stress as a natural part of human existence. The family is a complex, multigenerational system subject to internal and external demands. The reaction to such demands is considered to be the stress response, or "stress," and the demand itself is the stressor. Events themselves are not inherently stressful. The degree of stress experienced depends on the appraisal of the stressor and the ability to manage the situation to cope.

Each family system has its own repertoire of coping approaches, which may or may not be adequate to restore the family system to equilibrium. As the professional nurse employs the nursing process in the assessment of the family system, the focus is on the roles, rules, self-esteem, power, boundaries, and links between subsystems. Cues are provided for the formulation of nursing diagnoses and form the basis for planning coping strategies. The process needs ongoing evaluation to confirm its efficacy in helping the family deal with stress.

This chapter is designed to increase the nurse's knowledge of the concept of family coping and to suggest some specific strategies for management of potentially harmful levels of family stress. The goal of the intervention is to assist families to anticipate, recognize, and prevent stress from progressing into crises. The family is helped to regain or maintain functioning in such a way that strengths and resources are mobilized to cope effectively with stress.

THEORIES OF FAMILY COPING

The Coping Process

Since the mid 1970s, the concept of coping has been a component of models related to stress management. Lazarus and Folkman (1989) view coping as "constantly changing cognitive efforts to manage external and/or internal demands that are appraised as taxing or exceeding the resources of the person" (p. 179). This process-oriented approach indicates a difference between coping and automatic behavior: coping represents effort. Many behaviors initially require effort, yet eventually become automatic as learning occurs. Thus, coping refers to situations of psychological stress which call for mobilization and involve *all* efforts to manage regardless of outcome. Managing may include avoiding, denying, minimizing, tolerating, accepting the stressful situation, or striving for mastery.

Coping depends on how the event is cognitively appraised. A *primary appraisal* determines whether a stressful situation has potential for threat, harm/loss, or challenge. If this potential is present a *secondary appraisal* evaluates what might and can be done. *Reappraisal* is a third component and is based on new information. Appraisal processes may or may not be conscious (Lazarus & Folkman, 1989, p. 54). Effective coping has a number of functions; it is not simply problem solving. Lazarus and Folkman (1989) distinguish between coping that is directed at managing or altering the problem (problem-focused coping) and emotion-focused coping, which serves the purpose of changing the emotional response to the problem.

The family may decide to meet the situation head-on or to flee from the stressful environment. Efforts to manage the stress on the part of the family may include learning more information about the problem by reading, consulting experts, trying to increase their understanding of the problem, or direct problem solving. For example, a family with a toddler who won't eat could take direct action to reduce stress by reading about growth and development behaviors and using suggested strategies.

The second form of coping, *emotion-focused*, is used when appraisal indicates that nothing can be done to change environmental conditions of harm, threat, or challenge. Many of the management techniques discussed in the latter part of this chapter are emotion-focused because they reduce the affective, visceral, or motor responses to stress. For effective coping, people use a combination of the two modes. A family may continue to live in the stressful environment but may reduce their anxiety level by changing their expectations and focusing on their assets and strengths rather than needs.

A variety of coping strategies provides greater adaptability and flexibility for the family's use. This chapter will address a number of different strategies that can be used to increase the family's ability to cope.

Family Coping

Family coping is a complex process of adjustment and adaptation. It is the interactive efforts of family members working as a whole to achieve and maintain balance over time in response to stressors. All families experience stress, some of which is growth producing, however; when stressors exert unusual efforts on the family system, the family must cope to return to equilibrium. Stressors may be *internal* to the family system, such as developmental changes, or from *external* sources, such as social pressures (for example, the neighborhood becomes crime ridden).

The family coping factors include family culture, family communications, family resources, family cohesion, and flexibility (Olson, 1989). Because of internal and external social support, family perception, individual and family developmental stages, and the "pile-up" or amount of stress imposed on the family, coping efficacy varies considerably from family to family. Coping efficacy varies considerably and is influenced by culture, developmental cycles, and the time frame (Olson et al., 1983).

The Resiliency Model of Family Stress Adjustment and Adaptation (McCubbin & McCubbin, 1993), a revision of the Double ABCX model (McCubbin & Patterson, 1983), provides a framework for understanding the many factors involved in family coping. Another model, the Circumplex Model of Marital and Family Systems developed by Olson and his associates, facilitates family assessment in the domains of flexibility of family structure and the cohesiveness or emotional bonding of the family (Olson, 1989).

Families tend to use the problem-solving methods that have worked successfully in the past. These strategies may be effective for moderate stress, but in family crisis the pile-up of demands or the depletion of resources causes disorganization of the family structure. This disorganization requires changes in family roles, rules, goals, or patterns of interaction.

Pearlin and Schooler (1982) believed that three types of adaptive behaviors assisted the family coping process: changing the stressor event, controlling the family definition of the situation (reframing), and learning more functional coping strategies to control the stressful reaction. Using the first type of adaptive coping strategies, the family may pursue a solution to the problem that eliminates the stressor or that can decrease the pile-up of events that has depleted the family's resources. Increased understanding of the situation and acquisition of coping skills can bring about constructive change. The family may pull together and coordinate coping efforts, use social support networks as buffering agents to relieve distress, or interact with community supports as a way of balancing demands of stress with family resources. A grieving family who has lost a source of financial support will use job services to retrain and search for new employment opportunities while mutually supporting one another to prevent the loss of self-esteem and to maintain family morale.

Using the second type of adaptive coping, *reframing,* the healthy family controls the meaning of the stress by the way they perceive the situation and the relative importance of the threatened loss (Olson, 1989). Because of the importance of their values, a religious family may be devastated when an adolescent member rejects the religious practices of the family, whereas another family may think of it as a phase of adolescent development and take it in stride. Families have the potential to neutralize the stressfulness of an event by viewing the meaning relative to the situation at hand. Families may use *positive comparison* to control the meaning of stress by participation in community network or self-help groups. The hardship is reduced by sharing the notion that "we are all in this together" or "compared to others we have much to be thankful for." *Selective ignoring* is another coping strategy where family members look for the good within the situation. A woman recovering from mastectomy surgery told her nurse how lucky she was that her malignancy was discovered in such an early stage.

The third type of adaptive coping is an attempt to control the reaction to the stress. The family is passive and accepts the stressful situation without being overwhelmed by it. This more passive approach may be based on the belief that good-natured forbearance will have its rewards. Olson et al. (1983) define this type of behavior as *passive appraisal.* This form of adaptive behavior may include controlled reflectiveness, passive forbearance, helpless resignation, optimistic faith, or other strategies that will help to minimize the discomfort of the problem. This behavior can be effective for an out-of-work situation but ineffective when dealing with relationship issues such as parenting. Some families who are moderately cohesive and remain flexible during time of stress are more hardy than others. Family hardiness is the ability of a family to recover or change in response to major stress or crisis situation. Hardy families have strengths that include an internal locus of control, having a sense of the meaning of life, as well as feeling involved with community and committed to the process of growth (McCubbin & Thompson, 1987).

Healthy families adapt to stressful situations by mobilizing their resources and repertoire of many and varied coping strategies. According to McCubbin and Figley (1983), there is little research evidence about which coping strategies are most effective. However, Curran (1985) found that the stress-effective family "(1) views stress as a normal part of family life, (2) shares feelings as well as words, (3) develops conflict-resolution and creative coping skills, (4) makes use of support people and systems, and (5) is adaptable" (p. 61). The effectiveness of coping strategies varies depending on the uniqueness of each family, the developmental stage, and the choices made.

Healthy families have formed positive attachments that are not hostile nor that contain extreme emotional content (Doane et al., 1991). Healthy families are flexible and capable of changing structure to learn new coping behaviors when the initial problem-solving methods prove ineffective. One study of expectant couples found that those with greater flexibility were able to adapt to the changing family structure more successfully (Dietz & Omar, 1991). McCubbin and Patterson (1981) found that the intervening variables that helped families successfully adapt to stress included open and supportive interactions both within the family system and between the family system and the community. They found that the community provided families with social support and a variety of resources. Both internal and external resources and the ability to use them were instrumental to a successful outcome.

External coping strategies are often used by families to ameliorate the effects of stress. These strategies include the informal or formal support systems of members within the family system, neighbors, extended family, mutual self-help groups, and social institutions such as the health care system. In a study of 1000 families, Olson et al. (1983) reported that the most effective coping strategies were spiritual support and reframing, followed by informal support. The formal support systems were least used. Significant differences exist in the coping styles specific to each gender. Women are more likely to mobilize social support than men while men use organization to cope with role strain. Women, especially those with children, are more likely to use compartmentalization, cognitive restructuring, and limiting of vocational activities (Schnittger & Bird, 1990).

The family that deals most effectively with stress is often the family who is well integrated in terms of commitment to the group and to collective goals; the members possess inner strengths and they pull together to become cohesive. They can nurture each other and use the resources necessary for maintenance of the family unit and growth of the individual members.

Family Coping Resources

The manner in which the family copes is dependent on the resources available to them and the constraints present within the context of their situation. Additional examples of resources are positive beliefs, problem-solving skills, social skills, and social support.

Boss (1987) distinguished between the coping resources of the family and the process of coping. The coping resources are those sociologic, economic, psychological, or physical assets of the family that can be mobilized in coping. Health, family cohesiveness, economic security, open communications, or intelligence are all examples of resources. However, the family may fail to recognize their strengths or fail to use them during a stressful situation. In such a case, a family nurse can work with the family to assist them to see their full range of options, to acknowledge their strengths and chances for successful outcome, to teach new coping skills as necessary, and to follow through with the appropriate actions.

Ineffective Coping

Ineffective coping interferes with vital family functions so that needs of family members are left unfulfilled. For example, if a hospice nurse is assisting a family to cope with a dying grandparent in the home, he or she assesses how capable the family is in meeting the affective needs of its members. During this period of stress, are coping skills effective, or does the nurse see signs of psychological or physiological stress, such as somatic illness?

Ineffective coping fails to reduce or control the stress and may in itself produce undesirable consequences or risks. Boss (1987) believed that ineffective coping behaviors tended to be automatic rather than rationally planned. Some of these patterns of behavior may be a function of social learning from early family modeling. The phenomenon of child abuse is such a case. An abusive parent may respond to the stress of the fatigue and incessant crying with anger, lashing out to strike the crying infant. The rapid move from emotional reaction to behavioral response without the primary appraisal of the consequences is the ineffective aspect of this coping method.

According to Minuchin (1974) ineffective coping occurs when families respond to internal or external stress without acknowledging the need to change. Rather than developing a new level of functioning, the rigidity of the family structure is conveyed through stereotyped functioning. Some of the responses to the stressors themselves create greater internal stress for the family. Behaviors that indicate ineffective coping may be agitation, depression, hostility, guilt, intolerance, abandonment, desertion, neglect, and psychosomaticism.

NURSING PROCESS AND FAMILY STRESS MANAGEMENT

The role of the family nurse is to facilitate family self-care behaviors that prevent or aid in coping with stressors and to promote health. Through use of the nursing process, the nurse aids the family in identifying strengths and enhancing adaptive mechanisms. The major goals of the nurse are to promote wellness; to assist family members to anticipate, recognize, prevent, reduce, manage, or adapt to stressful high-risk situations (to cope); and to help the family to experience a feeling of satisfaction and closeness from working on a problem together. Coping skills can be taught as the nurse helps the family to "re-create" or to move toward wholeness as a unit.

If the network of family support has been disconnected, members may hesitate to call on other members for help. The nurse can encourage the family to reestablish their emotional support system within both the immediate and the extended family.

In times of relative stability, the nurse can use anticipatory guidance to assist the family to develop a plan to prevent stress or to cope effectively. The family, as client, must be an active participant in developing this plan. The nurse's role is to assist, not control, the process (Pender, 1987).

Assessment of Family Stress and Coping

Early assessment of family stress and strain is important to the prevention of problems with family function (Marsden & Dracup, 1991). A structural, functional approach to family assessment is very useful (Friedman, 1992). The nurse examines roles of family members, power structure within the subsystems of the family, boundaries, and communication patterns. As discussed in Chapter 8, because communication is the interaction within the family system that links the members, this is a vital part of the assessment and includes both verbal and nonverbal behaviors. The use of observation and interview techniques are recommended to help the nurse assess communication patterns such as openness, emotional bonding, use of space, active listening, respect, and willingness to meet each other's needs. The nurse will identify whether communications are open and direct and whether the meaning is clear. Does the communication system support and affirm family members? Does it build self-esteem?

Keeping in mind the variables in the Resiliency Model of Family Stress, Adjustment, and Adaptation, the nurse assesses both the stressors and the coping process. The significance of the stressor depends on the values of the family within a cultural and social context, the pile-up of stressors, the previous family life events, and the amount of change demanded by the stressor. To assess family coping, the nurse examines family and community resources as well as how effectively the family mobilizes them. What is the developmental stage of the family, and what is their experience in use of various coping strategies?

Family inventories are valuable tools both for family research and as assessment tools for measuring variables related to family stress and family coping. *The Family Inventory of Life Events* (FILE, shown in Chapter 10), (McCubbin et al., 1985) reflects common family pile-up variables across the family life span. *The Family Crisis Oriented Evaluation Scale* (F-COPES) (McCubbin et al., 1985) measures family coping behavior (see Table 14–1). The subscales of the instrument integrate the perception of stressors within the system and

TABLE 14–1. FAMILY CRISIS ORIENTED PERSONAL SCALES (F-COPES)

WHEN WE FACE PROBLEMS OR DIFFICULTIES IN OUR FAMILY, WE RESPOND BY:	Strongly Disagree	Moderately Disagree	Neither Agree Nor Disagree	Moderately Agree	Strongly Agree
1. Sharing our difficulties with relatives	1	2	3	4	5
2. Seeking encouragement and support from friends	1	2	3	4	5
3. Knowing we have the power to solve major problems	1	2	3	4	5
4. Seeking information and advice from persons in other families who have faced the same or similar problems	1	2	3	4	5
5. Seeking advice from relatives (grandparents, etc.)	1	2	3	4	5
6. Seeking assistance from community agencies and programs designed to help families in our situation	1	2	3	4	5
7. Knowing that we have the strength within our own family to solve our problems	1	2	3	4	5
8. Receiving gifts and favors from neighbors (e.g. food, taking in mail, etc.)	1	2	3	4	5
9. Seeking information and advice from the family doctor	1	2	3	4	5
10. Asking neighbors for favors and assistance	1	2	3	4	5
11. Facing the problems "head-on" and trying to get solution right away	2	3	4	5	
12. Watching television	1	2	3	4	5
13. Showing that we are strong	1	2	3	4	5
14. Attending church services	1	2	3	4	5
15. Accepting stressful events as a fact of life	1	2	3	4	5
16. Sharing concerns with close friends	1	2	3	4	5
17. Knowing luck plays a big part in how well we are able to solve family problems	1	2	3	4	5
18. Exercising with friends to stay fit and reduce tension	1	2	3	4	5
19. Accepting that difficulties occur unexpectedly	1	2	3	4	5
20. Doing things with relatives (get-togethers, dinners, etc.)					
21. Seeking professional counseling and help for family difficulties	1	2	3	4	5
22. Believing we can handle our own problems	1	2	3	4	5
23. Participating in church activities	1	2	3	4	5
24. Defining the family problem in a more positive way so that we do not become too discouraged	1	2	3	4	5
25. Asking relatives how they feel about problems we face	1	2	3	4	5
26. Feeling that no matter what we do to prepare, we will have difficulty handling problems	1	2	3	4	5
27. Seeking advice from a minister	1	2	3	4	5
28. Believing if we wait long enough, the problem will go away	1	2	3	4	5
29. Sharing problems with neighbors	1	2	3	4	5
30. Having faith in God	1	2	3	4	5

Source: Family Crisis Oriented Personal Scales (F-COPES). From H.I. McCubbin & A.I. Thompson. (1987). *Family Assessment Inventories*. Madison, Wisconsin: University of Wisonsin-Madison. Reprinted with permission.

use of resources, both internal and external to the family system. The instrument also measures coping that involves direct action and the more palliative modes of coping.

The subscales of the instrument measure the perception of stressors, the use of family resources, and the coping behaviors used by families. The internal coping strategies include the confidence of the family in active problem-solving methods as well as more passive methods such as reframing the family's perspective or passive appraisal. The external strategies used by families include the use of resources such as church or religion; the support of the extended family, friends, and neighbors; and the use of resources available through community organizations.

Scoring the instrument is done by summing the numbers circled for items in each subscale, except for items 17, 26, and 28, which are reversed. The subscales are social support (1, 2, 5, 8, 10, 16, 20, 25, 29); reframing (3, 7, 11, 13, 15, 19, 22, 24); spiritual support (14, 23, 27, 30); mobilizing the family to acquire and accept help (4, 6, 9, 21); and passive appraisal (12, 17, 26, 28). A total coping score is the sum of the subscales and has a possible range from 29 to 145. The mean scores reported (McCubbin & Thompson, 1987) range from 91.24 to 95.64, and standard deviations are from 12.06 to 14.05. For information on permission to use F-COPES, as well as for detailed instructions and norms for adults and adolescents, consult McCubbin & Thompson (1987).

Nursing Diagnosis of Family Stress

The next step in the nursing process is the development of a nursing diagnosis of family stress.

Family stressors that are included in the accepted nursing diagnosis catagories of the North American Nursing Diagnosis Association (NANDA) are extensive because stress affects the family structure and ability to function as well as the health of the individual family members (Gordon, 1991). Consequently, stress as an etiologic factor may affect all 11 of the functional health patterns shown in Table 14–2.

Problems the nurse identifies related to family coping, family communication, and family process are significant because they are mechanisms the family uses in dealing with stress and will limit the family's adaptability. Ineffective coping is compromised or disabling coping of the family or coping with the potential for growth (Carpenito, 1991). Nursing diagnoses related to the ability of the family to adapt to stressors are included in the accepted nursing diagnosis categories of NANDA. In a sense, each of the diagnoses can be viewed as a continuous moving from health to illness, that is, possible problems moving to disabling problems. Descriptors shown in Table 14–3 indicate the degrees of coping.

Family Stress Management Plan

The next activity in the nursing process is to develop, in collaboration with the family, a family plan to manage the stress. The plan should include:

1. Identification of willingness of family members to work on the problem, and where possible, a commitment of all family members to participate. For example, if a spouse has decided that the marriage is not worth working on, he/she will not be ready to risk

TABLE 14–2. EXAMPLES OF NURSING DIAGNOSES RELATED TO FAMILY STRESS

FUNCTIONAL PATTERN	NURSING DIAGNOSIs	FAMILY STRESSOR
Health perception/Health management	Health management deficit: Untreated medical condition	Single parent with role overload
Nutritional/Metabolic	Alteration in nutrition: Obesity	Unfilled intimacy needs
Elimination	Alteration in bowel elimination: Diarrhea	Repressed anger–Marital conflict
Activity/Exercise	Diversional activity deficit	Workaholic parent
Sleep/Rest	Sleep-pattern disturbance	Transition into parenthood
Cognitive/Perceptual	Decisional conflict	Death of spouse
Self-perception/Self-concept	Powerlessness	Rigid/Autocratic family structure
Role/Relationship	Alterations in socialization	Parental conflict over use of discipline
Sexuality/Reproductive	Altered sexuality patterns	Marital relationship problems
Coping/Stress tolerance	Ineffective family coping: Compromised	Chronic disease of child
Value/Belief	Spiritual distress	Alienation of family from source of spirituality

Data from Gordon, M. (1991). *Nursing Diagnosis: Process and Application* (3rd ed). St. Louis: Mosby.

TABLE 14–3. NURSiNG DIAGNOSIS: INEFFECTIVE FAMILY COPING

MODIFIER	INTERPRETATION
Possible	The nurse identifies a problem that may be present but more assessment is needed
High risk	The nurse identifies what may be a stressor depending on the family context but without evidence of characteristic signs and symptoms of stress
Potential for growth	Adaptation has occurred, and family is moved to a higher level of function
Compromised	Usually adaptive family lacks the adequate skill experience to cope with a stressor
Disabling	Coping behaviors absent or cause increased distress, preventing adequate coping

the changes needed. Or, if a child believes he/she will soon be out of the family, the energy devoted to the family plan will be lessened.

2. A discussion of approaches that have been used in the past to resolve previous stressors. How were these helpful or not helpful? How could these be modified to meet the current stress?
3. Brainstorming of possible plans. Brainstorming means that all opinions are accepted without judgment until a list of possibilities is available.
4. Discussion of the possible outcomes of each brainstormed plan. What are the positive/negative aspects of each? Can some be combined?
5. Initiation of a plan to cope. This may present increased anxiety to some members who view change as undesirable and frightening. As a result, supportive enactment of the plan by each member needs to be encouraged by the nurse.

At this point, nurses have the opportunity to teach stress management approaches that include new coping skills and behaviors that decrease stress and enhance interpersonal relationships.

Evaluation of Family Coping

The evaluation of nursing care for a family undergoing crisis or stress is an ongoing process. The nurse assesses the response of the family to the stressor event(s), the newly learned coping and adaptation behaviors, and the use of adaptive resources both within the family and in the community.

The evaluation phase includes determining the affective function of the family, the interaction and communication patterns, the function and coping style used, and the physical health of the family members. The affect of the family can be used as a thermometer to measure the progress of recovery. Is the family capable of sharing feelings of happiness, hopefulness, confidence, optimism, and satisfaction with their lives? Are there feelings of unresolved loss or grief in the family? If the

recovery is progressing too slowly, there may continue to be evidence of feelings such as anxiety, tension, fear, depression, despair, or low self-esteem.

The evaluation of family function is an important part of the ongoing assessment. Is there greater productivity on the part of the family? Are the family members resuming their role functions? Is the family meeting the needs of the members according to community standards? Is there less dependence on health care services? Does the family reflect a desire to recover, and do family members strive to be healthy?

The nurse assesses the health of family members. Are there fewer somatic symptoms, less dependence on medications, fewer alcohol and drug abuse problems, and fewer episodes of infectious disease? Is there an increase in energy and a sense of physical well-being within the family?

The final part of the evaluation of the family is to determine the adaptation and coping activities. Has the family learned new coping skills? Do they consistently use problem-solving approaches rather than denial to deal with stressful situations? Do they clearly and realistically identify sources of stress for the family? Is their locus of control within the family, or do they rely on an individual family member to handle stressful situations for them?

The progress of the family is evaluated within a specific social- cultural context set by family values. It is important for the nurse to evaluate the success of the plan of care within a developmental framework. The healthy family should evolve higher levels of function and acquire a rich variety of new skills for future encounters with stressors.

FAMILY STRESS MANAGEMENT APPROACHES

Some families cope effectively with stress, and other families proceed into crisis and disorganization. Boss (1987) suggests that the family's value orientation in terms of fatalism versus mastery is critical to how (or if) a family copes. The term "fatalism" means acceptance rather than mastery. A family with a mastery orientation may believe that it can control or handle the situation and is more likely to take action. One must use caution in assuming that the active strategy is more effective than the passive approach. A fatalistic belief system may be best when nothing can bring about a change. Families who cope well may be those who select what they will be fatalistic about and what they will master or control (Reeder, 1991).

The ability to manage stress is in part dependent on how one explains events (explanatory style). Research findings from a series of collaborative longitudinal studies show that men who were generally optimistic in college are healthier in later life than were those who had a pessimistic outlook (Peterson et al., 1988). Pessimists are likely to believe that negative events came about because of personal inadequacies that cannot be altered. Optimists are more likely to respond to stressful experiences by creating an action plan or requesting help. An explanatory style can be recognized and can be changed from that of the pessimist to the healthier state of an optimist. Since a change in one member affects the entire system, these findings have implications for work with the family—that is, the client. The nurse who can use cognitive change methods can act as a coach and a guide.

The crucial variable appears to be the *meaning* of the event for the family and for the individuals within it. The meaning is related to the perception of the situation and is mediated by the context (Boss, 1987). Human beings have the power to change their perception of an event and to alter its meaning. Thus, they can modify their attitudes and responses. One can decide to accept a certain situation as a learning opportunity and a challenge or to view it as a disaster.

Curran (1985) suggests that healthy families view stress as normal rather than as a sign of weakness or failure. Such a family is adaptable and has developed conflict resolution and creative coping skills.

In order to bring about and maintain constructive changes for stress management and health promotion, it is necessary to use a holistic approach that is individualized for the specific family. Because unhealthy lifestyles and generations of cultural patterns of coping have brought about many "disorders of living," the potential need frequently is for lifestyle changes. It is necessary to take into account existing capabilities, knowledge and skills, values, beliefs, and cultural background of the family. The plan should be flexible, with realistic expectations and time frame. Change is gradual. This can be presented to the family as an approach to living, a process rather than a destination. This helps the members to develop a sense of direction and a feeling of efficacy, hope, and some control over their lives.

The experience of "stress" is a personal event; each member of the family can learn to identify their own stress warning signals. These are cues to the early symptoms of stress. As stress rises, the symptoms increase in severity, thus adding more stress and beginning a negative feedback loop. The family can be taught to identify "stress warning red flags" and to choose a preventive strategy. It is often difficult for the person experiencing severe stress to identify the problem; both physical and psychic energy is "bound-up" and not available for healthy functioning. A compassionate approach from other family members can often help the person to identify feelings, explore options, and feel less overwhelmed.

Every family has the potential for becoming more self-actualized and more competent in the promotion and management of health. The family nurse can assist in this move toward wellness by providing information, serving as a catalyst for desired behavior modification and lifestyle changes, and providing clients with skills for continued growth and maintenance of healthy behaviors.

Stress management approaches for families are proposed in Table 14–4. Change is never easy, and barriers can arise from internal and external sources (Pender, 1987). However, change is often difficult because *one does not know how to behave differently*. Approaches to change involve learning and practicing new habits. The role of the nurse is to facilitate new patterns of family coping and to work with the family in the development of family goals. Once the family is committed to making changes, the nurse uses a systematic approach to plan how those goals can be met over time using a variety of family stress management techniques (see Table 14–4). Change can occur, but it requires time, effort, and commitment. The process of adopting new patterns of coping with stress can be facilitated by use of self-care contracting, as discussed in Chapters 2 and 10.

The first steps in stress management are prevention of stressors, recognition of stressors, anticipation of stressors, and elimination or avoidance of possible stressors. If families use these first steps, they are less likely to reach crisis in many situations. In addition, individual approaches to stress management affect the family system's quality of health. Some of the many approaches that have been documented to be effective in coping with stress include relaxation (Borysenko, 1987; Cohen & Jaffe, 1990; Davis et al., 1988; Hoblitzelle & Benson, 1992; Travis & Ryan, 1988), innate biofeedback (Ennis, 1992), imagery (Epstein, 1989; Hendricks, 1979; Hoblitzelle & Benson, 1992; Rossman, 1990), nutrition (Benson & Stuart, 1992; Pender, 1987), minimal use of drugs and alcohol (Benson & Stuart, 1992).

Problem Solving

When a problem arises in a family, it is important that the members recognize it and accept the reality of its existence. Denial of the problem is

TABLE 14–4. FAMILY AND INDIVIDUAL STRESS MANAGEMENT APPROACHES

FAMILIES AND INDIVIDUALS
Anticipation of stressors
Prevention of stressors
Elimination or avoidance of stressors
Recognition of stressors
Problem solving
Cognitive restructuring
Conflict resolution
Role sharing
Communication strategies
Time management
Intimacy
Family centering/meditation
Spirituality
Humor
Negotiated housekeeping standards
Family recreation

INDIVIDUAL STRESS MANAGEMENT
Relaxation
Biofeedback
Imagery
Good health habits
Music
Time alone

not a healthy alternative. However, the family may decide to avoid the problem or to eliminate the problem when possible. Active problem solving by family members is often an appropriate intervention.

According to Curran (1985), every study related to healthy families suggests that these families are "good problem-solvers." Nurses, taught to use a problem-solving approach in the nursing process, may assume that everyone knows the steps of gathering data, defining the problem, generating alternatives, finding solutions, and evaluating results. In actuality, many persons have not developed this creative process. Nurses can teach this skill as a coping strategy. The role of the family nurse is to teach clients a general coping strategy so that clients can more effectively control their own lives.

An effective approach may be to write down, in two separate columns, the positive aspects of an approach and the negative aspects. One can even "weigh," or rank, the positives and negatives. Often, just the simple act of making concrete positives and negatives provides data that the family can use to problem solve.

Cognitive Restructuring

Before a family member can focus on more adaptive thoughts or learn new coping skills, negative patterns of thought that sidetrack coping efforts need to be interrupted. Self-defeating thoughts, negative self-talk, and irrational beliefs

can evoke emotional and physical arousal that results in stress and has a profound impact on our moods, behavior, and health.

The Harvard Negotiation Project (Fisher & Ury, 1992) advocates "four basic steps in inventing options" (p. 70). They are identification of what is wrong, analysis of possible causes and barriers, brainstorming of possible approaches, and generation of specific actions that might be used to solve the problem. Cognitive restructuring is the conscious thought process of redefining or relabeling beliefs or thought patterns (self-talk). Self-talk is a part of every individual's personality, the way that person interprets the world. The thought patterns and beliefs are often illogical or distorted (Ellis, 1988). The interpretation of internal and external conditions may or may not be based on fact. Internal self-evaluation leads to messages of reward or punishment that affect the daily functioning of the individual (Davis et al., 1988).

It is possible to change patterns of self-talk, which can lead to reduction of stress. One approach is rational-emotive therapy (RET) (Ellis, 1988). This approach assists the person to critically evaluate the illogical nature of the self-talk and to understand that the way a person perceives or evaluates a situation determines his or her emotional reaction. All people develop sets of beliefs based on their experiences, and these beliefs mediate or determine their responses in a given situation. However, expectations or beliefs that are irrational or based on false assumptions create problems and increase stress. Cognitive theorists have identified that people often "awfulize" events by irrational self-talk. Breadwinners who have lost their jobs may muse that they are stupid for losing the position or may, in fact, feel that there are better positions waiting for a person with their talents. The process of self-evaluation and self-talk begins in the child at an early age and can aid in the development of self-esteem and healthy growth or can give rise to a harsh internal critic and feelings of inferiority. Parental verbal and nonverbal behaviors have an important role in this process. If the child hears "you are bad," "you are lazy," "you are stupid," this may be internalized to "I am bad, lazy, and stupid." Family members might be told to substitute a statement such as "that behavior was not skillful; I can change that to something more useful." This gives the message that growth is possible.

Changing internal messages and replacing negative, illogical self-talk with supportive statements based on realistic beliefs is a coping skill that, in essence, creates a new self-support system. Changing self-talk involves:

1. Identification of the self-talk and the situation
2. Evaluation of whether messages are rational or irrational

3. Replacement of the messages with supportive statements
4. Integration into daily life.

Imagery, an ancient practice, can be used to empower positive attitudes and change behaviors (Hoblitzelle & Benson, 1992). Imagery is useful to facilitate practice in altering self-talk. Encourage the individual or the family to imagine a problematic situation and then use positive self-statements, to imagine mastery within the event. Implementing these changes takes time and practice. The nurse is in a position to encourage, to support, and to empower the family to relabel or redefine individual family stressors.

For example, when the family nurse observes that the mother functions with the belief that she must be loved and approved of by all and that any open expression of anger is dangerous, the plan of action might include a family discussion of the results of this behavior on other family members, as well as on the mother. It could be suggested that no one can be loved and approved of by everyone and that appropriate expression of anger is acceptable. The mother could be encouraged to examine her self-talk when she perceives no one loves her and to restructure her beliefs about anger. Perhaps reframing an angry situation as "discussing differences" would be a more positive approach.

Conflict Resolution

Fisher and Ury (1992) report that "conflict is a growth industry. Everyone wants to participate in decisions that affect them" (p. xi). Conflict situations related to issues of power, use of resources, relationship needs, and differing value systems arise in families. Whatever the cause, the result is usually increased stress until the conflict is resolved. However, conflict as a concept characterizes a wide continuum of behaviors from quiet arguing to quarreling to aggression. Most therapists agree that it is healthy to have a degree of conflict in relationships, recognizing that if no disagreements are evident, one person in the relationship may be too submissive and/or may be stock-piling hurts and discomforts. Conflict can be healthy if it promotes open communication. However, conflict resolution is vital to the health of the family. A conflict that is ignored tends to go "underground," where it rises periodically in a new guise or issue, causing increasing dysfunction in the family.

Family life education programs offer training to help couples air disagreements and fight therapeutically (Burr, 1990; Renick et al., 1992). Conflict resolution demands active listening, effective communication, willingness to address underlying issues, commitment to the family relations, and use of negotiation skills. Fisher and Ury (1992) recognize that most conflict falls into one of three categories: perception, emotion, and communication. These authors recommend "(1) separate the people from the problem, (2) focus on interests, not positions, (3) invent options for mutual gain, and (4) insist on using objective criteria." (p. 15).

A communication technique that often needs to be taught and that is useful in conflict resolution is the communication skill of *claiming* feeling when upset (e.g., "I feel angry when you overspend our budget"). This approach clearly claims the emotion as a part of the person and allows the other to respond cognitively to the message and to the emotion expressed.

In contrast, a *blaming* message communicates that the other person is responsible for the individual's feelings (e.g., "You make me so angry when you overspend our budget"). The result is usually a defensive reply and little cognitive awareness of the source of the emotion. In addition, "we-statements" may be helpful "when a person wants to turn a problem they 'own' as an individual into a problem that is 'owned' by the relationship" (Burr 1990). By using a we-statement, such as "as a family, we don't show much affection" or " we don't seem to have much time for fun," the problem becomes a family group problem. However, one must be careful to note that a broad statement, such as "the checking account is very low," could be heard as a personal attack. It is important to point out that other people cannot control our feelings. Individuals make choices of emotional responses from a diverse set, depending on background, self-esteem, and previous learning. As a result of different perspectives, arguments or quarreling ensue. Arguments start with a current issue and focus on the sides taken by each party in the discussion, such as an argument about how the finances should be budgeted and by whom. Resolution is usually accomplished by a form of compromise, and the issue is settled. Quarreling and high levels of marital conflict have ramifications that are much more serious (Bowman, 1990). Quarrels attack the other person's values and usually represent unconscious needs and deprivations of the attacking person. Insults and personal attacks hurled in the anger of a quarrel fan the flame of retribution and cauterize the spirit. The result can only be incineration of the relationship. Techniques for preventing quarrels are (1) recognition of times when such quarrels are more likely to occur, (2) awareness of the danger signals of impending upsets, and (3) self-awareness of elements that trigger the response. In cases of extreme dysfunction, family therapy by a qualified family nurse therapist or family counselor is recommended. The role of the family nurse is to encourage the use of good communication and to reduce and settle conflicts in the family.

Role Sharing

Role sharing has evolved in response to societal and family system changes, that reflect almost two-thirds of women into the workforce accompanied by a decrease of nearby extended family (Hochschild, 1989). "Role sharing refers to participation of two or more persons in the same roles even though they hold different positions" (Friedman, 1992). In contrast, role specialization denotes that one person in the family fulfills a particular family function.

Although mothers continue to do the majority of infant care (Jones & Heermann, 1992), there have been changes in the masculine-feminine roles in society in which the roles of mother as nurturer and father as breadwinner are affected. Parents share child care and socialization activities. In addition, the role of father has become more loving and less focused on discipline; the role of mother has developed more parental authority, extending into disciplinary tasks.

However, these role transitions are not without stress for family members and can affect the homeostasis of the family for varying periods of time. The knowledge and skills needed to assume new roles is often lacking. In addition, some roles within the family give additional or less power for the role taker. When power is related to greater resources (money, possessions), the ability to influence others is increased. However, when a family member determines that a new role is necessary either developmentally or socially, the result often is confusion on the part of other family members. If a mother decides to go back to school or return to work, the roles of homemaker, such as nurturer, healer, chauffeur, and cook become available to other family members, and in fact must be assumed for family stability. Or when the wage earner, perhaps the father, becomes ill or unemployed, what happens to the role of resource provider?

As the nurse enters a system in which role inadequacy or dissonance is present, it is important to assess the normative system of what is expected to be done by whom. Assisting the family to evaluate roles enacted in the family system and to negotiate and communicate feelings regarding these roles is conducive to stress reduction. For example, a family conference that discusses the rights and responsibilities and feelings about each person's role can be helpful. If role inadequacy is diagnosed, role playing or contact with persons who successfully assume this role can provide support. If role dissatisfaction is the problem, negotiation with other members can often help with sharing or transferring this role. Often the family system falls into disarray when children or parents have not carried out the tasks assigned to maintain family functioning. At the family conference, discussion of the meaning and impact of the behavior can decrease stress. One successful method of task assignment is the development of a task assignment sheet for the week or month. But coupled with this, there needs to be an operative description of what each task entails. For example, one child may be assigned the task of taking out the refuse nightly. The operative description would include:

1. Take refuse to garbage can in garage.
2. Replace cover on can to decrease insects.
3. Reline the kitchen receptacle with plastic liner.
4. Close the cupboard door.

This process reduces argument and stress because it clarifies the totality of the assignment. A clear and effective role assignment coupled with good communication can result in more effective family stress management.

Communication Strategies

Although family communication has been discussed at length in Chapter 8, the following section includes specific approaches suggested to relieve family stress.

Communication in families is a powerful force that can foster or destroy relationships, egos, trust, growth, and joy. Satir (1982, p. 30) declared that "communication is the largest single factor determining which kinds of relationships he (the person) makes with others and what happens to him in the world about him." In the family, communication accomplishes bonding, conflict or harmony, decision making, task allocation, role enactment, and role delineation. And yet, clear communication is one of the most difficult processes to accomplish successfully.

Family members occasionally feel interpersonal stress but may feel unable to define clearly a specific cause. A strategy called "sculpting" provides a mechanism to give nonverbal expression to these feelings. The process consists of each family member taking his or her turn at:

1. Arrangement of all family members, including the sculptor, in "frozen-tag" positions that symbolize the attitudes and group relationships, as perceived by the sculptor.
2. Discussion of the meaning of the tableau with all family members. What does each position represent in the emotions of the relationship?
3. Reinforcement that each sculpting is neither right nor wrong but is simply the view of the family's emotional relationships by the sculptor.

Papp et al. (1973, p. 197) described the benefits of family sculpting as "literally worth a thousand words, revealing aspects of the family's inner life that have remained hidden. Vague impressions and confused feelings on the periphery of awareness are given form through physical spatial expression." Because of the nonverbal nature of the process, sculpting cuts through the defense mechanism of intellectualization, defensiveness, and blame, and each member is assisted to communicate in more depth (Mealey, 1977).

A number of family education programs have been developed to build family strengths, especially communication skills (Duncan & Brown, 1992; Renick et al., 1992). In most instances, awareness of communication patterns is so tied to self-esteem and acceptance that the impact of the patterns is outside the awareness of the person. Nursing intervention is directed toward helping family members recognize dysfunctional patterns of communication, practice empathic clarification of messages, and provide elicitation of feedback from each other. Supportive encouragement from the nurse is often needed by the family in initiation of change in communication; however, recognition of the value of successful change reinforces the change.

Time Management

Time, a relative concept, is viewed both subjectively and objectively. Culture influences the latter. Time is not a resource that can be increased, decreased, or borrowed, but management of time can structure family activities in a way that decreases the stress of time pressure. Poor time management brings about a constant sense of feeling overwhelmed and rushed. For many persons, the feeling of having too many tasks they must do and not enough time for the things they want to do is a major stressor. In a family situation there is often a frustrating attempt to cram a number of activities into an unrealistic amount of time. Members role model for each other and can be caught up in the trap of frantic, nonsatisfying, and nonproductive ways of being. When one member of the family feels overwhelmed and anxious, there is a ripple effect felt by all. Children often have difficulty managing time, and pressure for them may be manifested by emotional, physical, and behavioral disorder.

Behavior changes can be initiated that will assist individuals in the family to use time more effectively and thus enable the entire family to function in a more satisfying manner. Techniques to aid in this process have been described in the literature (Lakein, 1989; Davis et al., 1995; Young, 1985). Lakein (1989) is a pioneer in time management. Three concepts fundamental to his methods are (1) the goals statement, (2) the "to-do" list, and (3) the schedule. These skills can be taught to the family as a group.

Approaches summarized by Davis et al. (1988, p. 155) follow:

1. Set priorities that list most important goals.

2. Make time by realistic planning, and omit low-priority tasks.
3. Learn to make decisions based on identified goals.

Begin by keeping a log for time analysis, and note and record how time is used for a period of several days. Write down every activity and the length of time required. Compile this information. This analysis alone may give immediate feedback leading to decisions about better use of time.

The next step is to examine goals and values, the central concerns of each person's life. Make a list of general categories of importance such as personal, spiritual, work, community, and material (financial). Ask the following questions in every category, and write brief goals for each.

1. What would I like to accomplish in my life? (lifetime goals)
2. What would I like to accomplish in three years?
3. What would I like to accomplish in six months?
4. If I had only six months to live, what would my goals be?

This information helps one to sort out values and goals and to establish priorities. Use this list to create a blueprint for action. Choose the most important goals to begin to work on now. Add to this a list of specific tasks to accomplish, and break these down into realistic steps. Even young children in the family can be assisted to formulate their own "blueprint." When feeling pressured, one can say "I have all the time I need;" a self-statement such as this helps one to remain calm and complete the task at hand.

It is helpful to have a daily "to do" list and to decide into which order of importance the activities fall: A, B, or C. "C" items can wait or be eliminated. Focus on accomplishing the most important things each day. Plan and organize *every* day. It is helpful to set mimi-deadlines, do least favorite things first, learn to say "no," delegate, and decide how much time an activity is worth. Set a boundary or a time limit for a task and stick with it. Learn to break work into small "chunks" that can be finished and later recombined. Practice making decisions and move to overcome procrastination. Plan some time each day for quiet time for relaxation and renewal, and build some rewards for self into the action plan.

Time needs to be set aside for the family to meet as a group to share information and to formulate mutual plans for time management. A family calendar can be created, with input from each member, that provides information about activities, schedules, needs, and desires. Priorities can be set as each person participates and determines what is to be included on the calendar. Time for play and recreation is as important as time for study or work. A plan may be developed with modifications for each age group. According to Hymovich and Hagopian (1992), the nurse needs to consider culture time orientation, social class, sense of time, perception of time, and scheduling of time as unique within each family. The nurse can assist the family with this task. Implementation of a successful time management plan may open the door to better communication, greater intimacy, more time to spend with loved ones, or in solitude when it is the perceived need.

Intimacy

Intimacy refers to a moment in time or an ongoing relationship in which persons focus on each other. It is a process that can be close or at times distant. Lerner (1989) identifies the goal as to "have relationships with both men and women that do not operate at the expense of the self, and to have a self that does not operate at the expense of the other" (p. 4).

Issues around intimacy often arise in relation to the increased need for emotional support in times of stress. At these times, each member of the family feels the stress and needs support and yet has little to give to others. All ages have a need to relate and a desire to connect with others. Each individual can experience the other's uniqueness, and often, in a mutual exchange, feels perceived, loved, and wanted. There are many kinds of intimacy: intellectual, recreational, sexual, emotional, conflictual, and spiritual. People may experience more than one type, which offers an added means of nurturing a relationship. Conversely, each form has hazards to be navigated. Some of the barriers to intimacy are fears of conflict, rejection, hurt, control or "engulfment," as well as cultural gender differences and lack of a sense of identity. A person with a strong sense of identity and a feeling of self-worth is able to give in a relationship without fearing loss of self. Intimacy implies the ability of people to share feelings. It is correlated with equality of power and not with a hierarchy of leadership. As a result, each person is more comfortable expressing inadequacies and fears. According to Burns (1989, "Communication is more important to a healthy marriage than sex, money, or a microwave" (p. 41).

Intimacy is often a threat to individuals. The roots of this difficulty may be traced to a lack of bonding/attachment in a healthy relationship with a primary caregiver in early childhood. It is then that the infant develops a sense of self. If caregivers are unable to experience or to share emotional closeness, the child may never develop the confidence and ability to trust, to relate, or to reach out to others. Separation and individualization are problematic, and the individual may have lifelong problems with primary relationships.

Ghoulston (1988) describes men's fear of intimacy, and cautions caregivers to help parents stay firmly linked with each other and to view their marital relationship as primary. He provides specific steps to better understanding where men's need for independence and women's need for intimacy clash. Intimacy is reciprocal and is manifested as a rhythm. If the rhythm stops or gets stuck, problems can occur. Couples and families can be taught to be aware of the cycle, of the need to refocus on the "other," to renew and maintain the rhythm. They can set aside a special time in which to concentrate on each other, to touch, to listen, to look, and to be present in mutual sharing. A mother could take her teenager to lunch or plan a special one-to-one activity with a younger child. A father might take Mom out for a night or a weekend away from the children. A single parent could create special time for self-care activities. Interventions can be directed toward helping each member to have a stronger sense of self-worth, and appreciation of his/her uniqueness. Each person is valued. Family members can be encouraged to make clear statements of their beliefs, values, and preferences, to state differences and accept those of the "other." This is to take a position for self. Both strengths and vulnerabilities may be shared (Lerner, 1989). Health care providers need to encourage parents to stay linked firmly with each other and view their relationship as primary. For many men, fears of intimacy and needs for independence often clash with women's needs for intimacy. An approach to better understading and management of this behavioral pattern is described by Goulston (1988a, 1988b). The nurse can model messages and an approach that acknowledges the competencies of each member of the family. This affirms and empowers the family and helps restore their faith in their own abilities.

Family Centering/Meditation

Stressful experiences often bring about feelings of tension and anxiety that evoke a sense of being out of balance, an inability to feel a solid integration of mind and body, a lack of feeling connected ("grounded") in the environment. Thoughts are scattered, making it difficult to focus attention. This lack of harmony can be experienced within the family system as well as within individual members. In contrast, to feel centered is to experience one's psychologic center of gravity, to have a sense of balance and integration, which contributes to feelings of calmness and relaxation. Centering is the experience of turning within; of stilling the body and the mind; of focusing and maintaining attention on a part of the body, an object, or a thought. This process is that of passive concentration, "letting it happen" rather than making it happen, and needs to be experienced to be understood. It is possible to develop a feeling of family centeredness, or a feeling of unity within a family group (Hendricks, 1979). The feeling of being centered will be gained and lost and gained again. Hendricks (1979) says that being centered is a process of losing centeredness as well as getting it back again and that the sense of harmony will improve as the family uses good problem-solving strategies and opens up improved channels of communication.

A variety of participatory activities may be used to aid in the process of centering. A number of simple techniques suitable for use by the family group and for members of all ages are described by Hendricks, 1979 and Hendricks and Wills, 1975. Meditations and simple visualizations provided by Garth (1991) are designed to help children feel secure and cared for. A simple exercise that can be taught to the family group is to pause and focus awareness on an area of the body about 2 inches below the umbilicus. Each person concentrates on this area, sends thoughts and feelings there, and breathes deeply into this center. Another relaxation and centering exercise that enhances a feeling of closeness, love, and caring within the family unit is described in Table 14–5.

Centering is a useful technique to use with "everyday hassles" as well as in moments of high stress where it can aid in regaining self-control. It is often a necessary component of other relaxation exercises. The nurse can serve as a model as he or she facilitates a practice session for the family. The involvement and enthusiasm of the nurse, combined with verbal rewards for the family, can be potent reinforcers for new behaviors. It is helpful to give a handout with written instruction for general activities.

Spirituality and the Family

The spiritual dimension of individual existence integrates and transcends the other dimensions. This dimension permits one to individually experience and explore the meaning of existence in ways that exceed one's ordinary limits (Carson, 1989). "Spirituality may be viewed as the integrating or unifying factor, that which gives meaning and purpose" (Nafai-Jacobsen & Burkhart, 1989, p. 19). When spiritual needs are met satisfactorily, the person is free to function with a meaningful identity and purpose and to relate to reality with hope and confidence.

Religion as a correlate of family strength has received increased emphasis in the Social Sciences. Religion refers to an organized way of approaching worship, faith, and proscribed rituals that can serve as a vehicle for expression of spiritual needs. Religion has been a source of meaning and commitment for many. The National Council of Family Relations opened a section on Family Religion in 1984, and many recent writings include chapters on religion as a force in family health.

When family stress levels are high, a period of meditation may have a calming effect on family members. Family prayer has been advocated by numerous religious groups. Many believe the adage "The family that prays together, stays together." By sharing hopes, fears, and worries and by praying for each other, families may find strength and enhanced cohesiveness. Families may choose a special time to meditate or use regular prayer before meals to develop family unity.

Churches and groups within churches provide a source of social support, counseling for family and individual problems, and classes on parenting and marriage. Mutual support groups such as singles groups, older adult groups and couples groups are often formed in churches. Spirituality includes more than religious activities such as prayer, church activities, and church attendance.

TABLE 14–5. FAMILY CLOSENESS EXERCISE—THE FAMILY TREE

Instructions: "Quietly now, gather in a circle, and stand without touching each other. Let your arms hang loosely at your sides as you relax your body—just be loose and limp, like a rag doll. Close your eyes. Take a deep breath through your nose, and feel the air go down to your chest and on down to your stomach—find the place in your body that is *your* center. This is usually right below where your navel (belly button) is. Breathe again, and feel the air go to your center and all the way to your fingertips and toes. Feel them tingle. Now, let all the air out. Notice how your body feels more relaxed as your breath flows out. Feel your breath move gently in and out." (pause) "Now, imagine yourself standing firmly on the ground, like a tree. Send your roots down into the ground. Now, lift your arms up and stretch them high over your head like the branches of a tree. Like a tree, you can bend in the wind and not break. Imagine the wind blowing through your limbs but not breaking them. You are safe, and secure, and strong. Now, gently bring your arms down to your sides. Let your body relax and let go." (pause 5 seconds) "Now, join hands in the circle. Take another deep breath, and imagine a warm golden light filling your whole body. You feel its energy moving in and through you . . . and going to every person in this room. Feel this wonderful energy . . . and the energy coming to you from those in this circle. Send this energy to the person on your right." (pause 5 seconds) "You are now connected to every person in the circle. This feels good. Feel the love and the strength being shared now among the members of your family. Gently give a little squeeze to each of the hands you are holding, then let go. Slowly open your eyes, and move forward into the middle of the room for a special group hug."

Source: Haroldyne Richardson

Spirituality also includes such activities as communion with nature, artistic processes, journal writing, songs and chants, self-care of the body, loving relationships with others, reading, social gatherings, and service to others.

A holistic nursing approach to facilitating family stress management includes encouraging the family to use a variety of spiritual activities to adapt to life's stresses (Stiles, 1990). Consult Chapter 11 for more detail on family spirituality and approaches to assess religion in families.

Humor

Humor is an inexpensive, available, and powerful stress management technique. Often the family perspective of a situation is key to successful coping (Reeder, 1991). Being able to laugh at the incongruities of life interrupts the stress-worry cycle (Pasquali, 1991). Worry and stress are antithetical to humor. When a level of mirth is operating, research had shown increased levels of catecholamines in the body and endorphin release is stimulated; circulation is stimulated and ventilation increased. In the immune system, T. lymphocyte cells are stimulated, blood pressure and muscle tension decreases, and learning and memory are enhanced (Pasquali, 1991; Cohen, 1990).

How can a family most effectively bring these benefits to its members? The methods are numerous. Create regular times for enjoying humor, such as joke telling at dinner. (At the U.S. Naval Academy, midshipmen must bring a joke to meals to build family morale in the highly demanding atmosphere.) Cut out favorite cartoons and put them on desks or refrigerators or tuck them in lunch bags. Rent a funny videotape, and plan a family viewing. Write humorous notes to family members to convey serious messages. Give silly gifts. Dress up in ridiculous outfits for a family dinner. The objective is for the family to take themselves less seriously and take time to enjoy each other.

Negotiated Housekeeping Standards

Housekeeping standards and tasks not completed can frequently become a source of stress. Often, differences in standards between spouses are points of friction; one is usually extremely clean, the other less so. Cultural norms are also quickly absorbed from television as companies portray the efficient housewife painting in a slinky formal. The disparity between the ideal and the reality is shattering.

Family planning for equitable sharing of household duties is stress reducing. By weekly assignment of tasks to individuals, the responsibility is shared, as well as the stress. However, increased stress can result if the standard of carrying out the assignments becomes a source of argument. In order to avoid this trap, it is essential to have operational definitions of the assignments, as discussed earlier in this chapter.

Another element that needs to be addressed is an assessment of the total demands on the family at any specific time. If mother is working parttime or attending college, the children are in sports, and dad is president of a service club, it may well be that an agreement needs to be reached concerning vital housekeeping chores. Do the beds need to be made daily? Does dust on the table indicate a slovenly family? A conscious family effort to reduce the demands of perfect housekeeping and to share in the tasks that need to be done can reduce stress. In addition, more time can be provided for family and individual recreation and relaxation.

In the past, women attempted to play superwoman to keep dual roles as career woman and homemaker. Hochschild (1989) advocated that men and women negotiate a more equalitarian ideal, one that helps prevent the stress and frustration of role overload upon women. In today's world both men and women find themselves involved in conflicts between the time spent with work and family. Families are learning to manage in a variety of ways: by cutting back on involvement at work, with family commitments, or with personal needs. These need to be carefully balanced to maintain healthy families.

INDIVIDUAL APPROACHES TO MANAGE STRESS

Resources that discuss individual approaches to manage stress are numerous and readily available in lay and professional literature. If individual family members cope effectively, they will be more effective in coping with family stress. As discussed previously, as a system the family influences the health of its members and is influenced by the health of individual members. There is strong evidence that when high levels of family stress are present, a person's health can be adversly affected. Associated costs of this may result in severe illnesses and grater use of health care resources (Parkerson, et al, 1995). Family members who cope effectively also may be resources when the family experiences crisis. For example, a family member with skill in problem solving may help the family resolve a problem. A member with cognitive restructuring skills may encourage the family system to relabel a stressful event as a challenge rather than as a problem. The family nurse might use Figure 14–1 to encourage family members to evaluate the priorities in their lives in the professional, personal, spiritual, financial, and community realms. Clarification of values and their orientation or goals in life may be very useful in reducing stress.

GOALS: LIST IN EACH CATEGORY	PROFESSIONAL	PERSONAL	SPIRITUAL	FINANCIAL	COMMUNITY
Lifetime					
5 years					
6 months					
If you had only 6 months to live					

FIGURE 14–1. Put in Motion the Power within You. (Data from Lakein, A. (1973). *How to Get Control of Your Time in Life.* New York: Signet.)

CHAPTER HIGHLIGHTS

Each family system has its own repertoire of coping and stress management, which may or may not be adequate to restore family equilibrium during stress or crises.

Factors influencing family coping include culture, communication, resources, cohesion, flexibility, variety of coping strategies, social support, family perception, individual and family development, family and individual developmental stages, accumulation of stress, and the family coping efficacy.

The family coping processes may include changing the stressor event, reframing, control of reactions to the stressor, or ineffective coping.

The role of the family nurse in family stress management is the assessment of family coping; assisting family members to anticipate, recognize, prevent, reduce, manage, or adapt to stress; and facilitating the family to experience a unity from problem solving together.

A family stress management plan is developed in collaboration with family members.

Family stress management approaches may include problem solving or emotion-focused coping, cognitive restructuring, conflict resolution, role sharing, functional communication, time management, intimacy, family centering/meditation, spirituality, humor, negotiated housekeeping standards, and coping by individual family members.

HOLISTIC FAMILY STRESS MANAGEMENT

Family stress management includes all aspects of family health promotion that are included in Units II and III of this text. As with individual stress management, family stress management is a dynamic lifelong process. It is different at each developmental stage. Family nurses can assist families to understand their stress by teaching them the developmental tasks for the family system and individuals. In addition, because each family is unique, the strategies used to cope with stress will differ. Families should be encouraged to explore various coping approaches. In addition, they should be taught that stress is ever present. Whether stress influences the quality of family health is directly related to the piling-up of stressors, family strengths, resources, and coping.

REFERENCES

Benson, H., & Stuart, E.M. (1992). *The Wellness Book.* New York: Birch Lane Press.

Bigbee, J.L. (1992). Family stress, hardiness, and illness: A pilot study. *Family Relations: Journal of Applied Family and Child Studies,* 41(2), 212–217.

Borysenko, J. (1987). *Minding the Body, Mending the Mind.* Reading, MA: Addison-Wesley.

Boss, P. (1987). Family stress: Perception and context. In M. Sussman & S. Steinmetz (Eds.), *Handbook on Marriage and the Family* (pp. 695–723). New York: Plenum.

Bowman, M.L. (1990). Coping efforts and mental satisfaction: Measuring mental coping and its correlates. *Journal of Marriage and the Family,* 52, 463–464.

Burns, M. (1989). *Getting in Touch: Intimacy.* Greenville, MI: Empey Enterprises.

Burr, W.R. (1990). Beyond I—statements in family communication. *Family Relations,* 39(9), 266–273.

Carpenito, L.J. (1991). *Handbook of Nursing Diagnoses.* New York: J.B. Lippincott.

Carson, V.B. (1989). *Spiritual Dimensions of Nursing Practice.* Philadelphia: W.B. Saunders.

Cohen, M. (July, 1990). Caring for ourselves can be funny business. *Holistic Nursing Practice,* 4(4), 1–11.

Cohen, J., & Jaffe, D.T. (1990). Holistic health. In C.L. Edelmann and C.L. Mandle (Eds.), *Health Promotion through the Life Span* (2nd ed.). (pp. 245–246). St. Louis: Mosby.

Curran, D. (1983). *Traits of a Healthy Family.* Minneapolis, MN: Winston Press.

Curran, D. (1985). *Stress and the Healthy Family.* Minneapolis, MN: Winston Press.

Davis, M., Eschelman, E.R., & McKay, M. (1995). *The Relaxation and Stress Reduction Workbook* (3rd rev.). Oakland, Ca: New Harbinger Publications.

Dietz, C., & Omar, M. (1991). Couple adaptation in step families, and traditional nuclear families during pregnancy. *Nursing Practice,* 4(3), 6–10.

Doane, J.A., Hill, W.L., & Diamond, D. (1991). A developmental view of therapeutic bonding in the family: Treatment of the disconnected family. *Family Process,* 30(2), 155–214.

Duncan, S.F., & Brown, G. (1992). RENEW: A program for building remarried family strengths. *Families in Society: The Journal of Contemporary Human Services,* 73(3), 149–158.

Ellis, A., & Grieger, R. (1988). *Handbook of Rationale Emotive Therapy* (Vol. 11). New York: Springer.

Ennis, M.P. (1992). Tuning into your body, tuning up your mind. In E. Benson & E.M. Stuart, (Eds.), *The Wellness Book* (pp. 69–102). New York: Birch Lane Press.

Epstein, G. (1989). *Healing Visualizations.* New York: Bantam Books.

Fisher, R, & Ury, W. (1992). *Getting to Yes: Negotiating Agreement without Giving In.* Harrisburg, VA: R.R. Donnelly & Sons.

Friedman, M.M. (1992). *Family Nursing: Theory and Practice* (2nd ed.) Norwalk, CT: Appleton & Lange.

Goulston, M.S. (1988a). How to help males who fear intimate relationships with women. *Behavior Today,* 14(45), 8.

Ghoulston, M.S. (1988). Men's fear of intimacy linked to loneliness of their mothers. *Behavior Today,* 19(45), 4–6.

Gordon, M. (1982). *Manual of Nursing Diagnosis*: St. Louis: Mosby.

Halpern, S., & Savery. (1985). *Sound Music.* New York: Harper and Row.

Hendricks, G. (1979). *The Family Centering Book.* Englewood Cliffs, NJ: Prentice-Hall.

Hendricks, G., & Willis, R. (1975). *The Centering Book.* Englewood Cliffs, NJ: Prentice-Hall.

Hoblitzelle, O.J., & Benson, H. (1992). Eliciting the relaxation response. In H. Benson & E.M. Stuart (Eds.). *The Wellness Book.* New York: Birch Lane Press.

Hochschild, A. (1989). *The Second Shift.* New York: Avon Books.

Huston, J.L. (1991). Guest editorial humor and stress: The workplace connection. *The Journal of the American Medical Record Association.*

Hymovich, D.A., & Hagopian, G.A. (1992). *Chronic Illness in Children and Adults.* Philadephia: W.B. Saunders.

Jones, L.C., & Heermann. (1992). Parental division of infant care: Contextual influences and infant characteristics. *Nursing Research,* 41(4), 228–234.

Kanfer, F.H., & Goldstein, A.P. (Eds.). (1991). *Helping People Change* (4th ed.). Needham, MA: Allyn & Bacon.

Lakein, A. (1989). *How to Get Control of Your Time and Life.* New York: Signet.

La Vee, Y., McCubbin, H.I., & Patterson, J.M. (1985). The double ABCX model of family stress and adaption: An empirical test by analysis of structural equations with latent variables. *Journal of Marriage and the Family,* 46(4), 811–825.

Lazarus, R.S., & Folkman, S. (1989). *Stress Appraisal and Coping.* New York: Springer.

Lee, B.S. (1990). "Human relations" for nurse manager in the positive physiologic and psychologic benefits of laughter. *Nursing Management,* 21(5).

Lerner, H.G. (1989). *The Dance of Intimacy.* New York: Harper & Row.

Marsden, C., & Dracup, K. (1991). Different perspectives: The effects of heart disease on patients and spouses. *Critical Care Nursing,* 12(2), 285–292.

May, B.J. (1990). Principles of exercise for the elderly. In J.V. Basmafian & S.L. Wolf (Eds.), *Therapeutic Exercise* (5th ed.). (pp. 279–298). Baltimore: Williams & Wilkins.

McCubbin, M.A., & McCubbin, H.I. (1993). Families coping with illness: The resiliency model of family stress, adjustment and adaptation. In C.B. Danielson, B. Hamel-Bissell, & P. Winstead-Fry. (Eds.), *Families, Health and Illness.* (pp. 21–63). St. Louis: Mosby.

MCubbin, H.I., Cauble, A.E., & Patterson, J.M. (1982). *Family Stress, Coping, and Social Support.* Springfield: Thomas.

McCubbin, H.I., & Figley, C.R. (Eds.) (1983). *Stress and the Family: Coping with Normative Transitions* (Vol. 1). New York: Brunner/Mazel.

McCubbin, H.I., & Patterson, J.M. (1981. Broadening the scope of family: An emphasis on family coping and social support. In N. Stinner, J. DeFrain, K. King, P. Knaub, & G. Rowe (Eds.), *Family Strengths: Roots of Well-Being* (pp. 177–194). Lincoln: University of Nebraska Press.

McCubbin, H.I., Larsen, A., & Olson, D.H. (1985). *Family Inventories: Inventories Used in a National Survey of Families Across the Family Life Cycle* (rev. ed.) (pp. 120–136). St. Paul: University of Minnesota.

McCubbin, H.I., & Patterson, J.M. (1983). Family stress and adaptation to crisis: A double ABCX Model of family behavior. In D.O. Olson and B.C. Miller (Eds.), *Family Studies Review Year Book* (Vol. 1), Beverly Hills: Sage.

McCubbin H.I., & Thompson, A.I. (Eds.). (1987). *Family Assessment Inventories for Research and Practice.* Madison, WI: University of Wisconsin.

Mealey, A.R. (1977). Sculpting as a group technique for increasing awareness. *Perspectives in Psychiatric Care,* 3, 118–121.

Minuchin, S. (1974). *Families and Family Therapy.* Cambridge, MA: Harvard University Press.

Nafai-Jacobson, M.G., & Burkhardt, M.A. (1989). Spirituality: Cornerstone of holistic nursing practice. *Holistic Nursing Practice,* 3(3), 18–26.

Olson, D.H. (1989). Circumplex Model of Family Systems VIII: Family Assessment and Intervention. In D.H. Olson, C.S. Russell, & D.H. Spenkle (Eds.). *Circumplex Model: Systematic Assessment and Treatment of Families.* New York: Haworth Press.

Olson, D.H., McCubbin, H.I., Barnes, H.L., Larsen, A.S., Muxen, M.L., & Wilson, M.A. (1983). *Families: What Makes Them Work?* Beverly Hills: Sage.

Papp, P., Silverstein, O., & Carter, E. (1973). Family sculpting in preventive work with well families. *Family Process,* 2(12), 197–204.

Parkerson, G.R., Boardhead, W.E., & Tse, C.J. (1995). Perceived family distress as predictors of health-related outcomes. *Archives of Family Medicine,* 4, 253–260.

Pasquali, E.A. (1991). Humor: Preventive therapy for family caregivers. *Home Health Nurse,* 93, 13–17.

Pearlin, L.I., & Schooler, C. (1982). Family stress, coping and social support. In H.I. McCubbin, A.E., Cauble, & J.M. Patterson (Eds.), *The Structure of Coping.* Springfield: Thomas.

Pender, N.J. (1987). *Health Promotion in Nursing Practice* (2nd ed.). Norwalk, DT: Appleton & Lange.

Peterson, C.M., Seligman, M.E., & Vaillant, G.E. (1988). Pessimistic explanatory style is a risk factor for physical illness: A thirty-five year longitudinal study. *Journal of Personality and Social Psychology,* 55(1), 23–27.

Reeder, J.M. (May, 1991). Family perception: A key to intervention. *Clinical Issues in Critical Care Nursing,* 2(2), 188–194.

Renick, M.T., Blumberg, S.H., & Harkman, H.J. (1992). The prevention and relationship enhancement program (PREP): An empirically based prevention program for couples. *Family Relations,* 41(2), 141–147.

Rossman, M. (1990). *Healing Yourself.* New York: Simon & Shuster.

Satir, V. (1982). *Peoplemaking.* Palo Alto, CA: Science and Behavior Books.

Schnittger, M.H., & Bird, G.W. (1990). Coping among dual career men and women across the Family Life Cycle. *Family Relations,* 39(2), 199–205.

Stiles, M.K. (1990). The shining stranger: Nursey-family spiritual relationship. *Cancer Nursing,* 13 (4), 235–245.

Travis, J.W., & Ryan, R.S. (1988). *Wellness Workbook* (2nd ed.). Berkely, CA: Ten Speed Press.

Wynd, C.A. (1992). Relaxation imagery used for stress reduction in the prevention of smoking relapse. *Journal Advanced Nursing,* 17(3), 294–302.

Young, B.B. (1985). *Stress in Children.* New York: Arbor House.

ADDITIONAL READINGS

Dossey, B.M. (1988). Imagery: Awakening the inner healer. In B.M. Dossey, L. Keegan, C.E. Guzzetta, & L.G. Kolkmeier (Eds.), *Holistic Nursing: A Handbook for Practice.* Rockville, MD: Aspen.

Ellis, A. (1988). *How to Stubbornly Refuse to Make Yourself Miserable about Anything—Yes Anything!* New York: Carol Publishing Group.

Figley, C.R., & McCubbin, H.I. (Eds.). (1983). *Stress and the Family: Coping with Catastrophe* (Vol 2). New York: Brunner/Mazel.

Garth, M. (1991). *Starbright: Meditations for Children.* San Francisco: Harper.

Hill, L., & Smith, N. (1990). *Self-Care Nursing.* Norwalk, CT: Appleton & Lange.

McCubbin, H.I., & McCubbin, M.A. (1987). Family stress theory and assessment. The T-double ABCX model of family adjustment and adaptation. In H.I. McCubbin & A.I. Thompson (Eds.), *Family Assessment Inventories for Research and Practice* (pp. 3–34). Madison, WI: University of Wisconsin.

McCubbin, H.I., Patterson, J.M., & Wilson, L.R. (1985). Family inventory of life events and changes. In D.H. Olson (Ed.), *Family Inventories: Inventories Used in a National Survey of Families across the Family Crisis Life Cycle* (rev. ed.). (pp. 120–136). St. Paul: University of Minnesota.

Reiss, D., & Oliveri, M.E. (1983). Family paradigm and family coping: A proposal for linking the family's intrinsic adaptive capacities to its responses to stress. In D.H. Olson & B.C. Miller (Eds.), *Family Studies Review Yearbook* (Vol.1). (pp. 113–126). Beverly Hills: Sage.

Steiger, N.J., & Lipson, J.G. (1985), *Self-Care Nursing: Theory and Practice.* Bowie, MD: Brady.

SLEEP AND THE FAMILY

ELLA KICK

The beginning of health is sleep

Irish Proverb

OBJECTIVES

On completion of this chapter, the reader will be able to:

1. Identify stages of normal sleep
2. Explain normal sleep needs of family members at various developmental stages
3. Discuss selected sleep disorders
4. Develop a family sleep history
5. Explain the importance of circadian rhythm to sleep habits
6. Comprehend the role of the family health nurse as it relates to family sleep patterns

INTRODUCTION

Both the family and the family health nurse should be aware of the effects of sleep on family functioning. The family health nurse's knowledge of sleep and its effects on the family may be used during family assessment and in assisting the family to develop a healthful lifestyle.

The family is the learning arena for its members. They learn about developing relationships within the family as well as outside the family. Family members also learn acceptable and unacceptable behavior norms. They learn the values that are associated with their own life and the life of the family. Learning health behaviors also occurs in the family. A major health behavior that must be learned early in life is sleep. What infants and/or children learn about sleep and sleep rituals may stay with them for a lifetime. For this reason, it is necessary to establish healthful sleep habits early in life.

The space allotted for sleeping in the family house may be 50% or more of the entire space, depending on the size of the family. The allocation of sleeping space may be a source for much family discussion. Sleeping space usually dictates personal space or territory for individual family members.

Many theories exist related to the function of sleep. These theories include the energy conservation theory, which states that sleep is necessary for rest to reduce metabolic requirements of the body; the restorative theory, which states that sleep is a period of recovery when functional states that have been depleted in the wakeful hours can be restored; the learning theory, which states that there are beneficial effects of sleep on memory retention; the humoral theory, which states that there is a build up of a chemical toxin during the wakeful period which causes tiredness and sleep; and the restitution theory, which states that wear and tear of the body occurs during wakefulness and repair and tissue growth occur during sleep (Hodgson, 1991).

PHYSIOLOGY OF SLEEP

Rechtschaffen and Kales (1978) developed the sleep classification used today. They divided sleep into two categories: rapid eye movement (REM) and nonrapid eye movement (NREM). Their premise in developing the system was that wakefulness, REM sleep, and NREM sleep are different levels of consciousness. They used the electroencephalogram (EEG) to measure levels of consciousness.

NREM is called slow wave sleep and is divided into four stages: light sleep, transition sleep, and two stages of deep sleep. REM is called fast wave sleep and is not divided into stages. Physiologic changes occur during both NREM and REM sleep. During NREM sleep, the pulse rate, basal metabolism rate (BMR), temperature, respirations, blood pressure, cardiac output, heart rate variability, and muscle tone are decreased. There is a decrease in regional cerebral blood flow, even though there is a slight rise in pCO_2. This is different from the vasodilator effect of carbon monoxide during regular wakefulness. Growth hormone, promoter of protein synthesis and enhancer of amino acid transport into cells, is secreted from the anterior pituitary during NREM (Moorcroft, 1989).

REM sleep is divided into tonic and phasic periods. The phasic period includes short episodes of rapid eye movement and muscle twitching. Irregular breathing with short periods of hyopnea and apnea occurs. The heart rate is variable, and blood pressure may increase. It is thought that the excitation of the cardiac system during phasic REM may initiate heart attacks. The tonic period is very much the opposite of the phasic period. There is no movement, and a near paralysis of muscles occurs. Cerebral blood flow increases significantly, and vasoconstriction occurs in skeletal muscles. The brain temperature increases, which may indicate that there is increased brain metabolism during REM sleep.

During REM, thermoregulation does not occur; sweating and shivering are absent, and the temperature of the body moves toward the environmental temperature. Penile erection occurs in adults as well as in infants. Respirations are changed due to changes in the system. The diaphragm maintains activity while the intercostals and many upper airway muscles are hypotonic, and reaction to O_2 and CO_2 stimulation may be altered. It is thought breathing during REM is not controlled by chemoreceptors or metabolic needs but by REM-related processes (Rosenburg, 1991).

REM sleep is important for memory, learning, psychologic adaptation, and review and categorization of the day's activities so that information can be stored. Gastric secretions are increased. Dreams occur and problems may be solved during REM sleep. During periods of psychologic stress, there is a greater need for REM sleep (Peter et al., 1991).

Stage I of NREM is a period of very light sleep where persons may be easily aroused, may still be aware of the surroundings, but not be aware that they are asleep. They may feel very relaxed and dreamy but may experience some involuntary jerking which may arouse them. This stage lasts only a couple minutes, but physiologic altera-

tions are already beginning. Stage II sleep is a transition sleep; it is somewhat deeper than Stage I, but the subject remains easily aroused. This stage lasts five to ten minutes, only slightly longer than Stage I.

Stages III and IV, sometimes called delta sleep, are the stages of deep sleep. During this period, which lasts about 10 to 25 minutes, the body's energy is restored. During Stage III, temperature and pulse rate decrease and muscles relax. Body movements are likely absent, and arousal is very difficult during Stage IV (Peter et al, 1991).

Sleep occurs in cycles of the above described stages of NREM and REM sleep; however, each stage does not occur in each cycle. Most people experience four to five complete sleep cycles each night. Eighty percent of total sleep time is spent in NREM, and the remaining 20% is spent in REM sleep. The first period of REM sleep occurs 70 to 90 minutes after the onset of sleep. It lasts for only five minutes, and it is the least intense period of REM sleep during the night. Children frequently do not experience this first REM period.

The second cycle begins with State II NREM and has less delta sleep than the first cycle. The second REM period begins about three hours after falling asleep and lasts for ten minutes. After the second REM sleep period, 90-minute cycles containing only Stage II NREM and REM sleep occur until morning. During these cycles, REM becomes increasingly intense and longer. Although REM periods may last as long as 90 minutes, the mean length of time is 15 minutes.

Clinical Sleep Recordings

The electroencephalogram (EEG) is used to record brain activities during sleep. An EEG recording is made of tracings that are described in terms of amplitude and frequency. Amplitude describes the verticle height of the tracings, which denotes the amount of energy expended for each impulse and is measured in microvolts. Frequency is the means by which to measure the speed of impulses and is reported in Hertz (Hz) or cycles per second (cps).

EEG tracings during wakefulness are frequently used as a contrast to sleep tracings. During alert wakefulness, tracings are of low amplitude with a frequency of 13 to 35 Hz. When an awake person is relaxed, a frequency of 8 to 13 Hz is seen.

Stage I NREM sleep is made up of the waves with a frequency of 3 to 7 Hz and lasts from a half minute to seven minutes. Late in the stage, lower frequency and higher amplitude are seen. This stage makes up only 5% to 10% of total sleep.

Stage II is sometimes called "spindle" sleep because of the spindlelike tracings on the EEG. These spindles occur in bunches of 12 to 14 Hz lasting one half to two seconds. A K-complex, a high amplitude negative wave followed immediately by a slower positive wave, also occurs during this stage. The K-complex is usually related to auditory stimuli. This stage makes up 45% to 55% of total adult sleep time.

Stages III and IV sleep are frequently called "delta" sleep due to the slow delta waves of 1/2 to 2 Hz with an amplitude greater than 75 microvolts (peak to peak), which is considered to be high. The two stages are differentiated only by the percentage of slow waves. During Stage III sleep, slow waves appear in 20% to 50% of total adult sleep time. In Stage IV, slow waves appear in more than 50% of the tracings. In most adults, Stage IV occurs during the first third of the night, and most of the Stage III delta-wave sleep occurs later in the night.

REM sleep is made up of mixed-frequency, low-voltage waves, with some sawtooth waves. REM sleep periods become longer as the night progresses. REM sleep makes up about 20% of adult sleep.

SLEEP REQUIREMENTS

Infants and Children

Sleep classification in very young infants is difficult because the EEG is not useful in differentiating sleep stages. Variables observed when studying the sleep patterns of infants include facial and body movements, respiratory patterns, heart rate, and electro-oculogram (EOG). By age four or five months, the appearance of spindles on the EEG helps to distinguish Stages I and II NREM sleep.

Newborns sleep approximately 16 to 18 hours of every 24-hour period. The newborn spends 50% of sleep time in REM. In the first three weeks of life, sleep periods are distributed evenly over the 24-hour period. The length of each sleep cycle is shorter in infancy than in older children. REM periods recur every 50 to 60 minutes in infants.

Sleep for infants in the first six months of life progressively occurs more in the night than in the day. Stages of sleep also change from an almost even amount of NREM and REM sleep to a predominantly NREM sleep, with REM latency gradually getting longer. At the end of the first year, the infant has gone from sleeping 16 hours with two 8-hour periods of NREM and REM sleep to 12 hours of sleep. At one year, REM sleep time is four hours, or 25%. This percentage is maintained throughout most of life.

Newborns depend on an adequate amount of sleep to meet the needs of their rapid growth. Further, pituitary growth hormone is excreted during periods of deep sleep. While asleep, infants make many noises, such as sighing, gurgling, and coughing. Each infant develops a unique sleep pattern that changes as the nervous system develops.

Two- to three-month-old infants are beginning to sleep through the night. They will take from two to four naps during the day. As the infant continues to grow and develop, nighttime sleeping becomes well established, and daytime naps begin to get shorter and fewer. From 6 to 12 months, the infant sleeps 10 to 12 hours nightly, with two to three daytime naps. From 12 to 18 months, the infant sleeps 8 to 12 hours nightly and takes one to two daytime naps. Periods of wakefulness may occur during periods of teething or when the infant experiences dreams (Balsmeyer, 1990).

Toddlers have great energy needs for growing, playing, and learning. Their needs for rest and sleep are equally great. Toddlers will sleep 8 to 12 hours nightly and have one daytime nap. The daytime nap usually lasts 30 to 60 minutes. When the child does not want to nap in the daytime, a rest period should be provided. A quiet time when listening to music, lying quietly with a favorite stuffed animal, or listening to a book being read may serve as a quality rest time. When rest or sleep is not accomplished in the daytime, the child may become fatigued and irritable and may have restless nighttime sleep.

Preschool children usually have an established bedtime ritual that was begun in their toddler period. This ritual may include bedtime prayers, reading or storytelling by the parent, or putting a favorite stuffed animal to bed. An important aspect of the bedtime ritual is the child's own involvement in the ritual. It should not include sucking on a bottle or being rocked to sleep. When these activities are included in the ritual, the infant is unable to resume sleep independently if he or she should waken during the night. The child should be placed in the bed and be expected to stay there until morning. During periods of illness, of course, the child may need attention during the night.

Preschoolers more than toddlers are apt to prolong the bedtime ritual. They may continue to call the parents to perform favors, such as putting the light on, getting a drink of water, or getting another toy to place in bed (Sheldon et al., 1992). Parents should remember that they are helping the child to develop habits, and when the parents relent to such demands of the child, a major family disruption occurs.

Age is a major factor in sleep needs. The 4-year-old requires 10 to 12 hours, and the 10-year-old requires 9 to 10 hours. During adolescence, the need drops to about 7.5 hours, and the decline thereafter is very gradual, to about 6.5 hours in the elderly.

Stage IV NREM sleep in the infant and young child slowly declines from 30% to 20% to 15% during adolescence. Infants and children have larger amounts of slow-wave (NREM) sleep in the first sleep cycle than adults. It is very difficult to awaken a child in the first third of the night. Children rarely awaken during the night unless there is an illness.

Optimum sleep cycles are attained around age 10 to 12. Most children at that age sleep soundly; for 9 to 10 hours, awaken, and are very alert all day. They usually get sleepy spontaneously, awaken spontaneously, and may not use a clock (Sheldon et al., 1992).

Adolescents

Although sleep needs and patterns vary, most adolescents sleep seven to eight hours each night. A common occurrence in adolescents is to want to go to bed later and sleep later in the morning. They also have periods of drowsiness and sleepiness in the daytime. This is thought to be due to the many physiologic changes taking place. Energy needed for growth as well as for the many activities in which adolescents are involved may have an effect on their sleep needs.

The adolescent body and mind are in such a period of change that much energy is expended on maturational needs. Therefore, it would seem that more sleep would be necessary to restore these energies. Although it is thought that the adolescent needs an average of 7.5 to 8 hours of sleep, many do not actually spend this much time in sleep. They spend so much time exploring themselves and the world around them that they are unaware of their sleep needs. Their usual pattern is to go to bed late and sleep late. During the school term, it is not always easy to sleep late because of the school schedule. Their desire to sleep late and their usual sleepy feelings in the morning often cause stress in the family.

The parent who takes on the responsibility of seeing that the adolescent gets to school on time spends many mornings being frustrated. This frustration carries over into other interactions with the adolescent as well as with other family members.

Adolescents usually fall asleep soon after going to bed. They rarely suffer sleep latency. They spend about 50% of their sleep in NREM Stages III and IV and 25% in REM sleep. When they spend seven to eight hours in sleep, they are usually very well rested and require no daytime naps. Sleep is very necessary to the adolescent if he or she is to do well in school.

Adults

Stage I NREM sleep, the transition between waking and sleeping, gradually increases with age. Stage II NREM sleep also increases with age. Delta sleep, Stages III and IV NREM, gradually decreases from childhood to old age.

Early in the night, adults and elderly have less slow-wave sleep than young people. Stage IV NREM sleep is reduced to 6% or less in middle age and is almost nonexistent in persons over 60 years of age. Although REM sleep makes up 20% to 25% of adult sleep, the length of episodes of REM sleep decreases.

In the middle years, from 35 to 65 years of age, sleep needs are the same as those of younger adults: six to eight hours. However, some adults nearing the end of the period retire from their regular working schedule, and their sleep needs and habits change. They may expend less physical energy and thus have decreased sleep time at night. These people, as well as those who maintain a full work schedule, may find that they need a daytime nap. Working people often take a later afternoon or early evening nap for 30 to 60 minutes. That short nap gives them the energy necessary to function well in the evening.

Time in bed and total sleep time are equal until age 35. Thereafter a gradual increase in time in bed occurs, and sleep time decreases to present an unequal ratio. Elderly people have more and longer periods of wakefulness and body shifting during the night. They also experience more periods of daytime drowsiness. In sum, sleep efficiency (the ratio of total sleeping time to time in bed) and the restorative quality of sleep decline with age.

Older persons, over 65 years of age, sleep about five to six hours during the night. They sleep very lightly and are easily aroused. Falling asleep is sometimes problematic to older persons. There is a sleep onset latency period of about 10 minutes until age 60; after that time the latency period lengthens to about 23 minutes for those age 70 to 79 and to 26 minutes later. Many periods of wakefulness occur in the aged sleeper. Naps in the daytime increase with age.

Sleep disturbances increase with age, and the kind of disturbance changes also. Young adults complain of difficulties falling asleep, but they remain asleep after onset. It takes longer, but older people have little difficulty falling asleep; however, they have difficulty maintaining sleep. Sleep apnea and nocturnal myoclonus increase sharply after middle age (Biddle, 1990).

COMMON SLEEP DISTURBANCES

Interruption of Biologic Rhythms

Biologic rhythms may be classified as circadian, occurring in approximately 24-hour cycles; ultradian, occurring in cycles less than 24 hours; and infradian, occurring in cycles more than 24 hours. The human body, for the most part, operates on a circadian rhythm. Each system and cell has its own rhythm, and each rhythm is synchronized with other internal rhythms as well as with the external environment. The cyclical harmony that occurs assures that all hormones, neurotransmitters, and so on occur at the right time for maximal use and efficiency.

When the human eats and sleeps on a regular schedule, it contributes to maintaining the body's internal rhythm. When the body is out of rhythm or desynchronized, such as in jet-lag, the person may experience dysphoria, inability to sleep, and other physical complaints. When a person shortens or lengthens the day by travel, the usual activities of living are altered, but those internal functions over which the traveler has no control continue to perform on the old schedule.

Persons who must change hours of work interrupt their circadian rhythm, which, in turn, affects their sleep abilities. "Evening" people, those with infradian cycles, usually adapt to shift rotation better than the ultradian or circadian types. Most people can adapt well to a shift of two hours in either direction, but most shift work requires a shift of eight hours. Most people find it easier to stay up later and sleep later than to go to bed earlier and get up earlier. This is noticed in travelers. It is easier to travel from east to west than from west to east (Tepas & Carvalhais, 1990).

Persons working in jobs where they must rotate day, evening, and night shifts are continually disrupting their circadian rhythm. Workers get the least sleep while working night shift and the most sleep while working the evening shift. Many working the night shift get their sleep in periods of two to four hours through the day. These naps do not parallel the usual NREM/REM sleep cycle, which is customary for a day worker. Not only does this change in circadian rhythm change the sleep of the worker but it also changes the rhythm of the physiologic functions of the body. When the shift rotation progresses from nights to evenings to days, the worker usually gets more sleep than when the progression is in the other direction.

Sleep Deprivation

Everyone will lose sleep from time to time and recover in a few days. However, people who suffer prolonged sleep deprivation experience symptoms of disorientation, perceptual disturbances, irritability, fatigue, attention difficulties, feelings of persecution, and transient neurologic symptoms such as hand tremors, horizontal nystagmus, and weakness of neck flexion. When permitted to sleep after a period of deprivation, the subject will sleep for a longer time than usual and have increased Stage IV NREM and REM sleep.

Persons deprived of REM sleep only, due to drugs or to being aroused during this period, may be continually fatigued; lack powers of concentration; and have perceptual difficulties, confusion, paranoia, hallucinations, anxiety, and short-term memory impairment. When these persons return to regular sleep, they experience increased amounts of REM sleep, which is termed "REM sleep rebound." Persons with coronary artery disease have more difficulty with "REM sleep rebound" than others. They experience more arrhythmias because REM sleep places heavy demands on the heart. Cardiac patients have more pain and heart failure from 4:00 AM to 6:00 AM,

when the majority of REM sleep is experienced (Reilly, 1990).

PHYSIOLOGIC SLEEP DISORDERS

Classification System

The study of sleep disorders is very recent. The Association of Sleep Disorders Clinics (ASDC) was organized in October, 1975 to standardize patient evaluation and to classify sleep disorders. The classification system that was developed contains four categories of sleep disorders: (1) DIMS—disorders of initiating and maintaining sleep (insomnia), (2) DOES—disorders of excessive somnolence (excessive daytime sleepiness), (3) disorders of sleep-wake schedules, and (4) parasomnias—dysfunctions associated with sleep, sleep stages, or partial arousals.

Subjects classified as DIMS need physiologic as well as psychological assessment. Insomnia may be transient and situational, lasting only three weeks, or it may be chronic. Insomnia is associated with several psychological disorders, such as depression, phobias, and schizophrenia. DIMS may also be due to prolonged use of drugs or alcohol or the withdrawal from these substances (Leibenluft & Wehr, 1992).

Insomnia

Insomnia is not a single disorder, but is made up of several disorders, including psychophysiologic disturbances, psychiatric disorders, drug and alcohol dependency, sleep-related respiratory problems, sleep-related myoclonus, and medical or environmental problems, as well as child-onset DIMS. It is important that a differential diagnosis be made so that proper treatment may be used.

Insomnia may be transient and situational, lasting three weeks or less, or it may be chronic. The transient or situational type may be due to acute stress, a life crisis, or loss. Although this type is situational, it is often recurrent when the precipitating situation is again experienced.

Psychiatric problems that are frequently related to insomnia include personality disorder, affective disorders, and functional psychoses. Chronic use of drugs or alcohol or the withdrawal from these chemicals may cause insomnia.

Sleep Apnea

Persons who have sleep apnea usually snore or gasp, complain of being sleepy in the daytime, and experience sleep attacks. The snoring is caused by vibrations of the soft palate. As air is brought in through the mouth and passes through a passageway that is narrowed by relaxed upper airway muscles, a noise called snoring is generated. In addition to snoring, other symptoms include choking sensations during the night, profuse body movements, morning headaches, and enuresis. Although sleep apnea may occur in young people, it occurs most frequently in men over age 50 and in postmenopausal women (Westbrook, 1990).

Sleep apnea is divided into three categories and may be defined as a period of apnea that lasts at least ten seconds and occurs 30 or more times each night. Central apnea is the cessation of airflow and lack of respiratory effort. It occurs in any age, weight, or sex, and the subject may also have daytime breathing problems. It is frequently associated with a damaged respiratory center in the brain. Obstructive apnea is also a cessation of airflow, but respiratory effort is present. It is the most common of the sleep apneas and occurs more frequently in men than in women. It is more prevalent in obese persons, although it may occur in thin persons. Mixed apnea is merely a combination of the above two types of apnea and is the least common type.

Sleep apnea may be treated with weight reduction, a soft collar around the neck to prevent flexion, or by surgery if tonsillar or other tissue is causing the obstruction. Pharmacologic treatment of this disorder has not been completely successful. Persons with sleep apnea should be instructed not to take sedatives, hypnotics, or alcohol because these drugs are central nervous system (CNS) depressants and may cause an increased number and length of apneic episodes. Use of oxygen for sleep apnea is not recommended because it depresses respirations and lengthens the apneic episode. Permanent tracheostomy is performed as a last resort. Sleep apnea must be differentiated from narcolepsy, since both problems include excessive daytime sleepiness and sleep attacks (Westbrook, 1990).

Narcolepsy

Narcolepsy is a sleep disorder with an onset at age 15 to 30. It is made up of four identifying characteristics: sleep attacks, cataplexy, sleep paralysis, and hypnagogic hallucinations. Any of these characteristics may occur alone or in combination with any of the others.

Sleep attacks occur throughout the day with periods of uncontrollable sleepiness and periods of sleep attacks that last from 30 seconds to 15 minutes. These attacks are uncontrollable and may occur while an individual is driving a car, eating, or participating in athletics. The person usually sleeps normally at night. The amount of nighttime sleep has no influence on the number of sleep attacks or periods of drowsiness the subject may experience in the daytime. This problem is usually treated with drugs such as amphetamines.

Cataplexy is a sudden weakness and loss of muscle tone without a loss of consciousness. The loss of muscle tone may involve the entire body or just a part of the body, and it lasts for only a few seconds. These attacks are usually precipitated by a sudden emotional experience such as joy, sorrow, laughter, or anger. A sudden intense movement or the use of amphetamines for the treatment of sleep attacks may also precipitate an attack. Cataplexy is thought to be caused by an abnormal occurrence of REM in the wakeful state and is usually treated with imipramine.

Sleep paralysis is also thought to be due to a REM aberration. It occurs when a person is either falling asleep or waking up. It is manifested in sudden muscular paralysis where the individual is unable to move any muscle; the muscles of respiration are unaffected however. The paralysis lasts a few minutes and ends spontaneously or by being touched or spoken to by someone. During the attack, muscles are flaccid and areflexia.

Hypnagogic hallucinations occur while the person is falling asleep but is still conscious. The hallucinations last 1 to 15 minutes and are very vivid and bizarre. It is thought that the dream component of REM sleep is occurring during wakefulness (Williams, 1988).

Sleep-Related Myoclonus

Persons who have nocturnal myoclonus are often unaware of its existence. They usually complain of not sleeping well and of being sleepy in the daytime. This complaint is due to the three or more episodes of myoclonus each night. The episode is made up of abrupt contractions of leg muscles causing a leg jerk, extension of the big toe, and partial flexion of the ankle, knee, or hip and may last from a few minutes to an hour or more. These contractions may occur in one leg at a time or both legs. They occur in a definite pattern where there are several leg jerks in each pattern with a period of 20 to 40 seconds between each jerk.

Another sleep disorder involving the legs is "restless leg syndrome"; it often occurs in conjunction with nocturnal myoclonus. This problem presents as an uncomfortable dysesthesia that interferes with sleep. The etiology is unknown, but at least a third of persons who have the problem report that it is familial. Like nocturnal myoclonus, it becomes more severe with aging.

Parasomnias

Parasomnias are a group of disorders experienced by people who do not complain of sleep or wakefulness processes. The most commonly known parasomnias are sleep walking, sleep talking, nightmares, night terrors, enuresis, and bruxism. This category also includes conditions brought on by sleep onset, such as some cardiovascular symptoms, enuresis, asthma, epilepsy, and gastroesophageal reflux.

Sleepwalking and night terrors, disorders of arousal, are more prevalent in children than adults. They usually begin in late childhood or early adolescence and cease in late adolescence. There is usually a family history of these disorders, which have the same pathophysiologic origin. Children with these disorders frequently experience them following a febrile episode. Adults who have these disorders frequently experience them during periods of extreme stress. Sleepwalking is a mild disorder that includes mild confusion and minor physiologic changes. Night terrors is a much more severe experience and may include intense terror, confusion, and profound physiologic changes.

Sleepwalking and night terrors occur early in the night during Stages III and IV NREM sleep. Subjects have low-level awareness, low-level motor skill, and low-level ability to react. When they awaken, they are amnesic of the event. Night terrors are much more exaggerated than sleepwalking. The subject experiences excessive autonomic discharge, intense panic, extreme vocalization and motility, and very little or no recall on awakening.

Sleepwalking and night terrors are more serious in adults than children because during the episode an adult may try to drive a car or perform other functions that may be dangerous. Parents of children who have these disorders are warned to take necessary safety precautions to prevent injury to the child and to give the child reassurance when episodes occur. Adults who have these disorders may be treated with diazepam 5 to 20 mg at bedtime, since this drug suppresses Stage III and IV NREM sleep. However, it is recommended that a psychiatric evaluation and relevant treatment be done on adults with these problems, since there is frequently an underlying psychiatric disorder (Daws, 1989).

Nightmares are different from night terrors. Nightmares are episodes of intense anxiety and fear associated with a vivid, emotionally charged dream. Nightmares have less anxiety, vocalization, and motility, and the subject has vivid recall. Nightmares occur during REM sleep and night terrors occur during Stages III and IV NREM sleep. Nightmares usually occur between ages four and six. Nightmares may be associated with febrile episodes. However, because febrile episodes have a tendency to suppress REM sleep, the nightmares usually occur at the end of the febrile episode when there is "rebound REM" or increased REM due to the loss during the febrile state.

When the onset of nightmares occurs and persists after adolescence, a psychiatric evaluation is recommended. Data from Minnesota Multiphasic Personality Inventory tests revealed that adults with nightmares have specific personality patterns, including alienation, estrangement, distrustfulness, oversensitivity, and overreaction (Moorcroft, 1989).

Drugs that suppress REM sleep may cause nightmares since subjects experience "REM rebound" when these drugs are discontinued. The "REM rebound" causes an increase in the intensity of dreaming and the possibility of nightmares. Persons who experience nightmares usually have a higher incidence of other sleep disorders, especially insomnia.

Excessive Daytime Sleepiness

Several conditions with presenting complaints of excessive daytime sleepiness have been discussed. These conditions cannot be classified exclusively into one of the four classifications of sleep disorders. A differential diagnosis is necessary. For this reason, a detailed sleep history is imperative.

Excessive daytime sleepiness may be related to a transient psychophysiologic problem due to a sudden life change, such as entering a nursing home. Some conditions that may be related to transient excessive sleeping may include reactive depression, acute stress, and other factors that may disrupt the normal sleep-wake pattern of the subject. The problem may manifest itself by spending long periods in bed, getting up late, taking several naps in the daytime, or going to bed excessively early. If the condition lasts more than three weeks, a psychiatric evaluation is needed. Bipolar depressed persons frequently have this disorder. These persons usually have reduced Stages III and IV NREM sleep and short REM sleep latency.

Other causes of excessive daytime sleeping include long-term use or withdrawal from CNS stimulants and long-term use of depressants. Such pathology as hypothyroidism, hypoglycemia, and selected neurologic disorder may also cause excessive daytime sleeping. Some women have recurrent periods of hypersomnolence associated with the menstrual cycle (Reilly, 1990).

FAMILY DEVELOPMENT AND SLEEP HABITS

The New Family

The newly married couple faces many adjustments. To make this period of their life enjoyable and meaningful, adequate sleep must be attained. Because each of the partners in marriage comes from a different family background, each may have different sleep habits. It is necessary to bring these individual sleep habits to the marriage with the thought that a melding may occur in such a way that each partner will have to make as few adjustments as possible.

Not only will the new couple make changes in their sleep habits, but they will also make changes in their sleep environment. It is possible that each

---

person had slept alone in a single bed before marriage, and now they have chosen to sleep together. This brings up questions such as: What size should the bed be? Who will sleep on the right or left side of the bed? Will the bed coverings be light or heavy? Will the temperature of the room be warm or cold? Will the window be left open or closed? Will the air conditioner be used during sleep? Will the mattress be firm, or will a water bed be used?

Having made the necessary environmental decisions and adjustments, getting accustomed to sleeping with another person may be problematic. Some persons move about in bed with much gusto, and others may move without causing disturbance. Some snore or grit teeth. Some insist on having all the covers, and others may want no covers at all. It may take a few weeks of adjusting to another person in the bed. During this time, the subjects may experience increased periods of wakefulness during the night, which will precipitate increased periods of drowsiness in the daytime. These problems may be overcome by talking about them and making decisions together to solve the problems.

Decisions about wearing apparel also need to be made. What will be worn to bed? Because sexual interactions enjoyed by couples often occur in bed, sleeping apparel and bed linen may be an issue to be discussed. The time for sexual activity may have to be adjusted. For some it acts as a sedative, but for others it causes wakefulness. Self-comfort, needs, and desires of one's partner must be considered.

The couple who marries late in life seems to have more difficulty with adjustment than the young couple. Older people naturally have more wakeful periods in bed and much more body movement during the night. Older couples frequently opt for twin beds because adjusting to sleeping with another person is too difficult. On the other hand, some older couples are willing to put up with some disturbances in the night in order to have the benefits of having someone near.

The Emerging Family

During pregnancy, sleep habits change due to the physiologic changes occurring in the body. Early in pregnancy the woman feels tired and sleepy in the daytime regardless of the amount of sleep she gets during the night. If possible, naps of 30 to 60 minutes should be taken to relieve the drowsiness and to provide renewed energy.

During pregnancy, women sometimes experience heartburn, backaches, or other discomforts that make sleeping difficult. What is a comfortable sleeping position for one person may not be comfortable for another. The body should be maintained in alignment, and body parts should not rest on each other and interfere with circulation. Lying on the side with knees flexed, with a pillow placed between the legs to prevent the knees from resting on each other and a small pillow under the abdomen is a position many pregnant women find comfortable.

In the last trimester of pregnancy when the weight of the abdomen is much greater, the expectant mother experiences increased wakefulness. She may have to adjust to sleeping in different positions, and each time she moves her body during the night it is an effort. She may or may not be aware of awakenings during the night. However, it is periods of wakefulness along with carrying the added weight that make the pregnant woman more tired than usual. Daytime naps often refresh her and increase the quality of nighttime sleep.

New Members in the Family

Infants

A new baby in the house always causes environmental changes and adjustments. A major decision is the location where the infant will sleep. The infant usually takes a place in the parents' bedroom for the first couple of months until a pattern of sleeping through the night is established. Thereafter, the infant may have his or her own room. In some families where there are many children and few bedrooms, the infant may sleep in the parents' room until he or she has established a pattern of sleeping at least 12 hours a night. The baby may then be placed in the room of a sibling. Whether the baby sleeps in a bassinet or in a crib in the first few weeks, the mattress should be firm. Early in life, infants sleep on the abdomen or on either side until they are old enough to move their bodies into a different position. They are not placed on their backs for sleeping because of possible regurgitation in that position.

The crib should be checked for safety. Unleaded paint should be used, and the spaces between the rungs should be narrow enough that the infant's head could not be lodged between them. One soft cuddly stuffed toy could be left in the bed. Too many toys in the bed may eventually lead the child to believe that the bed is a play area. The bed should always be viewed and treated as a place where sleep occurs. This view helps children to develop good bedtime behaviors.

The birth of a baby causes a shift in routine. The mother's sleep-wake cycle is upset during the first two months of the infant's life. The mother should take an afternoon nap while the baby sleeps. Too frequently, mothers think they should get their housework done while the baby sleeps. Mothers who breastfeed are unable to get a reprieve from the nighttime feeding unless they pump their breasts and allow the father to feed the baby during the night on occasion. It is especially important for these mothers to get a daytime nap.

If other children are in the family, they should be encouraged to nap or at least rest in the afternoon while the baby sleeps. This will contribute to the mother's time for sleep or rest. While resting, the mother should put her feet up to ensure quality circulation. It is also important for new mothers who report back to work to get an afternoon or evening nap, especially if they must get up during the night with the newborn. Family members would have to plan time to assure that the mother could have at least 30 to 60 minutes to renew her energy.

By the time the infants are two to three months old, they should be sleeping through the night. The parents should begin to lengthen the time between the nighttime feedings, beginning as early as four weeks of age. Even if the time is lengthened only 10 or 15 minutes each night, by the time the baby is two or three months old, it should be sleeping a period of at least six to seven hours during the night. Removing the night feedings helps to establish the baby's circadian rhythm, so that eating occurs in the daytime and sleeping occurs during the night.

When the infant is two to three months of age, the parents may decide to move him or her from their bedroom. If parents fear they will not hear the infant, they may purchase a communication device that will relay the infant's sounds to their bedroom.

Adopted Children

When a family decides to adopt a child or children, many inherent adjustments must be made. Because sleep is such a necessary function for quality living, adequate sleeping arrangements must be made even before the new member of the family arrives. If the new member is an infant, the sleeping arrangements should be similar to those made for an infant who is not an adoptive member of the family. However, if the new member is beyond infancy and there are other children in the family, the adjustments may be more difficult.

Because every member of the family is new to the adoptive child, the child may have difficulty expressing his or her feelings. It is especially important to spend time with the child at bedtime. He or she is in a strange place and has many adjustments to make. The child may experience vivid dreams, enuresis, or even nightmares in the beginning. Continued reassurance and love should be provided during this sometimes stressful period. If the adjustment lasts more than a couple of weeks, limits may have to be set at bedtime so that the child does not develop poor sleep habits. New parents often are unsure of themselves, and consequently they permit the child to dictate evening routines in the family. After the parents are assured the child is safe and they have provided a warm good-night ritual, they should allow the child to put himself or herself to sleep.

Older Adults

People are living longer. The average age is well into the eighth decade. As people age they experience many losses including the loss of spouse and functional ability to care for themselves in their own home. This frequently results in the decision to live with one of the children.

Children who take their parents to live with them are usually in midlife and have children of their own who also need them. This midlife generation is frequently called "the sandwich generation" because they are caught in the middle of caring for others' needs and their own needs.

When the parent or parents are brought to live with the family, many adjustments must be made in the environment. One of the children may have to give up his or her room. Things may have to be put in storage, or the rec room or family room may be changed into a bedroom. One of the children may have to share his or her room with the grandparent. This latter change is the most difficult since older people have such different sleeping patterns from young people.

Older people usually like a very warm bed and sometimes insist on a higher room temperature than is customary in the family. This may be worked out by providing more blankets rather than adding more heat to the room. Older people usually go to bed earlier than young people. Therefore, their sleeping room should be protected from loud noises. A major complaint of old people who live in a family with teenagers is the teenager's loud music. Older people usually get up much earlier in the morning than young people, and they have more frequent awakenings during the night. Therefore, lights should be left on in the bathroom and hallways so that the older parent will be safe when getting up.

Older people sometimes get up during the night because they can't sleep. They should be permitted to have a place outside the bedroom to do quiet monotonous work. Or, they should be given a purposeful activity such as baking biscuits for breakfast. On the other hand, they will need to take a daytime nap when everyone else in the house may be up and involved in activities around the house.

Blended Families

When two families merge to become one, there are always adjustments that must be made. Planning a sleeping arrangement that will be satisfactory is a major objective of the newly formed family. This may be difficult if the children have been accustomed to sleeping in a bed and room alone and now must share a bed and/or room. It is always best to give a child a bed of his or her own if at all possible. This is especially true if a child has enuresis. For many children, the bedroom is not only the place where sleep occurs, but it is also where their treasures are kept. It is a place where privacy may be had when the need arises. Therefore, compatibility is a must when two children from different families of origin are made to share a bedroom.

When the blended family is formed, it may be necessary to experiment with different sleeping arrangements until a satisfactory plan is accomplished. When the children are permitted to keep their bed from their previous sleeping arrangement, fewer problems are encountered. When this is not possible, the child should at least be part of the decision-making process that will dictate sleeping arrangements. It is not uncommon for sleeping problems to occur for several weeks to a couple of months following the blending of families. Parents should give children assurance and spend more time with them during the period of adjustment.

COMMON DISRUPTIONS TO THE FAMILY'S SLEEP HABITS

Work Schedules

Parents and older children who work frequently have different work schedules. Some members of the family may even work swing shift and must change their sleeping pattern from one week to the next. This kind of schedule can, of course, be disruptive to family routine and sleeping habits.

Efforts must be made to plan family activities so that the work and sleep schedules of everyone will be respected. Because this is not always possible, decisions regarding various family activities must be made in such a way that all members have input. Certain chores that are usually done by specific family members may have to be done by others because work schedules prevent usual routines. Above all, each family member must get the required sleep needed to function. When this does not occur, anxiety, stress, and other behaviors are experienced, which put a strain on the entire family.

Illness

An ill family member may be able to care for his or her own needs during the night without causing disruption to the family. On the other hand, some illnesses, such as food poisoning, may attack most or all family members at the same time. Times like this can be very disruptive to the sleep of all members.

Frequently, the family is aware that fluid and nutritional needs must be met during periods of illness, but they often are not aware of sleep needs. The person or persons who are ill may

spend much time just "lying around" and find it difficult to fall asleep at bedtime. One way to handle the problem is to get some form of appropriate exercise, both mental and physical, during the day. If the illness is such that the person may go outside, another family member should accompany him or her on an outing. Frequently, a change in environment and fresh air influences the ability to sleep. It is important for the family to enhance the ill person's ability to sleep at night because one person's insomnia could keep the entire family up.

Another sleep problem that often occurs in families is sleep deprivation of the caregiver. The caregiver, like the new mother, thinks certain chores must be done while the ill person is sleeping. The caregiver should take naps in the daytime to help compensate for lost sleep during the night.

In families where a member is experiencing a chronic illness, such as cancer, or where an elderly member is chronically debilitated, members should cooperate in sharing responsibilities of caregiving. Frequently, one member takes on the role of caregiver, which predisposes that member to sleep deprivation. Nighttime caregiving is what really needs to be shared. If this is not possible, the caregiver should be given opportunity for daytime or evening naps. On the other hand, the family should recognize when it cannot handle the problem alone and get outside help.

When outside help is brought in for nighttime caregiving, the first few nights may be disruptive to the family. Having another person in the house moving around during the night could cause increased periods of wakefulness. Other stresses, such as worrying about the condition of the ill person, questioning if the outsider is doing a good job of caring, and perhaps having guilt feelings that the family was not self-sufficient may keep members awake.

Co-Sleeping

Co-sleeping occurs when children share a bed with their parents on a part-time or full-time basis. This practice may be based on the desires of the child or on the desires of the parent or parents. Nevertheless, it is the parent who permits it to happen.

The habit may be started when the child is an infant. The mother may place the infant in bed with her during breastfeeding, fall asleep, and permit the infant to stay there indefinitely. The infant becomes accustomed to this arrangement and cries when he or she is expected to sleep alone. The crying bothers the mother, so she allows the infant to remain in bed with her. The habit begins insidiously but, is difficult to break.

A parent may encourage co-sleeping when he or she is home alone during a spouse's absence for a short or long period. Parents may be lonely during the absence of a spouse and find the nearness of the child quite comforting and satisfying.

Some parents deliberately plan for the "family bed." They believe children feel wanted and develop good self-esteem when they are permitted to be close to the parents at all times. The family bed is used for parents and all preschool and early elementary school-aged children. These parents usually permit the child to initiate the move from the family bed, which usually occurs around the age of seven or eight years.

Children may insist on sleeping with parents when they are experiencing illnesses, fears, or anxiety. Examples of such times are during thunderstorms, the night before going to school for the first time, when a death occurs in the family, and during parental divorce proceedings. Children want a feeling of security during these times and sleeping with a parent provides that security.

There are very little data to support the benefits or the dangers of co-sleeping (Forbes & Weiss, 1992). Studies related to immediate and future problems caused by co-sleeping do not exist. However, popular literature marketed to parents usually warns against permitting co-sleeping.

Proponents of co-sleeping state that it demonstrates love and sharing in the family, gives children a feeling of belonging, and strengthens their self-esteem. Those who denounce co-sleeping claim sleep is not restful for the parents because children have many movements during sleep, thus causing the parents to get little sleep. Since sexual activities of parents usually occurs in their bed at night, many believe it would be disturbing to children and, in fact, may cause children to believe something "bad" is happening. Further, they believe co-sleeping may permit the child to see the parent in various stages of nudity, which may cause the child to have unwanted sexual feelings or may entice a parent to engage in an incestuous relationship with a child.

Parents who permit co-sleeping when a spouse is absent usually have difficulty when the spouse returns. The child usually wants to continue sleeping with the parent. For this reason, parents should discuss co-sleeping and make a decision about it before it has a chance to occur. This mutual decision should be respected by both parents.

NURSING CARE OF FAMILIES WITH SLEEP NEEDS

The family health nurse is in a position to be very helpful to families with sleep needs. Regardless of setting—school, clinic, nursing home, hospital, community/home health agency, occupational health setting, or hospital—the nurse has access to families or family members for the purpose of promoting and maintaining health and preventing disease. Frequently, the nurse

sees the family or family members during periods of illness when the family wants to focus on the illness. Such emphasis may be placed on illness therapy that health behaviors are not addressed. However, the nurse may be very helpful to the family not only by focusing on the illness but also by addressing health behaviors such as sleep.

Assessment

Assessment of the family's sleep pattern must begin with a sleep history (Table 15–1). The history should be developed with all members present to gain a full picture of when and how sleep occurs in the family. The time spent developing the history will meet two objectives: (1) a valid sleep history will be gained, and (2) family members will gain knowledge about other members' sleep habits, needs, interruptions, and so on that were never brought to the family's awareness before. For this reason a family history session, in itself, may be therapeutic to the family.

In cases where only the parents are having difficulty sleeping because of interpersonal problems, it would not be necessary to bring children in for the history. However, in such a case, the nurse may find that sleep patterns and sleep environments are not the problem and may refer the couple for marital counseling.

Nonliving Environmental Factors

The environment for sleep is usually assessed first. Changes in the environment are frequently easier to make than changes in personal habits or circumstances. Such environmental factors as noise, mattress and bedding, temperature, and bedrooms will be discussed.

NOISE. Noise is problematic to some and not to others, so it is important to elicit information from each family member about the level of noise he or she can tolerate during hours of sleep. Not only is the level important but the frequency or consistency of noise must be assessed. For example, does the clock chime every hour, thus waking a family member each time it chimes? Or does the noise from the typewriter of a student disturb the sleep of a parent? Does the family live on a busy highway where truck traffic is constant and varied in loudness? When does noise awaken the person? Early or late in the night, or does it not make a difference? Even though all family members are living in the same house, they may be in different bedrooms and hear different noises. Likewise, some persons in the same bedroom may report awakenings due to noise, and others do not. However, those who do not report awakenings may experience them but do not remember them. Whether memory of noise is present or not, the awakening can affect daytime functioning (Williams, 1988).

TABLE 15–1. SLEEP HISTORY

Instructions: The following topics and questions may be used as a guide in developing the sleep history. Some parts of the history may be developed with the entire family present, and some may be done with individuals. Open-ended questions should be used as much as possible to permit family members to be open. When you suspect that a family member needs privacy for specific information, you should discreetly allow him or her the freedom not to speak in the group and then speak with that member later.

NONLIVING ENVIRONMENT

Noise:
1. List all noises that are constant (hum of an air conditioner).
2. List all noises that are constantly intermittent (refrigerator motor).
3. List all noises that are outside the house (jets or truck traffic).
4. List all noises caused by family members (snoring, T.V.).

Mattress and Bedding (Information must be gained from each family member):
1. Is the bed size adequate?
2. Is the mattress comfortable?
3. Is the pillow adequate and comfortable?
4. Do the sheets and blankets feel comfortable?
5. Are the blankets light or heavy enough?
6. Are electric blankets or bedwarmers used? At what setting?

Temperature:
1. What room temperature is maintained in the summer? In the winter?
2. Is a whole-house humidifier in use? A room humidifier?
3. Is whole-house air-conditioning used? Room air-conditioning?
4. Are fans used in the bedroom?
5. Are windows left open in the bedroom in the summer? In winter?

Bedrooms:
1. List location of bedrooms. Away from activity centers such as kitchen and family room?
2. Are rooms insulated for noise?
3. Are rooms decorated for noise control? Carpet? Drapes? Wall covering?
4. Is a light left on in the bedroom? In the bathroom? In the hallway?
5. Is there a smoke alarm in the bedroom area?

LIVING ENVIRONMENT

Demographics:
1. How many family members live in the house all the time?
2. How many family members live in the house intermittently?
3. List the family members who sleep in each bedroom.
4. List the family members who share a bed.
5. List the family members who get out of bed during the night. One time? Two times? More than two times? For what purpose does each member get up?
6. List family members who sleep at a time other than at night. For what reason?
7. List all members who nap in the daytime. List the daytime naps taken.

Individual Family Members (elicit the following information from each family member as applicable).
1. Age?
2. Usual sleep pattern:
   Has the pattern changed recently? In the past 5 to 10 years?
   Time to bed?
   Time to get up?
   Does sleep occur shortly after going to bed?
   Sleep ritual?
   Awaken during sleep? How many times a night?
   What are sleep awakenings associated with?
   After awakening do you go back to sleep easily?
   Same sleep pattern on weekends as during the week?
   Do you nap in the daytime? How long? What time?
   Do you feel rested in the morning?
   Are you attentive throughout the day?
   Are you sleepy or drowsy during the day?
   Do you feel irritable, restless, lethargic, or listless during the day?
   Do you snore?
   Do you grind your teeth?
   Do you wet in bed?
   How frequently do you dream?
   Are your dreams vivid? Do they awaken you?
   Do you have nightmares? Night terrors?

TABLE 15-1. SLEEP HISTORY (continued)

3. Do you feel sleepy or drowsy in the daytime?
    What time of day?
    What do you do to relieve this feeling?
    Is it effective?
4. How much mental exercise do you get in the daytime? At what time of day?
5. How much physical exercise do you get in the daytime? At what time of day?
6. List all drugs (prescription, nonprescription, and illicit), dose, time taken, date of use of drug, when drug will
    be stopped.
7. Do you drink alcoholic beverages?
    What kind?
    How much/day?
    What time of day do you drink?
    How long have you drunk alcoholic beverages?
    Do you think alcoholic beverages interfere with your activities of daily living?
    What are your usual mealtimes?
    Do you eat before going to bed?
8. List caffeine substances used (coffee, tea, chocolate, soft drinks, drugs).
    How many cups of coffee/day? Tea? Chocolate? Soft Drinks? Drugs containing caffeine?
    What time of day do you drink caffeine beverages?
    How long have you drunk caffeine beverages?
    Dose and frequency of caffeine-containing drugs?
9. Do you smoke?
    How many cigarettes/day?
    When do you smoke?
    How long have you smoked?
10. List all sleep problems experienced in the past.
    When was it?
    What do you think caused it?
    How long did it last?
    How did it affect activities of daily living?
    What was done to relieve the problem?
11. List all sleep problems experienced at present.
    Give a full explanation of the problem.
    When was the last time you slept well?
    When did the problem start?
    What do you think caused it?
    What have you done to relieve it?
    Have you asked anyone else for help with this problem?
    How is it affecting your daily activities?
12. Do you have any other physical or psychologic problems? Are they being treated by a physician?
13. Are you experiencing any stress or anxiety in your life at present?
    Date of onset?
    What do you think is causing it?
    What are you doing to relieve it?
    Do you think it is affecting anyone else in the family? How?
14. Do you think anyone else in your family is having sleep difficulties?
    What makes you think this way?
    What do you think is causing it?
    Have you discussed it with that person?
15. Is there anything else you would like to discuss?

It takes more noise to awaken a sleeper from delta sleep (Stages III and IV NREM) than from Stage II or REM sleep. With REM sleep, the threshold may depend on the dream. Some noises are incorporated into the dream, and the sleeper is not aware of the outside noise. Awakening from noise also depends on the sleeper's sleep needs. As the need for sleep decreases, the sleeper will awaken more readily when noise is present. Frequently, a loud noise from a truck is more disturbing than a constant loud noise such as from an air conditioner.

MATTRESSES AND BEDDING. Some people like soft mattresses, and some like firm mattresses, and others prefer a water mattress. Some like satin sheets, others prefer percale; some want no pillow, others want one or two; some like an electric blanket, others prefer no blanket. What is best? In short, it depends on the likes and habits of the sleeper. It is important for the nurse to know if the family has changed any of their bedding recently. It may take a few nights to get used to a new mattress, but if it is essentially the same as the old mattress, there should be no problem. Persons who must sleep on a special mattress for orthopedic reasons may find more time is necessary to adapt. Also, persons who must have the head of the bed elevated because of hiatal hernia or breathing problems may need adaptation time. In these cases, the sleeper's partner may choose to sleep in another bed. When persons move from sleeping with someone to sleeping alone, they also find more periods of wakefulness until adaptation occurs.

TEMPERATURE. Temperature is another factor that depends on personal choice. Families that grow up together usually are accustomed to a set temperature; however, when a new member is added to the family, the new member may have to make adjustments. Temperature of the room, along with humidity, must be considered, but the temperature caused by the use of bed linen must also be considered. Some persons like to wear a lot of sleeping apparel, and others believe sleeping in the nude is more comfortable. Again, one's own preference should be considered so long as the wearing apparel is comfortable and safe. This is true for the amount of bedding; each person develops likes and dislikes that must be considered.

Weather has an influence on the temperature and humidity of the house, and heating and cooling systems are installed to maintain a livable, safe temperature and humidity. During times of weather change or when the heating or cooling systems are not operative, family members may experience sleep awakening, but this should be temporary. An excessively warm room is usually more disruptive to sleep than an excessively cold room. People usually have little trouble with extreme temperature early in the night because they are experiencing more NREM sleep, and their thermoregulation abilities are better. During the early morning when REM sleep is more prevalent, the thermoregulation is impaired, and extremes in temperature could cause awakenings.

BEDROOM. Most people sleep in bedrooms, the one place in the house that is intentionally meant for sleeping. The number of bedrooms needed is a great consideration when buying or renting a house. In fact, many moves are precipitated by the number of bedrooms in the present dwelling: either too many or not enough. Bedroom needs are usually based on the family's life style and the number, sex, and age of children in the family, as well as some projection on whether the family will be enlarging or decreasing in the near future.

The location of the bedrooms should be considered. It is best to have bedrooms away from activity and noise. Bedrooms are sometimes placed on a separate floor from the other rooms, or they may be placed on one end of the house away from kitchen, living room, and family room. The construction should be reviewed. Insulation for temperature purposes also may serve as a noise barrier.

Bedrooms, hallways, and rooms near the bedrooms should be carpeted since carpet absorbs noise better than other floor coverings. Drapes absorb more sound than plain curtains. Wallpaper is a better sound absorber than woodpaneled walls. Today, many houses are built with plasterboard walls that are fairly good sound absorbers. A smoke alarm should be located in the bedroom areas so that no one need fear that sleeping too soundly could interfere with family safety.

The bedroom often doubles for a place for young children to play or for students to do homework. In such cases, a place in the room should be designated for these activities. The child should be taught early that the bed is meant for sleeping. Further, when the room doubles for other activities, children must understand that during naps and nighttime they should be in the bed sleeping.

Some parents use the bedroom as a place to send the child for punishment. In these cases, the child should not be sent to "bed" for punishment but should be detained in the bedroom in a place other than on the bed. The child should not equate the bed with punishment. This could cause sleep-onset or sleep-awakening problems for the child.

Living Environment

Many things about families are constant, but many things can be changed to improve the quality of life for the family. Quality of life is greatly affected by how well sleep needs of each member are met.

Some things that cannot be changed are the age and sex of family members. These factors are usually considered when sleeping rooms are assigned to family members. On the other hand, many things can be changed, but first they must be recognized. One major factor to recognize is that when one family member is having a sleep problem, it affects all family members. Because sleep has such a great effect on people's behavior and daytime activities, many problems may be solved by evaluating the sleep patterns of persons and families who are having problems. Frequently sleep is not recognized as a problem by the family, but during a nursing assessment it may become clear that a sleep problem is the basis for a bigger family problem. Two significant factors, demographics and individual family members, which must be considered in assessment will be discussed.

DEMOGRAPHICS. The first important piece of history information needed is how many people are in the family and sleeping with the family on a regular basis or an irregular basis? Children who go off to college and come home for the summer months can sometimes interfere with the sleep habits of their parents because the parents have adapted to sleeping without them in the house. Or independent children who decide they can't make it alone come home to live with parents after a period of absence. Parents moving in has been discussed earlier. All of these people and their sleeping and working schedules must be considered.

INDIVIDUAL FAMILY MEMBERS. A history of the sleep habits and past and present sleep problems of each family member must be taken. These histories may be taken individually to maintain privacy of family members.

Nutrition information must be taken because weight gain and weight loss affects sleep. Weight gain is associated with long, uninterrupted sleep, and weight loss is associated with short, fragmented sleep. People who have recently lost weight complain of frequent night awakenings, especially in the last half of the night. Insomnia is a common symptom of anorexia nervosa. Hyperthyroidism is associated with weight loss and short sleep periods with excessive amounts of delta sleep. Hypothyroidism results in weight gain and long periods of sleep but a decreased amount of delta sleep.

L-tryptophan, an amino acid that is a precursor of serotonin and inhibitory neurotransmitter, is thought to contribute to sleep. For this reason, many people recommend drinking warm milk or eating cheese and crackers at bedtime.

Caffeine, a stimulant and an ingredient in coffee, tea, and some soft drinks, contributes to sleep latency and increased periods of wakefulness. It seems to affect different people differently: Many people are able to drink 10 to 12 cups of coffee and sleep quite soundly, and others can drink only one cup early in the morning. Those who consume large amounts of caffeine often have difficulty sleeping when caffeine is withdrawn. However, for those suffering from insomnia, limiting the caffeine intake is a must.

Nicotine is another CNS stimulant that affect sleep. People who are heavy smokers have more periods of wakefulness. The combination of smoking cigarettes and drinking coffee contributes to insomnia.

Mealtimes and other times when food is taken in relation to sleep time may have an affect on sleepiness or wakefulness. Because drowsiness frequently occurs after a meal, some people eat before going to bed with the thought that it will induce sleep. It is known with certainty what the effect of food intake is on sleep, but many people have such a habit. It could be problematic if the family member decides to diet and cut out food intake at bedtime. If the pattern is to eat to induce sleep, dieting may lead to difficulty sleeping.

Moderate physical exercise in the afternoon or early evening may contribute to a good night's sleep. However, exercise immediately before going to bed increases sleep onset time. Exercise should be done on a regular basis to have an effect on sleep. Persons who perform extremely heavy exercises may not feel the sleep effects of the exercise until the second night, when they will sleep soundly (Reilly, 1990).

Stress and anxiety are two factors that have a severe effect on sleep. These phenomena are usually seen in more than one person in the family at the same time. However, they may be seen in only one member of the family. One member may be having difficulty at work or at school, which causes stress. Some family members do not share all of life's happenings with each other. However, in close families, other family members may detect early that another member is having a problem. When stress or anxiety exist, they usually cause delayed sleep onset, wakeful periods during the night, or, in severe cases, insomnia. In developing the history, the nurse should always try to determine if there are stresses in the lives of people with sleep problems.

Chronic use of alcohol will provide a prematurely aged sleep pattern. That is, there will be many wakenings, little or no delta sleep, and somewhat decreased REM sleep. These people, like old people, spend more time in bed and less time sleeping. They also show increased daytime sleepiness since their sleep-wake rhythm is blurred. During periods of heavy alcohol consumption, the person may get no sleep at all. They may then experience delirium due to sleep deprivation. Insomnia and REM rebound often occur during alcohol withdrawal. Heavy alcohol drinkers may suffer slow-onset sleep, fragmented sleep, and very little sleep for as long as two years after giving up alcohol. This may be due to permanent or irreversible damage caused by drinking. Some think it could be that the drinker always had sleep problems and started drinking to relieve them.

Many other drugs also cause sleep problems. Stimulants and the cessation of hypnotics cause insomnia. Many people become addicted to drugs during periods of stress. People who take amphetamines for weight reduction may also have an addiction that manifests itself in sleeplessness. Persons who are trying to withdraw from marijuana or cocaine also have sleep difficulties. Other drugs may give rise to sleep problems, therefore it is important to list all prescribed as well as over-the-counter and illicit drugs in use presently and in the past year.

Nursing Diagnosis

Following the development of the history with the family and family members, the nurse may want to review a recent physical examination report or may want to perform some parts of a physical examination on selected family members if the history warrants. Most information needed to make an adequate nursing diagnosis will be gained through a thorough health history.

The nursing diagnosis Gordon (1989) has assigned to sleep is sleep disturbance. She defines sleep disturbance as, "Disruption of sleep time causing discomfort or interference with desired life activities." Houldin et al. (1987) take a different approach to the nursing diagnosis related to sleep. They provide a health status statement that can be used for a well person. Their health statements include "Sleep pattern, adequate (to meet demands of daily living)" and "Sleep quality, duration, and frequency appropriate to support wellness." It is suggested that when the family or family member is having a problem, the sleep disturbance diagnosis could be used, and when there is no problem, one of the wellness health statements could be made.

The diagnosis is made after first identifying characteristics that contribute to a sleep disturbance diagnosis (Table 15–2). Some characteristics listed by Gordon are verbal complaints of difficulty falling asleep, early wakening, interrupted sleep, sleep pattern reversal, verbal complaints of not feeling well rested, reduction in performance, and increasing irritability. Others listed by Carpenito (1989) are fatigue on awakening or during the day, dozing during the day and mood alterations. All of these characteristics should be available in the health history.

Some etiologic factors listed by Gordon are family stress, environmental or habit change, and daytime boredom or inactivity. Carpenito categorized etiologies according to pathophysiology, treatment, and situation. She lists such etiologies as respiratory disorders, use of various drugs, and pain. These etiologic factors should also be available in the health history.

It is imperative for the nurse to make the proper nursing diagnosis in order to develop an adequate plan of care. When the nurse has difficulty identifying the characteristics of etiologic factors, additional information may be sought from the family members or another health professional, and assistance with the diagnosis may be gained from another nurse.

Care Plan

The care plan for the family and individual family members is best done together. Each individual member should have an opportunity to be heard and to have his or her suggestions considered. When a sleeping disturbance problem is affecting only one member of the family, that member may be seen by the nurse alone. However, when one person has a sleep problem, it usually affects all or most members. Therefore, the nurse

TABLE 15–2. COMMON DEFINING CHARACTERISTICS AND ETIOLOGIES BY AGE FOR THE NURSING DIAGNOSIS: SLEEP PATTERN DISTURBANCE

AGE	CHARACTERISTICS	ETIOLOGIES
Newborn	Crying	Physical discomfort (e.g., wet, hungry, too much food)
6–12 mo	Crying at bedtime	Physical discomfort
	Frequent awakenings	Established habit
1–4 yr	Refuse to take daytime naps	Established poor habit
		Environment unconducive to sleep
4–7 yr	Do not fall asleep soon after put in bed—call to parents for water, hugs, etc.	Established poor habit
4–10 yr	Sleep terrors	Stress, overtired, irregular schedule
4–12 yr	Awake during night	Enuresis
13–18 yr	Sleepy during day	Poor sleep schedule
18–25 yr	Sleepy during day	Poor sleep schedule
	Insomnia	Use or withdrawal from drugs
Pregnancy	Tired, sleepy during day	Physiologic need for more rest and sleep
	Frequent awakenings	Physical discomfort
36–65 yr	Delayed sleep onset	Stress
	Insomnia	Use of caffeine, cigarettes, drugs
	Fatigue in AM	
	Dozing during day	Rotating work schedule
	Mood alterations	Physical discomfort or disorders
		Lack of exercise
		Family stress
65–100 yr	Delayed sleep onset	Normal aging process
	Insomnia	Use or withdrawal of hypnotics
	Frequent awakenings	Need for urination
		Lack of exercise
		Stress

should take the opportunity to discuss sleep habits and lifestyle alternatives with the entire family, with the objective of providing knowledge in areas where it is lacking.

Knowledge deficit regarding how much the baby should sleep, what makes a good sleep routine, what to do when the baby won't sleep, and when to stop nighttime feedings is common among new parents. Most people have a knowledge deficit regarding use of sedatives and other prescribed drugs, over-the-counter drugs, and illicit drugs. Older adults usually lack knowledge regarding the normal sleep needs and changes that occur with aging. It is important for the nurse to elicit information from the family regarding their knowledge of these facts; assumptions should not be made. The nurse should especially elicit information regarding the family's knowledge of the etiologies that were identified in the nursing diagnosis.

The etiologies identified should be discussed in detail with the family. The nurse may provide them with literature on the etiology or suggest that they visit the local library to learn more about the subject. A written plan of behaviors the family should practice to overcome their problem should be developed and discussed. A list of common behaviors to overcome sleep disturbance problems is found in Table 15–3. The plan should state the practices to be followed by each member, when they should be done, and short- and long-term goals. It is important for every family member to agree to follow the plan, otherwise their objectives may not be met. The plan should be written at the level of reading and comprehension of most family members. Further, the nurse should sign it and ask each family member to sign it.

In addition to providing the family with a sufficient knowledge base and a plan of action, the nurse should ask the family to keep a sleep log or diary (Table 15–4). Each member should be asked to keep an individual diary. The diary should be kept simple, otherwise the family members may view it as an added burden. After a two-week period, the family and the nurse will review the diaries together.

Evaluation

The diaries will give the nurse information about each member's performance of activities that he or she agreed to perform in order to solve the family sleep disturbance problem. The nurse should give the family as much positive feedback as possible to encourage continuation of activities that have caused improvement.

After reviewing the diaries, a discussion should be held to allow the family members to verbalize their feelings about the past two weeks. They should be made comfortable to say what went wrong as well as what went right. Further, they should also be permitted to set new goals. It may be necessary for the entire family to continue maintaining a diary, or it may be necessary for only the member with the primary problem to keep a diary. Nevertheless, the nurse will continue to evaluate and work with the family until they feel their problem has been solved.

Family sleep needs and performance change over time as individual members change and experience different developmental levels. Anticipatory guidance is needed to encourage families to evaluate continually their sleep habits and the impact on the quality of family health.

TABLE 15–3. COMMON BEHAVIORS TO OVERCOME SLEEP DISTURBANCE

1. Set the temperature, humidity, and lighting at a comfortable level.
2. Check the mattress and bedding for comfort.
3. Provide sound barriers to all possible noises—wear ear plugs to bed.
4. Go to bed and get up at the same time daily, including weekends and holidays.
5. Limit use of caffeine and cigarettes: use caffeine only in the morning.
6. Develop a plan to stop taking sedatives, other hypnotics, illicit drugs, and CNS stimulants.
7. When sleep does not occur soon after going to bed, get up and do something monotonous. Do not lie in bed awake.
8. Perform adequate physical and mental exercise in the daytime.
9. Do not exercise immediately before going to bed.
10. Do not take alcohol before going to bed.
11. Use relaxation exercises such as deep breathing and contracting and relaxing various muscle groups, beginning with the feet and moving up toward the head.
12. Do not take fluids three to four hours before bedtime; empty bladder immediately before going to bed.
13. Provide soft music.
14. Share room/bed with compatible roommate.
15. Take daytime naps.
16. Do not take daytime naps.
17. Relieve physical discomforts.

TABLE 15–4. SLEEP DIARY

Instructions: The diary may be kept in a looseleaf notebook or tablet. The following information should be kept for each day.

1. List all drugs, dosage, and time of use.
2. Time went to bed.
3. What activities you performed in the hour just before going to bed.
4. How long did it take you to fall asleep?
5. What did you do if you did not fall asleep soon after going to bed?
   What did you think about while you were waiting for sleep?
6. How many awakenings did you experience during the night? What do you think caused them?
7. What kind and how much physical exercise did you do during the day?
8. What kind and how much mental exercise did you do during the day?
9. Describe any stress or anxiety you experienced during the day.
10. Did you get out of bed during the night? What time was it? What did you do while out of bed? How long did you stay up?
11. What time did you get up in the morning?
12. Did you wake up spontaneously?
13. Did you feel rested when you got up?
14. Did you feel sleepy during the day? How did you overcome this feeling?
15. Did you feel fatigued during the day? Did it interfere with your work or other activities?
16. List any behaviors not already addressed that you agreed to perform to solve a sleep disturbance problem in the family.
17. How do you feel about your sleep progress?

CHAPTER HIGHLIGHTS

Many sleep patterns and rituals are established in early family life.

Family sleep needs and patterns change over time as individuals and the family unit experience different developmental transitions.

Many family transitions disrupt family sleep patterns. Examples of such family transitions include changing work schedules, new family members, new infants, illness of a member, and changes in the environment.

Family nurses can facilitate healthy family sleep patterns by assessing sleep history and assisting the family to resolve problems such as co-sleeping with children, infant sleep patterns, insomnia, environmental influences on sleep, and lifestyle patterns.

REFERENCES

Balsmeyer, B. (1990). Sleep disturbances of the infant and toddler. *Pediatric Nursing,* 16(5), 447–452.

Biddle, C. (1990). The nature of sleep. *Journal of the American Association of Nurse Anesthetists,* 58(1), 36–44.

Carpenito, L. (1989). *Handbook of Nursing Diagnosis* (3rd ed.). Philadelphia: J.B. Lippincott.

Daws, D. (1989). *Through the Night.* London: Free Association Books.

Forbes, J., & Weiss, D. (1992). The cosleeping habits of military children. *Military Medicine* 157(4), 196–200.

Gordon, M. (1989). *Manual of Nursing Diagnosis.* St. Louis: C.V. Mosby.

Hodgson, L. (1991). Why do we need sleep? Relating theory to nursing practice. *Journal of Advanced Nursing* 16, 1503–1510.

Leibenluft, E., & Wehr, T. (1992). Is sleep deprivation useful in the treatment of depression? *American Journal of Psychiatry,* 149(2), 159–168.

Moorcroft, W.H. (1989). *Sleep, Dreaming and Sleep Disorders.* New York: University Press of America.

Peter, J.H., et al. (1991). *Sleep and Health Risk.* New York: Springer-Verlag.

Rechtschaffen, S., & Kales, S. (1978). *A Manual of Standardized Terminology, Techniques, and Scoring System for Sleep Stages of Human Subjects.* Los Angeles: UCLA Brain Information/Brain Research Institute.

Reilly, T. (1990). Human circadian rhythms and exercise. *Biomedical Engineering,* 18(3), 165–180.

Rosenburg, R. (1991). Assessment and treatment of delayed sleep phase syndrome. In P. Hauri (Ed.), *Case Studies in Insomnia.* New York: Plenum.

Sheldon, S., et al. (1992). *Pediatric Sleep Medicine.* Philadelphia: W.B. Saunders.

Tepas, D., & Carvalhais, A. (1990). Sleep patterns of shiftworkers. *Occupational Medicine.* 5(2), 199–208.

Westbrook, P.R. (1990). Sleep disorders and upper airway obstruction in adults. *Otolaryngologic Clinics of North America,* 23(4), 727–743.

Williams, R.L. (1988). Sleep disturbance in various medical and surgical conditions. In R.L. Williams, et al. (Eds.), *Sleep Disorders: Diagnosis and Treatment.* New York: Wiley.

ADDITIONAL READINGS

Catalano, E. M. (1990). *Getting to Sleep.* Oakland, CA: New Harbinger.

Golbin, A. Z. (1994). *The World of Children's Sleep: Parent's Guide.* Salt Lake: Michaelis.

Kryger, M. H., Roth, T., & Dement, W. C. (1994). *Principles and Practices of Sleep Medicine* (2nd ed.). Philadelphia: W. B. Saunders.

Thorpy, M. J. (1991). *The Encyclopedia of Sleep and Sleep Disorders.* New York: Facts on File.

ORGANIZATIONS

The American Sleep Disorders Centers
P.O. Box 2604
Del Mar, CA 92014

National Sleep Foundation
122 South Robertson Blvd., 3rd Floor
Los Angeles, CA 90048

Sleep & Behavioral Medicine Institute
Alexander Z. Goblin, M.D., Medical Director
4200 W. Peterson, Suite #109
Chicago, IL 60646

16

FAMILY RECREATION AND EXERCISE

DARLENE E. McCOWN

Family ties are precious things
Woven through the years
Of memories of togetherness
Of laughter, love and tears.

VIRGINIA BLANCK MOORE

OBJECTIVES

On completion of this chapter, the reader will be able to:

1. Develop an understanding of the concepts of recreation, leisure, and exercise
2. Discuss the basic principles of exercise
3. Analyze the impact of exercise across the life cycle
4. Identify variables associated with family recreation and exercise
5. Examine the nursing role in promoting exercise as a nursing intervention

DEFINITION OF KEY TERMS

Before beginning the discussion of family recreation and exercise, definitions of key terms used in this chapter will be presented.

Aerobic exercise is activity that focuses on the increased use of oxygen. It is sustained exercise that increases heart and respiratory rates.

Anaerobic exercise is physical activity of short duration, usually 60 seconds or less, and uses energy derived from metabolic adaptation (McArdle et al., 1986).

Cardiovascular fitness is the ability to perform aerobic exercise for 30 minutes at a heart rate of 60% to 80% of the calculated maximum (Jopling, 1992).

Exercise is simply action or activity of physical and mental exertion.

Isometric exercises are activities resulting in a contraction of the muscle without movement of the joint, and the muscle stays at the same length.

Isotonic activities involve muscle contraction and joint movement, such as weight lifting and calisthenics.

Leisure is free time during which individuals or families may choose to do as they wish. It provides opportunity for recreation, exercise, service, and personal growth.

Play is activity of the mind and body for the purpose of diversion, pleasure, and recreation.

Physical fitness is the ability to adapt to the demands and stresses of physical effort.

Recreation includes acts or experiences selected by individuals or families during leisure time that meet personal desires for satisfaction and that restore and refresh the participants.

RECREATION AND LEISURE

The American lifestyle has shifted dramatically from an emphasis on work and toil toward a more sedentous lifestyle and a focus on leisure and recreation. The classical work ethic has faded. This may be attributed to multiple factors, including the increase in mechanization in both the workplace and the home, a decrease in the average work week, and an increase in physical and financial resources. These social changes afford the American family more time and money to enjoy the pursuits of leisure time—namely recreation. As a result, Americans are bombarded with opportunities for their leisure time attention. The government has become involved and the U.S. Public Health Service has established goals for a healthy nation to increase daily physical activity to at least 30% of the population aged 10 and over.

A discussion of leisure, recreation, and exercise must begin by clarifying terms. "Leisure" is the most general concept. "Recreation" and "exercise" are more specific. The three can be related in the following way: Leisure time may be spent in recreation or exercise, but it does not follow that recreation is always leisure, or even that exercise is always recreational. To derive the greatest benefits from exercise and recreation one must both enjoy and feel rejuvenated by the activity; that is, exercise and recreation must function for the individual as leisure.

The selection of beneficial leisure and recreational activities is a challenge. The criteria in Table 16–1 provide guidelines for judging the recreational quality of an activity.

A truly recreative lifestyle attitude is one without goals, demands, or expectations, where individuals can develop fully physically and cognitively and where human bonding occurs (Geba, 1985). Recreation involves renewing bonds, feel-

TABLE 16–1. CRITERIA FOR SELECTING RECREATIONAL ACTIVITIES

RECREATIONAL VALUE	
LOW	HIGH
Participation forced	Participation voluntary
Contributes only to the individual	Contributes to group goals
Has artificial motivation	Stimulates interest
Leads to more of the same	Builds self-confidence
Avoids comparison of self to others	Stimulates evaluation
Is noncreative	Inspires creativity
Becomes routine	Challenges ingenuity
Is repetitive	Has intrinsic value
Purpose is reward only	Brings happiness
Activity is disliked	Contributes to health
Is unhealthy	Offsets tension
Produces tension	Enjoys long-term acceptance
Exploits others	Includes others in the plan
Arouses fear	Promotes a positive attitude

Data from De Angelis, E. (1983). Recreation, art, music and dance therapy and adapted physical education. In M. Levine, W. Carey, A. Crocher, & R. Gross (Eds.), *Developmental Behavioral Pediatrics* (pp. 1128–1133). Philadelphia: Mosby; and Nash, J. (1960). *Philosophy of Recreation and Leisure.* Dubuque, IA: Brown.

ing emotions, having fun, relieving tension, and improving self-confidence. The focus of true recreation is not on the selected activity but on the attitude of the participants. A lifestyle attitude essential for leisure and recreation is composed of two basic interrelated processes: (1) the natural and (2) the cultural symbolic (Geba, 1985). The natural realm constitutes the autonomic body functions such as circulation, respiration, and endocrine functioning. The cultural symbolic realm is the part of life that the individual person is in charge of living. The individual's ability to make a blend between the natural and the cultural or symbolic elements of life is critical to good health. The recreational lifestyle allows for relating to the world sensuously with the body and analytically with the intellect. It is precisely at the natural or bodily movement realm that exercise affects the recreational lifestyle attitude of the individual.

FAMILY LIFE, RECREATION, AND EXERCISE

From a systems approach, the family exerts the most immediate and formative influence on the lifestyle patterns of its members. It is from the family context that attitudes and practices related to health, recreation, and exercise are established. Spending time together in leisure and recreation provides opportunity for lifestyle values and patterns to be passed on to family members. Curran (1983) and Holman (1985) both report that in healthy families time and leisure are shared with family members. Furthermore, it is known that families who are involved in well-organized recreational activities express greater satisfaction and family unity (Smith, 1985). A survey of parents has shown that 40% to 50% reported not spending enough time with their children (Holman, 1985). Another study indicated that one-third of adolescents surveyed felt they did not spend enough time with their fathers (Holman, 1985). Research has also shown familial patterns of activity levels between parents and children (Moore et al., 1991) This is significant because the active involvement of parents, especially the father, is known to be critical to the success of family recreation (Smith, H., 1985) and ultimately of family health.

Recreation can be a beneficial force in the family. It can provide members with common goals and measurable experiences that strengthen bonds. On the other hand, it can also be a negative force if it draws members apart for extended periods of time if they participate in different individual activities. The choice of recreational activities is a matter of value judgment that is developed early in life and stems partially from the family of origin.

Because there is potential for family indecision and conflict over the use of leisure time, it is recommended that each family unit develop a philosophy or guidelines for leisure that address the following issues (Vander Griend, 1985; Wade, 1985). First, who will be involved in family recreation (friends, teammates, extended relatives, and so on)? Second, when will the family recreate? This question addresses the amount of time required for recreation. Third, where will the family go for recreation? Supervision is an important aspect of this question when the family has young children and teenagers. Fourth, why does the family seek recreation? This can be answered by the benefits accrued to its members in terms of cohesiveness, unity, fun, and sharing as well as renewal of love and energy. Fifth, how is the family able to provide for recreation? This deals with the amount of money, materials, and time available for recreational use. Seeking answers to these five questions will help the family to select appropriate and satisfying recreational experiences.

Theoretical formulations toward a theory of family recreation have identified variables affecting family recreation. Exchange theory appropriately sets the basis for participation in recreation and exercise by proposing that people engage in activities they find satisfying (profitable). Neal (1984) abridged the earlier work of Carlson (1979), and their formulation of the interrelated components of family recreation provides a theoretical model as well as propositions (Fig. 16–1).

The various propositions and components of the model representing family recreation are derived primarily from behaviorism and exchange theory and also are related to family decision making and cohesion. Specifically, the rewards associated with recreation influence the frequency with which a family selects and engages in particular recreational activities. Demographic variables such as socioeconomic class and reference groups affect the range of recreation available to children in a family. The degree of family participation in recreation is related to family integration and communication as well as the demographic variables of ages of members and size of family. Family participation in recreation is found to be positively related to marital satisfaction.

Family recreation propositions (Neal, 1984) are as follows:

1. The greater the net reward realized from a recreation activity or set of activities in the past, the more frequently that activity or set of activities will be chosen from among alternatives in the future.
2. The more often a recreational activity or set of activities results in a high net reward, the more frequently the activity or set of activities will be engaged in.
3. The greater the expectations of the individual exceed the alternatives available for a particular recreational activity, the more frequently the activity will be engaged in.
4. Given voluntary behavior, the more frequently a recreational activity is engaged in, the more likely a point of diminishing returns will be met, and net reward will decrease.
5. The greater the investments in a particular style of recreational activities, the narrower the range of alternatives available to an individual or group.
6. The more industrialized the society, the more regimented the time dimension of an individual's life.
7. The greater the rate of social change in other sectors of the society, the greater the likelihood of changes in attitudes and values toward work and leisure.
8. The greater the discretionary time and income in a society, the greater the recreational goods and services.
9. The higher the socioeconomic level of the family of orientation, the wider the range of recreational alternatives available to the members of the family.
10. The greater the opportunity to engage in a recreational activity or set of activities, the more likely that activity or set of activities will become a part of the individual's recreational choices.
11. The wider the range of recreational alternatives for parents, the more likely children will be socialized into a wide range of recreational activities.
12. The greater the number of nonfamily reference groups, the greater the possibility of socialization into a wide range of recreational activities.
13. The greater the family integration, the more likely a family will engage in recreational activities as a group.
14. The wider the range of common recreational activities engaged in by members of the family, the more frequent the consensual decisions about recreation.
15. The greater the communication in the family, the less the likelihood of accommodative recreation decisions.
16. The larger the family and the older the children, the less the likelihood of consensual decisions about recreation.
17. The more similar the social class backgrounds of the spouses, the more likely their recreational patterns will be family oriented.
18. The more frequent the consensual decisions regarding recreational choices, the greater the total family satisfaction from recreational activities.
19. A positive but unclear correlation exists between family recreation and marital satisfaction.
20. The more frequent the consensus in decisions regarding recreational choices, the more likely recreational activities will be engaged in as a family unit.

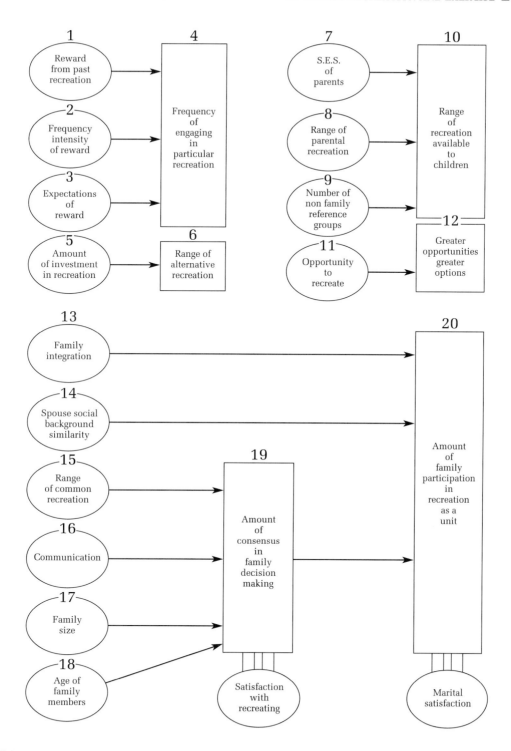

FIGURE 16–1. Propositions and factors related to family recreation.
Note: From "Family recreation: Trends, tenets, and model building" by L. Neal, 1984, *Journal of Physical Education, Recreation, and Dance,* October, 33–37. Reprinted by permission of the American Alliance for Health, Physical Eduction, Recreation and Dance, 1900 Association Dr., Reston, VA 22091
Adapted from: "The family and recreation: Toward a theoretical development" by Carlson J. (1979). In W. R. Burr et al. (Eds.), *Contemporary theories about the family,* Vol 1 (pp. 439–452). New York: Free Press.

GENERAL DISCUSSION OF EXERCISE

Less than one-fourth of Americans over 18 years of age exercise regularly at least 30 minutes (in light to moderate activity). This is an alarmingly low percentage, particularly because the benefits of exercise are well documented. *Healthy People 2000* (U.S. DHHS, 1990) developed objectives for the nation pertaining to fitness, which are presented in Table 16–2.

Benefits of Exercise

The effects of exercise include physiologic and psychosocial benefits across the life span. Physiologic benefits may be categorized as cardiovascular, biochemical, and morphologic. Because heart disease is a major health problem in the United States, let us first examine the cardiovascular changes associated with regular exercise (Allan, 1985; DeVries, 1986; Eckert & Montoye, 1984; Ferrara et al., 1991; Gordon & Gibbons, 1990; McArdle et al., 1986; Plowman, 1984; Rowland et al., 1991).

- Lowered resting and exercise heart rate
- Lowered blood pressure
- Increased cardiac output with exercise
- Increased cardiac circulation
- Increased pulmonary function
- Increased capillarization
- Decreased problems of cardiac rhythm in the elderly
- Increased adaptation to temperature in the elderly

Biochemical changes related to exercise include (Cooper, 1989; McArdle et al., 1986; NASA, 1984; Plowman 1984; Slemenda et al., 1991; Suominen et al., 1992):

- Lowered serum cholesterol
- Lowered blood sugar
- Increased high-density lipoproteins (HDL)
- Decreased bone mineral loss (osteoporosis in elderly)
- Increased blood volume and hemoglobin levels

TABLE 16–2. YEAR 2000 FITNESS OBJECTIVES FOR THE NATION

1. Reduce coronary heart disease deaths to no more than 100 per 100,000 people. (Age-adjusted baseline: 135 per 100,000 in 1987.)
2. Reduce overweight to a prevalence of no more than 20% among people aged 20 and older and no more than 15% among adolescents aged 12–19. (Baseline: 26% of people aged 20–74 in 1976–1980, 24% for men and 27% for women; 15% for adolescents aged 12–19 in 1976–1980.)
3. Increase to at least 30% the proportion of people aged 6 and older who engage regularly, preferably daily, in light to moderate physical activity for at least 30 minutes per day. (Baseline: 22% of people aged 18 and older were active for at least 30 minutes five or more times per week and 12% were active seven or more times per week in 1985.)
4. Increase to at least 20% the proportion of people aged 18 and older and to at least 75% the proportion of children and adolescents aged 6–17 who engage in vigorous physical activity that promotes the development and maintenance of cardiorespiratory fitness 3 or more days per week for 20 or more minutes per occasion. (Baseline: 12% for people 18 and older in 1985; 66% for youths aged 10–17 in 1984.)
5. Reduce to no more than 15% the proportion of people aged 6 and older who engage in no leisure-time physical activity. (Baseline: 24% for people aged 18 and older in 1985; 43% if aged 65 and older; 35% if disabled.)
6. Increase to at least 40% the proportion of people aged 6 and older who regularly perform physical activities that enhance and maintain muscular strength, endurance, and flexibility. (Baseline data available in 1991.)
7. Increase to at least 50% the proportion of overweight people aged 12 and older who have adopted sound dietary practices combined with regular physical activity to attain an appropriate body weight. (Baseline: 30% of overweight women and 25% of overweight men for people aged 18 and older in 1985.)
8. Increase to at least 50% the proportion of children and adolescents in grades 1–12 who participate in daily school physical education. (Baseline: 36% in 1984–1986.)
9. Increase to at least 50% the proportion of school physical education class time that students spend being physically active, preferably engaged in lifetime physical activities. (Baseline: Students spent an estimated 27% of class time being physically active in 1984.)
10. Increase the proportion of worksites offering employer-sponsored physical activity and fitness programs.
11. Increase community availability and accessibility of physical activity and fitness facilities, e.g., hiking, biking, and fitness trails, public swimming pools, and areas of park and recreational open space.
12. Increase to at least 50% the proportion of primary care providers who routinely assess and counsel their patients regarding the frequency, duration, type, and intensity of each patient's physical activity practices. (Baseline: Physicians provided exercise counseling for about 30% of sedentary patients in 1988.)

Data from *Health People 2000: National Health Promotion and Disease Prevention Objectives* (1990). Washington, DC: U.S. Dept. of Health and Human Services, Public Health Service.

- Decreased lactic acid buildup during sub-maximal work
- Increased tolerance for lactic acid at maximal work

The motivation for participating in exercising often is due to a desire for the morphologic changes resulting from exercise. These changes include (McArdle et al., 1986; Plowman, 1984; Voorrips et al., 1991):

- Decreased body fat and weight
- Increased size of cardiac chambers
- Increased muscle size
- Increased work performance due to increased strength
- Improved flexibility of joints

Psychosocial benefits from exercise incorporate both personal and societal rewards. Personal benefits are (Fort, 1978; McNeil et al., 1991; Norris et al., 1992; NASA, 1984; President's Council on Fitness, 1986; Reuter, 1980):

- Increased stamina
- Improved sleep quality
- Decreased reaction time in elderly
- Decreased stress level
- Tranquilizing effect of exercise
- Improved mood
- Improved self-esteem

Social benefits resulting from attention to physical exercise affects the work and school environments of participants in the following ways (NASA, 1984; President's Council on Physical Fitness, 1986):

- Improved attitude toward work
- Improved work performance
- Decreased absenteeism
- Improved classroom behavior in children
- Decreased emotional and physical disorders
- Fewer accidents

Environment and Exercise

Environmental factors exert an influence on exercise performance. High or low environmental temperatures pose a challenge to the exerciser whose body has a narrow range of temperature norms. Light, loose clothing that allows for rapid evaporation of perspiration is recommended. The symptoms of *heat exhaustion* are nausea, dizziness, mental confusion, and heavy sweating. Usually body temperature is near normal in heat exhaustion. The remedy includes discontinuing the exercise and replenishing fluids. For adults, a fluid intake of 200–300 cc of fluid every 15–20 minutes is recommended during high-level competition in hot weather (Johnson, 1982). Exercise heart rates remain lower in individuals who consume liquids during exercise (Wanner, 1982). *Heat stroke* is a more serious condition associated with hot weather. Indications of heat stroke are elevated body temperature and hot, dry skin. The victim's body temperature must be lowered by removing the person's clothing; increasing heat loss by cool cloths, ice packs, or cool bath; and increasing fluid intake. Immediate medical attention is recommended for heat stroke (Greenberg & Pargman, 1986). In contrast, cold temperatures require that the exerciser dress warmly with multiple layers. Gloves and hats are important for comfort and to prevent heat loss. Careful attention should be paid to protection from undue chilling and frostbite.

When the altitude is above 5,000 feet sea level, the body experiences reduced ability to carry oxygen to tissues. This means that endurance activities are more difficult in high altitudes. The first recognizable symptom associated with high altitudes is hyperventilation. Other symptoms are mental confusion, decreased vision, and sleep disturbances. The remedy is to decrease the extent of the activity and to return to lower altitudes.

Air pollution is the last environmental hazard to be considered. An adequate oxygen supply is essential during exercise. The amount of oxygen available in the air is compromised by pollutants such as carbon monoxide, nitrogen oxides, sulfer oxides, and ozone. During exercise, these pollutants are inhaled excessively as the rate and depth of respirations increase. These pollutants inhibit cardiorespiratory function (Greenberg & Pargman, 1986). The solution to this problem is to avoid strenuous exercise in areas with high pollutants (near freeways, on smog alert days with high pollutant levels, in congested areas). It is clear that in our contemporary society, environmental factors exert significant influence over the reaction and exercise patterns of individuals and families.

Exercise Programs

Components of an exercise fitness program include activities that address (1) endurance, (2) strength, (3) flexibility, and (4) body composition. Endurance usually refers to the body's cardiovascular/cardiopulmonary ability to supply oxygenated blood to the whole system. Aerobic exercises such as walking, swimming, jogging and bicycling, which require sustained work by the heart and lungs, increase the endurance capacity of the body. These types of exercise are appropriate for individuals of all ages and stress the cardiorespiratory system.

Strength exercises such as weight lifting are important in developing muscle mass and contribute to good physical appearance and posture. Results of strength exercises are more obvious in men because women cannot develop the same amount of muscle mass because of the lack of testosterone hormone. Across the age ranges, increased muscular strength results in less fatigue, increased stamina, and improved appearance in adults, children, and the elderly.

Flexibility training is another important aspect of any fitness program. Flexibility is the body's ability to move through the full range of motion at the joints. It involves lengthening and stretching of the elastic fibrous tissue surrounding and connecting the muscle, ligaments, and tendons. These structures may become stiff and shortened if not adequately stretched by a slow, continuous process of about 20–30 seconds' duration (Jopling, 1992). Stretching exercises are important for people of all ages and for the elderly in particular. Stretching should be a normal part of warm up prior to any type of physical exercise.

Body composition is the proportion of body organs, bone, fat, and muscle that makes up the human body. Body fat percentage varies with age and sex. Females carry more body fat than males. Also, the percentage of body fat increases with age. Exercise combined with calorie restrictions effectively assists with body fat and weight control. Norms for body fat composition and measurement techniques are readily available in the current literature (contact the President's Council on Physical Fitness and Sports, Washington, DC, 20001).

EXERCISE AND RECREATION ACROSS THE LIFE CYCLE

Leisure activities that involve the components of recreation and exercise will provide a wide range of positive effects at all stages of the life cycle. The literature is increasing in this field of study and seems to substantiate what the recreationalists and exercisers are already convinced of—it's good for us. If one can continue to approach leisure activities as activities that are intended to restore, replenish, and rejuvenate, their benefits will be apparent in healthy individuals. This section addresses specific issues related to children, young and middle adults, and the elderly.

Children and Exercise

As children grow up, they are constantly changing physically and functionally. Increases in structure (growth) are accompanied by increases in function (development). Being aware of these developmental stages will aid in selecting appropriate recreation, exercise, and sports activities for children. With this understanding, the risk of injury can be reduced, and positive emotional as well as physical development can be promoted.

Infants

In infants, the purpose of activity is to develop muscular strength and coordination for basic movements, such as rolling over, sitting, crawling, and eventually walking. The instinctive activity of an infant exploring his or her environment by reaching, scooting, and kicking often will provide the necessary exercise for optimal development.

Problems in this age group can arise with the extensive use of such devices as strollers, playpens, windup swings, and walkers. Because these may restrict an infant's movement, muscular activity and development can thereby be decreased. Windup swings, may encourage passive motion and cause the infant to lose the desire to move about and explore. Parents can encourage their child to use his or her arms and legs through stimulation and guided play sessions.

Toddlers and Preschoolers

Generally, the purpose of exercise with this age group continues to be the promotion of coordination and muscular development. Both groups are typically very active and need no directed exercise. Movement in toddlers is crucial to self discovery. In fact, because of the short attention span of toddlers and preschoolers, any attempt to introduce structured exercise may frustrate them and the teacher and promote a dislike for exercise.

Drowning is responsible for 15% of all deaths in children ages one to four. As a result, organized swimming classes have become quite popular. The author recommends that formal swimming lessons not be instituted until a child is at least 3 years old. It is believed that children younger than this are unable to be taught water safety or appropriate reactions to emergency situations. Furthermore, it is believed that such classes may give parents a false sense of security.

School Children

Development of muscular strength, balance, and coordination is an important purpose of exercise in the school-aged child. Many experts feel, however, that the psychosocial development may be even more important. They believe that team sports offer an opportunity for the school-aged child to learn to work cooperatively with others, to meet new friends, and to develop self-esteem and self-confidence.

It is during these school years that organized competitive team sports are introduced. There are basically three types of organized sports: noncontact, contact, and collision. Noncontact sports include swimming, gymnastics, and some track and field events. They are appropriate for children from ages six to seven. Contact sports include soccer, softball, basketball, and wrestling. It is recommended that participants be at least eight to ten years old. Younger children usually lack the necessary muscular development and have a greater chance of injury. The collision sports are typified by football, hockey, and rugby. They are recommended for post-pubescent children because it is only after most muscle growth has occurred that children are able to handle the associated physical trauma without serious injury.

Children and Sports

The American Academy of Pediatrics Committee on Sports Medicine and Committee on School Health (1989) provides recommendations regarding sports. They suggest that the preadolescent years are the time to develop an enjoyment of sports, physical fitness, positive self-image, basic motor skills, and a commitment to teamwork and sportsmanship. These attributes can be developed through participation in organized athletic programs. There is a dramatic increase in sports participation for both sexes and females in particular.

Some physiologic issues concerning children, training, and sports need to be answered. Is sports training harmful to the preadolescent epiphysis? Sports-related injuries are common; about one-half of all adolescent boys and one-fourth of all adolescent girls receive medical attention due to sports-related injuries (McKeag, 1991). Evidence suggests that recovery from epiphyseal injuries occurs without medical intervention in 98% of children (McKeag, 1991). Also, nutritional requirements for young athletes do not call for additional nutrients beyond an increase in calories to meet the extra energy demands. The pediatric athlete also has adequate thermoregulatory mechanisms to meet the demands of increased exercise. Training at moderate levels appears beneficial for children, but inadequate or excess physical activities are detrimental (McKeag, 1991). One of the long-term specific benefits of exercise in children is the long-term decrease in body fat composition as young adults and a stronger, more supple adult body physique (McKeag, 1991).

Proficiency in a sport takes time and work. About four and a half to five years of practice with a sport are required to become adept and to gain neuromuscular skill in the sport. Most children do not have the neuromuscular ability to train for a sport until five years of age. One exception to this is running. There also appears to be little effect of cardiorespiratory training on children until adolescence. Then at adolescence, cardiopulmonary efficiency decreases unless physical training is initiated for maintenance. The price children pay for skill at a particular sport is time in practice. Because time is limited, the child involved in sports will have less time for other activities and pursuits.

Young children, parents, and athletic directors alike all need to be informed that the need for fun in this age group has not changed. According to Nathan Smith (1985, p. 1) "The most important goal of sports in the lives of preadolescents should be to have fun and learn to share a pleasurable time with peers and friends; to enjoy some energy-expending exercise; to experience a low-keyed introduction to sports and sports skills; and to encounter and identify with new adult models." Smith goes on to say that preadolescents should be introduced to winning and losing only when they are mature enough to know that worthiness is not based on the outcome of an athletic performance or contest. These aims and goals must not be lost amid multiple practices, all-star teams, trophies, and award banquets. Children, parents, and other adults involved in sports for children can be helped with the understanding that what children need from sports and exercise changes with the child's age.

Sports and Physical Development

Although age is the most common basis for a child's participation in a specific sport, many experts suggest that it should be less important due to the vast differences in size and development in children. Thus, participation may be based on physical characteristics, such as height and weight (Siegel, 1985). A suitable test for evaluating muscle strength and flexibility in preschool through adolescent children is the Knaus-Weber Test (K-W). This test measures minimal performance and is easy to administer in less than two minutes. A complete review of the test can be found in *How to Keep Your Child Fit from Birth to Six* (Prudden, 1986). Not every child is suited to all sports. Basketball and football are generally geared to those with a larger, taller stature, and gymnastics, swimming, tennis, and some track and field events are generally suited to those with smaller statures. Directing a child to the sport to which he or she is most physically suited will help to assure that the child's experience will be a positive one.

Prepuberty

Before the onset of pubertal changes, few physical differences exist between young boys and girls in size and strength. Therefore, there is no reason why boys and girls should not compete against each other or play on the same teams. When girls begin their rapid growth and pubertal development about age 10 or 11, boys and girls should probably compete only against other children of the same gender. Boys generally are stronger and taller and have decided physical advantages that make mixed-sex competition unfair and unsafe after male puberty has been achieved.

Puberty

For most 11- to 14-year-olds (Tanner Stages 2 and 3) in junior high and middle schools, skeletal immaturity and large variations in body size and strength make collision sports such as football, hockey, and rugby inappropriate and potentially unsafe. In addition, weight/strength training should not be encouraged during this time as it will generally result in little increase in muscle size and strength (Smith, 1985). The child of this age who is entering the period of most rapid height increase is in the period of greatest risk for serious epiphyseal skeletal injury. Thus, competitive collision sports should be avoided.

Although an increase in weight during the adolescent period is associated with a measurable increase in strength, newly developed muscles are weak and limited in flexibility. Aerobic conditioning and weight/strength training with weights should be discouraged at all times as it carries a high risk of injury.

Physical Maturity (15–20 Years Old)

Muscular endurance can be achieved at physical maturity since there is the potential for increasing capillary numbers in response to physical training. Muscle phosphofructokinase has also developed by this time, allowing for anaerobic carbohydrate metabolism as an energy source. Muscular and skeletal maturity now permit a serious commitment to collision sports. Fortunately, fractures and lacerations are relatively infrequent injuries. Sprains and strains (stretching injury to tendons and muscles) account for about two-thirds of injuries in most studies. Football and wrestling lead the list of injuries occurring in high school competitive sports; swimming and tennis cause the fewest injuries.

Special attention must be given to the impact of exercise on women. It is recognized that exercise can affect menstruation, particularly among women involved in high-intensity training and competition in sports such as long-distance running, gymnastics, swimming, and dancing. For example, approximately one-third of female distance runners develop amenorrhea during their training and competitive seasons. The amenorrhea is due to a critical lean-fat ratio. Generally a weight gain restores the normal menstrual cycle. In the case of an adolescent, body fat levels of less than 17% may delay the onset of puberty. Parents, coaches, and athletes should be advised that a medical evaluation should be done to determine if secondary amenorrhea is a normal variation of athletic training, a pathologic problem, or a pregnancy. Fear of breast injuries are a common concern of female athletes; however, serious injuries to the breasts are rare. Tight-fitting "dancers" and sports bras are generally recommended to reduce discomfort and irritation for women participating in athletic activities.

Levels of iron in the blood of women have been found to be significantly decreased after heavy physical training; thus, female athletes, especially those who have heavy menstrual blood losses, may wish to consider supplementing their diets with extra iron. A note of caution is needed: Overdoses of iron can be toxic. Therefore, the athlete contemplating taking iron supplements should first consult a physician.

Weight training increases strength and muscle tone and may be advocated for females in sports activities, particularly for those engaging in sports that demand a great deal of strength. Wilmore (1974) found women could increase their upper body strength by 15% to 45% with minimal hypertrophy of muscles. Muscular hypertrophy is influenced by the male hormone testosterone. Therefore, weight training will not cause excessive bulging of the muscles in females.

Assessing Youth Fitness

A careful medical evaluation is a vital first step in the prevention of injuries in young athletes. The physical examination will help determine whether a child can participate safely in a particular sport or should be guided to another activity. The results of the examination may temporarily suspend the child's participation or may preclude certain sports altogether. For more information concerning the preparticipation examination of the young athlete, see Runyan (1983) and Smith (1985).

There are very few tests available to assess the physical fitness of children. Most physical fitness tests available are for children 16 years and older. The scarcity of current testing standards for children indicates more research is needed in assessing physical fitness in children.

The two most common youth fitness tests available are the President's Council on Physical Fitness and Sports test (PCPFS), and the American Alliance for Health, Physical Education, Recreation and Dance test (AAHPERD). However, some experts feel that these tests are based on a battery of tests that are motor-fitness related, not health related. Experts also feel that factors such as body build (shape and density), height, weight, body fat, style and efficiency of running, experience, and cardiovascular endurance (VO2 max) should be considered (Murphy, 1986; Rowland, 1981).

Various parameters are measured in the youth fitness tests currently available for determining physical fitness in children. These parameters include pull-ups or flexed arm hang and sit-ups to measure arm and abdominal strength. The sit-and-reach tests measure flexibility. Aerobic and anaerobic conditioning/endurance are determined by the 50 yard dash; shuttle run; and one-mile, 1 1/2 mile, and two-mile runs. Detailed standards are available in the literature (Murphy, 1986; Prudden, 1986, 1988; Rowland, 1981). Further development and refinement of youth fitness testing is currently taking place.

Research suggests that regular physical activity, begun in childhood, may help prevent degenerative diseases. Physical activity is necessary for a growing child and is well documented in terms of growth and fitness needs. Physical activity increases muscle tone, improves respiration and circulation, benefits digestion, aids in controlling obesity, promotes rehabilitation after illness and surgery, and stimulates proper growth and development. Physical benefits alone could be sufficient reasons for supporting physical exercise and education programs for children.

Recreation and Exercise for the Pregnant Adult

In recent years there has been an emphasis on physical conditioning and exercise during pregnancy. The emphasis has focused on the benefits to the pregnant mother as well as the developing fetus. Specific research studies have been undertaken to address this issue on a scientific basis (Clapp, 1991). Because of a variety of limitations inherent in these studies, their results must be used with caution. However, they do indicate an overall pattern: complications of pregnancy and delivery both for the mother and for the child are decreased in well-conditioned females. One study showed multiparas who exercised during pregnancy had more endogenous hormones, less stress hormones, and less pain on delivery (Varrassi et al., 1989). There is also evidence of increased risk of preterm labor for mothers who have jobs that require standing versus sitting (Teitelman et al. 1990). Further, women who were active during pregnancy delivered babies who had higher APGARs at 1 minute but who showed no difference in 5 minutes APGARs or birth weight (Rice & Fort, 1991.) A knowledge of the basic physiologic changes occurring during this reproductive time is essential. Beyond the information provided in this section, one may refer to the articles listed in the references for more information on this topic.

In the first trimester, some of the usual changes in a woman's body relate to nausea, vomiting, tenderness and growth of the breasts, and increasingly frequent urination. The major increase in blood volume occurs in this period with the plasma volume increasing from 40% to 90% (Bullard, 1981), leading to what is called a "hyperdynamic state." There is a concomitant increase in cardiac output and renal perfusion, leading to an increased glomerular filtration rate. Ventilation rate also begins to increase during this time due to an increased sensitization to carbon dioxide levels. This sensitivity often leads to the "breathlessness" described by many pregnant individuals (Mullinax & Edwin, 1986).

In the second trimester, the breasts continue to develop and the uterus rises out of the pelvis and into the abdomen. Bones and joints in the pelvis and low back begin to soften, often leading to low back pain. Decreased motility of the bowel potentiates problems with elimination and can often bring on hemorrhoids. As the uterus continues to grow and places increased pressure on the major veins coming from the legs, there are often problems associated with altered venous return. In the late second and early third trimester, cardiac output increases at a lessened rate due, in part, to the altered venous return (Mullinax & Edwin, 1986). Moderate exercise such as walking during this period contributes to increasing and improving venous return and general circulation.

In the third trimester, physiologic changes primarily involve growth of the uterus in the abdomen. Many of the other changes noted above continue to exist. Because of the enlarging uterus, problems associated with balance and center of gravity begin to appear. Exercise in the last trimester is thought to be associated with premature labor. The rowing ergometer, recumbent bicycle, and upper arm ergometer produce the least uterine activity (Durak et al. 1990). Increased ligamentation relaxation and joint mobility also result in potential for sports-related injuries (Warren, 1991).

When beginning an exercise program, the pregnant adult must keep in mind virtually the same cautions as the nonpregnant adult. If the individual is sedentary, activity must be chosen carefully to allow for a gradual conditioning. The special considerations to be taken by the pregnant adult should include the following:

1. Choose activities that do not place direct impact on the abdomen.
2. Protect the breast area with adequate support to avoid the problems associated with tissue breakdown. Use a well-fitted support bra.
3. Choose activities suited to the level of fitness and coordination of the pregnant individual. Problems related to coordination will be exaggerated during this period. Consider those activities that will be positively reinforcing.
4. Select attire and an environment where the pregnant individual can feel comfortable to perform the selected activities.
5. Avoid hot tubs and exercising in extreme heat because of the problems of hyperthermia for the pregnant adult as well as for the developing fetus.
6. Lower intensity exercises should be chosen. Any activity that employs large muscle groups in weight-bearing, repetitive action should be altered by decreasing intensity and decreasing the weight-bearing component. An example of such a modification

would be making a switch from walking or aerobic dancing to swimming.

7. All exercises on an anaerobic level should be avoided throughout the pregnancy (Mullinax & Edwin, 1986; Bullard, 1981).

8. Exercises that require a change in atmospheric pressure should be avoided (Barger, 1988).

9. Avoid scuba diving and high altitude activities.

Further, specific guidelines for exercise during pregnancy have been reported by The American College of Obstetricians and Gynecologists (Gauthier, 1986). These guidelines include the following recommendations:

1. The maternal heart rate should not exceed 140 beats per minute.

2. Strenuous activities should not last longer than 15 minutes.

3. Exercises in the supine position should not be done after the fourth month of pregnancy.

4. Pregnant women should avoid the Valsalva maneuver.

5. Sufficient calories and fluids should be ingested to cover the demands of both pregnancy and exercise.

6. Maternal core temperature should stay below 38 degrees C.

The Young and Middle-Aged Adult

This population of individuals seems to have the greatest appetite for recreation and exercise. However, this can be a double-edged sword. What was intended to rejuvenate and recreate all too often drains and frustrates the participant as he or she is unable to meet his or her goals. Though the young middle-aged are often familiar with basic exercise, they frequently have not acquired the ability to engage in regular exercise activity. The nurse's role in health promotion for the age group may be to motivate the adult to begin an exercise program. The middle-aged population needs to consider the following suggestions:

1. Create additional time for activities, other than planned exercise sessions, that will provide true rejuvenation.

2. Rethink present recreation activity/exercise involvements. Perhaps what is needed is something as simple as including someone else in the session to add the element of friendship and communication.

3. Evaluate the environment presently used for activity/exercise. Perhaps a simple change of place would help, e.g., inside to outside. Or, perhaps what is needed is a change from outside alone to inside with a group, e.g., a health spa.

4. Evaluate personal goals: Are they realistic given the present level of conditioning, age, and time constraints? It may be necessary to seek objective counsel to help in setting realistic goals.

A variety of available activities are classed in categories from low- to high-intensity activities. According to Pollock et al. (1984), low-intensity exercises for adults are defined as those that expend less than 5 Kcal/minute. Moderate-intensity activities expend 5–10 Kcal/minute, and those activities that expend 10–14 Kcal/minute are classified as moderate to high intensity. Any activity that expends 14 Kcal/minute or more is termed high-intensity activity.

In selecting activities, one may refer to the list in Table 16–3 as a general guideline. This list is a summary of research represented in Pollock et al. (1984).

TABLE 16–3. ACTIVITY ACCORDING TO INTENSITY LEVEL

LOW-INTENSITY ACTIVITY
Archery
Recreational basketball
Bowling
Fishing
Golf (using a power cart)
Horseshoe pitching
Sailing
Shuffleboard
Slow walking

MODERATE-INTENSITY ACTIVITY
Badminton
Bicycling (recreational and stationary)
Canoeing/rowing
Calisthenics
Dancing (recreational and aerobic)
Fencing
Swimming
Volleyball
Circuit training
Golf (walking)
Hiking
Walking/jogging
SCUBA diving
Skating
Skiing (downhill)
Soccer

HIGH-INTENSITY ACTIVITY
Squash
Snowshoeing
Cross-country skiing
Rope skipping
Racquet/paddle ball
Big game hunting
Handball
Running

Older Adults

The considerations for exercise, recreation, and leisure in this population involve much more than at any other time in life. Leisure time tends to take on a whole new meaning during these years. It is often difficult to decide what to do with all of the leisure time now available.

Following is a list of many of the needs that can be met by leisure and recreational/exercise activities during this phase of life (Moran, 1979).

1. Social group interaction. This is often used to replace what was previously taken up by work and friends in the preretirement setting. This may be important as well because of the void left by a deceased friend or partner.
2. Sense of status and achievement.
3. Development of positive attitudes toward leisure activities.
4. Incorporation of certain aspects of work, e.g., hobbies that create things to be sold. This reinforces the sense of usefulness and heightens the sense of self-worth.
5. Regular, organized activities that provide a sense of community and identity for the individual.

In addition, there are many social and physical factors that must be taken into account by the older adult. These would include financial considerations and physical limitations. Many activities are available that take these considerations into account. Groups like churches, retirement centers, country clubs, civic groups, YMC(H)A, and YWC(H)A often have a variety of activities for the older adult. The following are but a few activities that can be undertaken:

- Aquatic exercise
- Dances
- Walking clubs, e.g., shopping-mall walking groups
- Outings, e.g., camping, mini-trips, cruises
- Golf
- Hiking
- Exercise classes
- Bowling
- Badminton or tennis
- Croquette
- Deck or table tennis

The older adult is often more interested in the social factors involved in leisure activities than in fitness. It is important to provide for the needs of the older adult in the area of recreation and exercise. Recreation and exercise will keep the individual sharp, physically, socially, psychologically and mentally.

NURSING APPROACHES TO PROMOTE FAMILY RECREATION AND EXERCISE

The nurse's role in promoting recreation and exercise consists of modeling behaviors, providing an education and a knowledge base, and contracting for client self-care through the nursing process. As nurses increasingly become the primary providers for health teaching and preventive maintenance, their expanded role demands they serve as role models and become more informed in the health care of the well client or family member. To develop contracts related to active recreation and exercise, the nurse must assess and evaluate each family member's level of physical development and fitness potential. Guidelines from the American Heart Association (1990) and the President's Council on Physical Fitness (1986), as well as recent relevant research, serve as a basis for goal setting and decision making. Because most of the research has been completed under exercise conditions, this author will discuss active recreation and exercise as having the same guidelines and parameters throughout the remainder of this chapter.

The Nursing Process

Assessment

A primary question professional nurses need to address is whether to recommend that a family member have a physical examination and stress testing prior to initiating active recreation or an exercise program. The American Heart Association (1990) recommends that if the client checks one or more of the following items as positive, he or she should have a physical exam before starting these programs:

___ 1. High blood pressure
___ 2. Heart trouble
___ 3. Family history of early stroke or heart attacks
___ 4. Frequent dizzy spells
___ 5. Breathlessness after mild exertion
___ 6. Severe muscular, ligament, or tendon problems
___ 7. Other known or suspected diseases
___ 8. You are over 40 and not accustomed to regular exercise

A physical exam is recommended for all males over 45 and for all females over 50 who are not accustomed to vigorous exercise.

Fair et al. (1979) add that the risk factors for coronary artery disease include hypertension, smoking, diabetes, hyperlipidemia, and a family history of early atherosclerotic disease. The presence of these factors would modify exercise prescription, even in the younger than 45–50 age group. Chronic active health problems such as asthma, hyperthyroidism, chronic renal disease, chronic infectious processes, anemia, obesity, and back problems should be carefully evaluated in all family members before prescribing exercise. Previous injuries could also influence the type of aerobic exercise performed. Maximum blood pressure acceptable during exercise for adults is 240/120 mm Hg. Exercise should be terminated if the person reaches those levels (Cooper, 1990). More detailed information regarding exercise and hypertension is available in *Overcoming Hypertension* by Cooper (1990).

To evaluate general aerobic fitness, a one-mile walking test has been developed for persons between the ages of 30 and 69. Clients are advised to walk one mile as fast as they can and to time themselves. Then they should compare their results with the times in Table 16–4.

If family members are inactive but healthy, they should start with mile-long walks taking 20 minutes (three miles per hour) five times a week. Over the course of a month, they can increase their pace to a mile in 15 minutes, also five times per week. Studies show that "brisk" walking at speeds of $3\frac{1}{2}$ to $4\frac{1}{2}$ miles per hour produces cardiovascular benefits. Slow walking (two miles per hour) can be "advantageous to older people, cardiac patients, or people recuperating from illness" (*Walking: A Program for Life,* 1987, p. 6).

The one-mile walking test gives concrete evidence of the need for a fitness program and can serve as a guideline for initial fitness contracting between the professional nurse and the clients. The nurse acts as a resource person who offers guidance; the client or family has the responsibility for initiating and completing the program or contract.

Nursing Diagnosis

After a thorough assessment of the family's fitness needs, knowledge base, risk factors, and exercise capabilities, the nurse and family should agree on a nursing diagnosis. The most common nursing diagnosis that would call for an exercise or active recreation program would be "health maintenance alteration related to a sedentary or inactive lifestyle." Exercise may also be an intervention for additional diagnoses such as:

- Alteration in nutrition: more than body requirements related to excessive intake in relation to metabolic need
- Knowledge deficit related to the role of exercise in preventing coronary artery disease
- Knowledge deficit related to the role of active recreation and exercise in promoting health
- Altered growth and development related to lack of exercise and activity
- Alterations in cardiac output: decreased: activity intolerance secondary to myocardial ischemia
- Self-care deficit related to muscle weakness after prolonged immobility. (Carpenito, 1991).

Goal Setting through Mutual Contracting

The goals of an exercise or recreation program are to:

1. Increase the individual's or family's awareness of the need for physical activity
2. Teach family members how to safely achieve cardiovascular fitness
3. Assist clients to maintain the lifestyle change (Bulechek & McCloskey, 1985, p. 206).

For each of the above goals, mutual goal setting or contracting between the professional nurse and the family is most important for initiating and maintaining change. Brykczynski (1982, p. 27) states that the characteristics of good goal setting and good health contracting are "completely congruent." Both processes must be specific, measurable, attainable, and time limited. The belief that all persons have potential for change and growth and that the family is accountable and reasonable is the basis of the process. Open communication and flexibility are essential and must be promoted. Hill and Smith (1985) warn us that contracting requires much patience and work. A wide divergence may exist between clients' goals and goals the nurse would set for them.

Health professionals are encouraged to contract not only with active clients and families but also with the sedentary majority. The "Objectives for the Nation" for the year 2000 developed by the

TABLE 16–4. ONE-MILE WALKING TEST

CATEGORY	MALE (MIN:SEC)	FEMALE (MIN:SEC)
Excellent	Less than 10:12	Less than 11:40
Good	10:13–11:42	11:41–13:08
High average	11:43–13:13	13:09–14:36
Low average	13:14–14:44	14:37–16:04
Fair	14:45–16:23	16:05–17:31
Poor	More than 16:24	More than 17:32

Public Health Service propose that 30% or more of the population aged 19–64 should achieve the optimum goal of "vigorous physical exercise." The rest of the population should aim for exercising three times a week for the same frequency and duration but with less vigorous activities like walking.

Nursing Interventions

Fair et al. (1979) list six criteria that must be met if recreation and exercise interventions are to achieve their desired effect:

1–3. Describe the *duration, intensity,* and *frequency* of the conditioning exercise
4. Include a warm-up and cool-down period
5. Prescribe a training program that can be easily incorporated into the daily routine of the client
6. Determine methods for monitoring the exercise and conditions that would warrant discontinuing the program (p. 17)

Duration, Intensity, and Frequency

Certain active recreation and exercises are naturally very vigorous, aerobic, and need to be done at least 15 minutes three times per week. The activities that are considered conditioning for the cardiopulmonary systems are cross-country skiing, uphill hiking, ice hockey, jogging, jumping rope, rowing, running in place, and stationary cycling. Other activities are moderately vigorous but can be excellent conditioners if done for at least 30 minutes, three times per week. If done briskly, they also condition both the heart and the lungs. These are bicycling, downhill skiing, basketball, calisthenics, field hockey, handball, racquetball, soccer, squash, swimming, singles tennis, and walking. Sports that can help relieve tension, improve muscle tone, and increase coordination serve as excellent recreation but that do *not* condition the cardiopulmonary system include baseball, bowling, football, golf (on foot or by cart), softball, and volleyball (American Heart Association, 1990).

Cooper (1982) ranks the top five athletic activities that provide the best aerobic conditioning potential:

1. *Cross-country skiing* is the most aerobic because of the number of muscles involved and because it is usually done at high altitudes.
2. *Swimming* involves all the major muscles in the body and gives total conditioning effect. There are also fewer problems with injuries because the buoyancy of the water reduces exercise pressure on joints and bones.
3. *Jogging or running* has a low level of skill, but the injuries with jogging are high, especially if you do not warm up properly.
4. *Outdoor cycling* causes less wear and tear on the joints and muscles than jogging. The elderly and people with joint problems can greatly benefit.
5. *Walking* can be done anywhere by anyone but takes about three times as long to get the same aerobic effect as from running. The slower pace encourages conversation and companionship, which can be very beneficial for continued programs.

How hard should one exercise? For the average individual, the intensity recommended by the American Heart Association (1990) is between 50% to 75% of the maximum heart rate (220 minus age). Find the individual's age category in Table 16–5, and recommend training within the target heart rate. A common rule to remember is to exercise to the perspiration point while maintaining the ability to carry on a conversation (Jopling, 1992).

When beginning to exercise, aim for the lowest target zone (50%) during the first few months. Certainly those family members who fall into the poor to low-average categories on the one-mile

TABLE 16–5. ADULT TARGET EXERCISE HEART RATES

AGE YEARS	MAXIMUM HEART RATE	TARGET ZONE		
		50%	75%	85%
20	200			
25	195	98	146	170
30	190	95	142	165
35	185	93	138	160
40	180	90	135	155
45	175	88	131	150
50	170	85	127	145
55	165	83	123	140
60	160	80	120	135
65+	155	76	116	130

Data from President's Council on Physical Fitness and Sports (1986) and American Heart Association (1990).

walking test should aim for the lowest target zone initially. One study found that "90% of women, and two-thirds of the men" between ages 30 and 69 could achieve target training zone within 12 weeks by fast walking alone. Remember that the lower the fitness, the lower the exercise intensity required to induce a training effect (*Walking for Fitness*, 1986). Monahan (1986 p. 194) writes that "joints are more protected when muscles are toned, but become increasingly vulnerable when muscles are pushed beyond the point of fatigue." He further recommends a vigorous two- to three-month walking program prior to participation in sports or aerobic dance, particularly for both men and women over 40 years of age. After six months or more of regular exercise, individuals can exercise up to 85% of their maximum heart rate if they wish. However, it is not necessary to exercise that hard to stay in good condition (American Heart Association 1990).

To maintain fitness, one must exercise on a regular basis. After two weeks without training, the level of fitness decreases significantly. "After 10 weeks to 8 months, you may be no fitter than when you started training" (*Aerobic Exercise*, 1986, p. 6).

To check the target heart rate, take the pulse immediately after exercising. Using the carotid artery in the neck, count the pulse for 10 seconds and multiply by 6. If the pulse is below the target zone, one should try a little harder; if the pulse is above the zone, one should slow down. Cooper (1970) cautions that one should also check his or her recovery heart rate. The sooner the heart rate returns to a normal resting rate after strenuous exercise (usually one to three minutes), the fitter the person. "If it's still over 120, it's a sign that the exercise was too tough for a person in your condition. Ten minutes after exercise it should be back to 100. If it isn't, let up a little on your exercise program" (p. 42).

Warming Up and Cooling Down

Providing for a warm-up and cool-down period is of utmost importance. The American Heart Association recommends a 5-minute warm up (stretching and medium-paced activities), 15–30 minutes of exercising at your target zone, and 5 minutes of cooling down. The total exercise time, depending on the activity, would be 25–40 minutes. By cooling down, one slows down gradually—swimming less vigorously, progressing from running to walking, and so on. Stretching after exercise is included to loosen up muscles and to prevent stiffness (American Heart Association, 1990). Also, an abrupt drop in blood pressure can occur when vigorous activity is suddenly stopped. This blood pressure drop can lead to fainting and cardiac arrythmias in susceptible people. It has been found that the "immediate post-exercise phase can be one of enormous stress on your heart" (*After Exercise*, 1985, p. 2). Family members should be carefully instructed concerning gradual cessation of exercise.

Incorporation into a Daily Routine

Developing an exercise program that can be easily incorporated into one's daily life requires thorough self-care contracting with the family. Hill and Smith (1990) state that the criteria for a realistic plan include exercise that would (1) allow the family to participate near or at home; (2) be cost conscious—programs and equipment should be low cost (if necessary); and (3) fit into home routines with minor alterations.

Exercise programs do take time. Frequently, family members are too ambitious initially and do not set realistic and attainable goals. A realistic first goal may be to "complete the One-Mile Walking Test" (see previous paragraphs). Another example would be to walk ten minutes Monday, Wednesday, and Friday for the first week or to do stretching exercises five minutes every other day. Small, planned successes help to avoid discouraging failures.

Some families can set long-term goals immediately. For example, a walking program with five-minute warm up, five minutes of brisk walking, and five minutes of slow walking could also be a goal for the first week. Adding two minutes to the "brisk" walking time, three times each week for 12 weeks may be an agreeable long-term contract for some (American Heart Association, 1990).

There are exercise strategies useful for individual family members who are on the busy schedules. Parking the car a mile or two from work and walking rapidly to the destination gives a moderately good aerobic workout. Walking up flights of stairs rather than using the elevators, or devoting one-half your lunch hour three times a week to fitness, are possibilities. Stamford (1986) advises "not to engage in vigorous exercise for at least two and preferably three hours after eating" (p. 162). Therefore, the timing of meals should influence the time for exercise. Because the metabolic rate remains elevated after vigorous exercise, weight loss may be affected by the time of day chosen for exercise.

Conditions that Warrant Cessation of Exercise

The American Heart Association (1990) warns that prevention is the most powerful medicine for injuries. Caution must be taken to build up activity gradually over weeks and to adhere to the previously mentioned warming up and cooling down periods. Again, one should slowly build up to his or her target heart rate over weeks. An awareness of possible signs of heart problems is always necessary. Nurses should warn family members to stop exercising immediately and to seek medical attention at the first opportunity if they experience any of the following conditions (American Heart Association, 1990; Hill & Smith, 1990):

- Chest, neck, or arm pain
- A significant increase in shortness of breath
- Fainting, light headedness, or dizziness
- An irregular heart beat
- Nausea and vomiting during or following exercise
- Prolonged fatigue

Frequently people complain of a pain "below their bottom rib." The American Heart Association (1990) states that vigorous exercising may cause this "side stitch," and it is not the result of a heart problem. One must "listen" to his or her body for early warning pains. Excessive exercising can cause injuries to feet, joints, ankles, and legs. Minor strains and injuries to the muscles and joints should be treated immediately with rest, ice, compression, and elevation. A physician should be consulted if pain and swelling persist. Soreness need not make one stop but should lengthen the warm-up period and moderate activity (Myth: No Pain, No Gain, 1985).

Bulechek and McCloskey (1985, p. 213) report that a large number of all "pains and injuries suffered by runners, joggers, and walkers are related to a lack of shock absorption or lack of motion control. The body absorbs shock as the impact of a poorly padded foot on a hard surface transmits a force through the heel and leg." This, coupled with excessive flattening of the foot as it moves through the gait cycle, causes the most common running injuries: knee pain, shin splints, ankle pain, low back pain, arch pain, tendinitis,

and hip and calf pain. Both knee pain and shin splints are reported more frequently by female runners. Both symptoms are related to the intensity of running, and there is little fear of physical injury for individuals who jog or run 10 miles or less per week (Rudy & Estok, 1983).

For joggers, a careful selection of running shoes is mandatory. Shoes should be light-weight and yet provide maximum cushioning to prevent overstretching of muscles and tendons. A good arch support, a cushioned sole, and a one-inch heel should all fit well enough to keep the foot from slipping within the shoe (Bulechek & McCloskey, 1985).

Aerobic dance has become a popular form of recreation and exercise. A modified form of aerobic dance called low-impact aerobics has evolved. Low-impact aerobic exercise substitutes side-to-side marching or gliding movements, low kicks, and high-powered steps for the jolting up-and-down motion of high-impact aerobics. At least one foot remains on the floor, and the exerciser's arms are constantly moving above the level of the heart. Low-impact aerobic exercise has gained in popularity as a way to tone muscles and reap the benefits of aerobic exercise without subjecting the body to excessive stress and strain.

The low-impact approach assumes that jumpless dance steps, proper floor surfaces, and proper aerobic shoes will reduce the impact shock on muscles and joints. Studies have found that low-impact aerobic dance does have fitness benefits, and future studies will determine its effectiveness in decreasing injuries. To make workouts more challenging and still achieve optimum cardiovascular conditioning, 1/2- to 2-pound hand or wrist weights can be used during workouts.

TABLE 16–6. THREE-MONTH AEROBIC FITNESS WALKING PROGRAM

WEEK	MILE	MINUTES OF WALKING			
		< 30 YRS.	30–49 YRS.	50–59 YRS.	60+ YRS.
1	1.0	16	17	19	22
2	1.0	14	15	17	20
3	1.5	22	24	26	30
4	1.5	21	23	25	29
5	2.0	29	32	34	39
6	2.0	28	31	33	38
7	2.5	36	40	42	48
8	2.5	35	39	41	47
9	3.0	43	48	50	57
10	3.0	42.30	47	49	55
11	3.0	42	46	48	53
12	3.0	< 42	< 45	< 47	< 51

A walking program 4–5 times a week is encouraged for fitness. A minimal level of fitness may be achieved with 3 times a week (Cooper, 1990).

Data from Cooper, K. (1990). *Overcoming Hypertension*. New York: Bantam Books.

Contracting for Individual Family Members

Cooper (1988) has developed exercise programs for people "under 30 years of age," "30–49 years of age," "50–59 years of age," and "60 and over." These programs are included for almost all types of recreation and exercise from walking to swimming to stair climbing to racquetball. For an example of a typical program see Table 16–6.

For programs designed specifically for women, the reader is referred to *New Aerobics for Women* (Cooper, 1988). Multiple programs are available in every community and can be identified by contacting local community agencies.

Baldi et al. (1980) devised a form for self-contracting (Fig. 16–2) that could be adapted to assist the nurse and the family to develop and implement an exercise program. This form includes goal setting, environmental planning (in-

---

FAMILY CONTRACT

My Goals:

Short-term—by the end of six weeks we will . . . __walk for 20 minutes 4x a week__

Long-term—by the end of six months we will . . . __walk/run for 30 minutes 5x a week__

Environmental Planning: (all the steps we will take to reach our goal)

1. Buy good walking shoes
2. Set our alarm clock 30 minutes early
3. Set out our exercise clothes the night before
4. Find a pretty place to walk in
5. Keep a calendar on our refrigerator (star for each day we meet our goal)

Thoughts and Actions

Helpful thoughts: We really do sleep better when we exercise like this.	Helpful actions: We will compliment each others' physical improvement!
Non-helpful thoughts: It's more important that we get our rest today.	Non-helpful actions: Eating a heavy meal before our planned exercise time

My Reward (if we meet our goals) We will go as a family to Disneyland

The Cost: (if we fail to meet our goals) We will all clean the garage together

Reevaluation Date: 6 Weeks—7/30 6 Montha—11/13

I agree to help with this project:

_____
(Support Person)

We agree to strive toward this goal:

_____
(Your Signatures)   (Date)

FIGURE 16–2. Family contract. Format adapted with permission from Susan Baldi et al., *For Your Health: A Model for Self-Care* (South Laguna, CA: Nurses Model Health, 1980), p. 47.

terventions), helpful and nonhelpful thoughts and actions, rewards, costs, and an evaluation date. The contract is signed by both the nurse and the family members. The inclusion of an environmental planning section allows the family to list steps to take to reach their goal. Addressing nonhelpful thoughts and actions assists the family to replace negative thought patterns by more positive (helpful) thoughts and actions. This author has found that such contracts allow the nurse insight into the client's attitudes and into negative as well as positive "self-talk." Frequently these thoughts and attitudes need to be discussed before progress is made.

Evaluation

Planned evaluations are an integral part of the nursing process. Families should monitor the leisure, recreation, and exercise of their members at periodic intervals. The facilitators, barriers, and results of recreation and exercise programs should be identified as the family evaluates physical changes of its members and the impact on family relationships (Keller, 1988). Do family members

sleep better? Have they reached ideal weight? What factors hinder or help in a member's exercise program? What has been the effect of individual and family recreation and exercise on family relationships? Family patterns of recreation and exercise may need revision in light of individual and family life changes such as pregnancy, increased work demands, graduations, or illness (Hill & Smith, 1990).

REFERENCES

Aerobic exercise: How much, how often (1986). *University of California, Berkeley Wellness Letter, 2*(6), 6.

After exercise—cool it. (1985). *University of California, Berkeley Wellness Letter, 1*(10), 2.

Allan, J. (1985). Exercise program. In G.M. Bulecheck and J.C. McCloskey (Eds.), *Nursing Interventions* (pp. 198–219). Philadelphia: W.B. Saunders.

American Academy of Pediatrics, Committee on Sports Medicine and Committee on School Health. (1989). Organized athletics for preadolescent children. *Pediatrics, 84,* 583–584.

American Heart Association. (1990). *Exercise and your heart.* Dallas: American Heart Association.

Baldi, S., Costell, S., Hill, L., Jasmin, S., & Smith, N. (1980). *For Your Health: A Model for Self-Care.* South Laguna, CA: Nurses Model Health.

Barger, M. (Ed.). (1988). *Protocols for Gynecologic and Obstetric Health Care* (p. 128). Philadelphia: W.B. Saunders.

Brykcznski, K. (1982). Health contracting. *Nurse Practitioner, 7*(5), 27–31.

Bulechek, G.M., & McCloskey, J.C. (1985). *Nursing Interventions.* Philadelphia: W.B. Saunders.

Bullard, J.A. (1981). Exercise and pregnancy. *Canadian Family Physician, 27,* 977–982.

Carlson, J. (1979). The family and recreation: Toward a theoretical development. In W. Burr, R. Hill, F. Nye & I. Reiss (Eds.), *Contemporary Theories about the Family: Vol. I. Research-Based Theories* (pp. 439–452). New York: Free Press.

Carpenito, L. (1991). *Nursing Diagnosis* (4th ed). Philadelphia: J.B. Lippincott.

Clapp, J. (1991). Exercise and fetal health. *Journal of Developmental Physiology, 15*(1), 9–14.

Cooper, D. (1991). Year 2000 fitness objectives for the nation. *Clinics in Sports Medicine, 10*(1), 225.

Cooper, K.H. (1970). *The New Aerobics.* New York: Bantam Books.

Cooper, K.H. (1982). *The Aerobics Program for Total Well-Being.* New York: Bantam Books.

Cooper, K.H. (1988). *New Aerobics for Women.* New York: Bantam Books.

Cooper, K.H. (1989). Exercise: The first answer to osteoporosis. In K.H. Cooper (Ed.), *Preventing Osteoporosis* (pp. 39–49). New York: Bantam Books.

Cooper, K.H. (1990). *Overcoming Hypertension.* New York: Bantam Books.

Curran, D. (1983). *Traits of a Healthy Family.* Minneapolis: Winston Press.

DeAngelis, E. (1983). Recreation, art, music, and dance therapy and adapted physical education. In M. Levine, W. Carey, A. Crocher & R. Gross (Eds.), *Developmental-Behavioral Pediatrics* (pp. 1128–1133). Philadelphia: W.B. Saunders.

CHAPTER HIGHLIGHTS

Recreation as a family unit provides family members with common goals and measurable experiences that strengthen bonds.

Recreation and exercise promotes the well-being of individual members mentally and physically in addition to strengthening family ties.

In order to reduce the possibility for conflict over decisions about leisure time, negotiate and discuss member involvement, time, location, preferences, and cost of family recreation.

Contracting as a family is often a nursing strategy to facilitate family goal attainment in the area of individual and family recreation.

Exercise is often an individual activity that is health promoting for members during the family life course, but it can also be a family activity or family supported activity.

The role of the family nurse in family recreation is the assessment of family recreation, setting priorities and goals with the family, providing health teaching and resources that facilitate reaching their goal, and evaluation of a family's progress in recreation.

DeVries, H. (1986). Exercise and the physiology of aging. In H. Eckert, H. Montoye (Eds.), *Exercise and Health* (pp. 76–88). Champaign, IL: Human Kinetics.

Durak, E., Jovanovic-Peterson, L., & Peterson, C. (1990). Comparative evaluation of uterine response to exercise on five minute aerobic machines. *American Journal of Obstetrics and Gynecology, 162*, 754–756.

Eckert, H., & Montoye, H. (Eds.). (1984). *Exercise and Health* (American Academy of Physical Education Paper, No. 17). Champaign, IL: Human Kinetics.

Fair, J., Rosenaur, J., & Thurston, E. (1979). Exercise management. *Nurse Practitioner, 4*(3), 13–18.

Ferrara, L., Mainenti, G., Fasano, M., Marotta, T., Borelli, R., & Mancini, M. (1991). Cardiovascular response to mental stress and handgrip in children. *Japanese Heart Journal, 32*(2), 645–654.

Fort, J. (1978). *The Acute Effect of Aerobic Exercise on Measures of Stress.* (ERIC Document Reproduction Service, No. ED 228.204)

Gauthier, M. (1986). Guidelines for exercise during pregnancy: Too little or too much? *The Physician and Sportsmedicine, 14*(4), 162–169.

Geba, B. (1985). *Being at Leisure, Play at Life.* La Mesa, CA: Leisure Science Systems International.

Gordon, N., Gibbons, L. (1990). *Why Exercise? The Cooper Clinic Cardiac Rehabilitation Program* (pp. 129–145). New York: Simon & Schuster.

Greenberg, J., Pargman, D. (1986). Physical fitness: A wellness approach. Englewood Cliffs, NJ: Prentice-Hall.

Hill, L., Smith, N. (1990). *Self-Care Nursing.* Englewood Cliffs, NJ: Prentice-Hall.

Holman, T. (1985). How recreation can strengthen marriages and families. *Perspectives on Family Recreation and Leisure.* Centennial National Conference. American Alliance for Health, Physical Education, and Dance. Atlanta, GA, April, 1985. (ERIC Document Reproduction Service, No. ED 263-106).

Johnston, B. (1982). Influence of environmental factors on exercise and activity of cardiac patients. *Cardiovascular Nursing, 18*(2), 7–11.

Jopling, J. (1992). Physical fitness in children. In R. Hoekelman, S. Friedman, N. Nelson & H. Seidel (Eds.), *Primary Pediatric Care* (246–256). (2nd ed.). St. Louis: C.V. Mosby.

Lotgering, K., Raymond, D., & Long, D.L. (1984). The interactions of exercise and pregnancy: A review. *American Journal of Obstetrics and Gynecology, 149*, 560–568.

McArdle, W., Katch, F., & Katch, V. (1986). *Exercise Physiology,* Philadelphia: Lea & Febinger.

McKeag, D. (1991). The role of exercise in children and adolescents. *Clinics in Sports Medicine, 10*(1), 117–130.

McNeil, J., LeBlanc, E., & Joyne, M. (1991). The effect of exercise on depressive symptoms in moderately depressed elderly. *Psychology of Aging, 6*(3), 487–488.

Monahan, T. (1986). Should women go easy on exercise? *The Physician and Sportsmedicine, 14*(2), 188–195.

Moore, L., Lombardi, D., White, M., Campbell, J., Olivera, S., & Ellison, R. (1991). Influence of parents' physical activity levels on activity levels of young children. *Journal of Pediatrics, 118*(2), 215–219.

Moran, J.M. (1979). *Leisure Activities for the Mature Adult.* Minneapolis: Burgess.

Mullinax, K.M., Edwin, D. (1986). Some considerations of exercise during pregnancy. *Clinics of Sports Medicine, 5*, 559–570.

Murphy, P. (1986). Youth fitness testing: A matter of health or performance? *The Physician and Sportsmedicine, 14*, 189–190.

Myth: No pain, no gain. (1985). *University of California, Berkeley Wellness Letter, 1*(12), 8.

NASA Office of Occupational Health (1984). *Physical Fitness Program* (No. 426-598). Washington, DC: U.S. Government Printing Office.

Neal, L. (1984, October). Family recreation. Trends, tenants, and model building. *Journal of Physical Education and Dance,* 33–37.

Norris, R., Carroll, D., & Cochrane, R. (1992). The effects of physical activity and exercise training on psychological stress and well-being in an adolescent population. *Journal of Psychosomatic Research, 36*(1), 55–65.

Plowman, S. (1984). Effects of exercise on women from 20–50 years old. *Proceedings of the National Women's Leadership Conference on Fitness.* Washington, DC: The President's Council on Physical Fitness and Sports.

Pollock, M., Wilmore, J.H., Fox, S.M. (1984). *Exercise in Health and Disease: Evaluation and Prescription for Prevention and Rehabilitation.* Philadelphia: W.B. Saunders.

President's Council on Physical Fitness and Sports (1986). *Fitness in the Workplace—A Corporate Challenge* (No. 396). Washington, DC: Health and Human Services.

Prudden, B. (1988). *Teenage Fitness.* New York: Ballantine Books.

Prudden, B. (1986). *How to Keep Your Child Fit From Birth to Six.* New York: Ballantine Books.

Reuter, M. (1980). *The Effects of Running on Individuals Who Are Clinically Depressed.* Paper presented at American Psychological Association 88th Meeting, Quebec, Canada. (ERIC Document Service, No. ED 198-413).

Rice, P., Fort, I.C. (1991). The relationship of maternal exercise on labor, delivery and health of the newborn. *Journal of Sports Medicine & Physical Fitness, 31*(1), 95–99.

Rowland, T., Varzeas, M., Walsh, C. (1991). Aerobic responses to walking training in sedentary adolescent. *Journal of Adolescent Health, 12*(1), 30–34.

Rowland, T. (1981). Physical fitness in children: Implications for the prevention of coronary artery disease. *Current Problems in Pediatrics, 11*, 5–54.

Rudy, E.G., Estok, P.J. (1983). Intensity of jogging: Its relationship to selected physical and psychological variables in women. *Western Journal of Nursing Research, 5*(4), 325–326.

Runyon, D.K. (1983). The pre-participation examination of the young athlete. *Clinical Pediatrics, 22*, 10.

Siegel, B. (1985). Counseling and health screening for children entering sports and physical exercise. *Nurse Practitioner, 10*, 11–21.

Slemenda, C., Miller, J., Hui, S., Reister, T., Johnston, C. (1991). Role of physical activity in development of skeletal mass in children. *Journal of Bone & Mineral Research, 6*(11), 1227–1233.

Smith, H. (1985). What research is telling us about family recreation. *Perspectives on Family Recreation and Leisure.* Centennial National Conference American Alliance for Health, Physical Education and Dance. (ERIC Document Reproduction Service, No. ED 263-106).

Smith, N.J. (1985). *Sports Participation: Current Developmental Considerations in Childhood and*

Adolescence. (Children Are Different: Behavioral Development Monograph Series: No. 13). Columbus, OH: Ross Laboratories.

Suominen, H., Rahkila, P. (1992). Bone mineral density of the calcaneous in 70–81 year old male athletes. *Medical Science Sports Exercise,* 24(3), 401.

Stamford, B. (1986). What time should you exercise? *The Physician and Sportsmedicine,* 14(8), 162.

Teitelman, A., Welch, L., Hellenbravel, K., Bracken, M. (1990). Effect of maternal work activity on preterm birth and low birth weight. *American Journal of Epidemiology,* 131, 104–113.

U.S. Dept. of Health and Human Services. (1990). Physical activity and fitness. In *Healthy People 2000: National Health Promotion and Disease Prevention Objectives.* Washington, DC: Public Health Services.

Vander Griend, M. (1985, November). Developing a family philosophy of recreation. *Intermountain Leisure Symposium Proceedings* (pp. 15–16). Logan, UT.

Voorrips, L., von Staveren, W., & Hautrast, J. (1991). Are physically active women in better nutritional condition than their sedentary peers? *European Journal of Clinical Nutrition,* 45(11), 545–542.

Wade, M.G. (1985). *Constraints on Leisure.* Springfield, IL: Thomas.

Walking: A program for life (1987). *University of California, Berkeley Wellness Letter,* 3(5), 6.

Walking for fitness (1986). *The Physician and Sportsmedicine,* 14(10), 145–159.

Wanner, R. (1982). Physical performance as a function of liquid intake. In P. Komi (Ed.), *Exercise and Sports Biology.* Champaign, IL: Human Kinetics.

Warren, M. (1991). Exercise in women. *Clinics in Sports Medicine,* 10(1), 131–139.

Wilmore, J.H. (1974). Alterations in strength, body composition, and anthropometric measurements consequent to a 10-week training program. *Medical Science Sports,* 6, 133.

17 FAMILY SEXUALITY

KATHLEEN HEINRICH

Sex lies at the root of life, and we can never learn to reverence
life until we know how to understand sex.

HAVELOCK ELLIS

OBJECTIVES

On completion of this chapter, the reader will be able to:

1. Describe the psychological and sociocultural aspects of sexuality
2. Differentiate between sexual identity and sexual role behavior
3. Identify the role of the family in the development of children's sexuality and sexual identity
4. Describe the role of the family in development of sexuality in infancy, childhood, adolescence, adulthood, and old age
5. Describe relationships in the homosexual family
6. Define domestic partners and discuss the relationship to family life
7. Identify data needed to assess family sexuality
8. Identify nursing diagnoses related to family sexuality
9. Describe interventions to promote family sexuality
10. List criteria to evaluate interventions used to promote healthy family sexuality

INTRODUCTION

Sexuality can be defined broadly to include the physical and psychological energy that individuals expend in attaining warmth, tenderness, sexual response, and love. With this definition all of us can be seen as sexual beings from birth until death (Coleman, 1988, p. 119). To describe family sexuality requires a broader view of sexuality and its interactional aspects, and raises the questions, "How is sexuality lived out in this family? How

does the parent(s)' sexuality influence the children? How does the child's sexuality affect the parent(s)?"

Family life enhances personal and sexual growth and development. A stable family life provides children with security, love, and emotional nourishment that fosters healthy sexuality. In fact, parents are the earliest and most important influences on sexuality. White and DeBlassie (1992) believe that family patterns, especially communication skills and parenting methods, as well as family configuration, strongly affect children's sexual development.

Sexuality is a complex, multifaceted phenomena. Since families are systems, sexual issues will, to some degree, for better or for worse, affect all

The author wishes to express appreciation to Catherine Costin for her critique of the chapter and suggestions to make it more specific to healthy sexuality. This chapter is a revision of the chapter authored by Rosemary Hogan in the first edition.

members of the family. This chapter will focus on the biologic, psychosocial, and cultural aspects of sexuality as they relate to individuals and to families; on sexuality across the life span; on the effects of social change on families and variations in family sexuality; and finally on assessment, nursing diagnoses, intervention, and evaluation of family sexuality.

SEXUALITY AND FAMILY HEALTH

Sexuality is intrinsic to our being. Fonseca (1970) has described it as a quality of being human, all that we are as men and women. The term "sexuality," unlike the word "sex," encompasses biologic, psychological, sociocultural, and ethical components of behavior.

Sexual health, like health in general, is relative, and definitions include all aspects of sexuality. Maddock (1975) indicates that four factors must be considered: (1) congruence of personal and sexual behavior with gender identity and comfort with various sexual role behaviors; (2) ability to form interpersonal relationships with same or different sex individuals; (3) ability to respond to erotic stimulation with pleasure; and (4) ability to make mature judgments about sexual behavior based on one's values and beliefs. This definition can serve as a guideline, but a client is not necessarily "unhealthy" because one aspect is missing.

Family sexual health involves these individual aspects as well as the ability of the family to foster positive sexual self-esteem of its members, to validate each member's sexuality, and to maintain a gratifying sexual relationship between the parents. Parents with unresolved issues around sexuality may have difficulty fostering healthy sexuality of children.

Family sexuality is more than the sexual interactions of the adults; it is the pattern of same-sex and opposite-sex relationships that includes the quality of parental interactions, parent-children interactions, and sexual learning, usually unplanned, that occurs in the family. Consequently, the description of sexuality as having biologic, psychosocial, and cultural aspects is applicable to the family as a whole because it is through the interactions of all these aspects of sexuality in each of the family members that family sexual health occurs.

Illness and Family Sexuality

Because sexual response involves complex physiologic responses, pathology of the nervous system such as stroke, multiple sclerosis, spinal cord injury, or peripheral neuropathies may compromise sexual function. Pathology of the vascular system, such as arteriosclerosis that affects pelvic vessels and diseases such as diabetes and kidney failure, may be implicated in sexual dysfunction.

Surgery such as mastectomy, hysterectomy, and cancer and its therapy may cause body image disturbance as well as compromise physiologic response. As a result, the sexual relationship may suffer (Hogan, 1985). Even if pathology does not alter function, anxiety and fear that illness will be exacerbated may cause sexual partners to avoid coitus.

Family roles and relationships may also be strained. Husbands or wives may have to give up cherished roles or accept those that formerly belonged to the spouse. Anxiety, depression, or anger that follows may further disrupt the relationship. During these times of crisis, families must sit down together, share their concerns, and seek mutually agreed on solutions to problems.

Psychosocial Factors Related to Sexuality

Gender Identity and Sexual Role Behavior

The terms "gender identity" and "gender role behavior" are often confused. Gender identity is the conviction that one belongs to the female or male sex; it is a sense of self as female or male. It is formed in early childhood as a result of biologic factors (embryologic and central nervous system factors), genital anatomy, which signals to parents the child's sex, sex assignment, and childrearing practices.

Gender or sexual role behavior has two aspects. It is all that we do to disclose ourselves as male or female to others and the pattern of behavior identified as appropriate for each sex in a society. It is built up cumulatively through experience and through planned and unplanned learning. The greatest influence is the sexual value system of the family and the community. Even information that children receive from their peer groups, often the most frequent source of sexual information, is filtered through the parental value system.

The Family and Psychosocial Factors

From birth, parents and children reciprocally influence each other's sexuality (Friedrich et al., 1991). Mrazek and Mrazek (1981) suggest that families establish a "psychosexual equilibrium"—a synergistic interplay of parents' sexual adjustment, the child's developing sexuality and sexual development on the parental sexual adjustment, and the interaction that evolves when the child's sexual development stimulates parents to relive their earlier sexual development through memories and feelings.

Sexual self-esteem is characterized by acceptance of the value of self as a sexual being. Positive self-concept is formed and nurtured in the family where loving care by parents and siblings confirms children's worth. Positive body image, the internalized picture that individuals have of their bodies as satisfying and attractive, is also developed in the family (Pletsch et al., 1991; Roberts et al., 1990; Rauste-von Wright, 1989; Offer et al., 1988).

In addition to sexual self-esteem, family communication transmits attitudes toward sexuality as well as sexual knowledge, opinions, and beliefs (Sanders & Mullis, 1988). Adolescents are aware of their parent's sexual attitudes even when parents have not directly verbalized them. Parents' attitudes, expressed or unexpressed, can influence their children's sexual behavior.

The parental influence on children and adolescents' gender role socialization is less recognized. Research indicates that parental attitudes have a central influence on the adolescent gender role formation (Hertsgaard & Light, 1984). With the social changes that have swept the nation in the last thirty years, liberal sexual attitudes became associated with liberal attitudes in general, including liberal gender role attitudes (Fingerman, 1989). Children and adolescents of the 1980s and 90s are exposed to less traditional gender role and sexual attitudes. The fact that adolescent females grow up in a time when the role model of working women is the norm considerably influences their attitudes toward gender roles (Fingerman, 1989). Indeed, Fingerman (1989) found that daughters of mothers in professions traditionally considered to be male professions had more liberal views on sexual behavior. These views were linked to their liberal attitudes toward gender roles. Coles and Stokes's (1985) study found that although young women are permitted more intimate sexual behavior without censure from peers, there remains a significant degree of conservation—about one-half of the female respondents wanted to marry as virgins. Such findings indicate that traditionalism/liberalism may be shaped by variables beyond the mother's occupational choice, such as family configuration or religiosity.

Family Configuration

Miller and Bingham (1989) indicate that "aspects of family configuration, including both sibling constellation and parents' marital status, are related to adolescents' sexual intercourse experience" (p. 505). Parental divorce or separation has been correlated with adolescents initiating intercourse (Stewart, 1987). Research confirms that although healthy sexuality can and does develop in children of single-parent families, it is the stable relationship of two people that has the greatest potential for fostering sexual health (Schumm, 1985). Newcomer and Urdy (1987) explored how parental marital status is related to adolescent sexual behavior. They found that adolescent boys may sexually act out secondary to the emotional disturbance of losing their father and

that adolescent girls reared without fathers are more likely to become sexually active. As validation, they pointed to the recent increase in sexual activity in adolescents that parallels the rapid increase in the number of children being raised without fathers. Flewelling and Bauman (1990) also found a significant association between non-intact families and sexual activity.

Cultural and Ethnic Variables

The way in which sexuality is expressed is learned through culture, which defines sexual norms, ideals, and ideology. What is "normal" sexual behavior varies by ethnic groups and societies.

Religions are important subcultures that may have profound effects on sexuality. Religious beliefs of the family may influence children's behavior. Second only to the family, the church is a primary agent of socialization responsible for the transmission of values and standards of sexual behavior (Struder & Thornton, 1989). Studies show a strong correlation between adolescent sexual behavior and religious participation (White & DeBlassie, 1992). Thornton and Camburn (1989) found that young people who attend church frequently and espouse religious values have less permissive attitudes and are less experienced sexually. White and DeBlassie (1992) observe that both the Catholic and Protestant churches in the United States have denounced premarital sex and expressed views on other sexual issues. While these churches discourage sexual activity, the authors note that they offer little or no help for those adolescents who wish to use contraception if they are sexually active.

Religion and culture together appear to have an influence on urban black adolescent girls' level of sexual activity. Keith et al. (1991) found that the church and family, including the presence of the father, were associated with not being sexually active during early and middle adolescence. While they suggest that a strong family and participation in church can lead to more responsible sexual behavior, it is also possible that these factors inhibit adolescents from admitting the extent of sexual activity.

Some cultures permit premarital and extramarital sexual relationships, and other cultures view sex as a duty, and sexual intercourse is considered weakening or debilitating. In the Hispanic community, women may be protective of their traditional roles in a male-dominated society. In the American Navajo Indian family, however, the mother has the power and runs the family.

Mexican-American, Arab-American, and Oriental men do not usually participate during the birth of a baby. Birth is considered a woman's affair, and women may not want a man's involvement (Hogan, 1985).

Because of changing cultural and ethnic values and acculturation into the pluralistic American society, it is difficult to predict with certainty how ethnic background will affect sexual and family relationships. Careful assessment of the family attitudes toward sexuality and sexual behavior is more important than stereotyping behavior based on ethnic or cultural background.

FAMILY ROLE IN TEACHING ABOUT SEXUALITY

Although sex education experts agree that parents can be the ideal educators of their own children, many parents are ill-prepared or unable to deal with issues surrounding sexuality. In moving toward independence and identity development, the adolescent must separate from the family. Paradoxically, it is the family who has provided the adolescent with the moral and ethical foundation upon which to build his or her ethical code. Studies indicate that parents are often conflicted or ambivalent about giving adolescents information about sexuality. The findings of the studies that examine parental communication and adolescent sexual behavior are conflictual. According to researchers (Moore, Peterson & Furstenberg, 1986) "parental communication with teenage children is often recommended as a means of discouraging early sexual activity" (Moore et al., p. 781). The relationship of family communication to sexual behavior seems to vary with the gender of parent and child, and Fisher (1989) suggests that further research needs to account for attitudes of parents, the gender of the adolescent, and the source of information about sexual communication.

In a study by Sanders and Mullis (1988), parents had the greatest influence on adolescents' sexual opinions, beliefs, and attitudes, but were less influential than friends, school, and books as sources of sexual information. While nearly all the respondents preferred that parents teach them about sexual issues, only 15% noted that parents were a major source of this information.

Coles and Stokes (1985) found that most adolescents are likely to learn about puberty and reproductive physiology from school and parents, only 1 out of 3 is likely to learn about human sexuality from other sources. The researchers concluded that the issues adolescents struggle with most—contraception, sexual techniques, sexual orientation—are outside of the "acceptable" discussion topics for parents and adolescents. The findings of this study also indicated that most teens find it difficult to communicate with parents. Only 36% said they would turn to parents for desired sexual information.

Parents have a number of barriers to overcome in providing sexual information, including being ill-informed. Chilman (1990) offers additional reasons for parents' difficulty with discussing sexual subjects with their children. He observed that family dissatisfaction tends to reach its peak when children enter adolescence. Stresses at this middle stage of life may include a dwindling sense of marital unity, the adolescents' push for an independent identity; the parents' own unresolved parent-child conflicts, or changing gender role identities. As these stresses intensify, parents' self-esteem may decrease, and they may become either highly impulsive or overly controlling and rigid.

Adolescents' sexuality may also be very threatening to parents who are uncomfortable with their own sexuality or who have not resolved their own sexual issues. Grant and Demetriou (1988) note that as the prime socializers of their children, parents teach children a range of social skills. These same parents are generally uncomfortable in teaching a child how to be sexual and their input in this manner often involves teaching children not to be sexual. The authors give the example of masturbation, a natural behavior that offers a child bodily enjoyment, yet parents typically feel uncomfortable observing this behavior. Even the youngest child may sense a parent's discomfort about sexual issues and learns not to ask questions. In combination, Grant and Demetriou (1988) conclude that these stresses can induce high levels of anxiety and block communication between parents and adolescents. Findings by Hanson, Myers, and Ginsburg (1987) encourage parents to teach responsible behaviors in general, which in turn would have a more positive effect than simply teaching about birth control or providing sex education.

Education should enhance children's self-esteem, prepare them for marriage and parenthood, promote responsible decision making, and help them understand love as a basic component of sexuality. Since it is in the family where values are learned, Tucker (1989) recommends that parents need to be educated about sexual issues so they are better informed and feel more comfortable in instructing children and adolescents. Researchers have correlated negative parental attitudes with early adolescent sexual intercourse. Fisher (1989) found that adolescents who were taught by parents that sex is not healthy and normal were 38% more likely to have intercourse than those whose parents promoted healthier views (24%). Miller and Bingham (1986) found that either very strict parental discipline with too many rules or no parental rules resulted in the most sexually active adolescents. Their findings indicated that the most effective strategy was moderate parental discipline and reasonable, flexible limits. The nature and quality of parental communication is also important. Adolescents want more than prescriptions and admonitions for sexual behavior from their parents. Families who share mutual closeness, a consistent set of values, and an intact family structure are more likely to develop adolescents who delay sexual activity. Since schools have a role and a stake in this process, sex education in schools can supplement and augment, rather than diminish, parental influence. Families, schools, and communities need to shift from an avoidant or reluctant stance to a more open, celebratory attitude toward sexuality.

SEXUALITY ACROSS THE FAMILY LIFE SPAN

With the rapid social changes that have transpired over the last thirty years, parents, children, and professionals in health care are often unsure of what is "normal," healthy sexuality and development. Concern about normality is complicated by issues of right or wrong, good or bad, and healthy or unhealthy at all stages of the family life span. What has been accepted by one generation may be condemned by the next. There is no denying however, that one generation affects the sexuality of another. Parents influence the development of their children's sexuality, who in turn affect the sexual expression of their siblings (Friedrich et al., 1991).

Sexual Development: Infancy and Childhood

Sexual development begins before birth and is affected by complex biopsychosocial factors. Table 17–1 presents the stages and characteristics of normal psychosexual development. Each development stage is affected by earlier events in individuals' lives. Some believe that the nature and goals of adult sexual behavior are partially or completely determined by what happens as children move through various psychosexual stages. Sexuality at any age or stage of development encompasses more than sexual behavior in the physical sense, although infants' and children's sexual activity of the most benign types is probably the cause of more anxiety in parents than any other behavior.

Parents' responses to children's sexual behavior may more positively or negatively affect the achievement of healthy sexuality than the behaviors themselves. Childrearing practices and the family environment may have a greater impact than the biologic factors of anatomy and physiology.

Sexual identity, that is the feeling or belief that one is male or female, is shaped by biologic factors and by childrearing practices. Sexual role behavior, what individuals do to distinguish themselves as men or women (dress, for example), is not established at birth but is built up cumulatively through experience by interaction with family and peers. Biology may be a given, but the family has a pivotal role in development of sexuality.

Prenatal Factors and Sexuality

The fetus has the potential for developing into either sex, but after the seventh week, male or female characteristics develop depending on the constitution of the sex chromosomes. The sex of the child is determined by the type of sperm that fertilized the ovum. Genetic sex is determined exclusively by the sperm (Guyton, 1986).

The XY or XX chromosomes program the gonadal tissue, which is initially identical in both sexes, to become either testes or ovaries. If testes are formed, the androgen they secrete programs that fetus to become a male. In the absence of gonadal hormones, the fetus differentiates into an anatomic female. Various factors may interrupt or alter the process and adversely affect the fetus: a deficiency of maternal hormones, maternal stress, viral infections, nutritional deficiencies, or trauma.

Testosterone is essential to the differentiation of the male external genitalia. The ovaries are not essential for fetal development at this stage. If embryonal gonads are removed before the reproductive anatomy is formed, the embryo will develop into a female regardless of its genetic sex. Fetal androgens (male hormones) seem to organize the brain for masculine behavior and seem just as important as assignment of "male" sex to the infant in the development of sexual identity (Pardridge et al., 1982).

The study of differentiation has been stimulated by the discovery of relatively notable structural differences (structural dimorphism) in the brains of males and females. It is believed that steroid hormones may control other structural development, but study of the causative mechanisms is just beginning. Testosterone given in prenatal life or immediately after birth causes permanent changes in brain structure in animals. Androgens may also cause imprinting of the brain during fetal life (Bamford, 1980).

It seems likely that gender identity is influenced by genetic sex despite childrearing practices that are sometimes appropriate for the opposite sex. Biologic factors in prenatal life seem to influence gender identity and argue against the belief that environmental factors are the only determinants of sex differences. However, the exact role of prenatal hormones and postnatal socialization on male or female sexual identity and behavior must still be determined.

Birth to Two Years

No matter what the biologic inheritance, life experiences have a tremendous impact on the development of sexuality. The infant needs a warm, physical relationship with the mother (or other caregiver) if sensory and affectional development are to occur. Adults who were not given warm, physical contact in infancy are more likely to have

TABLE 17-1. NORMAL PSYCHOSEXUAL DEVELOPMENT

STAGE	CHARACTERISTICS
Prenatal	Differentiation of fetus into male or female after seventh week
Birth–2 years	Need for close physical contact
	Touching and exploring genitals
	Establishment of core gender identity
	Learning sexual role behavior
2 years	Neuromuscular coordination and control, bowel and bladder control
	Continued genital manipulation
	Sensual stimulation by hugging, kissing others
	Further sexual role development
3–5 Years	Further autonomy, independence
	Pride in genitals, exploration, exhibition of own or by others
	Development of relationship with parent of opposite sex
	Genital self-stimulation (masturbation)
6–12 Years	Final role identification
	Interest in differences between sexes
	Interest in opposite sex
	Beginning preoccupation with bodily changes
	Beginning independence from family emotional ties
13–19 Years (Adolescence)	Development of secondary sex characteristics
	Focus on body image, appearance
	Interest in sexual activity (petting to coitus) and/or relationship with opposite sex
	Increased ability to love
	Consolidation of sexual identity
20–45 Years (Early Adulthood)	Independence from family
	Choice of a marital partner or development of a sexual relationship
	Giving and receiving love
	Establishment of family
	Communication of sexual needs, feelings between partners
46–65 Years (Later Adulthood)	Opportunity for greater sexual freedom
	Menopause in women
	Male climacteric
	Freedom from family responsibilities
66 Years and Older	Decrease in intensity of sexual response
	Continued fulfilling intimacy if good health and interested and interesting partner

retarded sexual development, aggressive behavior, and socioemotional problems.

There is evidence that male and female infants are capable of sexual arousal, although there is no way of knowing the nature of their subjective experience since they cannot communicate verbally. Erection has been observed in utero during sonograms and may also be observed right after birth, but it is probably reflexive, mediated through the lumbosacral spinal cord and not dependent on higher brain centers associated with thought and emotion. It is not unusual, however, for infants to touch and explore their genitals, and parents should not be concerned about this normal developmental behavior.

Immediately after birth, psychosocial factors influence sexual development. Parental treatment of males and females may differ. Daughters are handled gently, and sons are treated more roughly by fathers. Mothers appear to be expressive and open in their affection to their daughters. Although this behavior may be unconscious, it may result in a form of covert imprinting when consistently repeated (Jacklin et al., 1984).

After birth of a male infant, the parents must make a decision about circumcision, the surgical removal of the foreskin that covers the glans penis. Circumcision is sometimes a religious practice, especially in Islam or in Judaism. In the United States it may be done primarily for hygienic and health reasons. Inflammation or infection of the glans and cancer of the penis are less likely to occur in circumcised men, and the evidence of cancer of the cervix is lower in spouses of circumcised men.

Those who oppose routine circumcision argue that there is no reason for the procedure, that penile injury may occur, that sexual sensitivity in the area is lessened, and that there is increased risk of premature ejaculation. It does not appear, however, that there is empirical evidence that circumcision affects male sexual function in any way

(Masters et al., 1982). Consequently, the decision for circumcision rests primarily on the religious and personal beliefs of the parents.

Two Years

By two years of age, children are developing neuromuscular coordination and control, are developing language skills, and are better able to explore their environment. Bowel and bladder control is a parental goal. Children often avoid accidents to obtain parental approval. However, toilet-training practices that include punitive measures, such as shaming the child or physically punishing for "accidents," may cause further conflicts that are related to giving and receiving.

Parents may also become anxious about and punish children's growing curiosity about the environment and their genitals. Parental anxiety about the behavior may be communicated to children, who may have difficulty during adulthood accepting sexual activity as normal, good, and right.

Two-years-olds may obtain sensual stimulation from hugging and kissing family members, friends, and toys as well as through rhythmic motor activities such as swinging. Although the "terrible twos" may cause parents to focus on coping with children's negative behaviors, parents must continue to promote children's sense of security that comes with being held, cuddled, and given other signs of affection.

Three to Five Years

At three to five years of age, children develop further automony and independence. Size increases dramatically but with little change in the genital organs.

Along with developing an increasing sense of privacy, children develop pride in their genitals and discover they can bring pleasure. Children may fondle their genitals, explore those of playmates, or exhibit their own.

The quality of the communication between parents and children concerning this behavior may affect sexual development. If parents are too strict and shame the child or if they are too encouraging, that is if they laughed at the child or show how to engage in this behavior, children may associate shame or guilt with the pleasure associated with the genitals. If parents threaten children with statements such as "we'll cut off your hand if you don't stop playing with yourself" or "your penis (or the euphemistic term used) will fall off," children may develop anxiety about losing something that is important, and major problems related to sexuality may develop later in life.

Masturbation or genital self-stimulation that results in sexual gratification, has no adverse bio-

logic or psychological consequences except those caused by guilt, anxiety, and fear. It is believed that most children masturbate by six to eight years of age in sexually permissive societies. Most genital manipulation is best dealt with by "benign neglect" and by explanation of the appropriate and inappropriate times and places for such activity.

Excessive masturbation is difficult to define because what is considered excessive is defined by the parent. Masturbation that becomes compulsive and is used to avoid social interchange or to ward off anxiety or feelings of distress and not as a release of sexual tension can be considered excessive and a sign of a deeper problem. Compulsive masturbation is not usually accompanied by any real pleasure or satisfaction.

Parents need to find ways to help children understand parental expectations without threats and misinformation. If parents recognize the normality of the behavior as a part of sexual development, they may be able to respond positively.

Parents should give children special attention when the children are *not* masturbating by involving them in other activities and by giving them the love, attention, tenderness, and closeness that fosters feelings of security about one's body and healthy sexual development.

During this stage of development, children also begin to develop a relationship with the parent of the opposite sex, laying the foundation for future healthy relationships with those of the opposite sex. While children 3 to 6 years old can be flirtatious, they are not able to understand the nature of sexual activity. Some have suggested that parental sexual activity (or that of others) should not be kept hidden from children who need to accept this activity as a part of relationships. To children, however, adult sex acts seem dangerous and aggressive, especially in the darkness or if the sounds accompanying sex are interpreted by children as being painful. Closed bedroom doors and/or privacy should be a prerequisite to adult sexual activity.

Casual nudity of the parent of the opposite sex, although not usually harmful, may be detrimental to the young child if it is seductive in nature or presented in a stimulating manner. When parents are insufficiently sexually satisfied and hostile toward each other, children may also develop a negative attitude toward sex that may persist into adulthood.

Children may become frightened when they see menstrual blood on pads, tampons, or clothing. Mothers should explain that they are not hurt or sick but that this is a normal part of being a woman. As in the earlier periods of children's lives, warmth, tenderness, and closeness provided by the family foster feelings of security about the body and are needed for the children's healthy sexual development. (See Resources for Teaching/Counseling at the end of the chapter.)

Five to Twelve Years

During this period, all children are in school where they have increased contact with peers of both sexes. Children from five to seven years of age develop increased interest in differences between the sexes, for example, beards on men and breasts on women. There is more interest in having a baby and playing house. Five-year-olds realize that they are to marry someone of the opposite sex and not from the family.

One in ten children around the age of five have their first sexual experience beyond autoerotic behavior, usually exhibiting the genitals or inspecting those of other children, often under the guise of playing doctor. Boys become more active than girls. There may be a great deal of lying on top of one another, but even when children undress, there is usually nothing more than genital opposition (Hogan, 1980). Sexual activities may be more advanced if one partner is older and more experienced. Parents may become concerned about this activity, but it is a reflection of children's natural curiosity to learn about themselves and the world around them rather than any precocious sexual arousal (Broderick, 1966).

Interest in reproduction continues by ages eight to nine, but sexual exploration is less common. Girls are interested in menstruation, and both sexes want to know about fertility, pregnancy, and birth. Both sexes begin to evaluate their physical attractiveness, but they begin to play separately, their interest in the opposite sex evidenced by peeping, sex jokes, and provocative giggling. They are inhibited, self-conscious about their bodies, and concerned with modesty. Kissing games or teasing about boyfriends or girlfriends may take place during mixed play.

By ages 10 to 12, there is increased preoccupation with body changes, especially those connected with puberty. Telling sex jokes may be a favorite pastime. Although there may be a facade of disinterest in the opposite sex in some, there is the beginning of romantic interest in others.

Sexual activities of the preadolescent male are generally group oriented. Activities such as genital exhibition, demonstration of masturbation, or group masturbation usually satisfy social needs rather than relieve sexual tension. At times, sex play may involve homosexual behavior with oral-genital contacts and attempts at anal intercourse. Kinsey et al. (1948) found that fewer than half of all males continued homosexual play into puberty.

Prepubescent girls confine sexual play to genital exhibition and touching. Sexual activity for the most part is harmless, although there is increasing parental concern about this activity.

The social and cultural impact of the environment is also felt. Through television, movies, and fiction, children learn about the adult sexual world, at least as portrayed by the mass media.

Moral values are learned. It is essential that children gain accurate information, yet information about sexuality is often inadequate and distorted so that it becomes mixed with fantasy life. Much information must be obtained and sexual learning augmented later in life to correct information obtained earlier (Hogan, 1980).

Ideally, children should learn accurate information about sexuality primarily from the parents. However, many parents, either because of discomfort with the topic and/or lack of information, are unable to teach clearly and unequivocally about sexuality. Peers are often the source of myths and misinformation that contribute to the distorted view of sexuality that is presented by the media and internalized by children.

Although parents may be poor purveyors of facts, they have a far more important role in the development of healthy sexuality. It is primarily in the family that children learn the importance of male-female relationships. Parents who are loving, tender, and respectful of each other teach children how to use their own sexuality so that it enhances their lives and those of succeeding generations.

Sexual Development: Adolescence

Puberty is marked by accelerated growth and development of secondary sex characteristics. In young women, menstruation is the obvious indication of puberty, although breast enlargement, growth of pubic and axillary hair, and widened hips precede menses by about two years. Young women may have ambivalent feelings toward their genitalia, negative feelings about menstruation, and various concerns about breast size, or lack of size, and general attractiveness. Current research supports the notion that girls tend to have less favorable notions of their bodies than boys (Offer et al., 1988; Roberts et al., 1990; Rauste-von Wright, 1989).

In adolescent males, growth of pubic hair and enlargement of the testes herald the start of puberty. Penile growth and ejaculation occur later. The first ejaculation may or may not contain viable sperm. A growth spurt is accompanied by increased muscle mass, body and facial hair, and a deeper voice. Penile size or lack of size, body build, and attractiveness cause similar concerns among adolescent boys. Research indicated that boys are more comfortable with and interested in matters of sex than girls (Offer et al., 1988; Pletsch et al., 1991).

Adolescent females are slower to awaken to sexual activity than adolescent males. Whether this is culturally determined or related to lower androgen levels is equivocal.

The adolescent girl is usually introduced to erotic feelings by petting, or stimulation by the man, rather than by masturbation. If the first intercourse takes place within an affectionate relationship and with mutual consent, the girl usually has more satisfaction and enjoyment with few feelings of guilt, shame, or anxiety.

In adolescent girls there is no sudden increase in sexual activity at puberty as experienced by adolescent boys. Women show steady increases in responsiveness that peak in their middle twenties to late thirties. Males show a quick upsurge in sexual activity and reach the sexual peak of their lives during adolescence and young adulthood. Masturbation is a fairly common sexual activity, beginning slightly before puberty, peaking during the middle teens, and dropping by the late teens.

Sex dreams are a very small part of sexual outlet for both sexes. If accompanied by orgasm and ejaculation in young men, "wet dreams" are said to have occurred. Sex dreams, although pleasant, may also frighten the adolescent.

Most adolescents engage in petting (erotic caressing without coitus). Early coital behavior of adolescent boys tends to take place in relatively nonserious relationships and is usually not followed by more than two or three repetitions with the partner.

"Sexuality is not unique to adolescence, but is a phenomena that spans the entire life cycle. What is remarkable about adolescence is the complex physical, cognitive, and psychosocial changes that affect how sexuality is expressed. Physical maturity and the ability to engage in sexual activity does not necessarily imply sufficient cognitive maturity to understand and anticipate the undesirable consequences of adolescent sexuality" (Grant & Demetriou, 1988, p. 1271). In Piagetian terms, cognitive development in adolescence is moving from concrete operational thinking to formal operational thinking. Using formal operational thinking allows adolescents to transform erotic thought into symbolic abstractions. When fantasies are recognized as such, they are not acted on, and potential guilt is alleviated. If adolescents have not developed formal operational thinking, they are unable to think through a decision-making based on the understanding of the potential consequences of certain behaviors. Concrete operational thinking or incomplete development of formal operations results in adolescents who see themselves as "omnipotent and infallible." Grant and Demetriou believe that this type of thinking results in excessive risk-taking in sexual behavior.

Adolescence may be described as a time of biopsychosocial ferment. In addition to profound bodily changes, adolescents must learn to establish relationships with peers of both sexes, integrate changing body image into the self-concept and sexual identity, and deal with new role expectations, responsibilities, and greater autonomy.

In early adolescence, male peer groups become important; in later adolescence, dating and "rating" become central. Much of male sexual activity is subject to peer review, with much of the language and activity focused on "scoring" or getting "points." Conversations may focus on sexual prowess and ability to surpass the "norms."

Adolescent girls' interactions with peers focuses on concerns about love, affection, and marriage rather than sexual ability. For both sexes, frequency of dating, popularity, and number of partners are subjects of intense interest.

One of the "risks" of adolescent sexuality that Hajcak and Garwood (1988) underline is that sex can be used in an attempt to satisfy emotional and interpersonal needs that have little or nothing to do with sex. Sexuality may be used to bolster a faltering self-concept. Adolescent girls may endure promiscuous and joyless encounters to gain or maintain popularity. Underneath the behavior is a defense against loneliness. Adolescent boys may engage in sexual exploits to protect against self-doubt about their masculinity (Hogan, 1985).

However, encounters with the opposite sex may go beyond the purely sexual and involve feelings of love and tenderness. Establishing an intimate relationship outside the family is a developmental task of adolescence and early adulthood. Sexual intimacy includes a blend of eroticism, emotional closeness, mutual caring, vulnerability, and trust, commonly referred to as commitment (Sarrell & Sarrell, 1981).

Some adolescents have little or no physical sexual contact and still complete healthy sexual development. The nature and quality of adult sexuality is not a function of how much or what kind of sex takes place in adolescence. It is predicated on a host of factors.

The family has an essential role in the development of adolescent sexuality since they hold a new set of expectations for adolescents. Greater autonomy, less supervision, and greater involvement with peer groups is permitted. Yet adolescent sexual activity is feared, ignored, or chastised by parents.

A double standard still may exist. Adolescent boys are usually given more freedom by parents than girls, so their conflict regarding independence and autonomy is not so prevalent. In contrast, girls have more restrictions placed on them. Conflicts may arise since sexual attractiveness but not sexual activity is valued.

Further conflict results from parents feeling that they must control adolescents' sexuality. Adolescents want to hear about sexuality but decry preaching or moralizing and may rebel against coercion. They want facts and information about contraception, sexually transmitted diseases, pregnancy, and sexual orientation. Sexual behavior puts adolescents at risk for unintended pregnancy and STDs (Gilchrist, 1991). In 1990, persons aged 12 to 19 represented 27.9 million, or nearly 12% of the U.S. population (Bureau of Statistics, 1990). Approximately 50% to 60% of adolescent girls and 70% to 75% of adolescent boys have had sexual intercourse by the time they graduate from high school (Alexander et al., 1991). Of more concern is the fact that growing numbers of teens report having sexual intercourse before age 13—in one study 53% of adolescents under 14 reported having had sexual intercourse (Orr, 1989). The National Adolescent Student Health Survey (1989) indicates that two-thirds of sexually active teens use no contraception. Almost 40% of adolescents who became pregnant choose to undergo abortions (Gilchrist, 1991). With the incurable strains of genital herpes and AIDS, the adolescent is especially at risk (Koyle et al., 1989; Shayne & Kaplan, 1988). The incidence of HIV infection in the adolescent population is rising at an alarming rate.

For adolescents who are grappling with their sexual orientation, the teen years can be particularly painful and confusing. Increased anxiety and fear can increase these adolescents' vulnerability to substance abuse, sexual acting out, pregnancy, HIV infection, homelessness, and suicide (Sanford, 1989).

In spite of easy access to contraception, more liberal attitudes toward contraceptives, and increased implementation of sex education curricula in schools, teen pregnancy rates continue to rise in epidemic numbers. The National Survey of Family Growth (1987) documented that pregnancy in teens results in disrupted education, reduced employment opportunities, low incomes, unstable marriages, and health and developmental risks to the children of adolescent mothers. Society pays a big price in government financial support (White and DeBlassie, 1991), health care, and special education for teenaged mothers and their children. Teenagers may become pregnant for various reasons: to have someone to love, to express dislike of school or of the home environment, to trap a man into a relationship, to prove femininity, to relieve loneliness and depression, or to get a man to marry.

Parents' confusion and ambivalence about sexuality results in girls having to interpret mixed messages. Society, which emphasizes adolescents' freedom, makes it difficult for parents to set limits. When pregnancy occurs, parents may feel guilty about their relationship with the daughter, causing further disruption in family relationships.

Parents who are able to share sexual information, who exemplify a positive sexual value system and lifestyle, and who show trust, love, and pride in their adolescents provide the best foundation for healthy sexual development.

Sexual Development: Adulthood

In adulthood, sexual maturation has been essentially completed. Choosing a marital partner or developing a sexual relationship with another is one of the tasks of this stage of the life cycle.

Premarital sexual activity has increased as both sexes and couples experiment more openly with different sexual practices. Positions for intercourse different than male superior, oral-genital contact, cunnilingus (with female genitals) and fellatio (with male genitals) is used in a larger proportion of sexual relationships than a generation ago. The duration of foreplay has increased.

Downey (1980) concluded in a further analysis of Kinsey's data (1948) that there seemed to be a gradual decline in moral considerations and less concern about feared emotional and physical results of various sexual behaviors. In contrast, Story (1982) found that university students tended toward more traditionally sanctioned sexual behavior in 1980 than in 1974.

It is usually during the adult years that the family is established. Adults learn to give and receive love in a stable relationship. Marriage combines the responsibilities of a sexual relationship with that of reproduction and socialization. The couple becomes parents and transmits the sexual values of the culture.

Traditionally, childrearing and housekeeping have been the responsibility of women. They now increasingly demand that men assume their fair share of these tasks so that wives can continue their careers. Role conflict may occur in women who are not committed to both career and family responsibilities and in men who have similar ambivalent feelings about dual responsibilities. Loss of self-esteem may occur if either partner perceives their assigned tasks as demeaning (Payne, 1985).

Sexual intimacy may suffer if couples are fatigued or anxious about their relationship or if work and achievement become more important than family relationships. The advent of children and the responsibilities of childrearing may also negatively affect sexuality. Women may feel they have to choose between love and children and work and accomplishment. Sexual relationships may also suffer when the women direct their attention and energy toward their children, and men feel that their sexual and other needs are being ignored (Hogan, 1985).

Perhaps the most important factor in achieving a satisfying family life in relation to sexuality is the partners' ability to communicate to each other their sexual needs, feelings, fears, and love and respect for each other. The most important variable affecting satisfaction with the relationship is the quality of the marital relationship. Women, especially, are more satisfied when they can express their needs and feelings to their partner (Schenk et al., 1983). This contributes to stable family relationships and provides the ideal environment for the further development of their own and their children's sexuality.

In later adulthood, anxiety about sexual performance and attractiveness may occur in both sexes. Depression in middle-aged women may be attributed to menopause or may be related to the "empty-nest syndrome," when children have grown and left home.

Fear of loss of sexual attractiveness may affect sexual responsiveness of one or both partners. Sexual self-esteem may suffer, and hormonal and emotional changes of menopause may reduce or halt sexual activity.

Male menopause may also contribute to family stress. Middle-aged men may describe increased irritability, fatigue, urinary irregularity, hot flashes, and decreased sexual interest and drive (Sheehy, 1995).

Between the ages of 40–50, men may conclude that they have not reached their potential, and dissatisfaction may lead to depression and decreased self-esteem. Solutions may involve extramarital sexual activity that may symbolize status and bolster self-esteem.

Some wives may resume careers interrupted by childrearing, and husbands, suffering through their own crises, may feel threatened and anxious. Couples must review their relationship and learn to resolve their problems as they did earlier.

Sexual Development: Age Sixty-five and Older

Sexual function may be compromised by illness or by decreased strength and vigor that accompanies aging, although with attractive and healthy partners, sexual activity may continue into the eighties or nineties. Women who have had little pleasure in intercourse before menopause are more likely to avoid sexual activity in later years (Pfeiffer & Davis, 1972). Many women report that they stopped activity after the illness or death of their husbands or after the husband lost erectile ability. Men report a higher level of sexual interest and activity than women, although the proportion engaging in sexual intercourse decreases with age.

As aging occurs, sexual response is less intense. Longer foreplay is necessary for vaginal lubrication in women. There may be thinning of the vaginal walls and narrowing of the vagina barrel.

Erections may be less firm, may take increased stimulation to be achieved, and may be lost more readily. The refractory period, during which another erection cannot be obtained, is longer, at times days rather than minutes or hours.

Martin (1981) suggested that a lower level of sexual activity in the aged was due to decreased motivation and that individuals generally maintained high or low patterns of sexual activity over their lifetime. Older people may also express their sexuality in more varied and diffuse ways: touching, cuddling, or holding (Starr & Weiner, 1981).

Children do not see their parents as sexually active at any age, and society assumes the attitude that the elderly should not be interested in sexual activity. If death of one parent occurs, grown children often react with horror if a widowed parent begins to date again, and many children discourage remarriage. Paradoxically, just as parents have had concerns about their children's developing sexuality, grown children have concerns about the sexual behavior of their parents.

In a long-standing marital relationship, old age may be the golden age of sexuality that has matured through the years, resulting in a close, fulfilling intimacy and concern for one another.

FAMILIES WITH ALTERNATIVE LIFESTYLES

In the 1990s, fewer than 27% of the nation's 91 million households fit the definition of the traditional nuclear family. That means only 1 in 19 families are composed of a wage-earner father, a mother who stays home, and two or more children. With changing sexual mores, rapidly increasing numbers of single parents, and a recessionary economy forcing more people to share households (Ames, 1992), the family must be broadly defined to include "a group of people who love and care for each other" (Seligmann, 1990). Various forms of families who fit this new definition include single parents, stepfamilies, and domestic partners. As the divorce rate has increased to one out of every two marriages, the incidence of remarriages and stepfamilies has also increased so that stepchildren make up 20% of all children in married-couple families. A term unheard of ten years ago, domestic partnerships refer to gay, lesbian, and heterosexual "cohabitants who have an intimate relationship and are financially dependent" (Ames, 1992, p. 62). The Census Bureau has counted 1.6 million same-sex couples living together (up from 0.6 million in 1970) and 2.6 million heterosexual couples sharing a household (up from a half a million in 1970). Reasons cited for these changes include divorce, delayed marriage, and the growth of the gay-liberation movement (Footlick, 1990). This section will focus on selected variations in family sexuality patterns, including gay and lesbian partnerships and heterosexual domestic partners.

Gay and Lesbian Domestic Partnerships

Homosexuality has occurred in all societies, and at present, one out of every ten individuals is homosexual (Sanford, 1989). In its broadest definition, homosexuality refers to strong erotic attachment to members of the same sex.

American society has traditionally discriminated against homosexual individuals by declaring sexual acts between same-gendered partners illegal, not recognizing gay marriages as legal, and denying custody or adoption of children to same-sex partners. Homosexual partners have no legal rights during illness, cannot cover one another with health insurance benefits, and cannot be listed as next of kin on records. Conservative political and religious groups oppose homosexual marriage and parenthood on the grounds that it is against the natural law, is intrinsically disordered, and is not in harmony with the purposes of male-female psychological and physiologic differences. Lesbians and gays are perceived as unfit to raise children and a threat to family life.

After twenty-five years of gay rights activism, there has been some movement toward mitigating discrimination based on sexual preference. In 1990, Footlick argued that gays, more than any other group, have benefitted from broader social acceptance of alternative lifestyles. Although the gay lifestyle of the 1970s and 1980s often involved multiple liaisons and short-term relationships, lesbians have traditionally developed monogamous relationships with life-long partners. In the post-AIDS era of the 1990s, many gay men as well as lesbian women are choosing to live in monogamous relationships. Many of these couples have formed domestic partnerships (DP), participated in marriage ceremonies, and have or are interested in having children as part of their family units. In the last several years some corporations, in response to employee pressure or because it will make them more competitive, and a few local governments have set up DP programs. These programs provide low- or no-cost items, like sick leave or bereavement leave, and some are even beginning to offer more costly items like medical and dental or relocation costs (Ames, 1992). In May 1990, San Francisco's Board of Supervisors passed the "domestic partnership" legislation recognizing homosexual and unmarried heterosexual couples as having the rights of married couples. In the summer of 1990 the New York State highest court expanded the definition to protect a gay survivor of a couple and set four standards for a family: (1) the "exclusivity and longevity of a relationship"; (2) the "level of emotional and financial commitment"; (3) how the couple "conducted their everyday lives and held themselves out to society"; (4) and the "reliance placed on one another for daily services" (Footlick, 1990, p. 18).

Strommen (1989) estimates that approximately 20% of gay men marry women and that half of their marriages produce children, so that 10% of these men are also fathers. The reasons gay men marry include (1) the belief that homosexuality is only incidental to identity or an unawareness of homosexual identity at time of marriage; (2) family pressure to marry; (3) the belief that marriage is the only way to achieve happiness, regardless of the sexual orientation; (4) the belief that marriage will help them overcome homosexual orientation; (5) the desire for children; and (6) love for their marriage partner (p. 44). No matter what the reasons for a heterosexual mar-

riage, the pull of homosexual erotic attraction is strong, and either divorce or bisexual relationships may follow.

Divorce may follow the announcement of the homosexual orientation. The reaction of children to the news a parent is gay is usually better than might be expected in most cases and usually better than that of spouses. Daughters are more accepting than sons (Harris & Turner, 1985/86).

If there are children, the issue of custody arises. Courts have given various reasons for awarding custody to the heterosexual partner, usually stated as "the best interests of the child." The courts' concerns are over short- and long-term consequences of a son or daughter being with a homosexual mother or father. The expected short-term problems include social stigmatization and confusion over sexual identity; the long-term problems include fear of the child's eventual homosexual orientation (Green et al., 1986). These fears appear to have little foundation, however. Contact with the heterosexual parent, parents of peers, and conventional family patterns portrayed in the media (television, movies, books) all model heterosexual behavior.

In spite of these attitudinal and legal impediments, permanent relationships are being established, and gay couples are raising children, usually from a previous heterosexual marriage of one of the partners. The quality of parenthood consists of love, care for the child, quality of time spent with the child, and ability to provide for and act in the child's best interest. The quality of parenthood is not affected by the sex of the parent's lover.

Green et al. (1986) compared two types of households: 50 homosexual mothers and children and 40 heterosexual mothers and children. No significant differences were found in general intelligence, core morphologic identity, gender role preferences, family and peer relationships, and adjustment to single-parent families in the boys and only a few in the girls. There was data to indicate that girls of lesbian mothers were less traditionally feminine in dress, in activity preference in school and at play, and in anticipated occupation. The literature suggests that gay parents are little different from heterosexual parents except in their sexual orientation, and that the children of gay parents are similar to other children.

A major health problem that affects homosexual families is AIDS. The majority of AIDS cases are among males with a mean age of 30 who are gay or drug users. This disease has catastrophic effects on the family due to exorbitant health care costs; the threat of death; and family conflict resulting from anger, grief, frustration, or despair. In addition to providing nonjudgmental holistic care, the nursing intervention should incorporate health teaching about AIDS and prevention (Tibler, 1987).

Heterosexual Domestic Partnerships

Given its prevalence, cohabitation is a "family status" that must be included with marriage if nurses are to understand family life in the 1990s (Bumpass et al., 1991). The number of Americans living together outside of marriage has increased 400% since 1970. Four percent of Americans 19 and older are cohabiting, 25% have cohabitated at some time, and unmarried couples account for 3 million of the country's 93 million households (Ames, 1992). The popularity of cohabitation may be attributed to two factors: Americans postponing marriage, and the social stigma against premarital sex diminishing (Larson, 1991). The large increases in the proportion of people in their early twenties who have never been married does not mean that young people are staying single longer, rather they are setting up households with heterosexual partners at almost as early an age as they did before the marriage rates declined. Bumpass et al. (1991) reported that the proportion of people living with a partner before marrying for the first time increased from 11% around 1970 to nearly 50% for recent first marriages.

Cohabiting relationships tend to be short-term arrangements. According to Bumpass and Sweet (1989), by the end of a year and a half 50% of cohabiting couples either marry or break up. Only 1 in 10 cohabit after five years without either breaking up or getting married. Since two-thirds of first cohabiting couples get married, there is little evidence that large numbers of cohabitants are rejecting marriage (Larson, 1991). Sweet (Larson, 1991) believes that fear of relationships not working out or not being economically viable is often the reason couples choose to cohabit.

Recent research has called into question a number of common myths about couples who live together. Cohabitation is often viewed as a new stage in the American courtship process and an important step prior to marriage that screens out "potentially incompatible mates more effectively than does traditional courtship" (Bumpass et al., 1991; DeMaris & Rao, 1992) and engagement. In reality, cohabiting relationships are much less stable than those that begin as marriages; 40% will disrupt before marriage and marriages that are preceded by living together have 50% higher disruption rates than marriages without premarital cohabitation (Bennett, Blanc & Bloom, 1988; Booth & Johnson, 1989; Bumpass & Sweet, 1989; Hoem & Hoem, 1992; Teachman & Polonko, 1990; Trussel, Rodriguez & Vaughn, 1992; Thompson & Colella, 1992). Attempting to explain this "cohabitation effect" (DeMaris and Rao, 1992), researchers postulate that cohabitation is a nontraditional lifestyle that attracts people who are more prone to unstable marriages (Booth & Johnson, 1988); less well-adjusted (Bumpass et al., 1992); perceive themselves or their relationship as a poor risk; define marriage in more individual than couple terms and view marital quality as more central to relationships (Thompson & Colella, 1992); and have a generally weaker commitment to the institution of marriage and are more likely to accept divorce as a solution (Bennett et al., 1988). In spite of the fact that the cohabitation effect is beginning to take on the status of an empirical generalization, future research is needed to explain the precise connection (Thompson & Colella, 1992).

The "diffusion theory"—that college students initiated the trend toward cohabitation in the 1960s, which then spread to the rest of the population in the 1970s and 1980s—is not accurate. It is the least-educated segment of society that led the trend (Bumpass et al., 1992), and cohabitation is most common among those who did not complete high school, grew up receiving welfare, or were raised in single-family homes (Thornton, 1991). In fact, cohabitation is more common among separated and divorced people than among the never married.

How do cohabiting couples with children differ from married couples with children? Cohabitating couples report lower levels of certainty about their relationship than do married couples. Raising children is one function that always defined the family. Individuals with alternatives, such as employed women who do not need marriage to raise children, are likely to delay marriage. Forty percent of cohabiting couples have children in the unit. Webster found that while cohabiting units look like a family, they function differently than families. For example cohabiting couples share the housework more equitably than married couples, but they share the child care less—the children usually belong to and are cared for by the woman (Riche, 1991).

NURSING PROCESS AND FAMILY SEXUAL HEALTH

Assessment and Diagnosis

Nurses who are comfortable with sexuality either grew up in families who were comfortable with sexual issues or had some life or educational experience that helped them sort out their feelings, experiences, and values. Between the contradictory messages from culture, media, religion, education, and families, it is not uncommon for nurses to feel uncomfortable with their own and with other's sexuality. Few nurses, particularly those who completed their education more than five years ago, have been taught in their nursing programs to include sexuality as part of their routine history taking. Some nurses have learned "on-the-job" to explore only those particular aspects of sexuality related to their specialty areas, for example, post-myocardial infarction patients' resuming sex after hospital discharge. They remain uncomfortable with issues beyond their narrow purview.

Before nurses explore sexual issues with families using the nursing process, it would be helpful for them to complete a self-assessment of their own values, experiences, and belief systems related to sexuality (Muscari, 1987). There are a number of ways for nurses to accomplish this task, such as (1) to list topics like abortion, masturbation, fellatio, and various forms of sexual expression (e.g., homosexuality) to surface nurses' feelings and attitudes toward particular sexual issues (Hogan, 1980); (2) to complete a sexual history on themselves (see Table 17–2); or (3) to explore gender identity (Muscari, 1987)—a creative way to do this is for nurses to reflect on their "gender role journey" (O'Neil). The gender role journey involves responding to the question, "What has it meant for you to grow up a girl/woman or boy/man in this society?" Nurses review their lives to remember the messages they received and the experiences they had with families, religion, school, and peers that shaped their femininity or masculinity. Sharing either the sexual history or the gender role journey with a colleague gives nurses empathy for the vulnerability involved in sharing the intimate details of one's sexual life with another individual. This would sensitize them to the importance of understanding, rather than judging, individuals' and families' views on sexuality.

Any of the preceding exercises can alert nurses to issues that might be uncomfortable for them to discuss with families. There are issues for each nurse that are difficult or impossible to maintain objectivity about. It is important for nurses to be aware of the issues they are sensitized to and to either work through their own issues in supervision or to refer the family with this issue to another nurse.

When taking a sexual history, nurses must realize that it is not taken out of the context of the individuals' or families' total being; it is part of the larger health history that obtains information about other functional health patterns. Obtaining an isolated sexual history is as meaningless as taking a "stomach history" or "heart history" (Belliveau & Richter, 1970). Table 17–2 summarizes data that should be collected from all clients and families, with additional information gathered as the situation suggests. Comprehensive outlines of sexual history information are not for all clients. Questions are chosen selectively as the situation indicates.

In assessing for problems related to sexual response, general demographic data is obtained (see the assessment tool at the end of the chapter). Clients' knowledge, values, and attitudes about sexual activity are identified. Nurses determine what the usual sexual practices are, if they are satisfying, and if the clients have moral reservations about certain types of sexual behaviors (e.g., masturbation, positions for intercourse, and so on) (Hogan, 1982). Nurses also identify if there is conflict between the parents because of different beliefs.

Once the nature of the problem is identified, nurses ascertain (1) if the client or family has already sought help, (2) the precipitating factors, (3) the sexual partners' knowledge of the problem and point of view, (4) the clients' family's proposed remedies and needs, (5) effect of the problem on the clients' lifestyles and the rest of the relationship, and (6) the personality assets and strengths (Alexander, 1981). Data from other health patterns are also analyzed to identify related factors.

The family's attitude toward sexual behavior such as nudity, openess to showing affection, beliefs about masturbation, and premarital sexual relationships is assessed by direct questioning of family members. Nurses do not probe and are careful not to communicate their own beliefs and values about sexuality. When a trust relationship

TABLE 17–2. DATA TO BE COLLECTED FOR NURSING HISTORY FOR FAMILIES

DATA	DATA
Ages of family members	Health problems, medical conditions, surgical procedures in past and anticipated in the future; medication therapy (for parents and children)
Sex of all family members	
Education, occupation of family members	
Quality of relationships with significant others: parent-children, spouse-spouse (affectionate, punitive, hostile)	Changes in role relationships and ability to carry out the usual sexual role (of both parents, sexual partners)
Interests, hobbies of individuals and family as a whole	Potential changes in ability to carry out usual sexual role (of both parents, sexual partners)
Spiritual/religious/philosophical beliefs, congruence among family members	Change in perception of self as male or female due to illness or life events
Attitude of family members about sexual behaviors (touching, nudity, masturbation, coitus, etc.)	Existing or potential sexual dysfunction of one or both parents, sexual partners
Teaching children about sexuality (knowledge level of parents, responsibility for content given)	Presence of family conflict because of difference in values and beliefs about sexuality and sexual behaviors

has developed between nurse and clients, information will be shared and sexual health promoted.

Pregnancy and the birth of a child may be a time of sexual distress for the partners as roles and relationships change and the family dyad is expanded. Early in pregnancy the nurse assesses the couple's knowledge of pregnancy and its effect on sexuality, their attitudes toward the pregnancy and the coming child, and the nature of the sexual relationship.

Common nursing diagnoses and related factors, sexuality and family health include:

- Sexual dysfunction, which may be related to physical abuse, harmful relationships, misinformation or lack of knowledge, values conflict, lack of privacy, lack of a significant other, altered body structure or function, or change in roles and relationships
- Ineffective family or individual coping related to sexual dysfunction
- Depression related to sexual dysfunction
- Self-esteem disturbances related to sexual dysfunction, loss of sexual role
- Fear, related to possible loss of sexual function and/or knowledge deficit
- Parenting alteration (potential or actual) related to lack of sexual developmental guidelines, support system deficit, physical or psychosocial abuse, family or personal stress
- Lack of information about sexuality
- Negative attitudes about sexuality (Gordon, 1991)

Intervention and Evaluation

When intervening to promote sexual health, nurses must be careful not to impose their own beliefs and values on patients/clients since the amount and kind of information shared can be affected by nurses' biases. Nurses need to avoid subtly and nonverbally communicating negative attitudes about sexuality when clients ask questions or bring up concerns (Hogan, 1985).

To be effective, nurses need to be tolerant of human differences in sexual behavior and accepting of clients who have a different sexual orientation or lifestyle as valued individuals. They do not suggest or urge sexual practices that violate the client's moral or ethical code and that if practiced by the client may cause value conflict or guilt (Hogan, 1982). If nurses believe that discussion of sexuality is wrong or inappropriate or if they are uncomfortable or embarrassed by the topic, it is better that someone else do the sexual counseling or teaching (Hogan, 1985).

At some point in interventions, the sexual partner must be included since there are relationship factors to be considered. There is no situation in which there is an uninvolved partner.

Lack of knowledge about the sexual response cycle and the need for adequate foreplay can be treated by counseling both partners and describing arousal techniques. Foreplay may include kissing, oral-genital stimulation (fellatio and cunnilingus), and tactile stimulation to erogenous zones (these usually include the breast, vulva, anus, penis, lips, mouth, and other areas from which individuals experience pleasure). Fondling, caressing, or light scratching of the sexual partner's body, and massaging with creams and lotions increases sensation.

Darkness, soft lights or full illumination, music, pictures or movies of others engaging in sexual activity, and sexual fantasies may be effective for foreplay and arousal. Individuals know what they find most stimulating and need to share this information with their sexual partners.

Nurses also suggest various positions for coitus besides the male superior (missionary) position. Female superior, side-by-side, rear entry, and sitting positions may provide variety and increase response. Couples need to communicate what is pleasurable or unpleasurable, and partners must be caring and considerate of each other. Nurses stress the importance of a loving word or glance and a nonhurried, private environment (Hogan, 1985).

When couples complain of the fatigue that accompanies childbearing and childrearing, nurses suggest different times and places for coitus: for example, in the early morning or the afternoon (if privacy can be assured) rather than late in the evening or after a hectic day's work. Getting away from home to spend a weekend together or having a relative take the children for an evening or day gives parents an opportunity for leisurely lovemaking, sharing of confidences, and keeping in touch with who they are and what they mean to each other (Smith, 1981).

Finally, if there is conflict because of change in sexual roles due to illness or other life events, the nurse can serve as a catalyst to increase the partner's communication about the fear, frustration, and anger he or she may be expressing.

Interventions during pregnancy also require teaching and counseling both partners. Sexual activity can usually continue throughout pregnancy, providing there is no bleeding or history of abortion. As pregnancy progresses, the female superior, side-by-side, spoon fashion, or rear entry positions are recommended to avoid pressure on the breasts and abdomen. Nurses counter myths and misconceptions by explaining that the fetus is not harmed by coitus and cannot hear or see in utero. Nurses also help prospective parents talk about their new roles and the activities and responsibilities that accompany parenthood. Alteration in parenting can be prevented by anticipatory guidance and counseling. Nurses also may discuss the resumption of sexual activity after the baby is born. Group or individual classes with both partners present are an essential component of post-partum care.

After delivery, the woman may experience decreased sexual interest due to fatigue, weakness, and vaginal discomfort. Breast or other discomfort and decreased vaginal lubrication may also limit sexual response, as does postpartum "blues" or depression.

If decreased vaginal lubrication exists because of steroid starvation, a water-soluble gel or a contraceptive cream or jelly can be recommended. If vaginal tenderness continues, the partners are instructed to rotate one or two fingers around the vagina to help it relax. If vaginal pain persists for four weeks after resuming sexual activity, the woman should return for treatment.

Kegel exercises are recommended to strengthen the pubococcygeal muscle that controls not only vaginal perception and response during coitus but also bowel and bladder function. The nurse also provides the couple with contraception information if they desire it.

The depression that may follow pregnancy is self-limiting, especially if the partner gives support and love. Role-relationship problems require mutual discussion and "working out" by the parents. The mother is reminded that she should not neglect the father to focus on infant care (Hogan, 1985).

Evaluation of interventions related to family health include the couples':

- Verbal report that they are satisfied with their sexual relationship.
- Resumption of sexual activity that both partners describe as satisfying.
- Ability to describe alternative positions for intercourse and different foreplay activities.
- Commitment to and satisfaction with parenting as observed by the nurse.
- Ability to identify the effects of fatigue, discomfort in sexual relationship, and ways to relieve these effects.
- Identification of the importance of communication and a loving supportive relationship to promote sexual health.

NURSING IMPLICATIONS: SEXUALITY ACROSS THE FAMILY LIFE SPAN

Assessment and Nursing Diagnoses during Infancy, Childhood, and Adolescence

Nurses are in an ideal position to teach and counsel parents and children about the normality of psychosexual developmental behaviors. Nurses assess the parents' beliefs and attitudes about these behaviors and their knowledge of normal psychosexual development. Observation is made of infants' and children's relationship with parents and as appropriate with peers and siblings. Finally, the nurse identifies any concerns the parents have about children's sexuality, behaviors, and relationships with others. Physical examination is done to identify biologic abnormalities.

Adolescents and their parents may be reluctant to seek help, so sexual problems may be identified during legal or medical treatment for other problems. Consequently, nurses, are alert to subtle signs of difficulties.

Data collected include the adolescent's level of psychosexual development and knowledge of sexuality, exposure to sexual activity, environmental pressures, family and other support systems, and general physical development and health (Hogan, 1985).

Intervention and Evaluation: Infancy to Adolescence

Parents need anticipatory guidance in teaching children the correct terms for anatomy and physiology, providing information appropriate to the child's developmental level, promoting positive attitudes toward body parts and gender roles, and acceptance of masturbation in infants and small children as normal. Assuring to parents that touching the genital areas and exhibition of genitals are normal activities of children is usually sufficient. Involving children in activities; giving love, attention, and creative stimulation; and teaching children that touching their private parts is to be done in private should be encouraged. Families with young children should be encouraged to provide an environment where sexuality and issues can be discussed in an open and comfortable manner. In order to protect children from sexual abuse and rape, they should be taught about inappropriate touching of their genitals by others and how to relate to strangers.

Adolescents should be given an opportunity to discuss their view of self and their feelings about the opposite sex. Developmental and cognitive stages of adolescence must be taken into account when counseling adolescents and families (Grant & Demetriou, 1988). Textbooks and articles dedicated to caring for adolescents typically recommend that nurses be nonjudgmental, honor confidentiality, and honestly appraise the implications of sexual activity (Alexander et al., 1991; O'Keefe, 1992). Nurses who work with families with adolescents need to be aware of and sensitive to adolescents' and family's religious and community attitudes and values. If the individual has been seen since childhood, then the nurse-patient relationship needs to be redefined at adolescence to accommodate confidentiality. At adolescence the adolescent replaces the parent as the primary historian and helps establish the agenda for visits.

Nurses need to communicate to adolescents that they are approachable, for example, by initiating sexual discussions and having sex educational materials in waiting rooms (Alexander et al., 1991).

Nurses can educate parents to discuss sexual issues with children and adolescents, to clarify values, to help them guide decision making, and appraise them of helpful resources in the community and recommended books. Parents are often relieved to find out that they do not need to be "sexperts" who have all the answers.

It is also important for the nurse to identify adolescents who are at risk for sexual acting out. Potential risk factors may include (1) parental divorce or separation; (2) vague future educational plans—the higher the level of intended education, the less likely early sexual intercourse is; (3) no religious affiliation—the more religious the adolescent, the less likelihood of sexual intercourse; and (4) negative parental attitudes or teaching—the more affirming the parental messages about sexuality, the less chance the adolescent is sexually active (Furstenberg et al., 1985). Nurses can emphasize that coitus should take place in a deep, lasting relationship, something different than infatuation, and that healthy sexuality is based on more than peer approval or ability to "score."

Although adolescents may seem to be sexually sophisticated, they are often ignorant about sexual development and response and prey to the myths and misconceptions of adults. Adolescents need information about anatomy and physiology of sexuality, reassurance that isolated homosexual experiences do not mean one is homosexual, and

information about developing friendships with those of the opposite sex.

Contraceptive information is given to adolescents who request it, whereas other adolescents need sources of support for their beliefs that sexual intimacy should be reserved for marriage and that it is all right to say no. The school nurse who initiates teaching programs is in a position to foster healthy sexuality. Classes should be held for student groups as well as for families (Hogan, 1985). Table 17–3 summarizes content of classes related to sexuality.

The unmarried adolescent girl who becomes pregnant needs help in deciding about abortion, adoption, or keeping the baby with or without marriage. Rather than suggesting solutions, nurses can help the girl identify these alternatives, their advantages and disadvantages, and come to a solution. No matter what the decision, the adolescent may experience guilt and depression and needs support to deal with feelings. The nurse also helps the father work through his feelings about the pregnancy and recognize his responsibility to the mother and child.

Evaluation of interventions related to childhood and adolescent sexual health include meeting the following criteria:

1. Parents describe normal psychosexual development of children and teach children accurate and factual information.
2. Parents state they are satisfied with their child's psychosexual development.
3. Parents show evidence of love and affection for children (praise them, kiss and hold them appropriately, etc.).
4. Adolescents describe biopsychosocial aspects of sexuality, and understand conception, sexually transmitted diseases, and AIDS.
5. Adolescents make an informed decision to have or not to have sex.
6. Adolescents identify and use contraception measures when needed.
7. Adolescents who become pregnant express reasonable satisfaction with their decision about the pregnancy.
8. Adolescents who become pregnant state they have worked through any guilt and/or depression about their decision.

TABLE 17–3. CONTENT OF EDUCATION ABOUT SEXUALITY

1. Male and female: anatomy and physiology, reproductive system
2. Responses of men and women to sexual stimulation: sexual response cycle
3. Information about growth and development: secondary sex characteristics, menstruation, wet dreams
4. Fertilization, pregnancy, childbirth, conception control
5. Sexually transmitted diseases: types, prevention
6. Alternative forms of sexual expression: masturbation, homosexuality, bisexuality
7. Married and family love, emphasis on sexuality as a basis of family life and committed relationships
8. Making a choice of sexual behavior
9. Interpersonal relations: socializing with the opposite sex
10. Factors affecting family life: economic and social mobility, depersonalization, media distortion of sexuality

Nursing Process during Adulthood

In addition to situations discussed earlier in the chapter in the section on Nursing Process and Family Sexual Health, the middle years may strain sexual relationships as individuals approach menopause or "change of life." Nurses assess women's and sexual partners' attitude toward and knowledge of menopause and its effects. Signs and symptoms such as "hot flashes," thinning of the vaginal wall, and decreased lubrication are identified.

Myths and misconceptions that sexual activity is not suitable or may be painful after menopause can be dispelled by nurses. If the female client has vaginal atrophy and decreased lubrication, nurses recommend use of water-soluble jelly, saliva, or insertion of the finger in the vagina to bring out secretions deeper in the vagina. Referral to physicians for estrogen therapy may be indicated (Hogan, 1985).

Teaching and counseling focuses on the role of hormones and the need for exercise of the pubococcygeal muscle and includes giving permission to be sexual. A healthy lifestyle, good nutrition, weight control, and maintaining friendships and activities promote postmenopausal zest (Caldwell, 1982).

If there is change in sexual interest, causes are determined. If due to illness, the underlying problem is treated. If due to monotony in the relationships, nurses suggest different times, places, and lovemaking techniques to increase sexual pleasure (Hogan, 1985).

Nursing Process during Older Age

Data is collected to help distinguish among illness, disinterest, or relational problems as causes of sexual problems. Information similar to that of adulthood assessment is obtained by nurses who must be careful not to communicate their own biases and misinformation about older persons' sexuality. Diagnoses similar to those in adulthood may be identified.

Interventions include teaching physiologic changes that accompany aging, the need for longer foreplay, supplementation of vaginal lubrication with estrogen creams or water-soluble lubricants, less strenuous positions for coitus such as side by side or female superior, and time of day when partners are more rested (early morning or afternoon).

Some couples and their families need the reassurance that sexual activity is normal during old age. Nurses also remind couples that lying together, holding each other, touching, and sharing expressions of love are forms of sexual intimacy. Coitus is not necessarily the final goal.

Evaluation of the interventions related to healthy sexuality in the elderly include meeting the following criteria:

1. The aging individuals describe biologic changes in the sexual response cycle that accompany aging.
2. The aging individuals identify changes in foreplay and coitus that increase their sexual satisfaction.
3. The older individuals express satisfaction in their sexual relationship.

4. The older individuals identify the importance of expressions of love and tenderness to maintain the relationship.

NURSING IMPLICATIONS: FAMILIES WITH ALTERNATIVE LIFESTYLES

Assessment and Nursing Diagnosis: Gay and Lesbian Domestic Partners

Assessment data collected from homosexual families are similar to that of other families. They have problems and concerns similar to those of heterosexuals: difficulty in finding a partner, vulnerability to sexually transmitted disease (particularly AIDS), interpersonal awkwardness, plus the added pressures that come from an often disapproving and discriminating society.

Children living with a homosexual parent may have to deal with society's negative attitudes toward the parent's sexual orientation (Willhoite, 1991; Newman, 1991), so nurses need to assess the children's coping ability and self-esteem. They may have had to deal with ridicule and desertion by friends. Nursing diagnoses similar to those of heterosexual families may be identified.

Interventions and Evaluation: Gay and Lesbian Domestic Partners

Nurses must be careful not to discriminate against the homosexual family or individuals because of ignorance and fear of homosexuality. Whether the nurse sees their lifestyle as moral or immoral, variant or deviant, gay and lesbian patients/clients and families are entitled to competent and loving care.

Parents of homosexuals may need support and the opportunity to discuss fears and concerns. In light of the epidemic proportions of AIDS in this decade among homosexuals (particularly men), nurses are encouraged to provide sensitive holistic nursing care that includes anticipatory teaching about prevention and guidelines for safe sex to homosexual domestic partners.

The individual's sex mate should be regarded as a significant other and allowed similar rights and privileges of family care. Many health care problems and family life issues are similar to those of other families, with the additional problem that a legal relationship does not usually exist, and nursing interventions and evaluation are similar. However, homosexual families have unique needs. To meet these needs, recent social and political changes have brought about numerous social support and community resources specifically for gay and lesbian families, in the area of health promotion, disease prevention, and coping with life crises. Nurses are encouraged to seek out these resources when working with homosexual domestic partners.

Assessment, Nursing Diagnoses, and Intervention: Heterosexual Domestic Partners

Assessment, nursing diagnoses, and intervention are similar to those of married couples. In nursing intervention for family lifestyle issues, transitions and crises for heterosexual families can be handled using the nursing process. Since each couple is unique, the nurse can work with the couple collaboratively in the resolution of developmental and situational issues.

RESOURCES FOR NURSES

The American Association of Sex Educators, Counselors and Therapists, The Sexual Information and Education Council of the United States (SIECUS), the National Committee for the Protection of Child Abuse, and the Planned Parenthood Federation of America can be contacted for information and resources for any particular area. The public library is an excellent source of books, audiovisual material, and pamphlets related to sexuality. Books are available that give information about the various consumer resources related to health, and these can be a guide to information that would be useful to the nurse, as well as to the client. The *Journal of School Health* has many excellent articles about sexuality, especially as it relates to children and adolescents.

Nurses have a pivotal role in helping families develop healthy sexuality. They must be knowledgeable, tolerant of human differences, and comfortable with their own sexuality. No matter what the setting, clients' age, or biologic sex, nurses teach, counsel, and give care that fosters and promotes healthy sexuality.

Family Sexuality-Assessment

I. Demographic Data
   A. Clients' age, sex, marital status
   B. Parents' age, sex, marital status, religion, education, occupation
   C. Other children, sibling's age, sex, assets, problems
II. Biologic Factors
   A. Satisfaction with sexual relationship, frequency, pleasure, types of activity, foreplay
   B. Problems: impotence, anorgasmia, painful intercourse, lack of interest (drive)
   C. Illness affecting sexuality: diagnosis, type of problem (body image disturbance, change in physiologic response, role change)

III. Psychosocial Data
   A. Parent's relationship: congeniality, demonstration of affection, feelings toward children, communication patterns, mutual decision making, satisfaction with sexual roles, well-defined self-boundaries
   B. Family and child's attitudes toward sexuality: degree of openness or reserve about sex, attitude toward sexual activity, religious beliefs about sexuality
   C. Siblings relationship: congeniality, affection, communication pattern
   D. Homosexual family: children's acceptance of relationship, fears and concerns
IV. Learning about Sexuality
   A. Parents' knowledge of and attitude toward sexual response, sexual relation-

CHAPTER HIGHLIGHTS

Sexuality includes the physical and psychological energy that individuals expend in attaining warmth, tenderness, sexual response, and love. Therefore, each person is a sexual being from birth to death.

Family sexuality is a complex, multifaceted phenomena that is more than the sexual interaction of adult family members and includes the unplanned parent-child interactions in everyday family living.

Family patterns, communication skills, parenting approaches, and family configuration strongly affect children's sexual development. Children learn values toward sexuality within families; therefore, parents should be provided with information and the skills to instruct children about sexual issues.

Sexual behavioral norms and relationships vary by culture, religion, and societies. Therefore, careful assessment of cultural, religious, and family attitudes and beliefs is important.

In the past decade, there has been an increase in the number of heterosexual and homosexual domestic partners, and professionals working with these families should provide judgement-free health care to families who choose this lifestyle.

Sexuality issues vary during the family life course and for members at different developmental levels.

Nursing assessment of family history is affected by how comfortable the nurse feels in discussing and teaching sexuality.

ships, sexual development (sex play, masturbation, pregnancy, birth, menstruation, nocturnal emission, venereal disease, homosexuality)
   B. Children's knowledge of sexuality (see A. parent's knowledge)
      1. Explanations, teaching done by parents
      2. Attitude of children about sexuality
Childhood/Adolescent Sex Activity
   A. Incest: nature of activity, person involved, willing or unwilling, form of rewards, feeling about activity
      1. Physiologic problems: bedwetting, venereal disease, cystitis, vaginal infection, trauma
      2. Psychosocial problems: runaway behavior, withdrawal
   B. Adolescent pregnancy: age of both parents, attitudes about pregnancy, familial support and attitudes, strengths and weakness of adolescents involved, acceptance or rejection of pregnancy, proposed solutions, plans for future, general health and development

REFERENCES

Alexander, B. (1981). Taking the sexual history. *American Family Physician, 23,* 147–153.

Alexander, B., McGrew, M.C., & Shore, W. (1991, October). Adolescent sexuality issues in office practice. *Adolescent Family Practice, 44*(4), 1273–1281.

Ames, K. (March 23, 1992). Domesticated bliss: New laws are making it official for gay and live-in couples. *Newsweek.*

Bamford, F.N. (1980). Sexual development in children. *Clinics in Obstetrics and Gynecology, 7*(3), 193–211.

Belliveau, F., & Richter, L. (1970). *Understand Human Sexual Inadequacy.* New York: Bantam.

Bennett, N.B., Blanc, A.K., & Bloom, D.E. (1988). Commitment and the modern union: Assessing the link between premarital cohabitation and subsequent marital stability. *American Sociological Review, 53,* 127–138.

Bolton, F.J. (1981). *The Pregnant Adolescent.* Beverly Hills: Sage.

Booth, A., & Johnson, D. (1988). Premarital cohabitation and marital success. *Journal of Family Issues, 9,* 255–272.

Bor, R. (1991). The ABC of AIDS counseling. *Nursing Times, 87*(1), 32–55.

Broderick, C.B. (1966). Sexual behavior among pre-adolescents. *Journal of Social Issues, 22*(5), 6–22.

Brunngraber, L.S. (1986). Father-daughter incest: Immediate and long-term effects of sexual abuse. *Advances in Nursing Science, 8*(4), 15–35.

Bumpass, L.L., & Sweet, J.A. (1989). National estimates of cohabitation: Cohort levels and union stability. *Demography, 26,* 615–625.

Bumpass, L.L., Sweet, J.A., & Cherlin, A. (1991). The role of cohabitation in declining rates of marriage. *Journal of Marriage and the Family, 53,* 913–927.

Caldwell, L.R. (1982). Questions and answers about menopause. *American Journal of Nursing, 82,* 1100–1101.

Campbell, J. (1984). Nursing care of families using violence. In J. Campbell & J. Humphreys (Eds.), *Nursing Care of Victims of Family Violence.* Reston, VA: Reston.

Chilman, C.S. (1990). Promoting healthy adolescent sexuality. *Family Relations, 39,* 123–130.

Coleman, E. (1988, Spring). Research in human sexuality: Its importance to family practice. *Family Practice Research Journal, 7*(3), 119–121.

Coles, R., & Stokes, G. (1985). *Sex and the American Teenager.* New York: Harper & Row.

Daughtery, L.R., & Burger, J.M. (1984). The influence of parents, church and peers on the sexual attitudes and behaviors of college students. *Archives of Sexual Behavior, 13,* 351–360.

DeMaris, A., & Rao, K.V. (1992). Premarital cohabitation and subsequent marital stability in the United States: A reassessment. *Journal of Marriage and the Family, 54,* 178–190.

Downey, L. (1980). Intergenerational change in sex behavior: A belated look at Kinsey's males. *Archives of Sexual Behavior, 9,* 267–317.

Fingerman, K.L. (1989). Sex and the working mother: Adolescent sexuality, sex role typing and family background. *Adolescence, 24*(93), 1–18.

Finkelhor, D. (1979). What's wrong with sex between adults and children? *American Journal of Orthopsychiatry, 49,* 492–497.

Flewelling, R.L., & Bauman, K.E. (1990). Family structure as a predictor of initial substance abuse and sexual intercourse in early adolescence. *Journal of Marriage and the Family, 52,* 171–180.

Fonesca, J.D. (1970). Sexuality—a quality of being human. *Nursing Outlook, 18,* 25.

Footlick, J.K. (1990). What happened to the family? *The 21st Century Family: Newsweek Special Issue.*

Friedrich, W.N., Grambsch, P., Broughton, D., et al. (1991, September). Normative sexual behavior in children. *Pediatrics, 88*(3), 456–464.

Gilchrist, V.J. (1991, March). Preventive health care for the adolescent. *Adolescent Family Practice, 43*(3), 869–878.

Gordon, M. (1991). *Manual of Nursing Diagnosis 1986–1987.* St. Louis: Mosby.

Grant, L.M., & Demetriou, E. (1988). Adolescent sexuality. *The Pediatric Clinics of North America, 35*(6), 1271–1289.

Gray, J.P. (1984). The influence of female power in marriage on sexual behaviors and attitudes: A holocultural study. *Archives of Sexual Behavior, 13,* 223–232.

Green, R. (1978). Sexual identity of 37 children raised by homosexual or transsexual parents. *American Journal of Psychiatry, 135,* 692–717.

Green, R., Mandel, J.B., Holveldt, M.E., Gray, J., & Smith, L. (1986). Lesbian mothers and their children: A comparison with solo parent heterosexual mothers and their children. *Archives of Sexual Behavior, 15,* 167–184.

Guyton, A.C. (1986). *Textbook of Medical Physiology* (7th ed.). Philadelphia: Saunders.

Hajcak, F., & Garwood, P. (1988). What parents can do to prevent pseudohypersexuality in adolescents. *Family Therapy, 15*(2), 99–105.

Hanson, S.L., Myers, D.E., & Ginsberg, A.L. (1987). The role of responsibility and knowledge in reducing teenage out-of-wedlock pregnancy. *Journal of Marriage and the Family, 49,* 241.

Harris, M.B., & Turner, P.H. (1985/86). Gay and lesbian parents. *Journal of Homosexuality, 12,* 101–113.

Herman, J., & Hirschman, L. (1981). Families at risk for father-daughter incest. *American Journal of Psychiatry*, 138, 967–972.

Hertsgaard, D., & Light, H. (1984). Junior high girls' attitudes toward rights and roles of women. *Adolescence*, 76, 874–853.

Hoeffer, B. (1981). Children's acquisition of sex role behavior in lesbian-mother families. *Journal of Orthopsychiatry*, 51, 536–543.

Hoem, B., & Hoem, J.M. (1992). The disruption of marital and non-marital unions in contemporary Sweden. In J. Trussell, R. Hankinson & J. Tilton (Eds.), *Demographic Applications of Event History Analysis* (pp. 61–63). Oxford: Clarendon Press.

Hogan, R. (1980). *Human Sexuality: A Nursing Perspective*. Norwalk, CT: Appleton-Century-Crofts.

Hogan, R. (1982). Culture and human sexuality. *Nursing Clinics of North America*, 17, 365–376.

Hogan, R. (1985). *Human Sexuality: A Nursing Perspective* (2nd ed.). Norwalk, CT: Appleton-Century-Crofts.

Jacklin, C.N., DiPretro, J.A., & Maccoby, E.E. (1984). Sex-typing behavior and sex-typing pressure in child-parent interaction. *Archives of Sexual Behavior*, 13, 413–428.

Johnson, V.E., & Masters, M.H. (1976). Contemporary influences on sexual response. *Journal of School Health*, 46, 211–214.

Kaplan, S.J., & Pelcovitz, D. (1982). Child abuse and neglect and sexual abuse. *Psychiatric Clinics of North America*, 5, 321–332.

Keith, J.B., McCreary, C., Collins, et al. (1991, Winter). Sexual activity and contraceptive use among low-income urban black adolescent females. *Adolescence*, 26(104), 769–785.

Kinsey, A.C., Pomeroy, W.B., & Martin, C.E. (1948). *Sexual Behavior in the Human Male*. Philadelphia: W.B. Saunders.

Kinsey, A.C., Pomeroy, W.B., Martin, C.E., & Gebbard, P.H. (1965). *Sexual Behaviors in the Human Female*. New York: Pocket Books.

Koyle, P., Jensen, L., Olsen, J., & Cundick, B. (1989). Comparison of sexual behavior among adolescents having an early, middle, and late first intercourse experience. *Youth and Society*, 20(4), 461–475.

Larson, J. (1991, November). Cohabitation is a premarital step. *American Demographics*, 20–21.

Levin, R.J. (1980). The physiology of sexual function in women. *Clinics in Obstetrics and Gynecology*, 7, 220–246.

Maddock, J. (1975). Sexual health and health care. *Postgraduate Medicine*, 58(1), 52–58.

Martin, C.E. (1981). Factors affecting sexual functioning in 60–79-year-old males. *Archives of Sexual Behavior*, 10, 399–420.

Masters, W.H., Johnson, V.E., & Kolodny, R.C. (1982). Human Sexuality. Boston: Little, Brown.

Miller, B., & Bingham, C. (1989). Family configurations in relation to the sexual behavior of female adolescents. *Journal of Marriage and the Family*, 51(2), 499–506.

Moore, K.A., Peterson, J.L., & Furstenberg, J. (1986). Parental attitudes and the occurrence of early sexual activity. *Journal of Marriage and the Family*, 48, 777–782.

Mrazek, D., & Mrazek, P. (1981). Psychosexual development within the family. In P. Mrazek & C.H. Kempe (Eds.), *Sexually Abused Children and Their Families* (pp. 17–32). New York: Pergamon.

Muscari, M.E. (1987, September/October). Obtaining the adolescent sexual history. *Pediatric Nursing*, 13(5), 307–309.

Myers, M.F. (1982). Counseling the parents of young homosexual male parents. In J.C. Gonsiorek (Ed.), *Homosexuality and Psychotherapy* (pp. 131–143). New York: Haworth Press.

Newcomer, S.F., & Urdy, J.R. (1987). Parental marital status effects on adolescent sexual behavior. *Journal of Marriage and the Family*, 49(2), 235–240.

Newman, L. (1991). *Heather Has two Mommies*. Boston: Alyson.

Offer, D., Ostrov, E., Howard, K.I., & Atkinson, R. (1988). *The Teenage World: The Adolescent's Self-Image in Ten Countries*. New York: Plenum Medical Book Company.

O'Neil, J. (Unpublished paper). The gender role journey: A context for the workshop. Storrs, CT: University of Connecticut.

Orr, D.P., Wilbrandt, M.L., Brack, C.J., Rauch, S.P., & Ingersoll, G.M. (1989). Reported sexual behaviors and self-esteem among young adolescents. *American Journal of Disabled Children*, 143, 86–90.

Pardridge, W.M., Gorski, R.A., Lippe, B.M., & Green, R. (1982). Androgens and sexual behavior. *Annals of Internal Medicine*, 96, 488–501.

Payne, J.M. (1985). Marital sex roles. In H. Feldman & M. Feldman (Eds.), *Current Controversies in Marriage and Family*. Beverly Hills: Sage.

Peterson, G.W., Rollins, B.C., Thomas, D.L., & Heaps, L.K. (1982). Social placement of adolescents: Sex-role influences on family decisions regarding the careers of youth. *Journal of Marriage and the Family*, 42, 674–658.

Pfeiffer, E., & David, G.C. (1972). Determinants of sexual behavior in middle and old age. *Journal of the American Geriatric Society*, 20, 153.

Pletsch, P.K., Johnson, M.K., Tosi, C.B., et al. (1991). Self-image among early adolescents: Revisited. *Journal of Community Health Nursing*, 8(4), 215–231.

Proper, S., & Brown, E.A. (1986). Moral reasoning, parental sex attitudes, and sex build guilt in female college students. *Archives of Sexual Behavior*, 15, 331–340.

Rauste-von Wright, M. (1989). Body-image satisfaction in adolescent girls and boys: A longitudinal study. *Journal of Youth and Adolescence*, 18(1), 71–83.

Riche, M.F. (1991, March). The future of the family. *American Demographics*, 43–46.

Roberts, L.R., Sarigiani, P.A., Petersen, A.C., & Newman, J.L. (1990). Gender differences in the relationship between achievement and self-image during early adolescence. *Journal of Early Adolescence*, 10(2), 159–175.

Roper, B.S., & Labeff, E. (1977). Sex role and feminism revisited: An intergenerational attitude comparison. *Journal of Marriage and the Family*, 39, 113–119.

Sanders, G., & Mullis, R. (1988). Family influences on sexual attitudes and knowledge as reported by college students. *Adolescence*, 23(92), 837–845.

Sanford, N.D. (1989, May). Providing sensitive health care to gay and lesbian youth. Health care issues. *Nurse Practitioner*.

Sarrell, L.J., & Sarrell, P.M. (1981). Sexual unfolding. *Journal of Adolescent Health Care*, 2(39).

Schenk, J., Pfrang, H., & Rausche, A. (1983). Personality traits and the quality of the marital relationship. *Archives of Sexual Behavior*, 12(1), 31–42.

Schumm, W.R. (1985). Importance of the family. In H. Feldman & M. Feldman (Eds.), *Current Controversies in Marriage and Family*. Beverly Hills: Sage.

Scott, R.L., & Stone, D.A. (1986). MMPI profile constellations in incest families. *Journal of Consulting and Clinical Psychology, 54*, 364–368.

Seligmann, J. (1990, Winter/Spring). Variations on the theme: Gay and lesbian couples. *The 21st Century Family: Newsweek Special Issue.*

Shayne, V., & Kaplan, B. (1988). AIDS education for adolescents. *Youth and Society, 20*(2), 180–201.

Sheehy, G. (1995). New Passages: Mapping Your Life Across Time. New York: Random House.

Smith, E.D. (1981). *Maternity Care: A Guide for Patient Education*. Norwalk, CT: Appleton-Century-Crofts.

Starr, B., & Weiner, M.B. (1981). *On Sex and Sexuality in the Mature Years*. New York: Stein and Day.

Stewart, D.C. (1987, March). Sexuality and the adolescent: Issues for the clinician. *Primary Care, 14*(1), 83–99.

Story, M. (1982). A comparison of university student experience with various sexual outlets in 1974 with 1980. *Adolescence, 17*, 737–748.

Strommen, E.F. (1989). *You're a What: Family Member Reactions to the Disclosure of Homosexuality. Homosexuality and the Family*. New York: Hayworth Press.

Struder, M., & Thorton, A. (1989). The multifaceted impact of religiosity on adolescent sexual experience and contraceptive usage: A reply to Shornack and Ahmed. *Journal of Marriage and the Family, 51*, 1085–1088.

Teachman, J.D., & Polonko, K.A. (1990). Cohabitation and marital stability in the United States. *Social Forces, 69*, 207–220.

Thompson, E., & Collela, U. (1992, May). Cohabitation and marital stability: Quality or commitment? *Journal of Marriage and the Family, 54*, 259–267.

Thornton, A., (1991). Influence of the marital history of parents on the marital and cohabitational experiences of children. *American Journal of Sociology, 96*, 868–894.

Thornton, A. & Camburn, D. (1989). Religious participation and adolescent sexual behavior and attitudes. *Journal of Marriage and the Family, 51*, 641–652.

Tibler, K. (1987). Intervening with families of young adults with AIDS. In M.L. Leahey & L.M. Wright, *Families and Life-Threatening Illness* (pp. 255–270). Springhouse, PA: Springhouse.

Troidan, R.R. (1979). Becoming homosexual: A model of gay identity. *Psychiatry, 4*, 362–373.

Trussell, J., Rodriguez, G., & Vaughn, B. (1992). Union dissolution in Sweden. In J. Trussell, R. Hankinson & J. Tilton (Eds.), *Demographic Applications of Event History Analysis* (pp. 38–60). Oxford: Clarendon Press.

Tucker, S.K. (1989, Summer). Adolescent patterns of communication about sexually related topics. *Adolescence, 24*(94), 270–278.

U.S. Bureau of the Census (1990). Current population reports (Series P-20). Hyattsville, MD: U.S. Government Printing Office.

Weeks, M.O., & Kanter, J.F. (1980). Sexual activity, contraceptive use and pregnancy among metropolitan-area teenagers: 1971–1979. *Family Planning Perspectives, 12*, 230–237.

White, S.D., & DeBlassie, R.R. (1992). Adolescent sexual behavior. *Adolescence, 27*(105), 183–191.

Willhoite, M. (1991). *Daddy's Roommate*. Boston: Alyson.

RESOURCES FOR TEACHING/ COUNSELING ABOUT SEXUALITY

Agencies

American Association of Sex Educators, Counselors, and Therapists, Suite 304, 1010 Wisconsin Avenue, N.W., Washington, D.C. 20016.

The Planned Parenthood Federation of America (most large cities have local offices).

Sexual Information and Education Council of the United States (SIECUS), 80 Fifth Avenue, New York, New York 10011.

Books/Journal Articles

Gordon, S., & Gordon, J. (1985). *Raising a Child Conservatively in a Sexually Permissive World*. New York: Simon and Schuster.

Gordon, S. (1987). *Facts about Sex for Today's Youth*. Fayettesville, NC: Edu-U Press.

Hendeman, J. (1985). *A Very Touching Book*. Durkee, OR: McClure-Hendman Associates.

Kelley, G.T. (1985). *Learning about Sex: The Contemporary Guide for Young Adults*. Woodbury, NY: Bauman's Educational Series.

McCoy, K., & Wibbelsman, C. (1986). *Growing and Changing: A Handbook for Preteens*. New York: Pedigree.

Newman, L. (1991). *Heather Has Two Mommies*. Boston: Alyson Publications.

Ratner, M., & Shamlin, S. (1985). *Straight Talk—Sexuality Education for Parents and Kids 4–7*. New York: Simon & Schuster.

Willhoite, M. (1991). *Daddy's Roommate*. Boston: Alyson Publications.

18

FAMILY HEALTH PROTECTIVE BEHAVIORS

KAREN K. SZAFRAN

The primary goal of health protection is the removal or avoidance of encumbrances throughout the lifecycle that may prevent the emergence of optimum health.

NOLA J. PENDER

OBJECTIVES

Upon completion of this chapter, the reader will be able to:

1. Differentiate between the concepts of health promotion and health protection
2. Discuss the role of the family in the development and practice of health protective behaviors
3. Discuss three age-specific risk factors for each stage of the family life cycle
4. Assess the adequacy of health protective behaviors currently practiced by an individual or family
5. Identify nursing roles that facilitate family health protective behaviors

The concept of health protection or prevention has been receiving increasing attention. The changing patterns of morbidity and mortality within the American population, coupled with the skyrocketing costs of medical care, have focused interest on measures that serve to prevent the occurrence of disease or disability. The major threats to health no longer come from disease-producing bacterial or viral agents but rather from chronic conditions produced and fostered by inappropriate lifestyle factors or environmental hazards. It has been estimated that at least half of the deaths in the United States each year are the result of health-damaging lifestyles (Pender, 1987, in press; USPHS, 1990).

The family plays a critical role in the development and practice of health protective behaviors. Health-related decisions regarding diet, location and quality of residence, health care use, and leisure time activities affect all family members. The health practices of children and adolescents are greatly influenced by the examples set by adults within the family. Inappropriate health habits,

such as overeating, lack of exercise, use of alcohol and tobacco, and ineffective coping patterns, are often established in early childhood and adolescence and carried into adulthood (Keltner, 1992). Bruhn et al. (1977) suggest that throughout life, the individual must learn health tasks as well as developmental tasks to maintain health. This lifelong process begins at birth, with the family providing the stimulus for incorporating health into the value system of its members.

This chapter focuses on health protective behaviors as they relate to the stages of the family life cycle. As the primary source of socialization, the family must assume responsibility for fostering and supporting the self-care activities of all family members. Through the practice of appropriate health protective behaviors at each developmental stage of the family life cycle, the family works to ensure the health and safety of all family members and establishes lifelong lifestyle patterns. The nurse, as an educator and facilitator, plays a vital role assisting families in the incorporation of these behaviors into their everyday life.

A DEFINITION OF HEALTH PROTECTIVE BEHAVIORS

The term *health protective behavior* was introduced in the literature by Harris and Guten (1979) and was defined as

any behavior performed by a person, regardless of his or her perceived or actual health status, in order to protect, promote, or maintain his or her health, whether or not such behavior is objectively effective towards that end. (p. 18)

Their exploratory study was unique in that it focused on a wide range of health behaviors beyond those normally defined as preventive or protective by medical professionals. Harris and Guten concluded that virtually everyone studied performed at least some regular, routine behaviors related to protecting or maintaining their health. These authors also empirically identified five dimensions of health protective behavior: personal health practices, safety practices, preventive health care, environmental hazard avoidance, and harmful substance avoidance.

Pender (1987) refined the concept of health protection by differentiating the terms *health promotion* and *primary prevention,* which are often used interchangeably in the literature. According to Pender, health-promoting behaviors are directed toward improving well-being and the expression of human potential; preventive or health-protective behaviors are stabilizing in nature and occur in response to potential or actual threats to health:

Prevention is a defensive posture or set of actions taken to ward off specific illness or their sequelae that may threaten the quality of life or longevity. Prevention is better described by the term *health-protecting behavior* because of its emphasis on guarding or defending the body from injury. (p. 42)

Although the terms *health promotion* and *health protection* are conceptually distinct, they are by no means mutually exclusive. Disease-preventive measures usually also promote or maintain health, and health promotion is an integral part of disease detection and management (Kulbock & Baldwin, 1992). For example, avoiding excessive dietary sodium and maintaining recommended body weight are health-promoting behaviors; for a young black adult with a strong family history of hypertension, these same behaviors are important health protective measures. Thus, some behaviors can be labeled as primarily health promoting or health protecting, but many health behaviors function in both capacities (Pender, 1987, in press).

Traditionally, prevention has been discussed in terms of the levels used to describe patient care: primary, secondary, and tertiary. Although the conceptualization of prevention levels may be useful in determining appropriate goals and interventions based on the presence or absence of a specific disease process, their meanings may become vague or confusing when considering health protective behaviors that are not disease specific or medically sanctioned. Nursing practice and the concept of health protection extend beyond a focus on disease prevention and detection to include concerns regarding lifestyle practices, developmental issues, and psychosocial aspects of health.

In this chapter, health protective behaviors will be defined as defensive actions initiated for the purpose of removing or avoiding actual or potential health problems that might jeopardize or diminish well-being or quality of life. Health professionals play a vital role in assisting individuals or families to identify potential threats to health and to develop effective plans for health protection.

HEALTH PROTECTIVE BEHAVIORS THROUGHOUT THE FAMILY LIFE CYCLE

Self-responsibility is an integral part of health protection. Self-care behaviors and lifestyle are the major determinants of individual health. Of the ten leading causes of death among American adults, five are directly related to habits or lifestyle factors controlled by the individual: diet, smoking, lack of exercise, alcohol abuse, and stress (U.S. Public Health Service [USPHS], 1990). Many lifestyle decisions are made in childhood or adolescence and are a product of socialization within the context of the family. Thus, to a certain degree, family values and practices largely determine the future health of the individual.

Duvall's (1977) stages of the family life cycle and critical family developmental tasks are often used in the study of family health. A family's ability to master the tasks appropriate to each stage of development determines how well that family is able to meet the individual growth and development needs of each member. This family life-cycle perspective is also effective when applied to the study of health protective behaviors. The major threats to family and individual health vary throughout the life cycle, depending on the developmental stage and the family's activities related to health promotion and health protection. Actions initiated by the family in response to these potential health risks significantly affect the health of all family members.

The following discussion provides an overview of the major areas of focus for health protection in each of the stages of the family life cycle. Topics such as nutrition, exercise, and safety covered in depth in other chapters of this book will be addressed only briefly here. Other topics, such as smoking or hypertension, which are important areas of focus throughout the life span, will be addressed only in those stages where health protective measures are thought to be most effective or crucial.

The Expectant Family

Health protection plays a vital role during the prenatal period. The 1990 report by the U.S. Public Health Service, *Healthy People 2000*, states that "no period of life is more important to good health than the months before birth" (USPHS, 1990).

The major threats to the survival and good health of the infant are low birth weight and congenital birth defects. Seventy-five percent of infant deaths in the first month and 60% of all infant deaths occur among low–birth weight infants (USPHS, 1990). Low birth weight is also associated with growth and development disorders, increased occurrence of mental retardation, and disorders of the central nervous system. Birth defects are responsible for premature deaths and continuing poor health. Reducing the incidence of low birth weight and congenital abnormalities through intervention with the mother before and during pregnancy is being given high priority by medical and public health leaders in the United States (McClanahan, 1992; USPHS, 1990).

Maternal nutrition, socioeconomic status, maternal age and marital status, use of alcohol or cigarettes, and use of prenatal health services all affect birth weight and the health of the mother and child (Klein & Goldenberg, 1990). Congenital abnormalities may be genetic in origin or the result of a severe environmental insult in utero or birth trauma. Not all risk factors are preventable, but many are directly related to the health practices of the mother before and during pregnancy.

The prenatal period presents an excellent opportunity for the modification of health behaviors. Many women are highly motivated at this time to follow health advice. Good health habits started during pregnancy, such as better nutritional intake or avoidance of alcohol or tobacco, may be continued throughout the rest of life given proper reinforcement and reward.

Areas of Focus for Health Protection

PRENATAL CARE. Proper prenatal care has been shown to make a significant difference in maternal health and the subsequent health of the infant. An expectant mother with no prenatal care is three times more likely to have a low–birth weight infant (USPHS, 1990). Emphasis is placed on the importance of beginning prenatal care in the first trimester. In 1986, only 76% of all U.S. infants were born to mothers who initiated prenatal care in the first trimester of pregnancy (McClanahan, 1992). Prenatal care is necessary for all pregnant women and

is especially important for women at increased medical or social risk. Studies show that the women at high risk of having low–birth weight infants make the least use of the health care system during pregnancy. Maternal characteristics associated with receiving late or no prenatal care include low socioeconomic status, less than a high school education, adolescent pregnancy, and substance abuse (Novello, Degraw & Kleinman, 1992). Every effort must be made to increase the availability, accessibility, and utilization of prenatal health care for all women, particularly the poor, racial minorities, and adolescents. One objective proposed in *Healthy People 2000* is to increase first-trimester prenatal care to at least 90% of all live births (USPHS, 1990).

MATERNAL NUTRITION. Nutrition is a critical component in the prevention of prenatal and intrapartal complications and the promotion of fetal health. Maternal weight prior to conception and weight gain during pregnancy are major determinants of infant birth weight. Minimum recommended weight gain during pregnancy is 21 pounds, with gain minimal during the first trimester (Worthington-Roberts & Klerman, 1990).

Adequate caloric and protein intake are of particular importance for proper growth and development of the fetus. Mineral intake, especially calcium and phosphorus, is also essential. Adequate iron and folic acid is beneficial in building and protecting maternal reserves and preventing anemia. Many physicians prescribe supplementary vitamins and minerals during pregnancy. Further information on the nutritional needs of the pregnant woman can be found in Chapter 13.

The effects of inadequate nutrition are most profound in the pregnant adolescent, whose growing body competes with the nutritional needs of the fetus. Women who have experienced several closely spaced pregnancies are also at greater nutritional risk (Worthington-Roberts & Klerman, 1990).

SMOKING. There is overwhelming evidence that smoking during pregnancy affects fetal growth. Women who smoke are twice as likely to deliver a low–birth weight baby. Smoking is estimated to be related to 20% to 30% of all low–birthweight births in this country (USPHS, 1990).

No correlation has been documented between smoking and congenital defects; however, smoking doubles the risk of spontaneous abortion and significantly increases the risk of many maternal complications, such as bleeding, abruptio placentae, placenta previa, premature delivery, premature and prolonged rupture of membranes, and overall perinatal mortality. Particularly alarming is the association between maternal smoking during pregnancy and sudden infant death syndrome (SIDS), the leading cause of death in the first year of life (Mullen, 1990).

Studies indicate that the greater the number of cigarettes a pregnant woman smokes, the lower is the birth weight of her infant. If a woman stops smoking for the duration of the pregnancy, her risk of delivering a low–birth weight baby is no greater than that of a woman who does not smoke (Mullen, 1990). It is readily apparent that the reduction or elimination of the use of cigarettes during pregnancy is an important health protective measure.

ALCOHOL. Ingestion of alcohol during pregnancy has been shown to have detrimental effects on the developing fetus. Drinking as little as 3 oz of liquor daily increases the chances of congenital defects, low birth weight, premature delivery, stillbirth, or spontaneous abortion (Mullen & Glenday, 1990).

Heavy use of alcohol during pregnancy results in a characteristic set of abnormalities called the fetal alcohol syndrome (FAS). Affected infants are often of low birth weight, are mentally retarded, and exhibit behavioral, craniofacial, limb, and neurologic abnormalities. Heavy paternal drinking may also be a factor in FAS. A safe amount of alcohol consumption during pregnancy has not been determined, although the adverse effects are associated primarily with heavy consumption during the first trimester (Mullen & Glenday, 1990; USPHS, 1990).

ENVIRONMENTAL HAZARDS. Major environmental factors that have the potential to damage the fetus are radiation, various pollutants, drugs (both prescribed and over-the-counter medications), infectious agents (rubella, toxoplasmosis, sexually transmitted diseases), and workplace and household exposures to toxic and teratogenic substances (USPHS, 1990). The period of greatest danger is in the early weeks of fetal development, before many women even realize they are pregnant; however, it is important to avoid these hazards throughout pregnancy as much as possible. Additional information on environmental health can be found in Chapter 19.

Families with Infants

The birth of an infant brings profound changes to the family unit. The newborn infant is totally dependent on others within the environment to meet all personal needs; thus, the parents must assume new roles and responsibilities. The intensity of the infant's needs necessitates major changes in lifestyle, and the family may experience a period of disequilibrium as it strives to assimilate the needs of the infant with those of the rest of the family.

The ability of the parents to assume new roles and the responsibility for the care of the infant depends largely on their own maturity, their relationship with each other, their values and philosophy of life, their perceptions of and experiences with children and other adults, and the life stresses they have experienced. Parental influence begins at birth and is the single most important factor affecting the child's physical, emotional, and cognitive development and health (Keltner, 1992).

Areas of Focus for Health Protection

PREPARATION FOR PARENTHOOD. Most young adults are not prepared intellectually or emotionally for the responsibility of parenthood. In today's mobile society, extended family is often unavailable for assistance or advice, but a wide variety of prenatal and postnatal classes is available to help prepare young parents for the birth experience and the transition to parenthood. Increased knowledge of and a sense of control during the birthing process promote and facilitate the early parent-infant bonding process. Competence in infant care skills and an understanding of normal growth and development can allay anxiety, eliminate unrealistic expectations, and bolster parents' confidence in their ability to master the new role.

The development of a healthy personality and psychological wellness is a lifelong process that begins in infancy, when the infant learns to trust that the world is a safe and secure place. Emotionally healthy parents and stable families provide a sound environment and support system for growing children. Consistent and predictable love from parents contributes significantly to the development of self-esteem and self-love. Educational measures that focus on preparation for parenthood and increase parents' understanding of normal child growth and development foster a healthy family environment and work to prevent problems of family violence or abuse (Hann & Osofsky, 1990).

BREAST-FEEDING. During the first year of life, physical growth is more rapid than at any other period of life outside the womb. This rapid growth causes infants to have the highest nutrient needs per unit of body weight of any other age group. In terms of the nutrients it contains and the immunologic benefits it confers, human breast milk provides ideal nutrition for the infant. Because of the host-resistant factors in human milk, breast milk offers many advantages to the infant. The newborn's immune mechanisms are immature, and his or her defenses are weak. Human breast milk contains maternal antibodies and other substances that help protect the infant against various types of infections. Breast milk is free of harmful bacteria when consumed directly by the infant. In developing countries where water supplies are contaminated or areas of extreme poverty, breast-feeding offers a hygienic method of protecting the infant until immunologic independence is achieved (Lawrence, 1994).

Breast-feeding has also been associated with the prevention of allergic diseases. Newborns cannot effectively break down proteins into amino acids. The absorption of partially digested or undigested protein triggers an allergic response. Breast milk is nonallergenic and is also thought to coat the intestinal tract and prevent the absorption of proteins. Allergies to cow's milk occur in approximately 7% of bottle-fed children and are known to cause problems such as recurrent rhinorrhea and bronchitis, colic, spells of diarrhea and vomiting, asthma, and eczema (Lawrence, 1994).

The *Healthy People 2000* objectives for the nation set as a goal that, by 2000, the proportion of women who breast-feed their babies should be increased to 75% in the early postpartum period and to at least 50% 5 to 6 months of age (USPHS, 1990). Recent trends indicate a rapid increase in breast-feeding at both hospital discharge and at 6 months of age, although the increase has not been as pronounced among the disadvantaged or minorities. In 1988, the reported prevalence of breast-feeding among low-income women 6 weeks after delivery was 32% for white mothers, 47% for Native Americans, 51% for Hispanics, and 25% for blacks (USPHS, 1990). Increased efforts are needed to encourage breast-feeding and to provide education and support for prospective mothers, especially the economically and educationally disadvantaged.

METABOLIC DISORDERS AND CONGENITAL ILLNESS. Screening procedures and prophylactic treatment at birth are utilized to protect the infant from potential metabolic disorders and congenital illness. Routine testing for phenylketonuria (PKU) and hypothyroidism is done in all states and the District of Columbia. Early detection and treatment of these disorders can prevent severe mental retardation (Stanhope & Lancaster, 1992). Instillation of silver nitrate drops or erythromycin ointment in the eyes of the neonate prevents the possibility of blindness from gonorrheal infection. Injection of 1 mg of vitamin K in the newborn is effective in preventing hemorrhagic disease due to a deficiency of Factor VIII production (U.S. Preventive Services Task Force, 1989).

IMMUNIZATION. Immunization provides an effective means of protecting the infant from certain infectious diseases. Immunization against polio, diphtheria, pertussis, tetanus, measles (rubeola), rubella, mumps, *Haemophilus influenzae,* hepatitis B, and varicella zoster is the most effective form of primary disease prevention available. The Committee on Infectious Disease of the American Academy of Pediatrics recommends standard immunization schedules to ensure maximum levels of protective antibody levels. Currently it is recommended that American infants receive 3 primary doses of a combination of diphtheria and tetanus toxoids and pertussis vaccine (DPT) and a *Haemophilus influenza* type b conjugate vaccine (HIB) at ages 2, 4, and 6 months. A fourth dose should be administered at 12–15 months. Trivalent oral polio (TOPV) should be administered at 2, 4, and 15 months. At 1 year, the infant should be given a tine test to detect possible tuberculosis. A measles, mumps, and rubella (MMR) combined vaccine

should be received at 12–15 months. The immunization series of hepatitis B vaccine can be initiated at birth, with subsequent injections at 2 and 15 months, or it can be given simultaneously with the DPT and oral polio vaccinations (Centers for Disease Control, 1995; USPHS, 1992). A major role of the family nurse is to educate parents about the importance of their child's obtaining immunizations and maintaining accurate records of when they were received.

SAFETY MEASURES. Injuries are the leading cause of death and disability for children over the age of 9 months in the United States (Jones, 1992). Use of regulation infant car seats has reduced the incidence of injury and death in motor vehicle accidents.

The majority of accidents for this age group occur in the home, and their number and severity are closely linked to the child's developmental stage. Falls, burns, and aspiration of foreign objects are common types of accidents. As infants develop increasing motor skills and hand-to-mouth activity by the end of the first year, they are extremely vulnerable to accidental poisoning. A 30-milliliter bottle of syrup of ipecac should be kept in the home in order to induce vomiting when indicated, in case of accidental poisoning (Brannan, 1992). Practice of age-appropriate safety measures can significantly reduce or prevent accidental injuries.

Family nurses play an important role in educating parents and caregivers on the developmental abilities of the growing child, the common hazards of early life, and specific anticipatory guidance for accident prevention (Stanhope & Lancaster, 1992). Additional information on safety measures can be found in Chapter 19.

HEALTH SUPERVISION. Periodic medical evaluations are an established form of preventive health care. Although there is some disagreement as to the needed frequency of physical examinations in the adult population, "well-baby checks" are an important protective measure for infants. The American Academy of Pediatrics recommends that the newborn infant be seen 2 to 4 weeks after birth, four to five more times within the first year of life, and then every one to two years through age 21 (U.S. Preventive Services Task Force, 1989).

The routine medical examination provides health care professionals the opportunity to monitor infant nutrition and growth, to assess developmental progress, and to administer routine immunization. It also affords an excellent opportunity to educate the parents about various aspects of normal development and disease prevention. A major role of the family nurse is to teach parents to manage early symptoms of common childhood problems such as upper respiratory infections, gastrointestinal illness, elevated temperatures, and infant colic and to recognize serious conditions that warrant physician attention. Increased knowledge develops parental confidence and helps them to use the health care system effectively.

Families with Preschool Children

The preschool phase places great demands on the family unit. The preschool child, typically very active and inquisitive, is emerging as a social being, and his or her world begins to expand beyond the family to include association with peers. The parents must learn to support and encourage more independent activity for the child in safe, supervised settings away from the home.

Preschool children experience a high frequency of acute illnesses, predominantly upper respiratory infections, although accidents remain the major threat to physical health. Nutritional and dental health needs are great during this period of rapid growth, and future adult mental health, to an extent, is determined by how well emotional needs are met during this stage of development (Novello et al., 1992).

Areas of Focus for Health Protection

ESTABLISHMENT OF HEALTH BEHAVIORS. The importance of lifestyle on the health of the individual cannot be overstated. Habits and decisions related to nutrition, personal habits, activity and exercise, and sleep affect longevity and the quality of health an individual will enjoy. The family plays a critical role in the development of health behavior. It is generally accepted that many health attitudes and practices are established in early childhood. Lifestyle behaviors adopted by parents both influence the child and establish patterns of health behavior that the child will follow throughout the life span (Keltner, 1992; Swinford & Webster, 1989).

The preschool period (ages 3 to 5 years) is considered an ideal time to teach protective health behaviors because parental influences have the greatest impact on the child. Healthy families can promote a healthful family lifestyle by encouraging an appropriate balance of activity and rest, fostering nutritionally sound dietary practices, and promoting regular exercise. Child health care providers have a responsibility to assist the family in developing these healthful characteristics that promote optimal health in the child and set the foundation for a lifetime of good health practices. Parents need to be aware that they are probably most influential when they practice what they preach. Parents who say that sensible eating and regular exercise are important but do the opposite are usually less successful in establishing these important protective health practices in their children.

DENTAL HEALTH. Protective dental care practices are an important component of personal hygiene and should be initiated early in life. Assuming normal development, a child will have 20 primary ("baby") teeth by age $2\frac{1}{2}$ years. Decay begins to attack the teeth shortly after they appear in the mouth. In the United States, the average child has 3.4 decayed or filled primary tooth surfaces by the age of 5 (Griffen & Goepferd, 1991). Elements of protective dental care are correct and thorough flossing and brushing, sensible food selection, use of fluorides, and regular professional supervision.

Independent toothbrushing should be started early in the preschool years, with parents supervising and checking all tooth surfaces after brushing. Children should be taught to brush after every meal, or at least twice daily, with flossing done daily by the parents until the child is old enough to master this skill.

Good nutritional practices such as choosing fruit or raw vegetables for snacks and the avoiding excessive sugar intake promote dental health. The relationship between diet and dental caries is complex; however, most research points to the frequency of exposure to high concentrations of sugars and the rate at which the sugar is cleared from the oral cavity as critical factors (Griffen & Goepford, 1991). Sugars with meals are less harmful than those consumed as snacks since concentrations are less and they are cleared from the mouth more quickly. Cheese, peanuts, milk, sugarless gum, and raw vegetables are relatively safe snacks. Food to be particularly avoided are sugared gum, dried fruits, fruit juices and sugared soft drinks, and candy items (Christian & Greger, 1988). Dental professionals recommend that sugar intake, particularly sticky sweets such as certain types of candy and dried fruits, be limited to the times that brushing and flossing can occur shortly after consumption.

The common practice of giving infants or toddlers a bottle of milk or juice at bedtime as a pacifier leads to the development of a rampant form of tooth decay in the primary teeth of preschool children known as "baby bottle tooth decay" (Barnes et al., 1992). This syndrome, also documented in breast-fed infants, is believed to occur when the child falls asleep with a nipple in his or her mouth for long periods of time. To prevent this problem, all nutrients, including liquids, should be consumed before bedtime. Bottle feeding beyond the age of 1 year should be discouraged. If a toddler still has a bottle, it should contain only plain water and should be eliminated as soon as possible (Barnes et al., 1992).

Public health officials credit the fluoridation of water as being "the single most effective and efficient means of preventing dental caries in children and adults" (USPHS, 1990). At present about two-thirds of the U.S. population lives in communities with either naturally or artificially fluoridated water. Fluoride is incorporated into the tooth enamel and increases resistance to decay. To be most effective, adequate fluoride intake should begin in infancy. The American Dental

Association recommends that children receive adequate fluoride from infancy until at least 12 to 14 years of age (Griffen & Goepferd, 1991). Sources of fluoride other than community water supplies are fluoride toothpastes, fluoride mouth rinses, dietary fluoride supplements, and topical applications by dental health professionals.

An initial visit to the dentist is recommended between 1 and 2 years of age. This visit serves to familiarize the child with the setting and instruments and provides the dentist with an opportunity to assess the child for potential problems, such as overcrowding of teeth or poor hygiene. Semiannual dental visits should begin at age 3 and continue throughout childhood and adolescence. Because of rapid developmental changes and the high rate at which decay can progress, the timing of these visits is critical for preventive measures. Prompt attention to decay or overcrowding in primary teeth is essential to protect the development and proper alignment of permanent teeth (Griffen & Goepferd, 1991).

DAY CARE. Increasing numbers of families with young children use day care programs. Changing economic and social trends have increased the numbers of employed mothers: 50% of all preschool-age children have mothers who work outside the home, and that number is expected to increase to 70% by the year 2000 (Kuhns & Holloway, 1992). The selection of a quality day care program or nursery school is an important protective task for parents.

Although economic considerations are often the determining factor, parents should also examine the convenience of location, the range and flexibility of hours and services available, the quality of the facility and staff, and the congruence of the center's philosophy of child care with that of the family (Kuhns & Holloway, 1992). A comprehensive program should promote physical health, proper nutrition, a positive self-concept, and cognitive and social skill development.

EMOTIONAL HEALTH. An important component of psychological development occurring during the preschool years is the emergence of self-concept. The family functions to give the child a sense of social and personal identity. Like a mirror, the family reflects back to the child a picture of who he or she is and how valuable he or she is to others. Positive reflections provide the child with a sense of satisfaction and worth (Swinford & Webster, 1989).

The development of a favorable self-concept and sense of autonomy is thought to have a positive influence on health practices. Pratt (1976) states, "Children raised by parents who stress democratic relationships, give unconditional personal regard, and encourage individuality and personal development show greater competence and resourcefulness in taking care of themselves" (p. 85). Families who strive to maintain a positive emotional climate by supporting individual growth and encouraging initiative and autonomy can have a favorable impact on children's future mental health and personal health practices.

Families with School-Age Children

For many children the school-age years are the healthiest time of their lives. Their energy levels are high and seemingly endless, and their ability to recover from illness or injury is rapid and relatively complete. The school-age child exhibits increasing physical and emotional independence from parents and is exposed to new ideas, attitudes, perspectives, and modes of behavior as contact with the world outside the family expands. The family's developmental tasks at this stage revolve around the major goals of reorganization and letting go in preparation for the expanding world of school-age children (Edelman & Mandle, 1986).

Areas of Focus for Health Protection

IMMUNIZATION. Immunizations are required for children entering school; however, it is estimated that one-fourth to one-half of preschool and school-age children are incompletely immunized (USPHS, 1990).

Diphtheria and tetanus toxoids combined with pertussis vaccine and oral polio vaccines need to be given as indicated. Children immunized as infants need a booster dose of DPT and OPV between 4 and 6 years of age. In 1989, the AAP recommended that all children receive a second dose of MMR. School entry laws vary from state to state with some requiring the second dose for entry to kindergarten (4–6 years of age) and others requiring the dose prior to entry to middle school (11–12 years of age). A booster dose of tetanus and diphtheria toxoids (Td) should be administered at 11–12 years of age (Centers for Disease Control, 1995).

DENTAL HEALTH. The school-age child is constantly losing or gaining teeth. The 6-year molars are the first permanent teeth that erupt, by age 7. The deciduous (baby) teeth are lost at a rate of four teeth per year for the next seven years, usually in the same order in which they erupted. A 13 year old should have 28 permanent teeth to replace the 20 deciduous teeth lost (Edelman & Mandle, 1986).

Dental caries remain a major health problem for the school-age child. Even proper brushing and use of fluoride is not always effective in preventing caries in the pits and fissures of teeth, particularly the molars. These areas can be protected by the use of sealants, which form a plastic film over the deep crevices and defects, thus reducing susceptibility to decay. This coating, when properly applied by dental professionals, is almost 100% effective in preventing pit and fissure caries. The major problem with the use of sealants is the cost, which makes it unobtainable for many families (Griffen & Goepferd, 1991).

School-age children should be responsible for their daily dental care, both proper brushing and flossing. The use of fluoride and regular professional checkups should continue. Parents should remain active in supervising the child's oral health care practices and helping the child to maintain an appropriate diet, low in refined carbohydrates and frequent snacks.

VISION AND HEARING. Physiologic development of visual capacity and auditory acuity is complete by the sixth or seventh year of age. It is estimated that 20% to 30% of school-age children do not have normal vision. Common visual problems in this age group are myopia, amblyopia, and strabismus or a combination of defects. Most of these conditions are usually easily corrected with glasses, but as many as 75% are not detected for a long period (Stanhope & Lancaster, 1992).

Hearing deficits are less common than visual defects among school-age children; however, 3% of children have some degree of hearing impairment that may cause significant delays in speech comprehension, articulation, and social development. Chronic serous otitis media is the most common cause of a hearing deficit in the school-age child (Feightner, 1990).

Ideally, screening for visual or hearing problems should begin with the newborn and should be included in routine well-child care. Visual impairments that occur in the younger child may be undetected and untreated until the child attends school. Regular vision and hearing screening is mandated by school systems to detect children whose learning ability may be impaired due to a sensory deficit.

LATCHKEY CHILDREN. The importance of quality day care for the younger child has long been acknowledged; however, recently increasing attention as been focused on the needs of school-age children. The phenomenon of latchkey children—those who return home from school and stay alone without adult supervision—is a growing concern of many parents and child health professionals. Although there are no data to determine exactly the number of children who regularly care for themselves, estimates for those younger than 13 years of age range from 2 million to 6 million (Graham & Uphold, 1992). The provision of appropriate after-school supervision is an important protective task for families. Many public schools are beginning to develop before- and after-school day care programs for older children. Alternatives that the family may consider are neighbors, relatives, older siblings, or day care homes.

Parents should carefully assess a child's readiness for being at home alone. Emotional maturity and sense of responsibility may vary widely among children of the same age. For the child who has independent time, specific guidelines should be outlined by the parents regarding the use of television, answering the telephone, appropriate activities, who (if anyone) can enter the house, and where the child may or may not go. Emergency measures should also be planned for problem situations that may arise, such as the child's losing the key, becoming sick, or needing help for one reason or another.

TV VIEWING. The average child between the ages of 6 and 11 watches approximately 27 hours of television a week. For the preschool child, the number is almost 33 hours; adolescents average about 24 hours of viewing each week. Throughout childhood and adolescence, television viewing consumes more time than formal classroom study. Television and movies have a powerful influence on a child's behavior and communication practices. Concerns of consumer groups and child health professionals center on the harmful effects of violent programming, the unrealistic world depicted, the passivity of TV viewing, and the advertising directed at children. Numerous studies have linked violent programming with increases in aggressive behavior (Comstock & Strasburger, 1990).

More recent concern has focused on the influence of television advertising directed at children. The leading products advertised during children's programs are toys, cereals, candy, and fast-food restaurants. More than half of the advertising focuses on food, much of it high in refined sugars and potentially harmful to teeth and overall nutrition. Although a large portion of TV advertising is inaccurate or misleading, a study of the impact of TV health messages (mostly commercials) on fifth- and sixth-grade children found that 70% of the programming was "believed." A conclusion of the study was that television viewing, as presently programmed, might be labeled as "hazardous to the health of future adults" (Story & Falkner, 1990; Taras et al., 1989).

The influence of television in the lives of children is undeniable; however, it has been demonstrated that this influence is sensitive to intervention by parents and teachers. The challenge for parents and teachers is one of countereducation. Parents should be encouraged to watch television with their children so they can explain and discuss what is viewed. Parents should also evaluate programming: whether it is age appropriate and promotes positive values or roles. It is important the amount of time spent viewing television be limited since other activities, such as schoolwork or physical recreation, may suffer (Strasburger, 1992).

ACCIDENTS. Accident prevention remains a major health concern for the school-age child. Accidents account for half of all deaths in childhood (Stanhope & Lancaster, 1992). Equally significant are the 17 million nonfatal childhood accidents that occur each year, most of them minor, but some resulting in lifelong problems. Motor vehicle accidents are the leading cause of death for schoolchildren, followed by drownings and fires. The popularity of bicycles, skateboards, and roller-blades among schoolchildren increases the risk of injury on streets. The leading causes of nonfatal injury among children ages 6 to 12 years were falls, sports, bicycles, and motor vehicle occupant (Jones, 1992).

Accident prevention begins in the home. Parents can promote safety by helping children to identify and avoid potentially hazardous situations. The school-age child is a good candidate for safety instructions. Increasing cognitive maturity, including the ability to learn from past experiences and to anticipate probable outcomes of contemplated actions, allows the child to take an active part in accident prevention (Edelman & Mandle, 1986).

An important element in safety promotion for this age group is education regarding risk-taking behavior. The school-age child needs to develop personal values related to health and an ability to make decisions about risk-taking behaviors and their consequences. The family can be very influential in teaching the child how to assess the risks involved for engaging in certain behaviors and the benefits to be gained from practicing more health protective behaviors (Graham & Uphold, 1992).

STRESS MANAGEMENT. An important developmental task of the school-age child is learning to cope with stress. Although many tend to view childhood as relatively carefree, the school-age child confronts many problems related to change, competition, frustration, and failures, which must be confronted and adequately dealt with. Stress levels within families tend to increase at this time. Activities for the school-age child broaden to include interests outside the home. Unfortunately, the child can become involved in so many activities that they become a source of stress for both the child and the parents. This situation intensifies when there is more than one child in the family and both parents work outside the home. Family schedules must be balanced to accommodate the needs of all family members. Studies indicate parental satisfaction with family life is lowest when the oldest child is between ages 6 and 13 (Olson et al., 1983).

Stress control programs for school-age children are not widely available, yet they are needed. Many of the health problems encountered in adolescence and young adulthood (reckless driving, suicide, alcohol and drug abuse, obesity, etc.) are related to stress and inadequate coping skills. Pratt (1976) identified "the tendency to actively and energetically attempt to cope with life's problems and issues" (p. 86) as a characteristic of healthy families that fosters members' personal health practices. Positive behaviors included in this approach are an openness to new ideas, information, and resources; taking the initiative in seeking out new resources and applying them to the solution of family and personal problems; creatively developing original solutions in re-sponse to changing needs; rationally selecting among alternatives; and planning, with long-term consequences taken into considerations. The family of the school-age child can play an important role in promoting mental and emotional health and equipping children with the skills necessary to cope with the outside world, thus, potentially preventing future health problems in adolescence and adulthood.

The Family with Adolescents

Adolescence has long been considered a critical period in human development. Throughout the teenage years, the adolescent experiences complex physical, emotional, cognitive, and social changes. Rapid and significant developmental adjustments create a variety of stresses and problems that affect adolescent health. Major health problems in this age group are violent death, injuries, and alcohol and drug abuse. Contributing risk factors are a lack of problem-solving skills, rigid and inflexible family values, conflicts between parents and children, and daredevil risk-taking attitudes (Stanhope & Lancaster, 1992).

Families must focus on the major developmental task of loosening family ties and allowing greater responsibility and freedom to the maturing adolescent. The overwhelming physical changes of puberty may seem inconsequential when compared to the social and psychological changes that take place during adolescence.

Areas of Focus for Health Protection

NUTRITION. Adequate nutritional intake assumes major significance during adolescence. For boys, nutritional needs are the highest of any other time in their lives; the nutritional needs of the adolescent girl will be exceeded only during pregnancy and lactation. Unfortunately, the adolescent lifestyle often includes irregular eating habits, with 25% of caloric intake coming from between-meal snacks (Christian & Greger, 1988). As the adolescent spends increasing amounts of time away from the home, parental influence over dietary choices and habits diminishes.

Poor nutrition and obesity are common among adolescents. Among adolescent girls, two problems of mounting incidence and gravity are anorexia nervosa and bulimia. These conditions create severe nutritional problems in that they starve the victims; however, the etiology is predominantly psychological and related to a distorted sense of body image. Additional information related to adolescent obesity and nutritional needs can be found in Chapter 13.

DENTAL HEALTH. Adolescents between the ages of 12 and 17 have a higher incidence of dental decay than any other group—an average of 6.2 decayed, missing, or filled teeth. Seventy percent of this group exhibits some degree of periodontal disease (Griffen & Goepferd, 1991). Adolescent dental problems are related to improper diet, poor oral hygiene, and the low frequency with which adolescents obtain regular professional dental services.

Periodontal disease is a major health problem of American adults. It strikes 95% of the population at some time and after age 35 is the chief cause of loss of teeth. The prevalence and severity of periodontal disease are inversely correlated to oral hygiene and professional prophylaxis. Periodontal diseases can be prevented, or their progression interrupted, by removing soft and hard deposits and keeping the teeth free of bacterial plaque (Greene, Louie & Wycoff, 1990).

Parents need to ensure that adolescents continue to receive regular professional dental care. As the adolescent assumes greater self-responsibility for his or her health, the importance of good dietary habits and daily dental hygiene must be emphasized.

SMOKING. Cigarette smoking among adolescents is a significant health problem. Despite the fact that smoking has decreased dramatically among adults since 1964, the number of adolescent smokers remains high. More than 3 million adolescents in the U.S. smoke cigarettes. Data from the ongoing annual survey of high school seniors show little change in smoking prevalence in recent years. The proportion of adolescent girls who reported smoking in the last month actually rose slightly from 8.7% in 1990 to 9.4% in 1992 (Ernster, 1993). Research indicates that the younger a person is when he or she starts to smoke, the more likely that person is to be a heavy smoker as an adult and to continue to smoke well into the adult years. The average age when smokers first try a cigarette is 14.5 years; the average age when they become daily smokers is 17.7 years (Elders, Perry, Eriksen & Giorano, 1994). The age of initiation of the smoking habit is known to be inversely associated not only with lung cancer mortality but with mortality related to heart disease, stroke, emphysema, and bronchitis (USPHS, 1990).

Among youth, more than half of eighth graders and nearly two-thirds of tenth graders report having tried cigarettes. More than 25% of tenth graders report having smoked a cigarette during the preceding month, and nearly 20% report smoking a pack or more in the preceding month (USPHS, 1990). Also of concern is the recent upsurge in the use of smokeless tobacco, particularly in young male adolescents and adults. The Centers for Disease Control's 1990 *Youth Risk Behavior Survey* reported that 19% of male high school students used smokeless tobacco (American Cancer Society, 1992). Results such as these indicate the importance of the adolescent years in the formation of health-related behavior. Smoking during adolescence not only places the nation's youth at risk for poor health in the future but also jeopardizes their immediate health.

The family environment has been shown to have a significant effect on the smoking behavior of children. Only 4% of teenagers from households of nonsmokers will develop the habit. When both parents smoke, there is a greater likelihood that a child will smoke than if only one or neither parent smokes. When an older sibling plus both parents smoke, a child is four times more likely to smoke than if the family contains no smokers (Winkelstein, 1992). Peer pressure also has been shown to exert strong influence on adolescent smoking behavior.

Nurses and health professionals must work to educate young people of the health hazards of smoking. Education beginning in the elementary grades may help to prevent the initiation of the smoking habit. For older children and adolescents, intervention should be focused on measures that increase their ability to resist peer pressure.

ALCOHOL AND DRUG ABUSE. Alcohol and drug use, like smoking, is a behavior with major implications for adolescent health. Data from 1988 indicate that 25.2% of adolescents between the ages of 12 and 17 had had a drink in the past month; the rate for those ages 18 to 20 was 57.9% (USPHS, 1990). Drug use, which was virtually unknown in the 1950s, now represents a major health problem among adolescents, with 60% of adolescents having tried marijuana and 20% having tried harder substances, such as cocaine and hallucinogens (Stanhope & Lancaster, 1992). Although recent surveys indicate that the levels of overall drug use, including alcohol, have declined steadily since 1977, they remain alarmingly high, due partly to an ever-lowering age of first use and the continued use of alcohol among high school students. In 1988, the average age of first use of alcohol was 13.1 years and for marijuana, 13.4 years (USPHS, 1990).

Patterns of drug use among adolescents vary widely. Many adolescents use drugs or alcohol once or on an infrequent, experimental basis; others use drugs on a more regular, periodic basis. A small percentage of adolescents are chemically dependent. Studies indicate that adolescents tend to consume alcohol less frequently (an average of once a month) than adults, but when they do drink, they tend to do so in large quantities and experience frequent episodes of intoxication. This pattern of behavior greatly increases the risks of violent behavior, motor vehicle accidents, and a variety of other injuries (Stanhope & Lancaster, 1992).

Primary prevention intervention for alcohol and drug use should begin in the school-age years. Recent educational efforts geared toward the school-age child, such as the national "Just Say No" campaign, have focused on the young person's individual responsibility for daily decisions affecting his or her health and have attempted to stimulate positive peer pressure for drug abstinence. During the adolescent years, health education regarding alcohol and other drugs should focus on the serious side effects and should help the adolescent formulate responsible behaviors and attitudes in their use.

Families should be aware of the early signs of drug abuse among children or adolescents: gradual and unexplained deterioration in scholastic performance, increasing difficulties with parents or peers, increased frequency of accidents, and unexplained absences from school (Stanhope & Lancaster, 1992). Early detection of alcohol- or drug-related problems and referral for counseling or treatment may help avert serious problems or injury at a later date.

SEXUAL ACTIVITY. Adolescents become sexually active for a variety of reasons, depending on their age and maturity. Young teenagers may use sexual activity as a method to bolster self-esteem or their image among their peer group. Others may experiment with sex out of curiosity or because of increasing peer pressure to conform. Of all age groups, adolescents are least likely to practice contraception (Fielding & Williams, 1990).

Many adolescents over the age of 15 are at least occasionally sexually active. The primary health hazards for adolescents related to sexual activity are unplanned pregnancies and sexually transmitted diseases (STDs). Approximately 1 million teenage girls in the United States become pregnant each year. In 1986, more than 40% obtained abortions, and over 470,000 gave birth, with 38% of those births to girls 17 years of age and younger. Although the rates of initiation and practice of sexual activity are comparable in the United States and other developed countries, the rates for adolescent pregnancy, abortion, and childbearing remain higher in the United States (Fielding & Williams, 1990). The psychosocial impact of adolescent pregnancy or abortion is as significant as the threat to physical health.

Sexually transmitted diseases (including gonorrhea, syphilis, genital warts, genital herpes, and chlamydia) are a major public health problem in the United States. Eighty-six percent of all reported STDs occur in 15 to 29 year olds, with adolescent females (15 to 19 years) having the highest incidence of gonorrhea, chlamydia, and pelvic inflammatory disease. It has been estimated that by age 21, approximately one of every five young people has required treatment for an STD (Alexander, 1992). Many STDs of lesser severity go unrecognized because of a lack of apparent symptoms or the reluctance of the adolescent to seek treatment. As a result, many of these diseases are responsible for chronic conditions detected at a later date.

Ideally, primary prevention related to sexuality begins in the home with the provision of accurate information and an open discussion of responsible sexual behavior. Many schools are now providing sexual education for adolescents. There is a consistent body of evidence that sex education is associated with more contraceptive use among sexually active teenagers. Both young men and young women need to understand the available methods of contraception, including their proper use and potential hazards. Adolescents also need to be educated regarding the potential hazards of STDs and the means of prevention, detection, and diagnosis. Prevention is primarily through the avoidance of sexual contact with an infectious person; however, a partner's state of infection may not be apparent or recognizable. Recent attention has focused on the use of condoms as a means of protection from STDs. Emphasis must be placed on the importance of prompt attention and diagnosis of signs or symptoms indicative of sexual diseases.

SUNBATHING. The link between excessive exposure to direct sunlight and the incidence of skin cancer is well documented. Approximately 400,000 cases of skin cancer occur annually in the United States (American Cancer Society, 1992). Sunbathing is a popular sport and recreational activity for adolescents and young adults. Participants in outdoor sports or other recreational activities may spend hours of leisure time in direct sunlight.

Protective measures related to sun exposure include educating the adolescent and young adult regarding excessive sun exposure and tanning, the use of sunblocking creams and lotions, and the signs and symptoms of early skin cancer.

SUICIDE. Suicide occurs at all ages, but incidence peaks are noted during late adolescence and among the elderly. There has been a growing suicide rate in the adolescent population of the United States and other industrialized countries. Over the past 30 years, the suicide rate for those 15 to 24 years of age has tripled, and suicide is now the third leading cause of death for that age group (Haynes, 1990). The high incidence of suicide in adolescence has been attributed to the increasing pressures in society and an inability to establish a clear identity with satisfactory self-esteem. Other adolescent behaviors related to an inability to deal with excessive stress are vandalism, shoplifting, running away, substance abuse, and promiscuous sexual behavior (Murray & Huelskoetter, 1991).

Studies indicate that adolescents who attempt suicide often exhibit a characteristic presuicidal history of an increasing inability to deal with stress, loss, or frustration (Haynes, 1990). Low self-esteem and poor self-image are characteristic of children on entry to junior high school. Adapting to the new environment with its academic challenges and teen culture can be overwhelming for children who are also trying to adjust to the physical changes of early puberty. As the adolescent matures, increased academic pressures coupled with parental expectations for achievement and career and vocational selection impose additional stresses. An adolescent with inadequate coping mechanisms and social support may attempt suicide (Haynes, 1990).

Prevention of suicide begins with the development of a positive self-image and effective coping mechanisms during early childhood and the elementary school years. During adolescence, intervention should focus on the identification of individuals under extreme stress and the initiation of measures to reduce stress or increase coping ability. Young people who exhibit severe depression or talk about suicide should be taken very seriously and referred to a trained counselor.

ACCIDENTS. Accidents are the leading cause of death among adolescents aged 12 to 17, with over half of adolescent fatalities the result of motor vehicle accidents (Mayhew, 1991). Mortality statistics only illustrate a portion of the health impact of accidents in adolescence: for every youth killed in an automobile or other unintended accident, hundreds more are injured, maimed, or incapacitated. Excessive risk taking or aggressive behavior and the use of alcohol and/or drugs are implicated in the majority of accidents (USPHS, 1990).

One of the major parent-adolescent struggles revolves around driving. For teenagers, driving represents a major step toward independence and maturity. Parents, cognizant of the inherent dangers, may feel it is necessary to set limits and restrict the adolescent's driving. Driver education classes, offered through many high schools, can teach teenagers traffic regulations and driving techniques, but this technical knowledge does not ensure that the adolescent will adhere to safety measures when in the company of peers (Mayhew, 1991). Parents must assess each teenager on an individual basis regarding maturity, level of responsibility, common sense, and ability to resist peer pressure and risk-taking behaviors. Age alone does not automatically determine readiness for such a high level of independence. Adherence to ground rules such as the mandatory use of seat belts and absolute abstinence from drinking when driving should be conditional for the use of the family car.

Sports activities play an important role in adolescence. They provide both valuable exercise and experience in competition and team effort, and they help develop a positive self-image. Unfortunately, there is a high rate of sports injuries among adolescents. Most prevalent are injuries to the head, spine, and extremities. An estimated 600,000 injuries occur in high school football alone in the United States each year. Lack of coordination, immature judgment, and incomplete ossification of the skeletal system are thought to contribute to the high injury rate (Edelman & Mandle, 1986).

Most sports-related injuries can be prevented by following reasonable safety precautions appropriate to the sport. Participants in group sports or other potentially dangerous sports should wear proper safety equipment and receive adequate instruction (Mayhew, 1991). Education related to methods that strengthen and condition the adolescent body aid in the prevention of injuries. Sports-related physical examinations should also be conducted to ensure that each participant is physically capable of meeting the demands of the sport.

Families with Young Adults

The launching phase is a time of transition for all family members: Parents must reexamine and redefine their roles with the young adult and with each other; the wife and mother may feel unneeded or lacking in purpose as the children leave the home; and the husband and father may need to redefine his career goals as he realizes he has peaked in his advancement opportunities. Financial and emotional stresses may result as well from the increased needs of aging parents in the extended family or the young adults as they prepare for college, marriage, or work.

The young adult too enters new roles of responsibility in relation to work, society, home, and self. Acceptance of responsibility for self-care has serious implications for the future health of the young adult. Independent health behaviors practiced as a young adult with respect to nutrition, exercise, sexual development, alcohol, smoking, drug use, and family life will largely determine the quality of life in the later years.

Areas of Focus for Health Protection

CANCER SCREENING. Although the peak incidence of the major forms of cancer does not occur until middle age, it is important for the young adult to begin screening for these problems and to continue the screening process throughout life. Simple but effective screening measures are available for the detection of breast, cervical, and testicular cancers. Early detection and treatment of these diseases has been shown to reduce mortality rates significantly. Nurses can play a vital role in educating young adults and encouraging the regular practice of these routine screening measures.

Breast cancer is the leading cause of cancer incidence and death for females in the United States (American Cancer Society, 1992). Following maturation of the breasts, young women should be taught how to examine them for early signs of cancer. A breast lump is the most common presenting symptom of breast cancer, though nipple retraction or discharge, palpable lymph nodes, and skin changes may also signal progression of the disease. Breast self-examination (BSE) is important because an estimated 90% of breast cancers are self-discovered (Swinford & Webster, 1989). It is estimated that overall breast cancer mortality could be reduced nearly 20% if all women undertook regular self-examination. Yet despite more than 20 years of promotion by the

American Cancer Society and health professionals, less than 20% of American women practice regular BSE (O'Malley, Fletcher & Morrison, 1990).

One of the oldest cancer screening procedures is the Pap smear, a preventive measure that has played an important role in reducing the incidence of cervical cancer. The American College of Obstetricians and Gynecologists recommends pelvic examinations and Pap smears to begin by age 18, even if the young woman is not sexually active. Some disagreement exists as to whether the traditional recommendation of an annual Pap smear for all adult women is necessary. More recent recommendations suggest that testing at a 3- to 5-year interval after an initial negative screening may be adequate for healthy women (American Cancer Society, 1992). Although all sexually active women are at risk for cervical cancer, the disease is more common in women of lower socioeconomic groups and in women with a history of multiple sexual partners or early onset of sexual activity (Woolf, 1990).

Testicular cancer is one of the most common cancers in young men between the ages of 17 and 35. Like most breast cancers, testicular cancer is most often discovered by the men themselves; an unusual nodule or lump is usually the presenting sign. Young men need to be educated in the importance of performing regular monthly examinations of the testes and penis. If this cancer is detected and treated early, there is an excellent chance for total cure (Swinford & Webster, 1989).

HYPERTENSION. Approximately 30% of adults in America have high blood pressure. Hypertension is a significant health problem for both males and females during later young adulthood, particularly young black adults. Government statistics indicate that blacks have a higher prevalence of high blood pressure than whites (38% versus 29%) (USPHS, 1992). Hypertension control is vital in the prevention of strokes, coronary heart disease and heart failure.

Protective behaviors related to the prevention of hypertension include a reduction of sodium levels in the diet, reduction of high stress levels, and maintenance of normal weight. Periodic screening of blood pressure levels is recommended for all young adults.

SEXUAL ACTIVITY. STDs are a major health problem for young adults, with 85% of reported cases of gonorrhea occurring in this age group. Between 1986 and 1989, the number of reported syphilis cases increased over 55%, to the highest level in the U.S. since the early 1950s (USPHS, 1990). Pelvic inflammatory disease (PID) occurs in 17% of all women who have been infected with gonorrhea and is a major cause of infertility in women of childbearing age. Other complications in young adults from STD are a greater incidence of ectopic pregnancy, abortions, stillbirths, cancer associated with human papillomavirus, and Bartholin's ab-

scess. An STD can have a profound impact on the unborn child. Birth defects, mental retardation, and fetal and infant deaths can be the result of maternal infection (Alexander, 1992).

The human immunodeficiency virus (HIV) has emerged as a major STD since 1980. Without treatment, approximately 50% of those infected with the HIV virus will develop AIDS within 10 years of exposure. At this time, no known cure exists; the disease is considered 100 percent fatal. In 1990, an estimated 1 million people were infected with HIV in the United States (USPHS, 1990). AIDS primarily affects young adults between the ages of 20 and 49. Groups at special risk are intravenous drug abusers and their sexual partners, people with multiple sexual partners, and homosexual and bisexual males and their female partners. Among the current AIDS patients, more than 75% are male, and 66% are male homosexuals and bisexuals. The most rapid increases in documented cases are occurring among intravenous drug users, women, and babies born to women in high-risk groups (USPHS, 1990). In 1992, heterosexual intercourse with infected partners was the major route of transmission of HIV, with 56.8% of the cases due to intercourse with an IV drug user (Centers for Disease Control, 1993). Because of this, women and infants and children are the fastest growing risk groups. AIDS was the leading cause of death in 20–40 year old women in New York City in 1992 and was predicted to become one of the leading causes of death in all women between the ages of 20 and 45 years (Guinan, 1992)

The most effective method of prevention of STD is avoidance of sexual contact with infected individuals. The proper use of condoms is thought to decrease risks. Early detection and prompt treatment of STD may help prevent more serious complications.

Controlling unplanned pregnancies is an important issue for many young adults. An unplanned pregnancy may interfere with a young woman's educational or career plans and have a significant impact on her future life. Those who choose to terminate a pregnancy with abortion face possible physical and psychosocial complications, including emotionally draining ethical dilemmas. Both married and unmarried young women need information regarding effective contraception. Nurses can play a vital role in educating young adults about the risks, side effects, and complications associated with specific methods of birth control and assisting the individual to choose a method appropriate to her needs (Edelman & Mandle, 1986).

ALCOHOL, DRUG, AND TOBACCO USE. Much of the same information on the use of drugs, alcohol, and tobacco that was presented in the section on adolescents is applicable to young adults. Drug and alcohol abuse is increasing in this age group and is frequently related to the high numbers of fatal accidents. Smoking remains a present and future threat to health. If these patterns of excessive chemical abuse are not altered during young adulthood, it may be impossible for changes to be made later in life. Preventive education for the young adult must be directed toward reducing the use of chemical agents and raising the individual's awareness of the physical and psychological complications that may arise.

STRESS MANAGEMENT. Stress plays an integral part in the young adult's life. Newly acquired responsibilities related to college, mate selection, marriage, childbearing, job demands, and social expectations can produce overwhelming stresses. Internal pressures to succeed and excel contribute to the potential risk to health.

Assisting the young adult to identify and reduce stress-producing behaviors or situations can be effective in preventing future health problems. Initiation of programs for exercise or nutritional improvement can boost the individual's ability to cope with high levels of stress. Utilization of several of the stress-reduction techniques described in Chapter 14 can also be extremely effective. In fostering good health habits that can be continued late into life, the family nurse has a vital role in teaching stress management to young adults.

IMMUNIZATION. Although the importance of childhood immunization is widely acknowledged, the establishment or maintenance of immunity throughout the adult years is largely ignored. Childhood immunization programs have significantly reduced the incidence of many of the common vaccine-preventable diseases; however, a substantial portion of the remaining morbidity and mortality from these diseases occurs in older adolescents and adults. Immunity to some diseases such as tetanus and diphtheria requires a periodic booster to remain effective. Other adults who have escaped natural infection or proper childhood immunization may be at increased risk for measles, mumps, rubella, or poliomyelitis, and their ensuing complications, as adults.

Recommendations for adult immunization include a booster dose of tetanus and diphtheria toxoids every 10 years. Adults who have never completed a primary series of tetanus and diphtheria toxoids will require two doses of the combined toxoids at monthly intervals, followed by a third dose 6 to 10 months later, and thereafter a booster dose at 10-year intervals. Persons born after 1956 should receive a measles vaccine unless they were immunized with live measles vaccine on or after their first birthday or have documentation of a natural infection. Women of childbearing age should be ensured of immunity against rubella. Pregnant women should not be immunized; susceptible pregnant women may be vaccinated immediately after delivery. Though not universally recommended for healthy adults under the age of 65, influenza vaccine may be administered to those who are at increased risk of exposure or transmission of infection, such as military personnel, college students, and health care professionals. Hepatitis B immunizations are recommended for susceptible individuals in high-risk groups, including homosexuals, intravenous drug abusers, and household and sexual contacts of hepatitis B carriers. Persons in health-related jobs with frequent exposure to blood should also be immunized (LaForce, 1990).

Families with Middle-Aged Adults

Middle adulthood is a period of social, psychological, and biological change. For many, this extended period after the children leave home is a time of maximum economic productivity and marital satisfaction. For others, the transition into middle life is as critical as adolescence and in some ways more difficult; it is a period of reexamination and reevaluation of life goals and adult roles. Health tasks for middle-aged adults focus on guarding against the onset of preventable chronic diseases through continued good health habits and early detection and treatment. The three major risk factors for chronic diseases are cigarette smoking, obesity, and sedentary lifestyle (USPHS, 1994). Health education regarding risk factors remains the key to preventing or delaying many serious illnesses.

Areas of Focus for Health Protection

CANCER SCREENING. The second most common cause of death among American adults is cancer, with lung, large intestine, and breast malignancies accounting for almost half of the cancer fatalities among this age group (American Cancer Society, 1992). The importance of breast and testicular self-examination and routine Pap smears was discussed in the section on young adults. These effective screening measures should be continued throughout the life span. Additional effective screening measures for the middle-aged adult include the mammogram and testing for occult blood in the stool.

The mammogram, an x-ray procedure, has been shown to be highly effective in detecting early nonpalpable breast masses. Although there is some controversy surrounding the use of mammography as a routine, periodic screening method for young women, for women over the age of 50, it is considered a valuable and highly recommended procedure. The American Cancer Society currently advises all women to perform BSE monthly. Women 20 to 40 years of age should have a breast examination every three years, and women over 40 should have a breast examination every year. A baseline screening mammogram is recommended by age 40. Regular mammograms should be performed every one to two years for those between ages 40 and 49 and annually for women age 50 and over (American Cancer Society, 1992).

Ninety-five percent of colorectal cancers are found in adults over the age of 45. Digital rectal examinations, screening the stool for occult blood, and proctosigmoidoscopy are recommended by the American Cancer Society to detect colon or rectal cancers in asymptomatic patients. Digital rectal examination by a physician is recommended annually after age 40 and annual testing for occult blood in the stool advised after age 50. Proctosigmoidoscopy is recommended every three to five years after age 50 (American Cancer Society, 1992).

Health education for this age group should focus on recognizing signs or symptoms of serious illness. Weight loss, fever, change in bowel habits, change in appetite, shortness of breath, and chronic cough are all conditions that should be evaluated by a medical professional. Prompt attention to early warning signs may facilitate the detection and treatment of potentially serious illness.

SMOKING. Cigarette smoking is recognized to be the single most preventable cause of death in the United States; the conclusive evidence linking tobacco use with disease, disability, and premature death is extensive. The American Cancer Society estimates that cigarette smoking is responsible for 90% of lung cancer deaths among men and 79% among women. Smoking is also associated with cancers of the mouth, pharynx, larynx, esophagus, pancreas, cervix, kidney, and bladder. Smoking accounts for 30% of all cancer deaths. In addition, smoking is a major cause of heart disease and is associated with conditions ranging from colds and gastric ulcers to chronic bronchitis, emphysema, and cerebrovascular disease (American Cancer Society, 1992).

There has been a dramatic shift in the smoking behavior of Americans over the past 20 years. More than 37 million individuals have quit smoking, and the proportion of adult smokers declined from 40% of the population in 1965 to roughly 29% in 1987. The most dramatic change has been noted in the proportion of adult males who smoke, which fell from 52% in 1965 to 32% in 1987 (American Cancer Society, 1992). Nevertheless, smoking rates remain high among blacks, blue-collar workers, and those with fewer years of education. Between 1966 and 1987 smoking rates declined 50% for college graduates and 20% for high school graduates but remained fairly constant for those who did not complete high school (USPHS, 1990).

The challenge for health professionals continues to be to educate the public regarding the dangers of smoking. Recent public awareness of the hazards of second-hand smoke has facilitated the creation of smoke-free areas in public places and has encouraged the development of many smoking cessation programs for adults. Unfortunately, many middle-aged adults may have smoked for 20 or 30 years, and quitting for them can be a very difficult process.

HYPERTENSION. Controlling hypertension has been shown to be one of the most effective means available for reducing mortality in the adult population. Research studies have conclusively demonstrated that cardiovascular morbidity and mortality are substantially higher in individuals with elevated blood pressure, at all ages and in both sexes. Hypertension is a major contributor to pressure-related events such as stroke, congestive heart failure, and ruptured aortic aneurysm. It also poses a significant risk factor for other types of coronary heart disease and occlusive peripheral arterial disease (Logan, 1990).

A 1985 national public awareness survey indicated a high level of awareness among the public in relation to hypertension. Eighty-six percent of the adult population had had their blood pressure checked at some point in the preceding year, by either a physician or self-testing. Between 1982 and 1985, visits to health professionals for high blood pressure screening and/or monitoring increased by 52.7%, while visits for other reasons increased only 4.8% (U.S. Department of Health and Human Services, 1986). Regular screening remains the most effective method for detection of hypertension.

The specific etiology of primary hypertension is not known, although much has been learned about the risk factors that contribute to its occurrence. A growing body of knowledge over the past 20 to 30 years has strongly indicated that lifestyle and health behaviors play an important role in the maintenance, and possibly the etiology, of hypertension. Behaviors that have been shown effective in the prevention and control of hypertension include limiting dietary intake of sodium to 2 grams of sodium daily, maintenance of or reduction of weight to within 10 pounds of normal, control of psychological stress, and participation in moderate exercise (Martin, 1990). If medication is required for hypertension control, strict adherence to the prescribed regimen is essential. Although surveys indicate that most adults with high blood pressure are aware of their condition, only about 25% to 33% of them have their blood pressure under control (USPHS, 1990).

GLAUCOMA. Glaucoma is the third leading cause of blindness in the United States. Although the exact cause is not known, it is associated with an increase in intraocular pressure, which damages the optic nerve and causes a loss of vision. Early detection of glaucoma is possible through measurement of tonometric pressure within the eye, a procedure that should be included in all routine ophthalmic examinations after the age of 40. Glaucoma is easily treated with medication or iridectomy; delay in treatment will result in blindness (Battista, Huston & Davis, 1990).

Families with Older Adults

The proportion of Americans 65 years of age and older rose from 4.4% of the population at the turn of the century to 12.4% in 1988. The elderly population is projected to rise to approximately 14% in 2010, accelerating to nearly 22% by 2030. As we enter the next century, there will be 35 million Americans over the age of 65. Significantly, the greatest increase will be in those over the age of 85. By 2010 they will comprise 15.5% of our population (Institute of Medicine, 1990).

Health protective behaviors take on added significance with the elderly population. Although today's elderly are healthier than in the past, studies indicate that 85% of older Americans suffer from at least one chronic degenerative disease, and multiple chronic problems are commonplace. The most frequent chronic conditions among non-institutionalized elderly are arthritis, hypertension, hearing impairment, heart conditions, sinusitis, vision impairments, and arteriosclerosis (Yurick et al., 1989). Considering that half of those who reach the age of 65 will live to be at least 80 years old, the importance of protective measures that work to maintain functional ability and limit the effects of disabling conditions cannot be overstated. Small gains in health promotion or even slight reductions in the rate of decline can make a significant difference in the quality of life and the degree of independence of the elderly person (Ruffing-Rahal, 1991).

Areas of Focus for Health Protection

DENTAL HEALTH. Although dental health in older adults is largely determined by the health behaviors practiced or ignored in younger years, it remains an important determinant of quality of life. Three-fifths of Americans 65 to 74 years of age have fewer than half of their permanent teeth; 24% of the edentulous elderly do not have false teeth or do not use the teeth they have been fitted with (Institute of Medicine, 1990).

Dental health plays an important role in the nutritional practices of the older adult. The individual with loose teeth or poorly fitting dentures may limit dietary choices to soft foods and avoid meats, fruits, and vegetables that require biting and chewing. Frequently, food eaten by those who are edentulous is inadequate and nutritionally deficient. A gradual decrease in taste sensation and saliva production may have a further impact on dietary practices (Yurick et al., 1989). Dental health also has important psychological implications. A functional and healthy mouth is directly related to smiling, the ability to communicate and socialize, and sexual pleasure. Lack of teeth affects articulation, jaw alignment, and general appearance and may have a profound impact on self-esteem (Institute of Medicine, 1990).

Good dental hygiene should remain an important component of the daily health practices of the older adult. Routine brushing, daily flossing, and periodic professional care are essential. If manual dexterity is limited, a rechargeable electric toothbrush and commercial floss holder or Water Pik device may be helpful. Daily oral hygiene is also important for the individual with dentures. Proper cleaning of dentures prevents bad breath and stains and is necessary for the removal of debris under the denture that may cause pressure and shrinkage of the underlying structures. Dentures should not remain out of the mouth for extended periods because the configuration of the gums can change, causing the dentures to fit improperly. If the older adult is unable to perform dental care adequately, it is important that the integrity of the mouth be maintained by a caregiver (Yurick et al., 1989).

EMOTIONAL HEALTH. The aging process requires continual adaptation to a multitude of physical, psychological, and social changes. To a great extent, the health of older adults is dependent on their ability to cope with multiple stress-producing life events, especially adjustment to retirement, the loss of loved ones, and changes in health and physical appearance. Adaptation to retirement includes not only adjusting to a new leisure lifestyle but also coping with profound changes in role, status, and income. The inevitable loss of spouse and close friends alters lifelong roles and relationships and may contribute to loneliness and social isolation. Physical limitations resulting from chronic illness may restrict mobility or independence and have a devastating effect on self-esteem. Considering that these overwhelming transitions often occur in rapid succession, it is readily apparent that the elderly are at high risk for emotional difficulties (Murray & Huelskoetter, 1991).

Depression is a significant health problem among the elderly and is usually related to the onset of rapid and repeated losses. Depressed elderly are often overwhelmed by a sense of hopelessness and discouragement, which has an impact on their daily lives. Social and emotional withdrawal may result, as well as suicide. In the United States, the highest rate of suicide is found among white, elderly males between the ages of 65 and 74 (Murray & Huelskoetter, 1991; Yurick et al., 1989).

Although many of the adjustments of old age cannot be avoided, the negative effects can be diminished through anticipatory guidance. Planning for expected stressful situations, such as retirement or relocation, can offset many potential problems. Family relationships are of central importance in later life because of emotional, supportive, and sometimes economic functions (Ruffing-Rahal, 1991).

The presence of a social support network is also beneficial. Older people need companionship and social interaction. Research has demonstrated that older adults living together have a greater survival rate and retain their independence longer than those who live alone. The frequent company of other people and the companionship of a household pet provide avenues for expression and response and add meaning and a sense of purpose to life (Murray & Huelskoetter, 1991).

SENSORY CHANGES. Alterations in visual and auditory acuity and tactile sensation are common with advancing age. Eyeglasses or contact lenses are worn by 92% of individuals over the age of 65, and 65% of the known cases of legal blindness occur among the elderly (Yurick et al., 1989). Decreases in visual acuity and reduction in adaptation to darkness or low illumination have important safety implications for the elderly. Falls are the leading type of fatal injury and a major cause of morbidity and disability among the elderly (Moss, 1992). Older clients should be cautioned about the risks of driving at night or in moving from brightly lit to dark areas. The home should be arranged to provide unobstructed passageways and the use of night lights encouraged. Scatter rugs should be avoided (Mayhew, 1991). Older adults should continue to have regular vision testing, including a check of internal eye pressures to screen for glaucoma (Beers et al., 1991).

Hearing loss is the most common infirmity of old age. Approximately 35% of individuals over the age of 75 have a significant hearing deficit (Beers et al., 1991). Impaired hearing can have a profound impact on communication ability and social isolation. Routine testing can determine the nature of the hearing loss and whether it is treatable with a hearing aid.

Changes in tactile sensation and temperature regulation also create hazards for the older adult. Perception of and reaction to painful stimuli may be decreased with age, resulting in the elderly person's suffering burns or frostbite before being aware of any discomfort. Caution should be used when applying hot water bottles or heating pads. To prevent hypothermia, the room temperature may need to be elevated, particularly at night. The use of extra blankets, caps, socks, and layered clothing is also helpful (Mayhew, 1991).

NUTRITION. Meeting the nutritional needs of the older adult remains an important health concern. Although caloric requirements continue to decrease with age, adequate amounts of protein, vitamins, iron, and trace minerals are still needed for good health. Individuals who have maintained sound dietary habits throughout life need to change little as they age; however, there are many factors that can affect the nutritional practices of the elderly. For example, dental health may be an important determinant of food choices; gradual loss of olfactory and taste sensations may contribute to a lack of desire for food; and problems with digestion, including heartburn or excessive gas, may have an impact on dietary habits (Yurick et al., 1989).

Socioeconomic factors strongly influence nutritional practices. Socialization is an important component of meals or nutritional intake, which is often lacking with the elderly. Studies have indicated that older persons who live alone often have less dietary intake and less variety in their meals, eat fewer foods requiring preparation, and are more likely to skip the evening meal (Rakowski, 1986). Limited income, lack of transportation, and housing conditions may also dictate which foods can be purchased and how they will be prepared. Community resources such as Meals on Wheels or nutrition sites that provide nutritionally sound meals and social interaction can be utilized to enhance the nutritional status of the older adult (Christian & Greger, 1988).

MEDICATIONS. Adverse drug reactions or overdoses are a significant health problem for the elderly. A decreasing metabolic rate and diminished renal function contribute to increased blood levels of medication. Overprescription of medications or complicated drug regimens can also lead to unexpected or dangerous drug interactions. Personal practices of the older adult, such as taking too much or too little of a medication, saving and taking old drugs, mixing over-the-counter drugs with prescribed medications, or taking incorrect dosages because of visual impairments also contribute to problems with medication (Institute of Medicine, 1990; Moss, 1992).

Education of the elderly regarding the safe use of their medications is an important protective measure that can help avoid accidental poisonings or reactions. All medications should be labeled and taken only according to directions. Nurses working with the elderly should encourage the older adult to know the name of each prescribed medication and to be aware of potential side effects. Old or used medications should be destroyed and expiration dates checked regularly. The elderly should be advised against the use of over-the-counter drugs or medications prescribed for other persons (Clark, Queener & Karb, 1990). The Committee on Health Promotion and Disability Prevention for the Second Fifty recommends that elderly patients have all their medications, both prescription and nonprescription, reviewed by their physician for appropriateness, potential adverse reactions, and continued need at least every six months (Institute of Medicine, 1990).

IMMUNIZATION. Immunization, though largely ignored, continues to be an important protective measure for older adults. Elderly persons have increased susceptibility to a number of infectious diseases, particularly those of the lower respiratory tract. Influenza and pneumococcal pneumonia are the most lethal of the major acute infections, with a mortality rate of 25% to 35% among those over the age of 65. The nation's health objectives for the year 2000 call for a 60% influenza and pneumococcal immunization rate. It is estimated that only 20% of elderly are immunized for influenza and 10% for pneumococcal disease (Holt, 1992).

All adults, including the elderly, should have completed a primary series of tetanus and diphtheria toxoids and should receive a booster dose every 10 years. Maintaining effective levels of immunity is especially important in relation to tetanus. More than half of reported cases of tetanus occur in persons over the age of 50 years, often following injuries not considered tetanus prone. Recent studies indicate that only 14% of older adults over the age of 50 have protective blood levels for tetanus immunity (Wesche & Overfield, 1992).

HEALTH SUPERVISION. Although some disagreement exists regarding the recommended frequency of routine examinations for healthy adults, it is generally acknowledged that examinations are needed more frequently in the older years (Beers et al., 1991). An important component of routine examinations is screening for common health problems among older adults, including hypertension, glaucoma, hearing disorders, diabetes, anemias, and nutritional deficiencies. Early signs of breast, colorectal, or prostate cancers are often detected through routine examinations or procedures. Counseling regarding nutrition, accident prevention, lifestyle, and adjustment to the problems of aging should be an integral part of professional supervision (U.S. Preventive Services Task Force, 1989). Early detection and treatment of health problems can help to minimize disability and allow the older adult to maintain maximum functional independence and quality of life.

FAMILY SELF-CARE

An important element of health protection is the ability of the family to meet the physical self-care needs of each family member. Recent attention has focused on the increasing role that knowledgeable individuals can play in their own health care and that of their families (Pickney & Pickney, 1989). Self-care classes, such as those initiated by Dr. Keith Sehnert, help individuals to accept more responsibility for their own care and that of their families; teach them the skills of observation, description, and handling of common illnesses, injuries, and emergencies; increase their basic knowledge about health problems; and help them to use health care resources, services, and medications more economically and appropriately (Stanhope & Lancaster, 1992).

Home Supplies

Family self-care can be enhanced through the proper use of medical equipment and supplies kept in the home. Utilization of these materials allows family members to assess and manage common health problems and to perform periodic screening as needed. If a physical condition arises that warrants medical attention, use of these materials enables family members to furnish the health care provider with accurate information related to the problem.

TABLE 18–1. HOME HEALTH CARE SUPPLIES

Thermometer	Antipyretics
Stethoscope	Sphygmomanometer
Cool mist vaporizer	Tongue blades
Tweezers	Watch with second hand
Flashlight	Otoscope
Vaginal speculum	Measuring tape
Hot water bottle/heating pad	Dental kits
Emergency stock of regular medications	In-home pregnancy kit as needed
First aid supplies	

From Hill, L., and Smith, N. (1990). *Self-Care Nursing: Promotion of Health*. Norwalk, CT: Appleton & Lange. Reprinted with permission.

Table 18–1 lists suggested materials that can be kept in the home for periodic screening, illness management, or minor emergencies. Basic equipment, such as tweezers, thermometer, vaporizer, hot water bottle/heating pad, and flashlight, need no special instructions. Other supplies, such as a stethoscope, blood pressure cuff, otoscope, or vaginal speculum, require basic education by a health professional before they can be used properly. Use of these instruments should be for preliminary screening only—to determine if a physical condition warrants professional care (Pickney & Pickney, 1989). Nurses should work to educate families in the proper use of the suggested medical equipment and in the signs and symptoms of conditions that warrant professional medical attention.

Health Care Services

The provision of adequate medical services and supervision is an important family health protective behavior. Selection of competent health care providers whose philosophies and services meet the needs of the family members is a critical task that is often overlooked or taken for granted. Individuals or families should not hesitate to seek out the services of other health care professionals if they are not comfortable or satisfied with their provider.

Family self-care can also be enhanced through an understanding of the health care system. Information related to common medical and surgical procedures, hospital services and routines, reasonable costs, and insurance reimbursement can assist families in making responsible decisions regarding their health care and may help to avoid needless costs or procedures. A variety of books that address these areas of concern are available for families—for example, *How to Raise a Healthy Child . . . in Spite of Your Doctor* by Dr. Robert Mendelsohn, *Medical Access* by Richard Saul Wurman, *Modern Prevention* by Isadore Rosenfeld, *Take This Book to the Hospital with You: A*

Consumer Guide to Surviving Your Hospital Stay by Charles Inlander, and *How to Choose a Doctor* by the People's Medical Society.

Self-Care Resources

Every community has many self-care resources available to assist families in meeting their health protection needs—for example, local chapters of organizations such as Planned Parenthood or the American Cancer Society, worksite health programs, neighborhood health centers, and school-based clinics. Table 18–2 outlines guidelines that families and nurses can utilize in locating local self-care resources.

Families seeking health information can consult a variety of sources: local libraries, hospitals and clinics, self-help groups, health information centers, national health organizations, and U.S. government clearinghouses and information centers. There is no shortage of information available to consumers. At least 400 popular health books are published annually by the major trade publishers and a host of small presses. Many local libraries and bookstores have developed consumer health sections that offer medical tests and lay books. Access to health information is facilitated greatly by the existence of a large number of health information clearinghouses, information centers, toll-free hot lines, and resource organizations that provide informational and educational services to the general public. For families whose local sources are limited or inadequate, a wealth of health information is available by telephone or mail (Rees & Hoffman, 1990) Local hospitals and clinics often sponsor workshops or lectures on a wide range of health topics. Table 18–3 provides a sampling of information sources available to health professionals and the general public.

THE ROLE OF THE FAMILY HEALTH NURSE

The family health nurse (FHN) plays a vital role in the development and fostering of health protective behaviors within the family setting. A family approach is particularly important in relation to health protection because many of the diseases or health conditions to be prevented have some genetic basis or are related to lifestyle practices. It is vital that the family as a whole address its potential risks and work together to implement protective behaviors (Bigbee & Jansa, 1991). Through the use of the nursing process, the FHN can assist family members to identify actual or potential areas of health risk, to establish health goals based on the family's needs and interests, and to develop an effective lifelong plan for health protection.

Assessment

Assessment of family health protective behaviors involves the collection of data from which family strengths, concerns, and actual or potential problems can be identified. An important component of health protection is the identification of health risks. Many clients and families place high priority on areas of health protection if the threat of illness is apparent and easily understood. Health-risk appraisal is commonly used by nurses and other health professionals as a means of assessing individuals and families and providing them with a realistic estimate of the major health hazards to which they are particularly vulnerable (Stanhope & Lancaster, 1992). Family members may be more amenable to recommended lifestyle changes if their potential for developing a specific chronic condition is moderate or high risk. Figure 18–1 presents a sample risk appraisal tool that addresses the categories of cardiovascular disease,

---

TABLE 18–2. GUIDELINES FOR LOCATING SELF-CARE RESOURCES

1. Use the telephone book. Many agencies are cross-referenced in both the general listing and the classified section.
2. Clinics and hospitals in the community have many services and programs that are not advertised. Call and ask for a health educator. These people are excellent resources for referrals within the community.
3. University or community college student health centers may offer community outreach programs or provide referrals.
4. Professional organizations such as the American Medical Association, American Nurses' Association, and the American Dietetics Association generally have local offices. Even if you do not require their specific services, the organization can be helpful in locating other health care services.
5. Local newspapers frequently have articles highlighting available local services.
6. Official health care agencies such as county health departments generally have compilations of local service agencies.
7. There are a variety of written resources. Many books are published with addresses and telephone numbers of the national offices of self-care organizations. Local addresses and numbers may be obtained from the organizations.
8. The nurse is encouraged to go to or call the resource before referring a client. This may reduce embarrassment or surprise due to cost, change of location, or procedures.

From Hill, L., and Smith, N. (1990). *Self-Care Nursing: Promotion of Health* (2nd ed.). Norwalk, CT: Appleton & Lange. Printed with permission.

TABLE 18–3. SOURCES OF HEALTH INFORMATION

1. **Health information centers** are independently funded and provide unlimited public access to medical information:

   Boston Women's Health Collective
   445 Mt. Auburn St.
   Watertown, MA 02172
   (617) 924-0271
   Salt Lake City, UT 84102

   Center for Medical Consumers
   237 Thompson St.
   New York, NY 10012
   (212) 674-7105

   Center for Consumer Health Education
   1900 Association Drive
   Reston, VA 22091
   (703) 476-3400

   Consumer Health Information Center
   East 600 South St.
   Salt Lake City, UT 84102
   (801) 364-9318

   Planetree Health Resource Center
   2040 Webster St.
   San Francisco, CA 94115
   (415) 923-3680

2. **U.S. government clearinghouses and information centers** are federal and federally sponsored health information resources that provide health information to health professionals and the general public:

   National Clearinghouse for Alcohol Information
   P.O. Box 2345
   Rockville, MD 20852
   (301) 468-2600

   Arthritis Information Clearinghouse
   P.O. Box 9782
   Arlington, VA 22209
   (703) 558-8250

   Office of Cancer Communications
   National Cancer Institute
   Bldg 31, Rm 10A-24
   9000 Rockville Pike
   Bethesda, MD 20892
   (301) 496-5583; (800) 4-CANCER

   Consumer Information Center
   General Services Administration
   Pueblo, CO 81009

   National Diabetes Information Clearinghouse
   P.O. Box NDIC
   Bethesda, MD 20892
   (301) 468-2162

   National Clearinghouse for Drug Abuse
   P.O. Box 416
   Kensington, MD 20795
   (301) 443-6500

   Food and Nutrition Information Center
   National Agricultural Library Bldg, Rm 304
   Beltsville, MD 20705
   (301) 344-3719

   National Health Information Clearinghouse
   P.O. Box 1133
   Washington, DC 20013-1133
   (800) 336-4797

   Center for Health Promotion/Education
   Centers for Disease Control
   1600 Clifton Rd., NE
   Atlanta, GA 30333
   (404) 329-3492

   Maternal & Child Health Clearinghouse
   38th and R St., NW
   Washington, DC 20057
   (202) 625-8410

3. **National health agencies and organizations** provide written literature and referrals to local doctors and support groups:

   American Cancer Society
   777 Third Ave.
   New York, NY 10017

   American Diabetes Association
   2 Park Ave.
   New York, NY 10016

   American Heart Association
   205 E. 42nd St.
   New York, NY 10017

   American Lung Association
   1740 Broadway
   New York, NY 10019

   American Red Cross
   17th & D St., NW
   Washington, DC 20006

   International Academy of Preventive Medicine
   10409 Town & Country Way, Suite 200
   Houston, TX 77024

   National Association for Mental Health
   1221 22nd St., NW
   Washington, DC 20037

   National Research Council
   Food and Nutrition Board
   2101 Constitution Ave., NW
   Washington, DC 20009

   National Self-Help Resource Center
   1739 Connecticut Ave., NW
   Washington, DC 20009
   810 7th Ave.
   New York, NY 10019

   Planned Parenthood
   810 7th Ave.
   New York, NY 10019

4. **Additional information from publications:** *Pathfinder: Toll-free Numbers for Health Information.* National Health Information Center, Office of Disease Prevention and Health Promotion. Washington D.C.: U.S. Department of Health and Human Services, July 1987
   Health Information Resources in the Federal Government. Office of Disease Prevention and Health Promotion. National Health Information Center. Washington, D.C.: U.S. Department of Health and Human Services, 4th ed, 1987.

In each row, place a check in the box that best describes your current life situation or behavior

Risk for Cardiovascular Disease

RISK FACTOR: ⟶ INCREASING RISK ⟶

Sex and Age		Female under 40	Female 40–50	Male 25–40	Female after Menopause	Male 40–60	Male 61 or over
Family History (mother, father, brothers, sisters)	High Blood Pressure	No relatives with condition		One relative	Two relatives		Three relatives
	Heart Attack	No relatives with condition	One relative with condition after 60	Two relatives with condition after 60	One relative with condition before 60		Two relatives with condition before 60
	Diabetes	No relatives with condition		One or more relatives with maturity onset diabetes		One or more relatives with preadolescent or adolescent onset	
Blood Pressure*	Systolic	120 or below	121–140	141–160	161–180	181–200	above 200
	Diastolic	70 or below	71–80	81–90	91–100	101–110	above 110
Diabetes*		No diagnosis	Maturity onset controlled	Maturity onset uncontrolled	Adolescent onset controlled	Adolescent onset uncontrolled	
Weight*		At or slightly below recommended weight	10% over-weight	20% over-weight	30% over-weight	40% over-weight	50% over-weight
Cholesterol** (mg/100 mg)		Below 180	181–200	201–220	221–240	241–260	261–280	Above 280
Serum Triglycerides* Fasting (mg/100 ml)		150 or below		151–400		401–1000	Above 1000
Percent of fat in diet*		20–30%		31–40%		41–50%	Above 50%
Frequency of Exercise*	Recreational	Intensive recreational exertion (35–45 min at least 4 times/week)		Moderate recreational exertion		Minimal recreational exertion	No recreational exertion
	Occupational	Intensive occupational exertion		Moderate occupational exertion		Minimal occupational exertion	Sedentary occupation
Sleep patterns*		7 or 8 hr sleep/night		More than 8 hr sleep/night		4–6 hr sleep/night	

*Indicates risk factors that can be fully or partially controlled.
**Serum lipid analysis is also recommended to determine low-density (beta) and high-density (alpha) lipoprotein levels. Evidence suggests that high-density lipoprotein (HDL) carries cholesterol from tissues for metabolism and excretion. An inverse correlation appears to exist between HDL and coronary artery disease.

FIGURE 18–1. Risk appraisal form. (From Pender, N. (1987). *Health Promotion in Nursing Practice* (2nd ed.). Norwalk, CT: Appleton & Lange.)

In each row, place a check in the box that best describes your current life situation or behavior

Risk for Cardiovascular Disease

RISK FACTOR: ———————→   INCREASING RISK ———————→

Cigarette Smoking*	No./day	Non-smoker	1–10/day	11–20/day	21–30/day	31–40/day	Over 40/day
	No. of yrs. smoked	Non-smoker	Less than 10 yr	11–15 yr	16–20 yr	21–30 yr	31 yr or more

Stress*	Domestic	Minimal		Moderate		High	Very High
	Occupational	Minimal		Moderate		High	Very High

Behavior Pattern* (Particularly males)	*Type B* Relaxed, appropriately assertive, not time dependent, moderate to slow speech			*Type A* Excessively competitive, aggressive, striving, hyperalert, time dependent, loud, explosive speech			

Air Pollution*	Low		Moderate		High	

Use of Oral Contraceptives* (females)	Do not use oral contraceptives		Under 40 and use oral contraceptives		Over 40 and use oral contraceptives	

Risk for Malignant Disease

Breast Cancer (Women) Age	20–29		30–39		40–49		50 or over

Race	Oriental		Black		Caucasian	

Family History (mother, grandmother, sister)	None		Mother, sister, or grandmother		Mother and grandmother		Mother and sister

Onset of Menstruation	Over 12 yr of age			Under 12 yr of age		

Breast Cancer Pregnancy*	Time	First pregnancy before 25		First pregnancy after 25		No pregnancies	
	No.	Three or more		One or two		None	

Weight*	0–40% Overweight			Above 40% Overweight		

Personal History	No evidence of dysplasia or previous breast cancer		Breast dysplasia		Previous breast cancer	

Lung Cancer Cigarette Smoking	No./day	Non-smoker	1–10/day	11–20/day	21–30/day	21–40/day	Over 40/day
	No. of yr smoked	Non-smoker	Less than 10 yr	11–15 yr	16–20 yr	21–30 yr	31 or more yr

*Indicates risk factors that can be fully or partially controlled.

FIGURE 18–1. *continued*

In each row, place a check in the box that best describes your current life situation or behavior

Risk for Malignant Disease

RISK FACTOR: ————————————→ INCREASING RISK ————————————————→

Occupational exposure to toxic chemicals*#	Length of exposure	Less than one year	1–5 yr	6–10 yr	11–15 yr	Over 15 yr
	Frequency and intensity of exposure	Low frequency and low intensity	Low frequency, moderate intensity (or vice versa)	Moderate frequency, moderate intensity	Moderate frequency, high intensity (or vice versa)	High frequency High intensity
Cervical Cancer Onset of sexual activity*		Before 16 yr of age	16–21		22–27	After 28 yr of age
No. of sexual partners*		Two		Three		Four or more
Marital status*		Single			Married	
Sexual partner		Circumcised			Uncircumcised	
Colorectal Cancer Age		Below 45 yr of age			Above 45 yr of age	
Personal history		No history of ulcerative colitis		Ulcerative colitis under 10 yr		Ulcerative colitis more than 10 yr
Fiber content of diet*		High		Moderate		Low
Weight* (men)		Less than 40% overweight			More than 40% overweight	
Rectal bleeding or black bowel movement		Never		Occasionally		Frequently
Uterine and Ovarian Cancer Age		Below 45 yr of age			Over 45 yr of age	
Weight*		Less than 40% overweight			More than 40% overweight	
Vaginal bleeding other than during menstrual period		Never		Occasionally		Frequently
Skin Cancer Complexion		Dark		Medium		Fair
Sun exposure (without protection)		Never or seldom		Occasionally		Frequently

Risk for Auto Accidents

Alcohol consumption*	Nondrinker	Occasionally small to moderate consumption	Frequently small to moderate consumption	Occasionally heavy consumption	Frequently heavy consumption
Mileage driven/yr-	Under 5000 miles/yr	5001–10,000 miles/yr		10,001–20,000 miles/yr	Over 20,000 miles/yr

*Indicates risk factors that can be fully or partially controlled.
#Chemicals such as asbestos, nickel, chromates, arsenic, chlormethyl ethers, radioactive dust, petroleum or coal products, and iron oxide

FIGURE 18–1. *continued*

In each row, place a check in the box that best describes your current life situation or behavior				
Risk for Auto Accidents				
RISK FACTOR: ————————→ INCREASING RISK ————————→				
Use of seat belt	Always	Usually	Occasionally	Never
Use of shoulder harness*	Always	Usually	Occasionally	Never
Use of drugs or medication that decrease alertness*	No use	Occasional use	Moderate use	Frequent use

Risk for Suicide

Family history	No history		One family member	Two or more family members
Personal history*	Seldom experience depression	Periodically experience mild depression	Frequently experience mild depression	Periodically experience deep depression	Frequently experience deep depression
Access to hypnotic medication*	No access		Access to small or limited dosages	Unlimited access to large dosages

Risk for Diabetes

Weight*	Desired weight	15% overweight	30% overweight	45% overweight	Above 45% overweight
Family history (parent or sibling)	None		Either parent or sibling	Both parent and sibling

*Indicates risk factors that can be fully or partially controlled.

FIGURE 18–1. *continued*

malignant diseases, auto accidents, suicide, and diabetes.

Assessment of family lifestyle and current health habits is also a critical component of health protection. Many identified health risks can be controlled through the modification of lifestyle or health behaviors. The areas of focus for health protection that have been addressed throughout this chapter for each of the developmental stages of the family life cycle form a basis for health protection assessment. Health protective behaviors that the family perceives themselves as practicing must be acknowledged as a family strength, and efforts should be directed toward strengthening and expanding those behaviors. Appendix A at the end of this chapter contains a comprehensive assessment tool related to health protection.

The assessment phase of the nursing process concludes with the formulation of nursing diagnoses. The diagnosis is an analysis of the family assessment, including a comprehensive analysis of family strengths and family needs. Examples of

approved nursing diagnoses that relate to health protection are presented in Table 18–4.

Controversy continues as to what are acceptable nursing diagnoses, particularly in relation to healthy clients and families for which no actual or potential problem is identified. Edelman and Mandle (1986) suggest that the definition of nursing diagnosis should be expanded to include not only actual or high-risk problems but also clients with no real problems who have a curiosity, interest, or desire to increase their knowledge and health practices to maximize their health potential. Nurses working with healthy families may wish to identify areas of need for health protection.

Planning

Planning involves the determination of a comprehensive plan of action based on an analysis of assessment data. For a health protection plan to be effective, the client must have an active voice in

TABLE 18–4. NURSING DIAGNOSES RELATED TO HEALTH PROTECTION

NURSING DIAGNOSIS	ETIOLOGY
Adjustment, Impaired	Inadequate or unavailable support systems Depression Loss (object, person, job) Adult: loss of ability to practice vocation, role reversal Elderly: normal physiological aging changes
Breastfeeding, Ineffective	Maternal ambivalence Inadequate nutritional intake Nonsupportive partner/family Lack of knowledge
Family Processes, Alterations in	Loss of family member Gain of new family member Relocation Economic crisis Change in family roles Family conflict
Growth and Development, Altered	Parental knowledge deficit Stress (acute, transient or chronic) Inadequate, inappropriate parental support Parent-child conflict School-related stressors
Health Maintenance, Altered	Lack of exposure to the experience Lack of motivation Changes in finances Lack of access to adequate health services Inadequate health practice Elderly: Effects of aging, sensory deficits

Health Seeking Behaviors	Role changes (parenthood, retirement)
	Lack of knowledge or need for:
	    Preventive behavior (disease)
	    Screening practices for age/risk
	    Optimal nutrition/weight control
	    Regular exercise
	    Stress management

Injury, Potential for
  Related to lack of awareness of
  environmental hazards
	Infant/child: Suffocation, poison, fire, falls
	Adolescent: Automobile, bicycle, alcohol, drugs
	Adult: Automobile, alcohol
	Elderly: Motor and sensory deficits, medication

Nutrition, Alterations in: Less Than Body Requirements	Depression, stress Social isolation Inability to chew (ill-fitting dentures) Lack of basic nutritional knowledge Adolescent: Anorexia nervosa Elderly: Altered sense of taste
Parenting, Altered	Adolescent or single parent Separation from nuclear family Lack of extended family Lack of knowledge Relationship problems Change in family unit
Self-Concept, Disturbance in	Divorce, separation, or death of significant other Loss of job or ability to work Obesity Pregnancy Infant and preschool: Deprivation Young Adult: Peer pressure, puberty Middle aged: Signs of aging (graying or loss of hair), reduced hormonal levels (menopause) Elderly: Losses (people, function, financial, retirement)

TABLE 18–4. NURSING DIAGNOSES RELATED TO HEALTH PROTECTION (continued)

Self-Harm, High Risk for	Adolescent: Separation from family, peer pressure, role changes, identity crisis, loss of significant support person Adult: Marital conflict, parenting, loss of family member, role changes Elderly: Retirement, social isolation, loss of spouse
Sexuality, Patterns Altered	Lack of knowledge Fatigue Obesity Alcohol ingestion/drug abuse Fear of failure (sexual) Fear of pregnancy Fear of sexually transmitted disease Ineffective role models Negative or absence of sexual teaching Aging (separation, isolation)

Data from Carpenito, L.J. (1992). *Nursing Diagnosis: Application to Clinical Practice* (4th ed.). Philadelphia: J.B. Lippincott.

TABLE 18–5. THE ROLE OF THE NURSE IN FAMILY HEALTH PROTECTION

STAGE	NURSING ROLE
Expectant Families	Counselor on prenatal nutrition Counselor on prenatal maternal habits Counselor on breast-feeding Teacher of child-care skills, normal growth and development, management of common childhood illness Coordinator with pediatric services Supervisor of immunizations Teacher of safety measures/accident prevention Referrer to social services
Families with Preschool and School-Age Children	Monitor of early childhood development; referrer when indicated Supervisor of immunizations Coordinator with pediatric services Counselor on nutrition and exercise Teacher in problem-solving issues regarding health habits Teacher of dental hygiene Counselor of environmental safety in the home Teacher of safety measures/accident prevention Facilitator in interpersonal relationships
Families with Adolescents	Teacher of risk factors to health Teacher in problem-solving issues regarding alcohol/drugs, smoking, diet, and exercise Facilitator of interpersonal skills with teenagers and parents Direct supporter, counselor or referrer to mental health resources Counselor on family planning Referrer for sexually transmittable disease
Families with Young or Middle-Aged Adults	Teacher in problem-solving issues regarding lifestyle and habits Screener for hypertension, Pap smear, breast examination, cancer signs, mental health, and dental care. Referrer for sexually transmittable diseases Counselor on nutrition and weight control Counselor on menopausal transition for husband and wife Facilitator in interpersonal relationships among family members
Families with Older Adults	Referrer for work and social activity, nutritional programs, homemaker services, and so on Monitor of exercise, nutrition, preventive services, and medications Supervisor of immunizations Counselor on safety in home Screener for hypertension, diabetes, Pap smear, breast examination, cancer signs, mental health, and dental care

From McCarthy, N.C. (1986). Health Promotion and the Family. In C. Edleman & C.L. Mandle (Eds.), *Health-Promotion throughout the Life span* (p. 213). St. Louis: Mosby. Reprinted with permission.

the planning process. Pender (1987) identifies nine steps in the health planning process that actively involve both the nurse and the client:

1. Review and summarize data from assessment
2. Identify the client's self-care strengths
3. Identify personal health goals and self-care areas for improvement
4. List possible behavior changes
5. Prioritize behavior changes based on the client's perceptions
6. Make a commitment to behavior change
7. Identify effective reinforcements and rewards
8. Determine barriers to behavior change
9. Develop a time plan for implementation

The nurse assists the client in health planning by providing information, counseling, reinforcement, and feedback; however, it is the client or family who ultimately determines which health protective measures to incorporate into everyday life. The ultimate purpose of the planning process is to select the most appropriate preventive or corrective course of action based on the family's priorities, goals, resources, and values (Logan & Dawkins, 1986). The development of a health promotion/protection plan is described in Chapter 2.

Implementation

Although the client and family are ultimately responsible for carrying out the prescribed plan of action, the nurse continues to play an active role in health protection. Nurses in a variety of settings—schools, worksites, ambulatory care centers, and acute care institutions—contribute to health protection through teaching, counseling, and coordinating of services. The role of the nurse in health protection varies according to the developmental stage and needs of the family. Table 18–5 presents some of the various roles of the nurse related to family health protection.

Evaluation

Evaluation, an ongoing process between the nurse and client, measures the progress that has been made toward goal achievement. Because most health protective measures are performed by the self-directed, self-responsible client, evaluation is largely based on the client's perception of progress. Periodic revision of goals and the plan of action may be necessary because of a client's mastery of target behaviors, changes in the client's values and priorities, or new options available to the client. This periodic updating of the health plan provides a systematic approach for movement of the client toward higher levels of health (Pender, 1987).

SUMMARY

Health protection is an essential component in the promotion and maintenance of individual and family health. The incorporation of health protective behaviors into lifestyle begins at birth, with the family functioning as the primary role model and motivator. The major threats to health vary throughout the life cycle depending on the developmental stage and the family's previous activities related to health promotion and health protection. Actions initiated by the family in response to the potential health risks significantly affect the health of all family members.

The family health nurse can play a vital role in the development and implementation of health protective behaviors. Through the use of the nursing process, the nurse can assist families in the identification of actual or potential health hazards and the development of an effective lifelong health protection plan.

CHAPTER HIGHLIGHTS

Many chronic health problems and family health problems are caused by inappropriate lifestyle or environmental factors.

The family plays a critical role in the development and practice of health protective patterns in family nutrition, health care use, leisure activities, health habits, and interaction across the family life course.

Key areas of focus for health protection for families across the life course are family nutritional practices, substance abuse, family processes (parenting, parental communication, intergenerational communication, conflict resolution, etc.), immunizations, dental and vision health, stress management, sexuality, anticipatory planning, family self-care practices, and growth and development issues.

Family nurses have a vital role in assisting individuals or families to identify potential threats to health and to develop effective plans for health protection for individual members and the family unit across the family life course.

REFERENCES

Alexander, L. (1992). Sexually transmitted diseases: Perspectives on this growing epidemic. *Nurse Practitioner, 17*(10), 31–42.

American Cancer Society. (1992). *Cancer Facts and Figures—1992.* Atlanta, GA: American Cancer Society.

Barnes, G., Parker, W., Lyon, T., Drum, M.A., & Coleman, G. (1992). Ethnicity, location, age, and fluoridation factors in baby bottle tooth decay and caries prevention of Head Start children. *Public Health Reports,* 107(2), 167–171.

Battista, R., Huston, P., & Davis, M.W. (1990). Screening for primary open-angle glaucoma. In R. Goldbloom & R. Lawrence (Eds.), *Preventing Disease: Beyond the Rhetoric* (pp. 333–340). New York: Springer-Verlag.

Beers, M., Fink, A., & Beck, J. (1991). Screening recommendations for the elderly. *American Journal of Public Health,* 81(9), 1131–1137.

Bigbee, J., & Jansa, N. (1991). Strategies for promoting health protection. *Nursing Clinics of North America,* 26(4), 895–913.

Brannan, J. (1992). Accidental poisoning of children: Barriers to resource use in a black, low-income community. *Public Health Nursing,* 9(2), 81–86.

Bruhn, J.G., Cordova, F.D., Williams, J.A., & Fuentes, R.G. (1977). The wellness process. *Journal of Community Health,* 2(3), 209–221.

Carpenito, L.J. (1992). *Nursing Diagnosis: Application to Clinical Practice* (4th ed.). Philadelphia: Lippincott.

Centers for Disease Control (1995). Recommended childhood immunization schedule—United States, 1995. *MMRW, 44* (RR-5): 1–7.

Christian, J.L., & Greger, J.L. (1988). *Nutrition for Living* (2nd ed.). Menlo Park, CA: Benjamin-Cummings.

Clark, J., Queener, S., & Karb, V. (1990). *Pharmacological Basis of Nursing Practice* (3rd ed.). St. Louis: Mosby.

Comstock, G., & Strasburger, V. (1990). Deceptive appearances: Television violence and aggressive behavior. *Journal of Adolescent Health Care,* 11(4), 31–44.

Duvall, E.M. (1977). *Marriage and Family Development* (5th ed.). Philadelphia: Lippincott.

Edelman, C., & Mandle, C.L. (1986). *Health Promotion throughout the Life Span.* St. Louis: Mosby.

Elders, M.J., Perry, C.L., Eriksen, M.P., & Giovino, G.A. (1994). The report of the surgeon general: Preventing tobacco use among young people. *American Journal of Public Health,* 84(4): 543–547.

Ernster, V.L. (1993). Women and smoking. *American Journal of Public Health,* 83(9): 1202–1203.

Feightner, J. (1990). Preschool screening: A review of the evidence. In R. Goldbloom & R. Lawrence (Eds.), *Preventing Disease: Beyond the Rhetoric* (pp. 43–51). New York: Springer-Verlag.

Fielding, J., & Williams, C. (1990). Unwanted teenage pregnancy: A U.S. perspective. In R. Goldbloom & R. Lawrence (Eds.), *Preventing Disease: Beyond the Rhetoric* (pp. 94–100). New York: Springer-Verlag.

Graham, M.V., & Uphold, C. (1992). Health perceptions and behaviors of school-age boys and girls. *Journal of Community Health Nursing,* 9(2), 77–86.

Greene, J.C., Louie, R., & Wycoff, S. (1990). Preventive dentistry. In R. Goldbloom & R. Lawrence (Eds.), *Preventing Disease: Beyond the Rhetoric* (pp. 231–246). New York: Springer-Verlag.

Griffen, A., & Goepferd, S. (1991). Preventive oral health care for the infant, child, and adolescent. *Pediatric Clinics of North America,* 38(5), 1209–1223.

Guinan, M.E. (1992). HIV, heterosexual transmission, and women. *Journal of the American Medical Association,* 23(4): 249–256.

Hann, D., & Osofsky, H. (1990). Psychosocial factors in the transition to parenthood. In I. Merkatz & J. Thompson (Eds.), *New Perspectives on Prenatal Care* (pp. 347–362). New York: Elsevier Science Publishing.

Harris, D.M., & Guten, S. (1979). Health protective behavior: An exploratory study. *Journal of Health and Social Behavior,* 20, 17–29.

Haynes, M.A. (1990). Suicide prevention: A U.S. perspective. In R. Goldbloom & R. Lawrence (Eds.), *Preventing Disease: Beyond the Rhetoric* (pp. 129–136). New York: Springer-Verlag.

Holt, D. (1992). Recommendations, usage and efficacy of immunizations for the elderly. *Nurse Practitioner,* 17(3), 51–59.

Institute of Medicine (1990). *The Second Fifty Years: Promoting Health and Preventing Disabilty.* Washington DC: National Academy Press.

Jones, N.E. (1992). Childhood injuries: An epidemiologic approach. *Pediatric Nursing,* 18(3), 235–239.

Keltner, B.R. (1992). Family influences on child health status. *Pediatric Nursing,* 18(2), 128–131.

Klein, L., & Goldenberg, R. (1990). Prenatal care and its effect on preterm birth and low birth weight. In I.R. Merkatz, & J.E. Thompson (Eds.), *New Perspectives on Prenatal Care* (pp. 501–529). New York: Elsevier Science Publishing.

Kuhns, C., & Holloway, S. (1992). Characteristics of caregivers that promote children's development in day care. *Journal of Pediatric Nursing,* 7(4), 280–285.

Kulbock, P., & Baldwin, J.H. (1992). From preventive health behavior to health promotion: Advancing a positive construct of health. *Advances in Nursing Science,* 14(4), 50–64.

LaForce, F.M. (1990). Immunization, immunoprophylaxis, and chemoprophylaxis to prevent selected infections. In R. Goldbloom & R. Lawrence (Eds.), *Preventing Disease: Beyond the Rhetoric* (pp. 33–42). New York: Springer-Verlag.

Lawrence, P.B. (1994). Breast milk: Best source of nutrition for term and preterm infants. *Pediatric Clinics of North America,* 41(5): 925–941.

Logan, A.G. (1990). Mild hypertension: Controversies in management. In R. Goldbloom & R. Lawrence (Eds.), *Preventing Disease: Beyond the Rhetoric* (pp. 412–421). New York: Springer-Verlag.

Logan, B.B., & Dawkins, C.E. (1986). *Family-Centered Nursing in the Community.* Menlo Park, CA: Addison-Wesley.

McClanahan, P. (1992). Improving access to and use of prenatal care. *Journal of Obstetric, Gynecological, and Neonatal Nursing,* 21(4), 280–283.

Martin, J.E. (1990). Exercise in the prevention and early control of hypertension: Efficacy and adherence issues. In K. Craig & S. Weiss (Eds.), *Health Enhancement, Disease Prevention, and Early Intervention: Biobehavioral Perspectives* (pp. 168–201). New York: Springer.

Mayhew, M. (1991). Strategies for promoting safety and preventing injury. *Nursing Clinics of North America,* 26(4), 885–893.

Moss, A. (1992). Are the elderly safe at home? *Journal of Community Health Nursing,* 9(1), 13–19.

Mullen, P. (1990). Smoking cessation counseling in prenatal care. In I. Merkatz & J. Thompson (Eds.), *New Perspectives on Prenatal Care* (pp. 161–175). New York: Elsevier Science Publishing.

Mullen, P., & Glenday, M.A. (1990). Alcohol avoidance counseling in prenatal care. In I. Merkatz & J. Thompson (Eds.), *New Perspectives on Prenatal Care* (pp. 177–192). New York: Elsevier Science Publishing.

Murray, R., & Huelskoetter, M.M. (1991). *Psychiatric Mental Health Nursing: Giving Emotional Care* (3rd ed.). Norwalk, CT: Appleton & Lange.

Novello, A., Degraw, C., & Kleinman, D. (1992). Healthy children ready to learn: An essential collaboration between health and education. *Public Health Reports,* 107(1), 3–10.

Olson, D.H., McCubbin, H.I., Barnes, H.L., Larsen, A.S., Muxen, M.J., & Wilson, M.A. (1983). *Families: What Makes Them Work.* Beverly Hills: Sage.

O'Malley, M., Fletcher, S., & Morrison, B. (1990). Does screening for breast cancer save lives? In R. Goldbloom & R. Lawrence (Eds.), *Preventing Disease: Beyond the Rhetoric* (pp. 251–263). New York: Springer-Verlag.

Pender, N.J. (In press). Health Promotion in Nursing Practice (3rd Ed.). Norwalk, CT: Appleton-Lange.

Pender, N.J. (1987). *Health Promotion in Nursing Practice* (2nd ed.). Norwalk, CT: Appleton & Lange.

Pickney, C., & Pickney, E. (1989). *Do-It-Yourself Medical Testing: 240 Tests You Can Perform at Home.* New York: Facts on File.

Pratt, L. (1976). *Family Structure and Effective Health Behavior: The Energized Family.* Boston: Houghton Mifflin.

Rakowski, W. (1986). Preventive health behavior and health maintenance practices of older adults. In K. Dean, T. Hickey, & B.E. Holstein (Eds.), *Self-Care and Health in Old Age* (pp. 94–129). London: Croom Helm.

Rees, A., & Hoffman, C. (1990). *The Consumer Health Information Source Book* (3rd ed.). Phoenix: Onyx Press.

Ruffing-Rahal, M.A. (1991). Rationale and design for health promotion with older adults. *Public Health Nursing,* 8(4), 258–263.

Stanhope, M., & Lancaster, J. (1992). *Community Health Nursing: Process and Practice for Promoting Health* (3rd ed.). St. Louis: Mosby.

Story, M., & Falkner, P. (1990). The prime-time diet: A content analysis of eating behavior and food messages in television program content and commercials. *American Journal of Public Health,* 80, 738–740.

Strasburger, V.C. (1992). Children, adolescents and television. *Pediatrics in Review, 13*(4): 144–151.

Swinford, P., & Webster, J. (1989). *Promoting Wellness: A Nurse's handbook.* Rockville, MD: Aspen.

Taras, H.L., Sallis, J.F., Patterson, T.L., Nader, P.R., & Nelson, J.A. (1989). Television's influence on children's diet and physical activity. *Developmental and Behavioral Pediatrics,* 10, 176–180.

United States Department of Health and Human Services, Public Health Service. (1994). Prevalance of selected risk factors for chronic disease by education in racial/ethnic populations—United States, 1991–1992. *Morbidity and Mortality Weekly Report, 43*(48), 894–899.

U.S. Department of Health and Human Services. (1986). *The 1990 Health Objectives for the Nation: A Mid-Course Review.* Washington DC: U.S. Government Printing Office.

U.S. Public Health Service. (1990). *Healthy People 2000: National Health Promotion and Disease Prevention Objectives.* DHHS Pub. No. 91-50212. Washington DC: U.S. Government Printing Office.

U.S. Preventive Services Task Force. (1989). *Guide to Clinical Preventive Services: An Assessment of the Effectiveness of 169 Interventions.* Baltimore: Williams & Wilkins.

Wesche, H., & Overfield, T. (1992). Tetanus immunity in older adults. *Public Health Nursing,* 9(2), 125–127.

Winkelstein, M. (1992). Adolescent smoking: Influential factors, past preventive efforts, and future nursing implications. *Journal of Pediatric Nursing,* 7(2), 120–127.

Woolf, S. (1990). Screening for cervical cancer. In R. Goldbloom & R. Lawrence (Eds.), *Preventing Disease: Beyond the Rhetoric* (pp. 319–323). New York: Springer-Verlag.

Worthington-Roberts, B., & Klerman, L. (1990). Maternal nutrition. In I. Merkatz & J. Thompson (Eds.), *New Perspectives on Prenatal Care* (pp. 235–271). New York: Elsevier Science Publishing.

Yurick, A., Spier, B., Robb, S., & Ebert, N. (1989). *The Aged Person and the Nursing Process* (3rd ed.). Norwalk, CT: Appleton & Lange.

APPENDIX A

FAMILY HEALTH PROTECTIVE BEHAVIORS

The nurse should indicate for each item whether the family member accomplishes the item according to criteria indicated in the columns. If an item or section does not apply, the points represented by that item should be so indicated by marking the "not applicable" column. In scoring at the end of each section, the category "total points possible" means the total number of points that could be attained if every item applied. The "total not applicable" category shows the total points for items or sections that do not apply to the family at this time; this number should be subtracted from the "total points possible" to obtain the "total applicable" score. When comparing "total applicable" with the "total points attained," the nurse and family can see the numerical difference in what should or could be achieved and what does exist at the present time.

	Yes (2 pts)	No (0 pts)	Not Applicable

I. Family Health Protective Behaviors
  A. The Expectant Family
    1. Expectant mother receives adequate prenatal care ____ ____ ____
    2. Adequate nutritional intake maintained throughout pregnancy ____ ____ ____
    3. Expectant mother abstains from alcohol, drug, or tobacco use throughout pregnancy ____ ____ ____
    4. Expectant mother avoids environmental hazards during pregnancy ____ ____ ____

    Total points possible   8
    Total not applicable ____
    Total applicable ____
    Total points attained ____

  B. Families with Infants
    1. Infant screened for inherited metabolic disorders ____ ____ ____
    2. Ongoing health supervision arranged for immunizations and growth and developmental assessment ____ ____ ____
    3. Parents actively seek information related to infant care skills, normal growth and development, and parenting ____ ____ ____

    Total points possible   6
    Total not applicable ____
    Total applicable ____
    Total points attained ____

  C. Families with Preschool Children
    1. Parents are aware of accident hazards ____ ____ ____
    2. Parents are aware of symptoms and management of common childhood illnesses ____ ____ ____
    3. Parents provide for and encourage:
      a. Good nutrition ____ ____ ____
      b. Adequate sleep ____ ____ ____
      c. Adequate exercise ____ ____ ____
      d. Dental health practices ____ ____ ____

    4. Parents provide for ongoing health
       supervision

    5. Immunizations completed prior to school
       entry

    6. Vision and hearing screening prior to school
       entry

    7. Preschool facility provides healthy environment
       a. Proper light
       b. Adequate heating and cooling
       c. Free of accident hazards
       d. Ample room for vigorous physical activity

    8. Preschool caregiver has philosophy congruent
       with that of family

    9. Preschool program promotes physical health,
       proper nutrition, and cognitive and social skill
       development

Total points possible   30
Total not applicable
Total applicable
Total points attained

D. Families with School-Age Children
    1. Family teaches safety and accident prevention
    2. Child demonstrates safe behaviors in play and
       daily activities
    3. Child demonstrates increasing responsibility
       for self-care
    4. Family provides for and encourages preventive
       dental care
    5. School has comprehensive health program
       a. Routine vision/hearing screening
       b. Health education
    6. School sports programs promote mental and
       physical wellness
    7. Working parents provide appropriate
       after-school supervision of child
    8. Parents monitor and limit television viewing
       by children
    9. Family effectively deals with everyday stress

Total points possible   20
Total not applicable
Total applicable
Total points attained

E. Families with Adolescents
    1. Adolescent assumes nearly total responsibility
       for self-care
    2. Adolescent is actively involved in physical
       fitness program
    3. Dietary patterns adequately meet the
       nutritional needs of the adolescent
    4. Adolescent is aware of the health hazards
       related to drug, alcohol, and tobacco use
    5. Family members are aware of the early signs
       of drug abuse among children or adolescents
    6. Family members discuss aspects of responsible
       sexual behavior
    7. Adolescent receives accurate information about
       contraceptive methods and where to obtain them
    8. Adolescent demonstrates effective problem-
       solving skills

10. Adolescent completes driver education course _____ _____ _____

Total points possible	20	
Total not applicable		
Total applicable		
Total points attained		

F. Families with Young Adults
   1. Young adult assumes total responsibility for self-care _____ _____ _____
   2. Reviews and updates immunization status _____ _____ _____
   3. If female:
      a. Performs regular BSE _____ _____ _____
      b. Obtains Pap smear as indicated _____ _____ _____
   4. If male, performs regular examination of the testes _____ _____ _____
   5. Engages in responsible, "safe" sexual practices _____ _____ _____
   6. Refrains from alcohol, drug, and tobacco use _____ _____ _____
   7. Obtains and records baseline blood pressure _____ _____ _____
   8. Develops effective decision-making skills for career, marriage, and parenthood _____ _____ _____

Total points possible	18	
Total not applicable		
Total applicable		
Total points attained		

G. Families with Middle-Aged Adults
   1. Performs monthly breast or testicular self-examination _____ _____ _____
   2. Obtains routine Pap smear _____ _____ _____
   3. Obtains mammogram as indicated _____ _____ _____
   4. Obtains screening for occult blood _____ _____ _____
   5. Performs visual inspections of body monthly for lumps and changes in moles _____ _____ _____
   6. Refrains from alcohol, drug, or tobacco use _____ _____ _____
   7. Obtains screening for diabetes _____ _____ _____
   8. Obtains screening for hypertension _____ _____ _____
   9. Obtains screening for glaucoma _____ _____ _____
   10. Modifies nutrition practices as necessary according to caloric needs _____ _____ _____
   11. Maintains physical exercise program _____ _____ _____
   12. Identifies normal changes due to aging and adapts accordingly _____ _____ _____

Total points possible	24	
Total not applicable		
Total applicable		
Total points attained		

H. Families with Older Adults
   1. Maintains good oral hygiene practices _____ _____ _____
   2. Plans for expected stressful situations such as retirement or relocation _____ _____ _____
   3. Family aware of potential accident hazards due to sensory and mobility changes _____ _____ _____
   4. Maintains good nutritional practices _____ _____ _____
   5. Practices safe use of medications _____ _____ _____
   6. Obtains recommended immunizations _____ _____ _____
   7. Obtains physical examinations as necessary _____ _____ _____
   8. Performs self-screening for cancer _____ _____ _____
   9. Maintains physical exercise program _____ _____ _____

    10. Obtains screening for diabetes   ____   ____   ____
    11. Obtains screening for glaucoma   ____   ____   ____
    13. Identifies normal changes due to aging and
        adapts accordingly   ____   ____   ____

Total points possible	26
Total not applicable	
Total applicable	
Total points attained	

I. Family Self-Care
    1. Family maintains appropriate medical equipment and supplies in the home
    2. Family members demonstrate knowledge of proper use of equipment and supplies
    3. Family members state signs and symptoms of physical conditions that warrant medical attention
    4. Family evaluates the credentials of health care providers
    5. Family considers personal characteristics and wellness attitude when choosing health professional
    6. Family seeks information on health services and reasonable costs
    7. Family effectively utilizes available self-care resources in the community

Total points possible	14
Total not applicable	
Total applicable	
Total points attained	

Assessment Tool Summary

	Subtotal points possible	Subtotal not applicable	Subtotal applicable	Subtotal points attained
I. Family Health Protective Behaviors				
A. The Expectant Family	8			
B. Families with Infants	6			
C. Families with Preschool Children	30			
D. Families with School-Age Children	20			
E. Families with Adolescents	20			
F. Families with Young Adults	18			
G. Families with Middle-Aged Adults	24			
H. Families with Older Adults	26			
I. Family Self-Care	14			

Total points possible	166
Total not applicable	
Total applicable	
Total points attained	

Adapted from Kandzari, J.H., and Howard, H.R. (1981). *The Well Family: A Developmental Approach to Assessment*. Boston: Little, Brown. Adapted with permission.

FAMILY ENVIRONMENTAL HEALTH

DOROTHY J. D. WILEY

The economic and technologic triumphs of the past few years have not solved as many problems as we thought they would, and in fact, have brought us new problems that we did not foresee.

HENRY FORD II

OBJECTIVES

On completion of this chapter, the reader will be able to:

1. Define:
   a. environment, as it applies to family, health and nursing practice
   b. occupational hazard
   c. paraoccupational hazard
   d. primary prevention
   e. secondary prevention
   f. tertiary prevention

2. State two or more physical characteristics or warning properties of occupational hazards/toxicants

3. Delineate one or more potential vectors for paraoccupational contamination of family members by members of the workforce

4. Discuss one or more threats to family wellness within the home environment

5. Explain assessment criteria, planning and intervention methods, and one or more evaluation criteria for a select family problem.

FAMILY HEALTH AND ENVIRONMENTAL STRESSORS

Environmental issues have generated a concern for the effect of the environment on family health. Carson (1960) in her book *Silent Spring* encouraged increased awareness and concern for the impact of environment on health. Her book was one of the first to advocate that laypeople should assume self-care responsibility for their environmental health. One need only listen to national television news programming, read current periodicals, or routinely sample radio newscasts to be aware of the diverse environmental concerns that exist in the United States and the rest of the world.

We all live within a sphere of occupational, avocational, and home settings. Each arena may impose a variety of physical and psychologic stressors on the individual or family unit, and each poses a new challenge to families and health professionals.

This chapter will focus on the impact of the environment on family health. Content includes a definition of environment, a brief overview of the current problems and issues in environmental health, hazards in the environment affecting the health of individuals and families, and the role of the nurse in family environmental health. Environmental influences on family health are multidimensional and often obscure. Data collection is often difficult.

Nursing's concern for the impact of environment on family health status began with Nightingale's concern for the sanitary environment of families and soldiers. In recent years, nursing models address in more depth the influence of environmental variables on the quality of individual and family health. Johnson's Behavioral Systems Model includes assessment of society relative to the environment that surrounds the individual (Lobo, 1985). Roy's Adaptation Model (Roy & Roberts, 1984) systematically accounts for environmental stimuli as input to the feedback loop. King's Open Systems Model considers the natural environment as a variable that needs to be assessed (King, 1981). Neuman (1982) describes the family as always in interaction with the environment, with flexible lines of resistance to stressors.

THE ENVIRONMENT: A MULTIDIMENSIONAL CONCEPT

The environment is made up of all that is visibly and invisibly surrounding us. Individuals contribute to the environment by their presence their activities, and the by-products of their actions. They encounter environmental stressors at work, home, and play that may be physical, biologic, or chemical in nature. The exposure may be primary to the individual or relayed to them from another family member.

Stratifying the problem by the risk of contacting an agent allows the family nurse to begin preventing contact, performing early screening and diagnosis, and/or offering appropriate rehabilitative measures. The intensity and duration of an exposure may be the best indicator of risk for illness. Technologic advances have allowed the potential for monitoring many individuals and environments but are frequently fraught with issues of cost, accuracy, and violations of personal privacy. Ignorance may complicate screening and research efforts, as many individuals are unaware of the myriad of substances contacted during the course of any given day.

Generally, acute and excessive exposure to stressors will cause a toxic reaction directly related to the properties of the agent. Physical stressors might directly damage tissue or vital organs, and biologic hazards may induce sudden infection. Toxicants may cause poisonous reactions that are attributable to their chemical properties.

Lead Exposure

Lead is one substance that can cause acute and chronic toxicity to workers, their families, and community contacts if it is improperly handled. As of May 1992, only 18 state health departments required mandatory reporting of elevated adult blood lead levels. Illinois, New Jersey, and New York, the only states with these available data, reported 10,118 blood lead level elevations among 4,406 persons in 1991 (Centers for Disease Control, 1991, 1993). Definitions of reportable cases vary by microgram per deciliter blood concentrations and by age. Laboratory surveillance, as opposed to clinical surveillance, of high-risk individuals such as lead battery workers is preferable due to the relative insensitivity of the latter and the preventability of illness induced by the agent across a wide range of exposures.

Chronic, low-level exposures generally do not produce acute, toxic human reactions. We generally associate these insidious exposures with diseases and conditions that frequently have a latency period and a more diffuse onset of symptoms. Examples of illnesses evidencing long latency periods between exposure and onset of complaint include occupationally and environmentally related cancers, chronic musculoskeletal disease, chronic heart and lung diseases (e.g., emphysema and other chronic obstructive pulmonary diseases), infertility, and adverse pregnancy outcomes.

Latency periods do not always reflect a smoldering disease state but may represent a period of time necessary to accumulate exposure to a number of necessary component causes that are sufficient for disease to manifest (Rothman, 1986). Some exposures may be sufficient in and of themselves to cause a diseased state. However, the current belief is that many diseases require either a single specific number of necessary causal exposures or a number of different but sufficient necessary causal exposures. Therefore, we can begin to think of disease latency as the time necessary to accumulate a sufficient number of exposures for disease. This model precludes long periods of smoldering undiagnosed disease and is probably more consistent with the majority of illnesses we deal with today.

Cancer

Cancer, for example, is a disease with both posited long latency and environmental causal factors. However, it comprises a number of organ-specific proliferative cellular disorders that escape immune surveillance and erode through the primary site's basement membrane to escape and seed distant body locations with rapidly multiplying and dysplastic cells. Typically, the cellular disorder is a series of acquired and/or inherited somatic cell mutations. We better understand the molecular biology of cancer today. We also believe that these diseases probably evolve from a number of exposures and along a number of different pathways. Therefore, the varying rates at which the population manifests disease may be due to modifying effects of protective and causal risk factors, as well as the rates and intensities of exposures.

Epidemiologic studies have indicated that cancers occur with different rates throughout the world and that individuals who migrate from one geographic region to another frequently evidence different rates of disease from those who do not leave the region. Though migrant studies point to an overall impact of environmental factors in oncogenesis, specific causal relationships frequently remain unclear (Ruddon, 1987).

Some malignancies strongly suggest inherited genetic factors. It must be stressed, however, that though most malignancies do not evidence simple family inheritance patterns, it is difficult to untangle the causal web of inherited genetic factors and shared exposures we frequently witness in families. We cannot preclude that inherited factors are not causally operating when environmental influences are clear.

Mutation, translocation, and deletion of specific genetic material are examples of mechanisms that play a part in oncogenesis (Institute of Medicine, 1992). These genetic factors may be inherited or somatic changes to the cell. For example, Li-Fraumeni syndrome, a rare germline mutation of the TP53 (i.e., p53) gene, is associated with a wide variety of both maturity and childhood tumors (Li & Fraumeni, 1969; Malkin, Li & Strong, 1990). Similarly, retinoblastoma and osteosarcoma have been linked to inherited deletions on chromosome 13 in some families (Institute of Medicine, 1992).

There is no simple inheritance pattern evident in the majority of malignancies. Acquired damage to a cell's genetic structure can lead to unchecked proliferation, progressively poor differentiation, and metastasis (Solomon, Borrow & Goddard, 1991). For example, Fearson and Vogelstein (1990) have proposed a multicausal model for colorectal cancer. They place a series of successive mutations or deletions on chromosomes 5, 12, 18, and 17 that combine with other cellular changes to produce a metastatic tumor. This "multi-hit" model proposes that normal epithelium is transformed, proliferates, alters cellular character, and later metastasizes through a series of alterations in the cell's molecular biology that are determined by the cell's genetic structure. Few tumors are unique associated with a specific agent, and few exposures are uniformly and totally associated with a single disease outcome. Therefore, this multi-hit model of disease implies both a number of different agents and a number of separate exposures over time.

Cause and effect are difficult relationships to untangle in regard to cancer. Some studies suggest genetic factors, while others link environment and behaviors. Therefore, how do health professionals evaluate the biological and epidemiologic evidence that malignancies, poor reproductive outcomes, and other human disease may have many causes? How does one distinguish between the role behavior, environment, and genetics each play in the development of disease? How does one take this knowledge and distill it so that patients are cared for properly and also receive information that is accurate, timely, and important to their daily lives?

If causation is narrowly defined as the direct and exclusive linkage of a putative exposure and a disease outcome, few exposures would be classified as causal agents. Diseases are generally due to a cascade of exposures and events. However, if causation is defined more expansively and likened to a pathway, then a number of different paths, each with a variety of composite parts, might lead to the same disease outcome. For example, lung cancer might arise from several biological pathways that each include a number of environmental exposures. Tobacco smoke and asbestos might be two such environmental exposures. Additionally, each pathway might be composed of one or more genetic precursors. Consequently, the expansive definition of causation would allow 100% of these pulmonary malignancies to be *caused* by environmental risk factors, while 100% were also associated with genetic causal factors (Rothman, 1986; Arnott, 1981). In essence, these proportions reflect the relative associations between an exposure and a disease that we are able to observe in human populations.

Agents thought to be oncogenic risk factors have been deduced from experimental animal studies, epidemiologic research, and case studies reported in the literature. Some exposures, such as cigarette smoking, have become generally understood to be risk factors for malignancy, while other exposures remain poorly understood. Marked differences between recognized carcinogens exist among professional and federal agencies and organizations. These may reflect differences in research methods, timing of review, and outcome definitions. We suggest the reader review lists currently compiled by agencies and organizations such as the American Conference of Government Industrial Hygienists, the Occupational Safety and Health Administration (OSHA), and the National Institute of Environment Health Science to compare similarities and differences in their appraisals and classifications of human carcinogens.

Musculoskeletal Impairment

Holbrook et al. (1984) estimate that approximately 9% of the U.S. population suffers from all types of musculoskeletal impairments. Low back pain appears to be the most frequently occurring disorder. The development of low back pain and other musculoskeletal maladies appears to be related to work and play activities causing pressure and impact, human habits, and psychologic variables (Kelsey & Hochberg, 1986).

Reproductive Hazards

Exposure to potential reproductive hazards poses a problem for both men and women. The range of expression for altered reproductive capacity includes changes in libido and potency; altered fertility; menstrual disturbances; alterations in sperm morphology, number, and chemical makeup; chromosomal disturbances; teratogenesis; fetal death; cancer; and developmental delays or disabilities (Barlow & Sullivan, 1982). Though much investigation has been devoted to the direct effect of toxic substances on fetal tissues, chemicals need not directly interact with those sites to produce malformations or fetotoxic effect. Interference with maternal physiologic systems may, in fact, be a more important source of teratogenesis than the direct (fetal) tissue-chemical interaction (Juchau & Fantel, 1981). Although women possess more potential for expression or adverse pregnancy outcome, men also remain vulnerable.

When evaluating reproductive studies, it is imperative to consider the number of problems that make scientific investigation of causation difficult. Few studies demonstrate an unequivocal relationship between agents or events and specific adverse reproductive outcomes. Some methodologic problems, not necessarily unique to reproductive studies, are:

- The need for large study populations due to the expected rarity of untoward outcomes in cohort or longitudinally designed studies
- The difficulty in assessing the true underlying base population at risk because of our inability to measure fully the number of conceptions and undetected early fetal losses in human populations
- The probably large number of causal relationships, frequently referred to as "background noise," that begin to obscure a single causal risk factor under investigation
- Study confounding (i.e., independent relationships between exposures and other known causal risk factors for the outcome of interest) that yields biased results
- Other forms of bias engendered by factors such as differences in recall, classification schemes used in data collection and analysis, and subject selection
- Difficulties in quantifying exposure and outcome states relative to time, dose, and degree of effect
- Changing definitions of poor pregnancy outcome states that have occurred over the past 30 or more years relative to our increased diagnostic sophistication and direct social and medical interventions (e.g., phenylke-

tonuria disease, fetal karyotyping, and differences in amniocentesis utilization relative to maternal age)

Other conditions demonstrating chronicity and prolonged clinical latency periods include heart disease, chronic lung disease, diabetes, digestive disorders, and hypertension. The environmental component of each of these diseases may be related to dietary intake, human habits, emotional and physical stressors, and toxicants. The causal relationship between any one factor and an outcome is difficult to detect and quantify.

Delineating risk can become difficult. The frequency and duration of contact with high-risk environments is a good first-line screening tool for risk of exposure. A thorough health history reflecting occupational, recreational, home, and community environmental exposures remains an essential nursing tool. It is important to note both the total time of potential exposure and the specific physical, biologic, and chemical stressors present within each environment. Most jobs, for instance, generally encompass one-third or more of a person's day. The time factor alone allows potentially prolonged interaction with a variety of environmental stressors. Each workplace further presents a specific set and quantity of substances or dangers to employees and their families. The duration of exposure and the availability of specific stressors may combine to increase risk for specific groups.

TYPES OF HAZARDS

Occupational Hazards

Most members of our society perform some type of work. Whether this is structured within a factory, a shop, an institution, or a home, most people spend a significant portion of their day in the performance of their vocation. More than 100,000 persons per year die prematurely due to occupational hazards. Another 400,0000 Americans develop some disease due to their work environment (U.S. Department of Health and Human Services, 1986). In 1988, 311.4 work loss days per 100 employed U.S. workers over 18 years of age were reported in household interviews assessing the effects of acute conditions (National Center for Health Statistics, 1990, p. 57). The data indicate that individuals younger than 45 years of age were more affected in all categories of illness, including injury, when compared to their older counterparts. However, we caution that these statistics may reflect a survivorship bias or healthy worker effect in the older age category (National Center for Health Statistics, 1990, p. 57).

Statistics gathered between 1974 and 1983 reflect a diminished number of workplace accidental deaths, work-related disabling injuries, annual lost workdays, and incidence of compensable occupational dermatitis. However, data indicate an upturn in each of these statistics and are cause for concern.

It may be incorrect to assume the workplace is the most dangerous source of injury to U.S. citizens. Data indicate that though Americans reported 4.5 workplace injuries per 100 person-years, they also reported 9.2 injuries per 100 person-years that occurred in the home (National Center for Health Statistics, 1990). However, we should remember that though these statistics are remarkably different, some persons are workers in the home and their injuries may have been misclassified as home based rather than work related.

If you consider that each U.S. worker is a member of a family system, the impact of illness or demise goes far beyond the industrial setting. Effects on the family may be in the form of lost wages and burdens of physical and emotional care. Premature death further imposes emotional loss to survivors.

Many hazards possess characteristics that make their presence more noticeable to the average person. Color, mist, vapor, taste, odor, and tactile properties may act as clues. Hazards common to the workplace include physical dangers such as mechanical, chemical, electrical, thermal, vibration, radiation, and auditory threats. Biologic dangers encompass exposure to viruses, rickettsia, bacteria, fungus, and parasites. Chemical dangers include naturally occurring toxins and synthetically manufactured toxicants. Work-related stress may be global or specific in nature, manifesting itself during work or leisure.

Mechanical Dangers

Mechanical dangers within the workplace relate to environmental hazards and work processes. Crushing injuries, for example, may be caused either by a machine or by an unsecured falling object. The teaching and monitoring of safety is crucial to the safety of individual health. The magnitude of illnesses and injuries secondary to mechanical damage is difficult to detect and may be best monitored and conservatively estimated through worker compensation claims.

Asbestos

Asbestos is a natural, fibrous mineral historically used for insulation and in the manufacture of textiles (Selikoff, 1986). Currently, asbestos may be potentially encountered at work, in some aging buildings, or in the ambient air. Fibrous particles may be detectable to the human eye, though the smaller microfibrils are responsible for chronic disease.

Diseases associated with asbestos exposure include asbestosis, lung cancer, and mesothelioma. Asbestosis, a chronic pulmonary condition, is characterized by diffuse fibrosis, a long latency period, and a variable course of illness. Approximately 5,000 workers were newly diagnosed with asbestosis in 1979 (U.S. Department of Health and Human Services, 1986). Physical disability secondary to asbestosis may cause the family to experience a loss in wages and job security, increased demands of physical care, and social stresses associated with illness behaviors.

Lung cancer associated with asbestos exposure typically develops after a prolonged latency period of 30 or more years. Smoking further modifies the risk of developing lung cancer, suggesting that asbestos exposure may not be an entirely sufficient cause for asbestos-related lung cancer. Mesothelioma is a rare neoplasm for which past asbestos exposure is most likely. It may be experienced even when exposure is relatively low, and it is fatal. Though of concern among workers, paraoccupational exposure among family members through transport of dangerous fibers into the home on clothing or body surfaces may be a risk factor for disease among family members.

Heat

Heat as a potential hazard may be directly transmitted by machinery or work processes used to manufacture goods. Humans and other mammals are homeothermic, or capable of maintaining their body temperature within narrow limits. Enzyme activity and body functions are dependent on this narrow range of normal internal body temperature. Significant elevation of core temperature may cause denaturation of enzyme systems, increased oxygen consumption, nervous system malfunction, and even death. Varying degrees of burns are also a common hazard from machines or processes that produce heat.

Vibration

Vibration may cause fatigue for workers and may, in turn, cause work-related injuries. Humans respond to increased mechanical vibration with increased oxygen consumption, respiratory rate, and cardiac output. Posture regulation and tendon reflexes are inhibited (Koren, 1980). Under severe or prolonged circumstances, body functions are taxed, and injury may result.

Sound

Sound at high decibel levels is injurious to health. The frequency of sound refers to the rate at which each sound wave cycles; amplitude is a measure of sound intensity or "loudness." Single, high-amplitude, high-frequency sound may cause pain and temporary or permanent hearing loss. "Noise" is generally a mixture of frequencies, intensities, pressures, and durations of sound waves. Protracted exposure to noise levels exceeding 90 decibels (dB) can cause immediate or latent hearing loss.

The National Institute of Occupational Safety and Health (NIOSH) has estimated that 13.3% of American workers are exposed to noise levels of 85 dB or more (U.S. Department of Health and Human Services, 1986). Noise-induced hearing loss, like many other chronic conditions, may have a latency period of 10 or more years between initial insult and manifestation of symptoms (U.S. Department of Health and Human Services, 1986). Statistics from 1975 indicate that approximately 462,000 cases of work-related hearing loss were experienced by American workers. Some evidence links chronic, systemic disease with severe noise-induced hearing loss (Talbott et al., 1985).

Radiation

Ionizing radiation is but one of many levels of energy in the electromagnetic spectrum. Human absorption may cause physiologic damage by excitation or ionization of body tissues. Radiation may either pass through the human body or become internalized by ingestion, inhalation, or surface absorption of radioactive particles. Nausea, fatigue, blood dyscrasias, intestinal compromise, alopecia, central nervous system disorders, and death are short-term sequelae of acute and toxic doses of ionizing radiation. Genetic mutation and malignancies are potential long-term side effects (Johnson, 1984; Koren, 1980).

Nonionizing radiation is another range of energy in the electromagnetic spectrum. Wavelengths are longer than ionizing radiation and include ultraviolet (UV) light, visible light, infrared, microwave radiation, and radio frequency radiation (Frank & Slesin, 1986). The biologic effects of nonionizing radiation are related to the energy source, duration of exposure, and penetrating power. Short-term effects of excessive UV light exposure include pigment changes, changes in cell growth, and burns. Acute toxic reactions to radio frequency and microwave radiation have been documented outside the United States (Frank & Slesin, 1986). Long-term adverse outcomes associated with excessive UV light include skin cancers.

Biological Hazards

Biological hazards exist where direct or indirect contact between workers and virus, rickettsia, bacteria, fungus, and/or parasites is possible. Common vehicle, contact, air droplet, and vector contamination are modes of transmission. The efficiency of the transmission and the likelihood of resultant infection are related to host characteristics and the directness of the inoculation. Blood splashing into the eyes or into an open wound of a worker is an example of direct con-

tamination. Needle sticks and mouth pipeting require an intermediate object (i.e., needles and pipettes) between the contaminated substance and the new host and are therefore considered indirect. The probability of infection diminishes as the contaminated body substance becomes more removed from the reservoir of infection. For this reason, fomite are relatively low-risk transmitters of most infectious agents.

Infections

The current epidemic of human immunodeficiency virus (HIV) and its related diseases has led to a heightened and warranted awareness of biologic hazards among health care workers. The Centers for Disease Control and Protection (CDC) has continued to recommend adoption of appropriate, routine precautions and personal protective devices to limit the contact between the (infectious) agent and a potential host (Centers for Disease Control, 1995).

Though HIV infection is of concern, it is not the only type of infection that may be transmitted to humans and result in significant illness or death. Precautions to prevent infection should extend to all persons who risk exposure to microorganisms. Persons who treat or handle animals, manage sewage waste, or process body substance specimens should avoid unprotected contact. Body substance isolation is one example of a systematic approach to avoiding direct or indirect contact between biologic hazards and workers (Jackson et al., 1987). The system requires appropriate personal protective devices or barriers between workers and potentially infected fluids. It assumes that all body secretions, excretions, and fluids are potentially infected with harmful agents. The diagnosis-independent form of isolation shifts traditional isolation procedures that depend on diagnosis of specific disease entities before protective procedures are enacted to a system driven by the potential for interaction between agent and host.

Other forms of infectious agent transmission present less severe risk of infection. Classical "common vehicle transmission" generally occurs when a group of individuals have common contact with a contaminated substance. Outbreaks are typically related to ingestion of contaminated foods or beverages. Airborne transmission occurs when contaminated droplets remain suspended in the air. Not only must the droplet remain suspended, but the host must then inhale a sufficient dose of infectious material to cause illness. Tuberculosis remains one of the few known hazards among health care providers that may be transmitted through droplets and is a renewing concern of the 1990s (Centers for Disease Control, 1992a, 1992b, 1994a).

Toxicant Exposures

Workers come into contact with a variety of synthetic and organic substances and may suffer toxicant exposure by way of inhalation, diffusion, or ingestion. Environmental dust, fumes, mists, vapors, and gases may be indicators of possible pulmonary contaminants. Liquid and solid toxicants may pose dangers to the worker if diffusion or direct ingestion occurs. To protect workers from harmful agents, warning signals may be used and may include labels, signs, and company policies or procedures.

The Agency of Toxic Substances and Disease Registry (ATSDR) implemented a limited, active, state-based Hazardous Substance Emergency Events Surveillance System in 1989 to monitor the public heat consequences of hazardous substance releases (CDC, 1994b). The ATSDR data indicates that 77% of the 3125 hazaradous substance emergency events reported by participating states during 1991–1992 were from fixed-facilities and 23% we related to transportation. Most emergencies occurred on weekdays between 6 A.M. and 6 P.M. Volatile organic compounds, herbicides, acids, and ammoniac comprised almost 58% of the reported hazardous substance releases. Though 3,500 injuries were reported to the ATSDR during the surveillance period, approximately 60% were reported as respiratory or eye irritation (CDC, 1994b).

The effects of toxicant exposure may include direct toxicity, mutagenesis, oncogenesis, or teratogenesis. The effects on a family may include altered reproduction, cancer, and acute development of disease. Early detection of known toxic exposure may minimize the effect and may guide families in decisions about lifestyle, reproduction, and health surveillance.

The biologic effects of toxic exposures may be reversible or irreversible in nature. For example, lead toxicity is an illness experienced by battery factory workers. It may produce classic symptoms of lassitude, hematologic disturbances, sleep disorders, and weight loss. Unlike some others, this disorder may be treated and reversed when discovered early. In contrast, prolonged occupational exposure to 1,2-di-bromo-3-chloropropane (DBCP), a nematocide, has rendered male factory workers infertile (Whorton et al., 1977; Whorton et al., 1979). Animal studies infer that the effects of DBCP may be related to both age and dose (Holmes, et al., 1991; Kaplanski, et al., 1991).

Stress

Occupational and nonoccupational stress are difficult to describe because of the difficulty of quantification. Stress may be either positive or negative and requires an organism or system to adapt within an environment (Neuman, 1982). It is crucial for nurses practicing in occupational health settings to recognize that whether primary or secondary to the work setting, hazardous stressors may induce illness or disability.

Information and Regulation

Workers may or may not have access to information about the potentially harmful agents within their environment. A model "right to know" legislation exists in California and requires that Material Safety Data Sheets (MSDS) be available for inspection. Though an important piece of legislation, its implementation has been fraught with confusion among administrators and workers. Interpretation of the information provided by MSDSs is difficult for many workers, and administrators fear that misinterpretation may breed distrust and unnecessary worry among employees. Those industries producing potentially toxic substances may additionally fear increased liability from workers exposed to their products. Disclosure of chemical makeup may also jeopardize commerce if trade secrets are revealed.

The regulation of the industrial environment has been a controversial issue since prior to the inception of the U.S. Occupational Safety and Health Administration (OSHA). The 1970 legislation aimed to ensure that no employee would suffer impairment as a result of occupational exposure. Regulations are enforced by consultation, inspection, and citation. Many states have developed individual occupational safety and health administrations, some of which hold industry more accountable than their federal counterpart.

The development of the National Institute of Occupational Safety and Health (NIOSH) has promoted workplace research, consultation, and standard setting. This branch of the government was created to complement OSHA. Though its mission is noble, the number of potentially harmful substances are many, and resources are limited. Recent history has demonstrated both successes and failures attributable to OSHA and NIOSH.

Paraoccupational Hazards

Paraoccupational hazards are related to indirect exposures of nonworkers to the hazardous substances present within a work setting. Children, spouses, and constant social contacts within the home may be at risk for disease development when hazardous dust, residues, liquids, and solids are transported outside the occupational environment. Diseases related to paraoccupational exposures are dependent on the dose received, the chronicity or acuteness of exposure, and the physiologic and genetic properties of the individual. Soiled clothing and skin residues are examples of vehicles that may transport an agent into the home that would need assessment and consideration.

One example of a growing concern for risk associated with paraoccupational exposures recently surfaced. OSHA has drafted regulations that seek to protect the family and social contacts of workers employed at Superfund cleanup sites (Fergus & Martin, 1985). The regulations require that decontamination of clothing and equipment be conducted on site. Personal protective equipment and decontamination procedures must be explained in detail to the worker and are designed to protect the worker, peers, and off-site contacts. Examples of these procedures might include disposable impermeable clothing, on-site showering, separate decontamination "rooms," and impenetrable gloves.

Though monitoring family members for illness is costly and cumbersome, it is imperative that specific industries assume some accountability for family health. However, caution and wisdom should be used when surveying an at-risk population because all illness may not be related to paraoccupational exposures.

Morbidity is not evenly distributed within our culture. Starfield et al. (1984) demonstrated that only about 15% of the child population experienced a high frequency of unrelated illnesses. This maldistribution may be related to genetic predisposition, barriers to health care, social and biomedical factors, and environmental factors. Patterns of illness, reproduction, and death within a target group should be broadly assessed and compared to the larger population. Significant variance from normative data may indicate either chance "clustering" of cases or cause for real concern. Nurses should become familiar with epidemiology, treatment modalities, and screening techniques to facilitate the goal of proper monitoring and intervention.

Avocational Hazards

Hazards that result from recreational activities are difficult to estimate. Toxicants may be found in hobbies such as leaded-glass window construction, model-airplane assembly, furniture refinishing, and automobile restoration. Safety controls are generally limited to user knowledge and general regulation of substances by government agencies. For example, the sale of toluene, a chemical solvent, is regulated in some states due to both its potential for abuse and its toxic properties. The more stringent controls and inspections related to OSHA and state regulations on industry are absent within the home and recreation setting.

Recreational activities may pose additional environmental threats. Injuries related to automobiles, motorcycles, and bicycles are ever present. The financial and emotional burdens individuals and families endure from such injuries are great.

Automobile crashes account for the single greatest cause of death for persons 5 to 32 years of age in the United States, and it is estimated that nearly half are alcohol related (National Highway Traffic Safety Administration, 1991a, 1991b). National focus on drunk driving has stimulated widespread public education and discussion.

Injury prevention is frequently addressed state by state. Use of preventive measures may be different within and across age categories and gender. For example, the Centers of Disease Control and Prevention (1992) reported that only 29.5% of female and 25.9% of surveyed male U.S. high school students reported using auto safety belts. However, while 41% of these nationally sampled females and 38.2% of males reported always using motorcycle helmets, only 0.9% and 1.2% of females and males, respectively, reported consistently using bicycle helmets when they cycled.

Government surveys have indicated risk for disability associated with injuries. Though the statistics are global, they act as broad indicators of risk associated with accidental impairment. Low-income families are at higher risk for intentional and unintentional injury (U.S. Department of Health and Human Services, Public Health Services, 1985; Blain, 1990; Durkin, et al., 1994; Harlon, et al., 1990). Additionally, 40% of accidental impairments occur within the home setting (DHHS, PHS, 1984). The studies further indicate that risk of a "bed disability" due to injury or illness is highest among those persons older than 45 years of age.

Though adults are at risk for recreational injury and illness, it is imperative that the nurse consider the environmental hazards associated with youth. Traditional safety measures have long been a part of home nursing practice and must be continued. Toxicant exposure of young children due to improper handling and storage of chemicals and preparations continues to be a problem in modern society. Fewer than 40 U.S. cities have developed regional poison control centers. Table 19–1 lists the centers recognized by the American Association of Poison Control Centers. Rural communities and those not served by an official poison control center are usually dependent on a less formal system of physicians and nurses practicing in ambulatory care centers, emergency rooms, and home settings. Health professionals practicing in these settings need to be cognizant of the resources of nearby centers and how to intervene when poisonings and accidents occur.

Recreational drugs are another environmental concern to contemporary society. Citizen groups actively lobby state and federal legislatures for stringent controls and punishments associated with drunk or intoxicated driving. Currently, many sectors of our society are involved in antidrug, antialcohol campaigns directed at diminishing illicit use of chemicals.

TABLE 19–1. AMERICAN ASSOCIATION OF POISON CONTROL CENTERS 1988 CERTIFIED REGIONAL POISON CENTERS

Alabama Poison Center
809 University Boulevard East
Tuscaloosa, AL 35401

Arizona Poison Control System
College of Pharmacy
University of Arizona
Tucson, AZ 85721

Component Centers
Arizona Poison and Drug
Information Center
Health Sciences Center, Room
3204K
Tucson, AZ 85724

Samaritan Regional Poison Center
Good Samaritan Medical Center
1130 East McDowell Road
Phoenix, AZ 85006

Blodgett Regional Poison Center
1840 Wealthy S.E.
Grand Rapids, MI 49506

Cardinal Glennon Children's Hospital
Regional Poison Center
1465 South Grand Boulevard
St. Louis, MO 63104

Central Ohio Poison Center
700 Children's Drive
Columbus, OH 43205

Children's Hospital of Alabama
Poison Control Center
1600 7th Avenue South
Birmingham, AL 35233

Delaware Valley Regional Poison Control Program
One Children's Center
Philadelphia, PA 19104

Duke Regional Poison Control Center
Box 3007
Durham, NC 27710

Florida Poison Information Center
Tampa General Hospital
Davis Islands
Tampa, FL 33606

Georgia Poison Control Center
80 Butler Street, SE
Post Office Box 26066
Atlanta, GA 30335

Hennepin Regional Poison Center
Hennepin County Medical Center
701 Park Avenue South
Minneapolis, MN 55415

Intermountain Regional Poison Control Center
50 North Medical Drive
Salt Lake City, UT 84132

Kentucky Regional Poison Center of Kosair Children's Hospital
P.O. Box 35070
Louisville, KY 40232-5070

Los Angeles County Medical Association
Regional Poison Center
1925 Wilshire Boulevard
Los Angeles, CA 90057

Louisiana Regional Poison Center
LSU Medical Center
P.O. Box 33932
Shreveport, LA 71130

Maryland Poison Center
20 North Pine Street
Baltimore, MD 21201

Massachusetts Poison Control System
300 Longwood Avenue
Boston, MA 02115

Mid-Plains Poison Center
8301 Dodge Street
Omaha, NE 68114

Minnesota Regional Poison Center
St. Paul–Ramsey Medical Center
St. Paul, MN 55101

Nassau County Medical Center's Long Island Regional Poison Control Center
2201 Hempstead Turnpike
East Meadow, NY 11554

National Capital Poison Center
Georgetown University Hospital
3800 Reservoir Road, N.W.
Washington, DC 20007

New Jersey Poison Information and Education System
201 Lyons Avenue
Newark, NJ 07112

New Mexico Poison and Drug Information Center
University of New Mexico
Albuquerque, NM 87131

New York City Poison Center
455 First Avenue
Room 123
New York, NY 10016

North Texas Poison Center
Post Office Box 35926
Dallas, TX 75235

Oregon Poison Center
Oregon Health Sciences
University
3181 SW Sam Jackson Park Road
Portland, OR 97201

Pittsburgh Poison Center
One Children's Place
3705 5th Avenue at DeSoto
Pittsburgh, PA 15213

Poison Control Center
Children's Hospital of Michigan
3901 Beaubien Boulevard
Detroit, MI 48201

Rhode Island Poison Center
593 Eddy Street
Providence, RI 02902

Rocky Mountain Poison and Drug Center
645 Bannock Street
Denver, CO 80204-4507

San Diego Regional Poison Center
UCSD Medical Center
225 Dickinson Street
H925
San Diego, CA 92103

San Francisco Bay Area Regional Poison Center
San Francisco General Hospital
1001 Potrero Avenue
San Francisco, CA 94110

Regional Poison Control System and Cincinnati Drug and Poison Information Center
231 Bethesda Avenue
ML 144
Cincinnati, OH 45267

Texas State Poison Center
University of Texas Medical
Branch
Galveston, TX 77550-2780

UC Davis Regional Poison Control Center
2315 Stockton Boulevard
Sacramento, CA 95817

West Virginia Poison Center
3110 MacCorkle Avenue, S.E.
Charleston, WV 25304

Environmental Hazards

The macroecosystem is enormous, and yet it is "shrinking" with every passing day. Problems that once affected only small populations in distant corners of the globe are now important to town-

ships, states, and nations. Distance no longer affords protection against environmental hazards.

Soil, air, and water, are potential vehicles for toxic substances. They are ubiquitous within the environment and are essential to society's existence. It is beyond the scope of this chapter to discuss all environmental problems. The following discussion is a brief overview of environmental hazards.

Soil Hazards

Soil is essential to plant growth, which in turn provides nourishment, oxygen, shelter, and beauty. Cultivation has been radically altered by modern technology and the use of chemicals for pest control and fertilization. In addition, modern manufacturing processes and chemicals may alter the soil. The leaking of chemicals and toxicants from landfills is a hazard to the safety of soil. In rural areas soil may be polluted by inadequate sewerage systems, leaking septic systems, and animal waste from pork and poultry farms.

Contemporary society does not favor the presence of pesticides in foodstuffs. This may be related to fears of both immediate toxicity and long-term, unknown biologic effects. Residues may result from internal treatments, external treatments, or the accidental contamination of soil by spillage or previous application. Acute, high-level exposures to pesticides typically occur with accidental contamination and produce a constellation of symptoms related to the toxocologic properties of the substance. Chronic exposure, generally associated with ongoing occupational contact, produces a more diffuse pattern of illness. Disease patterns related to incidental exposures (associated with food ingestion and occasional contact with pesticides) are more difficult to predict and track (Blain, 1990; Harlon & Parsons, 1990). Widely used insecticides include the organophosphates (malathion, parathion), carbamates (temik, carbaryl), organohalides (lindane, methoxychlor), botanicals, arsenicals, and phenolic compounds.

Families would potentially benefit from removal of pesticide residue from foods. Proper application of chemicals to home-grown vegetables and fruits, with adherence to manufacturer's suggested dose, application, and timing, would minimize potential exposures. Thorough washing of fruits and vegetables prior to use significantly reduces the amount of toxicant present (Awad & el Shimi, 1993).

Hanta-virus disease (a recently identified human pathogen) was identified in a southwestern U.S. population and rural regions. It was found to result from direct or indirect contact with excreta from indigenous rodents. Most disease occurs in adults and is associated with domestic occupational, or leisure activities that bring humans in contact with infected rodents. To prevent and protect family members from diseases carried by rodents and their waste products, families should be instructed to eliminate rodent infestations, reduce rodent food sources, and eliminate nesting sites within homes or outbuildings. Also, rodent infestation sites should be cleansed thoroughly using disinfectants and detergents while avoiding inhalation of dusts that may contain particles of excreta (CDC, 1993a).

Air Pollution

Contamination of the ambient environment with particular matter, gases, and vapors poses difficult questions to modern society. We have grown dependent on automobiles, factories, and power plants, yet we suffer the consequences of dumping enormous amounts of waste into our air. Smog, acid rain, and "dwelling" pollution are but three examples of environmental contamination of current concern.

Scientific consensus indicates that wet and dry deposition of sulfur dioxide and nitrogen dioxide within our air causes acid rain (U.S. House of Representatives, 1983). This phenomenon may be related to natural occurrences such as volcanic eruptions but may also be the result of fossil fuel combustion. Unlike other forms of air pollution, the substances causing acid rain are organic and not "foreign" to the environment. The problem varies from region to region, depending on manufacturing, natural sources, and the prevalence of emission control devices. A limestone multiple stage burner, for instance, is a technology that has reduced sulfur dioxide emissions from industrial sources as much as 50% (U.S. House of Representatives, 1983). Despite recent advances, the timetable and impact of emission control as well as the long-range transport of acidic substances are unknown.

Common air pollution, "smog," results from an accumulation of combustion by-products. Domestic and industrial heating, incineration, manufacturing, and auto emissions are thought to be the major contributors to unclean air. The chemicals commonly constituting smog are sulfur oxides, nitrogen oxides, hydrocarbons, led, cadmium, beryllium, asbestos, and ozone.

Human health effects from air pollution have been difficult to measure. Metropolitan area residents are frequently familiar with smog reports and warnings during summer months and periods where weather patterns cause inversion layers to form. Most localities advise that vigorous exercise be curtailed and that those with preexisting respiratory and cardiovascular disease limit outdoor activity during high smog periods. The National Ambient Air Quality Standards (NAAQS) establish the maximal dose for particulate matter, sulfur oxides, carbon monoxide, nitrogen dioxide, photochemical oxidants, and nonmethane hydrocarbons. Carbon dioxide values, for example, were developed through experimental design plotting the onset of chest pain among coronary artery disease patients exposed to the gas (Higgins, 1986). The NAAQS values are reviewed every five years and are available through the U.S. Environmental Protection Agency.

Air pollution within homes is related to a variety of activities and substances. Stoves, fireplaces, and cigarettes produce respirable particles, nitrogen dioxide, and carbon dioxide. Formaldehyde may be present wivhin public buindings and homes insulated with urea foam, and asbestos has been historically used in building construction as a fireproofing material. Organic vapors may be present in homes where solvents and resin products are used (Last, 1986; Kilburn, 1992).

The development of superior home insulation materials has brought but another "air pollution" problem to contemporary society. Highly insulated dwellings are less costly to heat in frigid areas of the United States. Without compensatory ventilation systems, though, limited fresh air circulation may allow the accumulation of toxic gases. Nitrogen dioxide, carbon monoxide, particulate matter, and formaldehyde may cause health problems for family members (Higgins, 1986).

Family members and nurses alike need to be aware of the possible risk of disease associated with air pollution both within and outside the home. Assessment of housing insulation, ventilation, sources of combustion, and a general awareness of ambient air conditions will generally heighten awareness. Persons living in high-risk circumstances should be assisted to secure risk assessment information, location and costs of rehabilitative services, and pertinent information regarding health risks. Examples of these types of intervention include descriptive information about industry type and distribution within a community, smog patterns, housing codes and regulations, local contractors, and the number of the air pollution control district.

Water Resources

Water is essential to life. Without clean and safe sources, plants and humans cannot continue to survive. The sources of water include rain, surface water, groundwater, oceans, and recycled water. Desalination of ocean water is costly and is therefore reserved for extreme circumstances. Rain is a difficult resource to collect for large populations but is vulnerable to suspended particulate matter and organic chemicals.

Surface water has been an easily accessible and economical resource for humankind. Historical maps illustrate how early settlements frequently developed along streams, lakes, and rivers. Early evidence of microbial epidemics also demonstrates the vulnerability of surface water and dependent populations. Humankind has learned that direct contamination of proximal waters may heavily influence the health of those consuming water downstream.The epidemic of cryptosporidiosis that occurred in Milwaukee, Wisconsin in 1993 is evidence of the excessive morbidity and mortality that can occur when water resources are contaminated with harmful agents (CDC, 1995b). More than 400,000 people became ill when fil-

tered, treated, public water supplies were contaminated. (CDC, 1995b)

Groundwater may be drawn from springs or wells, is more mineralized than rainwater, and is less vulnerable to direct contamination than surface water. Direct toxic discharges or leaching, however, may cause an aquifer to become polluted. If groundwater becomes polluted, it may take many years to recover naturally, if detoxification occurs at all (Okun, 1986).

Water recycling is a reasonably new technology. Sewage reclamation and water hyacinth purification techniques are two methods being explored. Communities may be apprehensive about reusing water for drinking purposes but may be receptive to using reclaimed water for irrigation.

The adoption of drinking water standards since the early part of the twentieth century has promoted potable water and prevented disease transmission. Federal controls were enacted in 1974 with the passage of the Safe Drinking Water Act. Additionally, Congress amended the Safe Drinking Water Act in 1986 to substantially increase the number of regulated substances in drinking water (Okum, 1992). Maximal contamination levels were established for a variety of inorganic and organic chemicals, trihalomethanes, microbial organisms, and radioactivity in communities numbering 10,0000 or more persons (Okun, 1992; CDC, 1993b). Chemicals affecting the aesthetic qualities of drinking water have been separately regulated. The microbial center of water is regulated by the U.S. Government Protection Agency through two regulations: The Total Coliform Role and Surface Treatment Requirements (CDC, 1993b). The maximum contaminant levels for total coliforms and the turbidity of drinking water are specified by these policies.

Though federal and state efforts have been directed at regulating and ensuring the public of a clean water supply, the shortcomings must be stressed. Water resources in communities numbering fewer than 10,000 are more vulnerable. Rural families may also draw their water directly from aquifers that are contaminated by toxic substances or pathogens. Use of indirectly reused water (i.e., wastewater, partially treated and discharged into surface water) may pose additional problems of transmitting heavy metals, toxicants, and pathogens: An example of the long-term effects of toxic substances is shown in the case study.

CASE STUDY

A Multidimensional Problem: Times Beach, Missouri

Times Beach, Missouri, an ecological "experiment," illustrates a relationship between primary pollution of land and the secondary contamination of streams and rivers. Dioxin, a toxic by-product, was produced by a pharmaceutical and chemical company in Missouri between 1970 and 1972. Storage at the plant site appears to have been safe, and direct detoxification conducted by the company followed recommended guidelines. Unfortunately, 18,000 gallons of the toxic oil was removed by a waste oil hauler and sprayed on eastern Missouri roads as an anti-dust treatment (Powell, 1984).

The immediate effect of dioxin spraying was truly disastrous. Shenandoah stables, the first site of documented human illness, was sprayed with approximately 6 pounds of dioxin (Powell, 1984). Many animals died or were destroyed, and one child was hospitalized shortly after the contamination.

Bubbling Springs, the Minker/Stout homesites, and Times Beach were three contaminated areas with multidimensional problems. Like the Shenandoah stables, each location was directly contaminated with dioxin. The Bubbling Springs site was excavated, and fill dirt was transported to the Minker and Stout sites. Soil erosion of the Minker homestead subsequently contaminated the nearby creek. Tissue samples of fish, collected at the junction of this creek and the Meramec River, were positive for dioxin (Powell, 1984).

Times Beach is further postulated to contain more than 60% of dioxin-contaminated soil in Missouri (Powell, 1984). It was first tested in early December 1982, and residents were ordered to evacuate shortly thereafter. Two natural floods have occurred in Times Beach since the evacuation, and yet no appreciable change in the Meramec River dioxin concentration has occurred. Erosion and flood still pose significant problems as they potentiate the transfer of stored dioxin from soil to potable water and river-bottom soil over time.

The long-term effects of existing and potential dioxin contamination in Times Beach, Missouri, are only postulated. This example, though, poses the question of the interaction between general soil contaminants and ground water pollution. Chemicals and waste products may also be transmitted to our water supply through purposeful or accidental spillage. Sewage treatment plants, manufacturers, small business, and agricultural enterprises all handle and dispose of toxic chemicals causative of water pollution. The long-term effects of low-dose exposure upon family health and well-being are speculative.

ENVIRONMENTAL HEALTH ACROSS THE LIFE SPAN

Childbearing and Childrearing Years

Many couples today express concerns about the effects of toxicants on the unborn. Whether within the home or work settings, direct effects on the fetus are frequently difficult to ascertain. Adverse reproductive outcomes are related to known and unknown risk factors. Reproductive history, age, parity, and preexisting medical conditions are known to be associated with poor pregnancy outcome. The influence of specific products or work settings is much more difficult to ascertain. The occupational settings that have been clearly linked to poor reproductive outcomes have had dramatic effects on specific, sizable groups of individuals over time (Whorton et al., 1977, 1979). Hemminki et al. (1983), for example, demonstrated an increased rate of spontaneous abortion

among textile workers in Finland. Futher, Kierkegaard & Kristiansen (1992) found textile workers showed a greater risk for sick leave due to threatening abortion, pelvic loosening, or pain in the locomotor systems than the other surveyed childbearing women. In general, advice to family during the childbearing years would include the seeking of early prenatal care and the avoidance of unnecessary pharmaceutical, toxicant, or pathogen exposures.

Primary prevention of adverse reproductive outcomes include public education programs and activities to prevent contact between hosts and harmful agents. Secondary prevention activities would seek to provide early screening, diagnosis, and treatment, and tertiary prevention would necessitate attempts to restore reproductive function.

Adulthood

Environmental effects on health reach far beyond the early developmental years. Health risks to adults include acute, chronic, or latent illness or injury. They may encounter a myriad of chemical, physical, or biologic conditions; some are innocuous, and some are hazardous to health. Factors to be considered when evaluating the effects of specific agents include the type of exposure, known associated toxicity and health risks, intensity and duration of exposure, and associated latency.

Environmental agents and conditions often affect individuals beyond their working years. Clients are a product of all previous experiences and exposures, genetic predispositions, and current circumstances. Many agents and conditions have long latency periods between exposure and effect. A thorough history of both work and nonwork environmental exposures is helpful in counseling, diagnosis, education, and treatment of the older person.

NURSING PROCESS

Whether family health nurses function within an acute care setting, ambulatory care clinic, or public health agency, their role must include the holistic assessment of family wellness. Usual practice dictates that a history of present and past illness, developmental milestones, family strengths and weaknesses, and goals be reviewed. Incomplete assessment may leave a nurse without key pieces to a complex puzzle. A complete nursing assessment must take occupational, paraoccupational, avocational, home, and general environmental variables into consideration. A total history of family member health and illness would be incomplete without information relating to potential toxicant and pathogen contacts, areas of residence, employment patterns, and toxicant exposures. Table 19–2 is

TABLE 19–2. OCCUPATIONAL ENVIRONMENTAL HEALTH HISTORY, ADAPTED TO NEUMAN'S SYSTEMS MODELS

IDENTIFYING DATA: MEDICAL RECORD

Name:
Address:
Telephone:
Social Security #:
Sex: Male   Female   (Circle)
Age: Date of Birth:

STRESSORS PERCEIVED BY THE PATIENT

I. Chief Complaint: This statement is to be in the patient's own words. It should reflect the reason why the patient is currently seeking health care information or services.

Key Questions

1. Describe the health problem or injury you are currently experiencing.
2. Does any other member of your family experience this problem? Any coworker? Any acquaintance?
3. Do you smoke (packs per day, years duration)? Use chewing tobacco? Consume alcohol (how much)?
4. Do you smoke while on the job? At home? Do your coworkers smoke while on the job? Do your family members smoke while you are in the room?
5. Have you missed work within the past six weeks? When did these symptoms begin? Have you been forced to stay in bed since the onset of this problem? Are you distressed by this level of disability?
6. Have you ever worked at a job/hobby that caused you to have this problem before? If so, describe the pattern of illness or difficulty. Have you ever found yourself short of breath, lightheaded, dizzy, with a cough, or wheezing while at work? After work? At the beginning of a work week? At the end of a work week? During the weekend?
7. Have you ever changed jobs, homes, hobbies due to a health condition?
8. Have you ever experienced musculoskeletal difficulties related to work, home, or play? (e.g., back pain, fractures, muscle strain)?
9. Name the chemicals and compounds you work with and the frequency of contact with each. Describe the chemicals or compounds you work with for which you have no name. Describe their use. Approximate the frequency of contact.
10. Describe your neighborhood. Map out the location of industrial areas, waste disposal sites, water sources, and waste disposal.
11. Are there any community environmental problems that have evolved in recent time? Toxic spills, sewage breakage, smog changes, NIOSH/OSHA investigations pertinent to the patient's condition?
12. Do you use pesticides, cleaning solutions, glues, solvents, heavy metals, or poisons at work or within the home? Tell me the names of these substances and the amount and frequency of use.
13. Type of heating and cooling within the home (electric, natural gas, other) and its impact on the (temporal) illness pattern.
14. Type of home construction, insulation, ventilation sources.

II. Lifestyle Patterns

Note changes in previously stated patterns. It is important to note changes within the living (physical) environment, occupational setting (of the client or other family members), and recreational environment.

Power and Authority: Does the client have power to effect change to own environment in workplace? Has company experienced any official intervention (e.g., OSHA, CAL-OSHA assessment and outcome of assessments)? Are advocacy groups evident (e.g., unions) that can pressure employers to change? Who makes decisions for the family? Is there a struggle for power within the family unit? Does this illness evidence possible impact on power distribution within family?

Allocation of Role/Division of Labor: Are occupational and home roles perceived by the client as appropriate? Do the roles meet the patient's needs? How are family chores and responsibilities divided among family members? Does the client perceive that this illness will affect the distribution of labor in any particular fashion?

Financial Resources: Note the income and the major outflow stressors. Will this illness cause any change within the home (physical) environment and/or location? Will this stressor cause perceived changes within the occupational and recreational spheres?

Spiritual Beliefs: What are the spiritual beliefs of this family? Do such beliefs have bearing on the physical environment?

Activities of Daily Living: Include information about dietary habits, transportation method and patterns, housekeeping patterns and products, care of ill and infirmed family members, sleep and rest patterns. Does the patient perceive any of these areas to be of major concern?

Process Characteristics: Note atmosphere within the home, methods of communication, developmental tasks, and use of extended family network. How does the family process information from the physical environment? How

TABLE 19–2. OCCUPATIONAL ENVIRONMENTAL HEALTH HISTORY, ADAPTED TO NEUMAN'S SYSTEMS MODELS (continued)

does the family or individual respond to adverse conditions within the occupational, recreational, or general environment? Are they able to act when the physical environment appears dangerous? When given advice about issues within their physical environment, are they able to process the information and make changes that diminish stressors?

Coping Patterns: What makes the symptom or problem diminish or go away? Temporal sequence—map out the correlation of symptoms with work time, play time, home time, and recreational habits of the patient and individuals within the family.

Availability of Resources: What resources are available from personal, local government, or national government assets to assess or treat this environmental stressor? Is the family able to act independently on advice to use services within the health care or general community, or must a professional assist? Is this stressor occupationally induced or exacerbated? If so, what resources are available through the employer to deal with this stressor?

Client Goals and Perceived Assets: What does the client perceive as his or her sphere of influence on this problem? Health beliefs and attitudes: observable wellness activities, fatalism, use of emergency rooms or clinics. Does the client evidence a primary provider of health care services or use of informal nonprofessional network of health care providers?

STRESSORS AS PERCEIVED BY THE CAREGIVER

List the major problems or stressors as perceived by the provider

Do these observations differ from the patient's perceptions? If so, how?

How have previous problems or stressors paralleled this situation? How did the patient treat the problem? What was the outcome?

What resources does the patient possess? What resources are missing? What available resources need augmentation?

What do you perceive the patient expects form the health care provider? What role will you play in their illness and recovery?

Impressions

1. Intrapersonal factors:
   a. physical factors
   b. psychosociocultural
   c. developmental
2. Interpersonal factors
   Summarize the resources of immediate and extended family, work environment, recreational environment.
3. Extrapersonal factors
   Summarize community resources, occupational, and state and federal programs that may facilitate resolution of this problem.
4. Problem statement
   Use nursing diagnosis to formulate your problem statement. Note target dates for reassessment, and state changes in stressors, intra-/inter-/extrapersonal stressors when reassessing a problem.

Adapted from Neuman, B. (1982). *The Neuman Systems Model.* Norwalk, CT: Appleton-Century-Crofts.

---

an occupational/ environmental health assessment tool, based on the Neuman Systems Model, which provides valuable data to assess individuals or families.

The Workplace

Neuman (1982) emphasizes the use of primary, secondary, and tertiary prevention as an integrative tool to attain and maintain client stability. Primary prevention of illness within the work setting ideally requires that contact between workers and hazardous substances be prevented (Last, 1992). Education, industrial hygiene, and safety techniques are classically used to promote primary prevention. Secondary prevention requires early diagnosis and screening for active disease

(Mausner & Bahn, 1974). Rehabilitation and promotion of worker reentrance into the employment setting are essential to tertiary prevention techniques (Last, 1992).

Members of the industrial hygiene team must be sensitive to known hazards present within the work setting. This includes active surveillance of the site, periodic and thorough review of the literature, and consultation with known experts. Though employed by the industry, nurses and other professionals have an ethical responsibility to develop and enhance worker awareness of safety techniques.

The assessment phase of primary prevention requires the professional to recognize potential hazards confronting the worker that are directly related to industry. It further requires the assessment of behaviors and risk factors unique to the worker that might potentiate illness. The care plan and nursing actions then focus on intervention aimed at preventing contact between the host and the hazard and maximizing personal behaviors that promote health and minimize risk for disease. Health promotion is the most critical nursing role in primary prevention in the realm of environmental health.

Health promotion techniques might include education in the use of personal safety equipment, smoking cessation programs, physical fitness activities for sedentary workers, and stress recognition and management. Families benefit from primary prevention programs when the health and fitness of wage earners are enhanced, stressors are minimized, and family wellness and integrity are promoted.

Nurses and industrial hygienists have a responsibility to develop worker awareness of safety techniques. Personal protective equipment provided within specific environments requires a knowledge of proper use, limitations, regulations, and protective qualities. For example, health professionals exposed to chemotherapeutic drugs within their occupational settings may be unaware that gloves exist that are impermeable to the harmful chemicals they use. More important, they may be using gloves that provide a false sense of security, thus indirectly increasing risk. Nurses and industrial hygienists have a responsibility to educate managers and advocate personnel policies that ensure worker safety. For example, magnesium foundry workers undergoing health and safety education may pay little heed when line supervisors fail to wear personal protective equipment in appropriate areas. Here, combined strategies of manager education and increased management awareness of liability for these behaviors may encourage change in a relatively nonthreatening manner.

Health teaching and anticipatory guidance by nurses provides a heightened awareness of vulnerability and alternative behaviors that may increase workers' adherence to proper technique and protective devices. Other aspects of primary prevention include conducting employee assistance programs; monitoring noise and dust levels, temperature variations, and levels of toxicants; assessing risk factors (smoking, overweight, absenteeism, hypertension); and assessing the impact of factory on the air, soil, and water of the community (Last, 1992). Nurses also serve to introduce new knowledge into the workplace. Vigilance of pertinent literature; participation in local, state, and national organizations; and advocacy for responsible regulation are all methods of providing managers and workers with complete and up-to-date information.

Secondary prevention requires early diagnosis and treatment of illness. Periodically, a thorough history and physical examination are essential to diagnosis of industrial diseases. Special attention should be paid to prior employment patterns, exposures, and illnesses associated with work.

The use of biochemical profiles to monitor vulnerability and illness among workers has resurged in recent years (Parkinson & Grennan, 1986). Special laboratory tests are of questionable value to detection of disease or measurement of risk for potential illness.

Screening programs may be expensive, and the yield of accurate information is limited, even in highly sensitive and specific lab tests (Ordin, 1992). Implementation of mass screening tests therefore should be undertaken with caution. Wilson and Jungner (1968) suggest that screening programs be implemented if:

1. The disease or diagnosis is of importance
2. An acceptable treatment for the condition exists
3. Diagnostic and treatment facilities are available
4. The condition exhibits early symptomatic changes evident of disease
5. A screening test is available and acceptable to the population
6. A natural history of the disease is known and understood
7. A policy for treatment of diagnosed cases is evident
8. Costs of case finding are economical and acceptable to the population

Wilson and Jungner further suggest that screening and case finding should be planned and continuous rather than singular or episodic in nature.

Parkinson and Grennan (1986) suggest that screening programs should limit themselves to tests that determine or implicate worker exposure to harmful agents and further stipulate that tests be developed that monitor the environment rather than the worker (Binsham, 1992; Ordin, 1992). This approach suggests primary prevention rather than waiting until some physiologic or psychologic abnormality develops within the individual.

Tertiary prevention seeks to maximize rehabilitative efforts and return the individual to work. This not only benefits workers but directly affects the economic outcome of their families. Injured or disabled workers are subject to compensation regulations, which vary from state to state. In California, for instance, temporary disability benefits may be awarded after a waiting period and are paid at a rate of two-thirds of a predetermined statewide wage. A maximum weekly disability payment is frequently far below the usual earning capacity of the worker. Wage loss may impose great stress on both the employee and other family members.

Rehabilitation of workers injured in the performance of their job requires both individual and industry commitment. Focus on physical and emotional rehabilitation, collaboration with and referral to vocational rehabilitative services, and maintenance of a link between industry and worker will enhance tertiary prevention. Public health nursing referral may enhance family coping and worker reentry through enhanced services and continuity of care.

The Home

The home setting is complex. It is the occupational environment of homemakers, the recreational setting for many family members at a variety of developmental levels, and the site of many potential paraoccupational exposures. Environmental family health nursing must focus on all three arenas of risk when evaluating family wellness and health promotion.

Biologic hazards within the home include transmission of communicable disease. Susceptibility to illness may depend on general health and well-being, immunization status, and directness of transmission. Examples of easily communicable diseases are measles, mumps, and rubella. HIV infection is an example of an infection with limited modes of transmission. HIV infection is an example of an infection with limited modes of transmission. *Salmonella enteritidis* infection is one example of enteric infection that disproportionately puts infants, the elderly, and the immunocompromised at risk for severe illness and death. Uncooked or undercooked eggs and egg products are frequently responsible, and cases are usually sporadic or are limited to family outbreaks.

A number of dangerous or potentially dangerous substances can be found in and around the home. Often, potentially dangerous products used within the home are handled more casually than in an industrial setting. Individuals may endanger their health in a variety of ways. For example, they may use hair coloring products without protective gloves or adequate ventilation. Malathion or other garden insecticides may be applied to yards and around foundations without proper skin protection or respiratory equipment. Ovens or other kitchen equipment may be cleaned without proper protection from caustic, defatting properties or cleansers that may be further complicated by application in poorly ventilated rooms where fumes may accumulate readily. Parents may fail to protect their children from ingesting nonprescription medications such as iron supplements, prenatal vitamins, and aspirin or acetaminophen, many of which are coated, flavored, or colored for easier or more palatable administration.

Substances used to paint, maintain, clean, and enhance our family dwellings contain toxic substances. Cleaning solutions and powders contain chemicals that frequently are toxic, abrasive, defatting, and caustic to eyes or mucous membranes. Most manufacturers label their products with warnings about potential dangers. Families should be encouraged to store solutions and substances properly, so that young children and other family members minimize their potential for illness.

Storage of substances within the home may require the family to use special door latches or locked cabinets. Adults should be encouraged to minimize the number of flammable substances stored in houses, garages, or outbuildings. Special care to avoid storing flammables close to water heaters or furnaces will minimize the danger of fire.

Instructions accompanying home care products should be read and followed closely. Rashes and abrasions may result when defatting of the subcutaneous tissue occurs. The skin may also serve as a portal of entry for toxic chemicals. Goggles may protect eyes from splattering of highly abrasive liquids, and masks may protect the upper airway and lungs from suspended particulate matter when activities such as sanding or fiberglass installation are undertaken. Poison ingestions are an ever-present danger when small children reside within a home. Poison control or clinic numbers should be available at every telephone, and parents should be instructed in the proper use of Ipecac.

Poor ventilation, peeling paint, unstable structures, and unfenced pools, lakes, and streams are examples of physical dangers present within the home environment. For example, drowning is the third most common cause of unintentional injury death in the United States (Centers for Disease Control, 1990). Lead toxicity is a danger that requires all levels of preventive activity. Aged structures with peeling paint should be a warning signal to the family health practitioner. Children who ingest paint chips during exploratory play may be at risk for elevated serum lead levels. Dust and soil among major traffic thoroughfares may also contain high concentrations of lead. Children playing in contaminated soil are also at higher risk for lead poisoning. The primary prevention strategy of converting automobiles from the predominant use of leaded gasoline to unleaded fuel will aid in diminishing the soil concentration of lead.

Noise pollution can be remedied at many levels. Communities seek to prevent excesses through legislation and regulation. Unlike the work setting, official agencies do not police most neighborhoods for possible violations of rules and codes. Instead, cities and townships rely on citizens to report or ameliorate excessive noise.

Nurses working in frigid areas should be aware of home structures that preclude adequate ventilation. The accumulation of toxic gases may put a family at risk for illness during periods of extreme cold or warmth when conservation demands tight closure of the dwelling. The nurse may wish to refer the family to rural or metropolitan power companies for advice and information about proper insulation and ventilation.

Aging structures present environmental risks related to physical dangers. Unstable dwellings may increase the risk of falls or crushing injuries to all family members. Nurses may need to advise clients who live in old, inner-city areas or in rural settings to assess their homes for dangers. Also, as nurses work with temporary or chronically homeless populations, they may need even greater awareness of the physical structures their clients use to seek shelter from the elements. All homes, new and old, may present dangers related to loose rugs, cluttered stairways, overloaded electrical circuits, and unstable furniture. Nurses should be keenly aware of the structural environmental dangers as each family contact occurs.

Water presents a danger to families with children. Unfenced pools, streams, and lakes may lure children to unsupervised play and increase the risk of drowning. Parents should be made aware of the need for proper fencing of pools and natural swimming areas. Adults should be encouraged to learn cardiopulmonary resuscitation in all circumstances but especially if the home has easy access to water. Though seemingly simple advice, adults should be cautioned to supervise dependent children constantly around family pools or lakes or during bathtime. The risk of drowning while unsupervised is heightened for toddlers, preschoolers, and children with significant developmental delays.

Paraoccupational exposures may be related to the transport of toxic or caustic substances from a worksite to home, automobile, or recreational settings. Adults who work in industries where dust, chemicals, or gases may contain toxic substances should be cautioned to launder work clothing separate from the family laundry. Showering prior to leaving work or on returning home may be advised for those working in high-risk industries. Some employers have adopted voluntary use of worksite-specific clothing and showering for workers. Federal regulations, for example, require that protective clothing and shower facilities exist where Superfund cleanup sites are established.

Recreation and Play

Environmental stressors present within the avocational setting may be related to personal behaviors or external factors. Individuals may choose recreational pastimes that increase their exposure to environmental threats. Weight lifting, home construction remodeling, and motorcycle riding exemplify only a few hobbies that may predispose individuals to physical dangers. Nurses should encourage clients to abide by safe conduct rules, follow regulations and codes, and avoid solitary work or play. Health teaching to parents should include teaching children of all ages safety rules for play, recreational equipment, and vehicles. In addition, parental role modeling of appropriate safety behaviors helps to foster patterns of safety

wellness behaviors in offspring (Kandzari & Howard, 1981).

Animal care, travel, and ordinary human contacts may pose an increased risk of infection. Up-to-date immunization will promote immunity against illnesses such as measles, mumps, rubella, polio, and diphtheria. Foreign travel may necessitate special vaccinations and should be undertaken with the knowledge of endemic diseases and risk-reduction behaviors. Animal handling should include proper personal protective equipment, knowledge, and appropriate pet vaccinations.

Wood refinishing, model airplane assembly, automobile restoration, and leaded-glass assembly are but three of a myriad of hobbies that may increase the risk of *toxicant exposure.* Adults and children should be encouraged to read and follow instructions closely. Those working with volatile substances should do so in well-ventilated areas where the danger of spark or fire is limited. Protective clothing, eyewear, and/or masks should be used when substances are abrasive, caustic, defatting, or irritating to mucous membranes. Users should be aware of the limitations of protective equipment they use. Gloves permeable to toluene, for instance, are of little use to the wearer during contact with the toxicant.

Interpersonal factors affecting families during recreation include the responsible conduct of others. Adults and children should be aware of dangers imposed on others when toxic substances are improperly used or stored. More global, extrapersonal variables might include locations of toxic dump sites near recreational areas, contamination of streams and lakes, natural disasters, and improper labeling and marketing of recreational products. These variables are characterized by their locus of control beyond the family and may represent significant danger. Families should be encouraged to use areas specifically marked for recreational use. Hikers should filter water for impurities and pathogens, and adults should have an awareness of weather conditions prior to embarking on their journey. Families may wish to purchase products that are well known to them and should be aware of any illness or discomfort experienced during their use.

The nurse's role may include education, information seeking, and advocacy. Public forums and individual instruction are tools the family health nurse must use to inform public, payors, and professionals. Nurses encounter many daily opportunities to influence families. Special attention should be devoted to the development of family-centered goals for health and wellness. Nurses should define with the client the behavior or outcome desired, negotiate a realistic interval for accomplishment, start small and build on success, and document progress.

Nurses in all areas of nursing practice would benefit by a greater awareness of problems, services, and experts within their communities. No single individual could realistically filter and store all information necessary to deal with each environmental threat. The key, though, is a clear understanding of available resources and methods of use that will benefit individuals, families, and communities the nurse serves. Table 19–3 defines the purpose and services offered by a select number of city and county agencies. Table 19–4 describes selected federal agencies.

General Environment

Nurses must practice and live within the global environment. They contend with similar stressors that affect their clients and must devise actions to minimize distress and illness. As health professionals, family health nurses have a responsibility to be advocates for the environmental health of individuals and families.

Nurses have access to concentrated and descriptive data. Professional networking among epidemiologists, toxicologists, and other medical personnel may provide critical links between daily practice and research frontiers. Patterns of illness and outcomes may be valuable information when global issues of environmental contamination are in question.

Nurses may also implement their role of client advocacy on a local, regional, or national basis.

The reader should review *Healthy People 2000: National Health Promotion and Disease Prevention Objectives* for an in-depth commentary and interim report on national progress toward the goal of health for all by the year 2000 (USDHHS, 1991).

Nurses should understand the environmental forces that affect personal and population health indicators. For example, one national goal is to reduce asthma morbidity to no more than 160 hospitalizations per 100,000 persons. Ethnic and age disparity are present. Children are more likely than the elderly to display asthma. Black children are more likely to be hospitalized than white children, though they are only at slightly greater risk for disease than white children. Additionally, death rates due to asthma among blacks is three times that of whites. These statistics most likely reflect potential differences in social settings, access to health care, and differences in residential and working conditions (USDHHS, 1991, p. 317).

The federal government has continued to undertake surveillance projects such as the CDC-sponsored Metropolitan Atlanta Developmental Disabilities Study and the NHTSSA's Fatal Accident Reporting System. These studies characterize specific types of developmental disabilities as well as acute and chronic injuries or illness in samples of our population and provide density measures as well as cumulative information about

TABLE 19–3. CITY AND COUNTY OFFICIAL GOVERNMENT AGENCIES

Animal Control (sometimes listed with "Dead Animal Removal")
These agencies will generally remove dead animals that are not the property of the caller. They will respond if stray animals appear diseased and will generally pick up stray animals.

Building Inspection/Building and Housing Department
These agencies have regulatory functions but also may become involved in disputes between landlords and tenants when housing is unsafe or not in compliance with health/building codes.

Board of Supervisors/City Council/Town Council
Elected body of local government officials who govern the municipality/county/town. This group is generally responsive to the electorate and may be especially instrumental in getting changes in local codes, regulations, and laws that pertain to environmental health and safety.

District Attorney
Official of local government assigned to prosecute offenders of the law.

Health Services/Health Department
This agency generally has a broad scope of practice. It generally monitors vital statistics, epidemiologic changes, drug and alcohol programs, adult and child health, tuberculosis, mental health, and environmental health.

Hazardous Materials Department
This department may be subsumed by the local health department under the division of environmental health. It generally responds to hazardous spills and emergency situations. It has some regulatory functions.

Noise Control/Noise Abatement
This department may be subsumed by the local health department or may be a separate entity. It monitors noise levels in accordance with local regulations/codes when requested. It does not generally investigate noise violations without complaint.

Permits Department
This department issues many types of permits as directed by local codes and regulations. Some of interest to the family health practitioner might include: refuse disposal, explosives, sewers.

Public Works Department
This agency generally includes flood control and drainage, construction inspection, sanitation/sewer, and solid waste disposal. Many municipalities have a variety of services under the title of public works.

TABLE 19–4. UNITED STATES GOVERNMENT OFFICES AND AGENCIES

LEGISLATIVE BRANCH:

The Senate. This legislative body is composed of 100 members, two from each of the 50 states. They act to synthesize and amend law and policy that governs this nation. Standing committees that pertain to environmental issues include:

Agriculture, Nutrition, and Forestry
Appropriations
Banking, Housing and Urban Affairs
Budget
Commerce, Science, and Transportation
Energy and Natural Resources
Environment and Public Works
Finance
Judiciary
Labor and Human Resources
Rules and Administration
Small Business
Address: **The Capitol, Washington, DC 20510**
           Telephone: 202-224-3121

The House of Representatives. This legislative body is composed of 435 representatives. Standing committees pertaining to environmental issues might include:

Agriculture
Appropriations
Banking, Finance and Urban Affairs
Budget
Education and Labor
Energy and Commerce
Interior and Insular Affairs
Judiciary
Merchant Marine and Fisheries
Natural Resources
Science, Space and Technology
Small Business
Ways and Means
Address: **The Capitol, Washington, DC 20515**
           Telephone: 202-224-3121

Library of Congress. The Library of Congress was established in 1800 and acts as the national library. Though many services are available to the public, those wishing information about science and technology may use the **Research and Reference Division.** Technical reports, bibliographical data, and informational reference guides are available. A list of titles is available: **Reference Section, Science and Technology Division, Library of Congress, Washington, DC 20504-5580. Telephone: 202-707-5522.**

Office of Technology Assessment. This office was established in 1972 and acts to provide congressional committees with assessments or studies that identify the consequences of policy choices affecting the use of technology. The consequences may be social or physical.
Address: **600 Pennsylvania Avenue SE, Washington, DC 20510-8025**
           Telephone: 202-224-9241 (Congressional and Public Affairs)
           or 202-224-8996 (Publications)

OFFICE OF THE PRESIDENT:

Council on Environmental Quality. This council was established in 1969 to synthesize and advise the president on national policies designed to promote improved environmental quality. The council reports to the President of the United States and is charged with analyzing environmental trends, conducting research, and reviewing federal programs that affect the ecosystem.
Address: **722 Jackson Pl. NW, Washington, DC 20506**
           Telephone: 202-395-5754

Office of Management and Budget. This office assists the President in government organization review, interagency cooperation, budget and fiscal management, and the formulation of regulatory reform, and it evaluates program performance and efficiency.
Address: **Executive Office Building, Washington, DC 20503**
           Telephone: 202-395-3080

TABLE 19–4. UNITED STATES GOVERNMENT OFFICES AND AGENCIES (continued)

Office of Science and Technology Policy. This office was established in 1976 and provides the president with information and analysis about science and technology. Priority areas include health and the environment.
Address: Old Executive Office Building, Washington, DC 20506
               Telephone: 202-456-7116

DEPARTMENTS:

United States Department of Agriculture. This government agency is charged with small community and rural development. Priorities include funding the projects that promote soil conservation, watershed protection and flood prevention, natural resource conservation and development, agriculture marketing and inspection, and food and consumer services. The Agricultural Research Service conducts research that seeks to promote improved plant and animal protection and production. Natural resources of forested areas, plains, river basins, and mines are administered by a division of this department.
Address: Fourteenth Street and Independence Avenue SW, Washington, DC 20250
               Telephone: 202-447-2791

United States Department of Commerce. This department contains an Office of Consumer Affairs and attempts to work with a business community on behalf of the consumer. The Bureau of the Census is also housed within this department, as is the National Technical Information Service. The National Oceanic and Atmospheric Administration is charged with exploration, management, and conservation of global ocean resources. This agency is also charged with disseminating information about natural events that may be destructive in the immediate or long-reaching future.
Address: Fourteenth Street between Constitution Avenue and E Street NW, Washington, DC 20230
               Telephone: 202-720-4419

United States Department of Energy (DOE). The DOE is responsible for the management of a variety of programs that influence the availability, regulation, and use of energy resources. High-risk energy research and technology development is a focus of this department. The Environment, Safety, and Health Office acts to ensure compliance with environmental safety and health regulations. Energy Research, Fossil Energy, Conservation and Renewable Energy, Nuclear Energy, and Civilian Radioactive Waste Management Offices are housed within this department.
Address: 1000 Independence Avenue SW, Washington, DC 20585
               Telephone: 202-586-5000

United States Department of Health and Human Services (DHHS). The DHHS is the cabinet-level department of the federal government most involved with the health and welfare of American citizens. The U.S. Public Health Service acts to promote mental and physical health through program development, policies, research, planning, and education (professional and general public). The National Institutes of Health (Alcohol Abuse and Alcoholism; Drug Abuse; Mental Health; Cancer; Heart, Lung, and Blood; Environmental Health Science; Allergy and Infectious Diseases; Diabetes; Digestive and Kidney Diseases; Dental Research; General Medical Sciences; Communicative Disorders; Stroke; Eye; Aging; Arthritis; Musculoskeletal and Skin Diseases; Center for Disease Control [including National Institute for Occupational Safety and Health] and the Center for Nursing Research) are included within the DHHS.
Address: 200 Independence Avenue SW, Washington, DC 20201
               Telephone: 202-619-0257

United States Department of Housing and Urban Development (HUD). HUD is responsible for programs that address housing needs and opportunities. The general development of the nation's communities is a focus of this federal agency. The Environmental Policy Act of 1969, in addition to other laws, mandated that the Assistant Secretary of HUD enact policies that address environmental problems, establish standards, and provide technical assistance to communities.
Address: 451 Seventh Street SW, Washington, DC 20410
               Telephone: 202-708-1422

United States Department of the Interior (DOI). The Department of Interior is charged with conservation of nationally owned public lands and natural resources. Preservation of national parks and historical landmarks is a major focus of this agency. Mineral resource assessment and development are carried out by the DOI. Assistant Secretaries of the DOI are responsible for Fish and Wildlife and Parks, Water and Science, Land and Mineral Management, Territorial and International Affairs, and a variety of other focus areas. The Bureaus of the U.S. Fish and Wildlife Service, National Park Service, and Mines are located within this federal department.
Address: 1849 C Street NW, Washington, DC 20240
               Telephone: 202-708-3171

United States Department of Justice. The Department of Justice is considered to be the legal counsel to the people of the United States of America. As the federal agency responsible for enforcing law, the department plays a major role in crime prevention and detection. Regional offices are located in Boston, New York, Philadelphia, Atlanta, Chicago, Dallas, Kansas City (MO), Denver, San Francisco, and Seattle.
Address: Constitution Avenue and Tenth Street NW, Washington, DC 20530
               Telephone: 202-514-2000, 202-514-4019

United States Department of Labor. The U.S. Department of Labor is charged with the development and promotion of the welfare of workers within this nation. It maintains many regulatory functions that focus on

TABLE 19–4. UNITED STATES GOVERNMENT OFFICES AND AGENCIES (continued)

workers' rights, wages, employee safety and health, pension, and unemployment/worker compensation insurance. The Occupational Safety and Health Administration (OSHA) and Bureau of Labor Statistics are housed within this federal department.

Address: **200 Constitution Avenue NW, Washington, DC 20210**
           Telephone: 202-219-5000

United States Department of Transportation (DOT). This federal department is responsible for national transportation policy. Railroad, highway, and aviation travel are major focuses. The Urban Mass Transportation Administration falls under the auspices of the DOT.

Address: **400 7th Street SW, Washington, DC 20590**
           Telephone: 202-366-0600

INDEPENDENT ESTABLISHMENTS AND GOVERNMENT CORPORATIONS

Nuclear Regulatory Commission (NRC). The NRC is charged with protecting public health and the environment through the licensing and regulating of (public) nuclear energy sources.

Address: **1717 H Street NW, Washington, DC 20555**
           Telephone: 301-492-7000

Occupational Safety and Health Review Commission. This quasi-judicial agency is charged with ruling on contested Department of Labor, Occupational Safety and Health Administration (OSHA) cases. Employers may dispute alleged violations, penalties, and time allotments proposed for correction of hazardous situations. The four regional offices are located in Atlanta, Boston, Dallas, and Denver.

Address: **1120 Twentieth St NW, Washington, DC 20036-3419**
           Telephone: 202-606-5100

Source: Office of the Federal Register. (1994). *1994/1995 The United States Government Manual.* (CFR 9.1). Washington, DC: U.S. Government Printing Office.

health. Policy makers need to be encouraged and urged to understand that health is more than access to health care when ill but also protection from environmental hazards.

Future needs include the monitoring of the nation's health, especially that of vulnerable high-risk groups of individuals. We need to provide adequately trained professionals to develop and implement interventions, educate citizens, and conduct research. We need to focus on evaluating the impact of substances such as pesticides, air pollution, and indirect cigarette smoke inhalation on acute and chronic human illness. Though much of the public assumes that low-level exposures are as harmful as acute exposures, data are sparse and sometimes inconclusive.

Periodic special surveys and large-scale annual surveillance of the public's health should be continued. We need measures against which to compare progress. Surveillance of vital records and other reporting systems is essential to monitoring changes in national mortality and morbidity patterns. A keen awareness of national direction may allow the family health nurse to anticipate sources of information.

Professionals practicing in areas where acute environmental pollution exists should be available to offer congressional and local testimony about health and safety issues pertinent to their client population. Awareness of environmental problems requires that the practitioner keep abreast of environmental changes that affect society. A heightened social awareness, political ac-

tion, and advocacy are important characteristics of family nurses.

FOSTERING SELF-CARE IN ENVIRONMENTAL HEALTH

Using the Neuman Health-Care Systems Model (Neuman, 1982), the nurse can encourage clients to determine intra-, inter-, and extrapersonal variables that affect personal and family health. Family environmental self-care is a dynamic process that requires the family to perceive vulnerability to accidents, injury, or illness and to use self-responsibility to prevent environmental stressors and to protect and promote the family's environmental health and safety. The family is required to recognize and anticipate potential and actual threats to their health from the environmental variables that exist in ecosystems.

Using the self-care perspective to assist clients to improve their environmental health requires that the nurse (1) assess with the family their potential and actual hazards; (2) plan with and educate families about the primary and secondary prevention strategies to minimize hazards in their environment; (3) and evaluate the outcome of their plan. Questions in Table 19–5 will help individuals and families to assess their environmental health in the home and occupational setting at the primary, secondary, and tertiary prevention levels.

TABLE 19–5. SELF-ASSESSMENT OF ENVIRONMENTAL HEALTH

PRIMARY PREVENTION

Occupational

1. Do I work with substances my employer, my doctor, official agencies, or I consider potentially hazardous to my health? frequency? duration?
2. Am I asked to use safety/personal protective devices while I work? why? when? where? who else?
3. Do I use the safety/personal protective devices my employer requires me to use while performing my job? If not, why not? If yes, when? where? with whom?
4. Do I notice any patterns of illness in my working peers or family members? What specifically? Does anyone consider this a problem? family? company?
5. In describing my workplace, is/are there clutter? vapors? liquids? dust? fumes? heat? vibration?
6. Do I feel that my work or workplace presents physical dangers such as falls, slips, or falling objects?

Home

1. What hobbies do I or family members participate in while in our home? What products are used? Are warning or special use labels present on any of these products?
2. Do we undergo regular checkups with our primary health care provider/doctor? Frequency? Has our health care provider advised us to change any personal or environmental factors present within our lives? If so, what?
3. Are all family members up to date on their immunization status?
4. What cleaning, home-maintenance, or home-repair products are used or stored within our home? Do package directions indicate proper use and storage? How are they used and stored? Does this comply with directions?
5. What type of insulation is used in my home? Are there known health hazards with this type of home insulation?
6. What type of heating is used in my home? Are there health hazards associated with this type of heating?
7. What source of water is used for my home? ground? surface? reclaimed? desalinated? rain? Are there any problems known to be associated with this water resource? Is water purified, filtered, and/or chlorinated prior to entering my home?

Recreational

1. List all playtime activities. List frequency and duration of the activity.
2. Are there any known dangers associated with these recreational activities?
3. Are there any substances/chemicals required to perform the recreational pastime? If so, what? Are directions for use and storage present? Do we/I follow them precisely?
4. Is safety equipment recommended for the recreational activity? If so, is it used? If recommended and not used, why not?

Environmental

1. Draw a map of known greenbelts, industries, dumps, housing patterns, and bodies of water.
2. Is my community targeted as a "high-risk" area for any toxic waste? radiation? If so, where? Do family members have any contact with resources from this area?
3. Are environmental problems suspected within my immediate neighborhood? If yes, what?
4. List your immediate concern when you think of environmental problems within your community.

Personal

1. Do I or other family members smoke?
2. How much alcohol consumption occurs during one week for each family member? Has alcohol ever been a problem in daily life (i.e., driving, business, school)?
3. Do I or other family members use recreational/illicit drugs? If so, which ones and how frequently?
4. How many sexual partners do individuals within family encounter within a month? year? Can you/they describe "safe sex" practices? Do they/you use safe sex practices?

Do any of the above risk factors combine to increase the risk of disease (e.g., tobacco smoking and asbestos mining)?

SECONDARY PREVENTION

Occupational

1. Have I experienced any changes in my health, possibly related to my job, that caused me or my family to worry during the last week? month? year?
2. Describe a typical work week.
   a. Do I feel better on the first day of my work week or the last day?
   b. Is there any change between the way I feel on weekends and during the work week?
   c. Are my coworkers showing signs of illness? If so, what signs?

TABLE 19–5. SELF-ASSESSMENT OF ENVIRONMENTAL HEALTH (continued)

   d. How much sick leave have I used this quarter? How many sick-leave days are spent in bed due to illness or poor health? How many days are spent off work and not in bed? When did I last see a doctor during a sick-leave period? What information did the doctor give me about my illness?

   e. Do I think I need to see a physician or health care provider soon? If so, who? why?

   f. During the performance of my work, am I at risk for physical injury or disease?

Home

1. If I work or play at home, have I become exposed to substances that cause detectable illness?
2. Are there any illnesses that have been experienced within the home by more than one family member? If yes, what disease or symptoms? Is there any pattern of association common to all members?
3. Are family members acutely or chronically ill? If so, what diseases or conditions? Are they transmittable? Are they detectable through screening tests (e.g., tuberculosis)?

Recreational

1. Have I experienced any injuries related to my playtime activities in recent months? years? If so, what? Do these injuries indicate a need to seek screening for disease or chronic injury (e.g., neurologic compromise due to falls or moving vehicle accidents)?
2. Do any recreational activities aggravate preexisting diseases or injuries?

Environmental

1. Is my community or neighborhood targeted for any screening for disease or disability?
2. Do any environmental conditions exist (historical or current) that would alarm health officials or family members and indicate need for screening for disease? If so, what conditions? what exposures (e.g., radiation, infectious disease, and so on)?

Personal

1. Are family members at high risk for AIDS or other sexually transmitted diseases (homosexual males, IV drug abusers, multiple sex partners, sexual partners of the aforementioned)? Do I have single or multiple sex partners? Do I or my partners practice safe sex? Is HIV screening and treatment available within my community? Am I/family member in a risk group that indicates the need for screening and early diagnosis?
2. Do I or family members have habits that may put me or them at risk for diseases (e.g., IV drug abuse, illicit substance abuse, alcohol abuse)? Are they wishing screening and treatment? What services are available for screening and treatment within our community? What is the price to be paid for screening and treatment?
3. Is a family member a smoker with recent unexplained weight loss? When was last physical examination? When was last chest x-ray?
4. Is there any personal history of exposure, such as radiation exposure, that might indicate a need for periodic screening?
5. Is there any endemic disease I should be regularly tested for due to lifestyle or location (e.g., tuberculosis)?

Do any of the above risk factors combine to increase the risk of disease (e.g., tobacco smoking and asbestos mining)?

TERTIARY PREVENTION

When illness is present:

Occupational

1. Do I feel better or worse when I am in my normal work environment? What circumstances or activities make me feel worse? make me feel better?
2. Does my condition require that my employer accommodate the activities and circumstances that make me feel better? Are the accommodations made? Do the accommodations impose hardship on coworkers?
3. Can adjustments of the environment or equipment be made to allow me to work? Is retraining (habilitation) feasible? Do I or my family wish me to change jobs/retrain?

Home

1. How does the illness affect my role within the family and the completion of my tasks within the home?
2. Can adjustments of the environment or equipment be made so that I may better complete my activities within the home?
3. Do any home chores or activities exacerbate my illness or condition? If so, which ones? Can they be modified?

Recreational

1. Are my recreational activities limited due to illness or disability? If so, which ones? Can they be altered to accommodate the conditions without causing an increase in symptoms or exacerbation of illness?
2. Do any recreational activities worsen my condition? If so, which ones? Have they been altered or avoided to diminish physical or mental stress?

TABLE 19–5.   SELF-ASSESSMENT OF ENVIRONMENTAL HEALTH (continued)

Environmental

1. Do environmental conditions exist within my community or home that exacerbate my condition (e.g., smog)? If so, are they alterable? If yes, how?
2. Describe the climatic and general environmental conditions that potentiate your wellness. Can they be achieved within your current locale? If not, why not? If so, how?

Personal

1. Do my habits worsen my illness or conditions (e.g., smoking and emphysema)?
2. Is there a personal behavior I can enact that will facilitate recovery or rehabilitation? If so, what? If so, what lifestyle changes or resources will be needed? If so, are the resources available? accessible? acceptable?

Do any of the above risk factors combine to increase the risk of disease (e.g., tobacco smoking and asbestos mining).

CHAPTER HIGHLIGHTS

Diverse environmental concerns influence or have the potential to influence the health of individuals and families across the life span.

Biological, physical, and chemical environmental hazards can be found in homes, workplaces, schools, and play/leisure activities.

Occupational and recreational exposure to chemical and biological hazards can result in genetic mutations, fetal malformation, exposure of other household members.

The family nurse's role in environmental health for individuals and families is preventing contact by anticipatory guidance and health teaching, performing early screenings and diagnosis, and offering appropriate preventive or rehabilitative measures.

Primary prevention of environmental hazards includes public and family education and activities to reduce contact between hosts and harmful agents.

Secondary prevention activities provide for early screening, diagnosis, and treatment of harmful environmental agents.

Tertiary prevention includes attempts to remove harmful agents from the environment and to restore the host to normal functioning.

REFERENCES

Awad, O.M., & el Shimi, N.M. (1993). Influence of different means of washing and processing removal of acetellic residue from spinich and eggplant and its in-vivo action on mice hepatic biochemical targets. *Journal of Egyptian Public Health Association, 68*(5–6), 671–686.

Arnott, M.S. (1981). Carcinogen metabolism. In C.R. Shaw (Ed.), *Prevention of Occupational Cancer.* Boca Raton, FL: CRC Press.

Bingham, E. (1992). Occupational safety and health standards. In

Blain, P.G. (1990). Aspects of pesticide toxicology. *Adverse Drug Reactions and Acute Poisoning Reviews, 9*(1), 37–68.

Carson, R. (1960). *Silent Spring.* Greenwich, CT: Fawcett/Crest.

Centers for Disease Control (CDC). (1987). Update: Human immunodeficiency virus infections in healthcare workers exposed to blood of infected patients and B-virus infection in humans—Pensacola, Florida. *Morbidity and Mortality Weekly Report, 36*(19), 285–299.

Centers for Disease Control (1990). Alcohol use and aquatic activities—Massachusetts, 1988. *Morbidity and Mortality Weekly Report, 39,* 332–334.

Centers for Disease Control (1991a). Tuberculosis transmission in state correctional institution—California. *Morbidity and Mortality Weekly Report, 41*(49), 927–927.

Centers for Disease Control (1991b). Behavior related to unintentional and intentional injuries among high school students—U.S. *Morbidity and Mortality Weekly Report, 41*(41), 760–771.

Centers for Disease Control (1992a). Surveillance of elevated blood lead levels among adults—U.S. *Morbidity and Mortality Weekly Report, 41*(17), 285–288.

Centers for Disease Control (1992b). Transmission of multidrug-resistant tuberculosis among immunocompromised persons in a correctional system—N.Y. *Morbidity and Mortality Weekly Report, 4*(28), 507–514.

Center for Disease Control and Prevention (1993a). Hantavirus infection—Southwestern United States: Interim recommendations for risk reductions. *Mortality and Morbidity Weekly Reports, 42*(No. RR-11), 1–12.

Center for Disease Control and Prevention (1993b). Surveillance for waterborne disease outbreaks-1991–1992, *Mortality and Morbidity Weekly Reports, 42*(No. SS-5), 1–5.

Center for Disease Control and Prevention (1994a). Guidelines for preventing the transmission of mycobacterium tuberculosis in health care facilities. *Mortality and Morbidity Weekly Reports, 43*(No RR-13), 1–16.

Center for Disease Control and Prevention (1994b). Surveillance of emergency events involving hazardorous substances—United States 1990–1992. *Mortality and Morbidity Weekly Reports, 43*(55-2), 1–6.

Center for Disease Control and Prevention (1995a). HIV transmission in a dialysis center-Columbia 1991–1993. *Mortality and Morbidity Weekly Reports, 44*(21), 404–406.

Center for Disease Control and Prevention (1995b). Assessing the public health threat associated with cryptosporidoisis. *Mortality and Morbidity Weekly Reports, 44*(No. RR-6), 1–3.

Durkin, M.S., Davidson, L.L., Kuhn, L., O'Connor, P., & Barlow, B. (1994). Low income neighborhoods and the role of severe pediatric injury: A small area analysis in North Manhattan. *American Journal of Public Health, 84*(4), 587–592.

Fearson, R.R., & Vogelstein, B.A. (1990). A genetic model for colorectal tumorigenesis. *Cell,* 61, 759–767.

Ferguson, J., & Martin, W. (1985). An overview of occupational safety and health guidelines for Superfund sites. *American Industrial Hygiene Association Journal, 46*(4), 175–180.

Frank, A.L. & Slesin, L. (1986). In J.M. Last (Ed.), *Maxcy-Rosenau: Public Health and Preventive Medicine* (pp. 714–725). Norwalk, CT: Appleton-Century-Crofts.

Frazier, C.A. (1986). Occupational health. In B.B. Logan & C.E. Dawkins (Eds.), *Family-Centered Nursing in the Community* (pp. 487–513). Menlo Park, CA: Addison-Wesley.

Harlan, L.C., Harlan, W.R., & Parrons, P.E. (1990). The economic impact of injuries: A major source of medical costs. *American Jornal of Public Health, 80*(4), 453–459.

Hemminki, K., et al. (1983). Spontaneous abortions in an industrialized community in Finland. *American Journal of Public Health, 73*(1), 32–37.

Higgins, I. (1986). Air pollution. In J.M. Last (Ed.), *Maxcy-Rosenau: Public Health and Preventive Medicine* (pp. 576–586). Norwalk, CT: Appleton-Century-Crofts.

Holbrook, T.L., Grazier, K., Kelsey, J.L., & Stauffer, R.N. (1984). *The Frequency of Occurrence, Impact and Cost of Musculoskeletal Conditions in the United States.* Chicago: American Academy of Orthopedic Surgeons.

Holme, J.A., et al. (1991). DNA damage and cell death induced by 1,2-dibromo-3-chloropropane (DBCP) and structured analogs in monolayer culture of rat hepatocytes: 3-amino benzamide inhibits the toxicity of DBCP. *Cell Biology and Toxicology, 7*(4), 413–432.

Institute of Medicine (1992). *Advances in Understanding Changes in Cancer.* Washington, DC: National Academy Press.

Jackson, M., McPherson, D., & Greenwalt, N. (1987). *Infection Prevention and Control Manual.* San Diego: San Diego Medical Center.

Johnson, C.J. (1984). Cancer incidence in an area of radioactive fallout downwind from the Nevada test site. *Journal of the American Medical Association,* 25(1), 230–236.

Kandzari, J.H., & Howard, J.R. (1981). *The Well Family: A Developmental Approach.* Boston: Little, Brown.

Kaplanski, J., Shemi, D., Waksman, J., Potashnik, G., & Sod-Moriah, U.A. (1991). The effects of 1,2-dibromo-3-chloropropane (DBCP) on general toxicity and gonadotoxicity in rats. *Andrologia.* 23(5), 363–366.

Kilburn, K.H. (1992). Pulmonary responses to gasses and particles. In J.M. Last & R.B. Wallace (Eds.). *Maxey-Roseneau-Last Public Health and Preventive Medicine* (2nd ed.) (pp. 474–475). Norwalk: Appleton-Lange.

Kierkegaard, O., & Kristiansen, J.L. (1992). Sick leave during pregnancy. *Ugeskrift for Laeger, 154*(34), 2305–2308.

King, I. (1981). *A Theory of Nursing: Systems, Concepts and Process.* New York: Wiley.

Koren, H. (1980). *Handbook of Environmental Health and Safety: Principles and Practices.* New York: Pergamon Press.

Kuhn, D. (1981). A safe place to work. In C.R. Shaw (Ed.), *Prevention of Occupational Cancer.* Boca Raton, FL: CRC Press.

Last, J.M. (1992). Scope and methods of prevention. In J.M. Last & R. B. Wallace (Eds.). *Maxey-Rosenau-Last Public Health and Preventive Medicine* (2nd ed.) (pp. 474–475). Norwalk: Appleton-Lange.

Li, F.P., & Frauemeni, J.F.J. (1969). Soft-tissue sarcomas, breast cancer, and other neoplasms. A familiar syndrome? *Annals of Internal Medicine,* 71, 747–752.

Lobo, M.L. (1985). Dorothy E. Johnson. In J.B. George (Ed.), *Nursing Theories: The Base for Professional Practice* (2nd ed.). Englewood Cliffs, NJ: Prentice-Hall.

Malkin, D., Li, F. P., Strong, L.C., et al. (1990). Germ line p53 mutations in a familial syndrome of breast cancer, sarcomas, and other neoplasms. *Science* 250, 1233–1238.

Melson, G.F. (1980). *Family and Environment: An Ecosystem Perspective.* Minneapolis: Burgess.

National Center for Health Statistics. (1984). *Health Characteristics by Geographic Region, Large Metropolitan Areas, and Other Places of Residence.* U.S. DHHS Publ. 84-1574. Washington, DC: U.S. Government Printing Office.

National Center for Health statistics. (1985). *Health Characteristics According to Family and Personal Income.* U.S. DHHS Publ. 85-1575. Washington, DC: U.S. Government Printing Office.

National Center for Health Statistics (1988). Current estimates from the National Health Interview Survey. *Vital and Health Statistics,* 10(173), 56–58.

National Center for Health Statistics (1990). Types of injuries by selected characteristics, U.S. 1985–1987. *Vital and Health Statistics,* 10(175), 32.

National Highway Traffic Safety Administration. (1991a). *Drunk Driving Facts.* Washington, DC: U.S. Department of Transportation.

National Highway Traffic Safety Administration. (1991b). *Fatal Accident Reporting System, 1990: A Review of Information on Fatal Traffic Crashes in the United States.* DOT-HS-807-794. Washington, DC: U.S. Department of Transportation.

Neuman, B. (1982). *The Neuman Systems Model.* Norwalk, CT: Appleton-Century-Crofts.

Okun, D.A. (1992). Water quality management. In J.M. Last (Ed.), *Maxey-Roseneau: Public Health and Preventive Medicine* (pp. 807–842). Norwalk, CT: Appleton-Century-Crofts.

Ordin, D. (1992). Surveillance monitoring and screening in occupational health. In J.M. Last & R.B. Wallace (Eds.) *Maxey-Roseneau-Last Public Health and Preventive Medicine* (2nd ed.) (pp. 552–558). Norwalk: Appleton-Lange.

Parkinson, D.K., & Grennan, M.J. (1986). Establishment of medical surveillance in industry: Problems and procedures. *Journal of Occupational Medicine,* 28(8), 772–777.

Powell, R.L. (1984). Dioxin in Missouri: 1971–1983. *Bulletin of Environmental Contamination and Toxicology,* 33, 648–654.

Rothman, K.J. (1986). *Modern Epidemiology.* Boston: Little, Brown.

Roy, C., & Roberts, S.L. (1984). *Theory Construction in Nursing: An Adaptation Model.* Englewood Cliffs, NJ: Prentice-Hall.

Ruddon, R.W. (1987). *Cancer Biology.* New York: Oxford University Press.

Selikoff, I.J. (1986). Asbestos-associated diseases. In J.M. Last (Ed.), *Maxcy-Rosenau: Public Health and Preventive Medicine* (pp. 523–544). Norwalk, CT: Appleton Press.

Solomon, E., Borrow, J., & Goddard, A.D. (1991). Chromosome aberrations and cancer. *Science,* 254, 1153–1160.

Starfield, B., et al. (1984). Morbidity in childhood—a longitudinal view. *New England Journal of Medicine,* 310(13), 824–829.

Talbott, E., et al. (1985). Occupational noise exposure, noise induced hearing loss, and the epidemiology of high blood pressure. *American Journal of Epidemiology,* 121(4), 501–514.

U.S. Department of Health and Human Services. Public Health Service. (1986). *The 1990 Health Objectives for the Nation: A Midcourse Review.* Washington, DC: U.S. Government Printing Office.

U.S. Department of Health and Human Services. Public Health Service. (1991). *Healthy People 2000: National Health Promotion and Disease Prevention Objectives.* DHHS Pub. 91-50212. Washington, DC: U.S. Government Printing Office.

U.S. House of Representatives Subcommittee on Energy Development and Applications. (1983). *Acid Rain: Implications for Fossil Research and Development.* Washington, DC: U.S. Government Printing Office.

Whorton, D., Krauss, R.M., Marshall, S., & Milby, T.H. (1977). Infertility in male pesticide workers. *Lancet,* 2, 1259–1261.

Whorton, D., Milby, T.H., Krauss, R.M., & Stubbs, H.A. (1979). Testicular function in DBCP exposed pesticide workers. *Journal of Occupational Medicine,* 21, 161–166.

Wilson, J., & Jungner, F. (1968). *Principles and Practice for Screening for Disease.* Public Health Papers No. 34. Geneva: WHO.

FAMILY HEALTH PROMOTION DURING TRANSITIONS

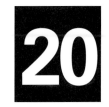

PATRICIA ROTH

If there is no struggle, there is no progress.

FREDERICK DOUGLASS

OBJECTIVES

On completion of this chapter, the reader will be able to:

1. Identify the various types of transitions that families experience as they move from one developmental phase to another

2. Analyze the corresponding role complex changes that occur in families experiencing transition

3. Explicate the key concepts and variables associated with the addition or loss of family members

4. Identify the sources of stress and family coping strategies associated with family role changes, chronic illness, and/or relocation

5. Incorporate variables concerning family adaptation to transitions into a nursing assessment

6. Develop effective strategies to mitigate the stress families experience during life transitions

7. Delineate researchable problems concerning the effects of transitions on the health of family members

---

Family development theory is the primary theory that deals with family change, traditionally describing family life over time as divided into a series of stages. Family development stages are identified using the criteria of a major change in family size, the development of the oldest child, and the work status of the primary provider. The scheme rests on an assumption of high member interdependence, necessitating a change in the rules for interrelating members each time one or more members are added or leave the family and each time the oldest child changes his or her own developmental stage. Although traditional family development theory has many important applications, it does not provide insight into the processes of developmental change by which families transform their interaction structures (Merderer & Hill, 1983).

The process of transition and adjustment is the major focus of critical transitions theory, which identifies the normal crises of transition experienced by all families bearing children, such as getting married, parenthood, deparentalization, leave taking, and retirement. Rapoport (1963) used crisis theory to account for the behavior of families, indicating that if the crisis is handled appropriately, the result is some type of maturation or development.

Hill (1973) operationalized the concept of critical transition, noting that the stages of development were marked by significant changes in the family's role complex. A major reorganization is required if multiple role complex changes occur. Three types of structural events were identified that could be stressful if they occurred within the same period of time, precipitating a critical transition and demarcating a new stage of development (see Fig. 20–1): changes in the number of family members, such as the addition or loss of spouses or children, including the return of adult children; age composition changes due to individual developmental status change and school status change; and major status changes such as marriage, parenthood, divorce, widowhood, location changes, changes in network affiliation, and changes in career status (Merderer & Hill, 1983).

Major life changes and role transitions are often identified as stressors that create a need for adjustment by the individual and the family. However, these transitions have a wide-ranging effect on mental health, an empirically supported variation that has produced several models in an attempt to explain the differential impacts of life events. One model attributes the impact of life events to differences in coping resources or strategies, ongoing dispositional qualities, or social locations, a model that has led to a research tradition based on the buffering effects of social support. A second model contends that events vary in stressfulness because of differences in such characteristics as undesirability, uncontrollability, unpredictability, and event magnitude. Wheaton (1990) compares these models with his own, which envisions life transitions as nonproblematic, or even beneficial to mental health, when preceded by chronic role problems. His findings suggest a need to specify social circumstances that determine whether a transition is potentially stressful and present a compelling argument against the presumption that life transitions are inherently stressful. Thus, life transitions have been conceptionalized as nonproblematic and even beneficial under certain circumstances or as inherently stressful.

This chapter explores various types of life transitions that families experience, with a major focus on the impact of these events on the family unit or the individual. Adaptation to specific life events will be examined, as well as implications for family adjustment or reaffirmation.

ADDITION OF FAMILY MEMBERS

Change in the number of family members is identified as one of the structural events that might be expected to be stressful, particularly if it occurs with other events, such as a major status change. The addition of a family member, such as a spouse or child, necessitates change in the predictable patterns of behavior among members in terms of their role structure. Decision making, affection, communication, and division of tasks must be renegotiated to meet the changing needs of the family and individual members. Marriage, parenthood, and remarriages are all major status changes that affect the number of family members and require considerable role alteration. Each of the transitions will be briefly explored in terms of stressors and role complex changes of family members.

Marriage

A critical role transition and central issue of adulthood is the formation of a partnership with another person in a committed relationship. A mature, intimate, committed relationship does not diminish a person's independent identity but rather reinforces it. The concept of intimacy involves a combination of a sense of mutuality, sensitivity to the needs of the partner, physical closeness, willingness to share, and openness or lack of defensiveness (Erikson, 1963). In an adult relationship characterized by true intimacy, each

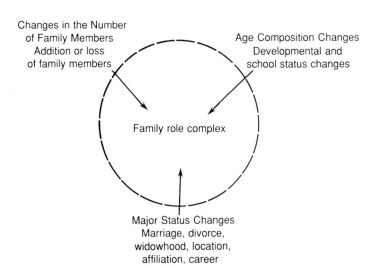

FIGURE 20–1. Critical transitions in family development. (Data from Merderer H., Hill, R. (1983). Critical transitions over the family life span: Theory and research. In H.I. McCubbin, M.B. Sussman & J.M. Patterson (Eds.), *Social Stress and the Family: Advances in Family Stress Theory and Research* (pp. 39–60). New York: Haworth Press.)

individual retains unique attributes outside the fusion of the two identities but is strongly committed to the bonds that join them. Intimacy, defined as mutuality, may characterize any relationship involving emotional commitments between two adults, not only those institutionalized through marriage.

The concept of mutuality may be further elaborated to provide greater specificity. A relationship characterized by mutuality has progressed beyond superficial role-based interactions to a high degree of intimate disclosure, knowledge of each other's personal feelings, and joint development of pair norms. Intimacy incorporates the process of open communication and strong commitment of both partners to one another and to the future of the relationship. The existence of mutuality in any relationship varies over time as growth toward or away from mutuality changes according to each partner's developmental status and factors within and outside of the relationship (Whitbourne, 1986).

Marriage constitutes the predominant framework of adult living in contemporary society, implying the formation of an intimate, committed relationship and the establishment of a common household with shared living and financial responsibilities and the interweaving of lifestyles into a single unit. Marriage is usually a critical role transition that involves disengagement from sibling and filial roles, a change in network affiliation, and the assumption of in-law status. In addition, it may involve a change in career status, school status, and residential status, leading to considerable stress for the couple and significant changes in role script (Merderer & Hill, 1983).

Role Adjustments

Several major adjustments characterize the transition from single person to married couple. Each person must continue to develop as an unique person while the partner also grows to greater self-awareness and acceptance. Second, there is the necessity of developing role patterns within the family, a process that redefines the behavioral patterns that each may have learned in the family of origin. The division of responsibility is another important area of adjustment. The couple must also establish effective communication patterns, developing styles of conflict resolution, decision making, and social interaction. Kimmel (1990) further emphasizes the importance of a commitment to the relationship and to working together as the relationship changes over time.

Both husband and wife continue to develop as adults during this transition to life as a married couple. Each must develop his or her own career goals while assuming responsibility for the support and management of the household. In addition, each must learn to communicate effectively and intimately with the other and develop compe-

tence in his or her sexual role. Other individual developmental concerns include establishing relationships with in-laws and engaging in mutual social activities. Together, the married couple also shares developmental tasks in maintaining a home, supporting themselves, allocating household responsibilities, establishing mutually acceptable roles, and maintaining motivation, even when obstacles arise (Duvall & Miller, 1985).

Establishing mutually acceptable roles involves defining the set of attitudes and behaviors a spouse is expected to demonstrate in the context of the marital relationship. Couples today are freer to develop male-female relationships than were their parents. Changing family patterns as a result of changes in women's roles, marriage of partners from widely different cultural backgrounds, and the increasing physical distance from families of origin place couples in the potentially stressful position of defining their relationship and their roles in nontraditional ways (Carter & McGoldrick, 1988). Traditionally, the husband assumes the provider role; the wife assumes the child care, housekeeper, and sexual roles; and both share the kinship and child socialization roles. In spite of greater opportunities to define role patterns creatively, Caycedo, Wange, and Bahr (1991) noted that in the 1980s, attitudes became more egalitarian, but behavioral changes in family roles appeared to be small.

The division of labor is an important area of negotiation and possibly an area of conflict resolution for young couples. Working out an acceptable pattern, consistent with both spouses' attitudes toward enacting roles, can be a considerable challenge. Kamo (1988) explored factors associated with a husband's involvement in domestic work. The amount of time husbands spend in domestic labor was positively associated with their education and egalitarian sex role orientation and negatively associated with their income. The wife's level of earnings and egalitarian sex role orientation were positively associated with the husband's participation in domestic work. Husbands did about 36% of the total domestic work, an amount that increased 5% to 7% if the wife was employed full time. Following a review of a decade of research, Caycedo et al. (1991) found no significant changes in the amount of time husbands spent in housework and child care. Such findings indicate that the division of labor may continue to be a problematic area in spite of more egalitarian attitudes among men and women.

Developing a strong sense of intimacy in the relationship is a function of commitment and effective communication to resolve conflict and to make decisions. Clear communication should focus on the problem at hand and permit maximum transmission of information. Burr (1990) recommends the use of "We Statements" rather than "I Statements" to communicate more effectively in some family situations and to identify a problem with a group or relationship. The use of we statements is more consistent with the connectedness, enduring intimacy, and emotionality that characterizes family relationships.

Ineffective communication patterns can lead to discord and marital dissatisfaction. Defensiveness, stubbornness, and withdrawal from interaction were identified as longitudinally dysfunctional, especially when exhibited by the husband. Disagreement and anger related to concurrent unhappiness and negative interaction were predictive of improved marital satisfaction over time (Gottman & Krokoff, 1989). Marital satisfaction is the result of several communication and interaction factors: validation of each spouse for the other, reciprocation of the positive effect, lack of negative verbal exchanges with accompanying negative nonverbal cues, and problem resolution that is satisfactory for both partners (Steggell & Harper, 1991). Clearly the development of effective communication patterns is essential to a successful marital relationship, a relationship that forms the basis for the family structure and the first stage in family development.

Marriage and Family Health

It is important at this point in family development to consider factors related to the health status of the couple and other potential family members. Mauksch (1974) has defined a concept of family health that focuses on the interdependence of the health of the family and the health of individual family members, referred to as the *family health estate*. Each family unit is a unique and distinct health behavior unit, representing a fusion of the properties that family members contribute to the family health estate. For example, each person in the couple relationship brings to the family an awareness of health-relevant knowledge and unique methods of introducing these factors into the emerging family unit within the context of his or her own culture. The emerging family, consisting of the founding members and the individuals who join the unit, develops health values, habits, and risk perceptions that are characteristic of that particular family. The family health estate also concerns the development of roles concerning the health status of the family and the allocation of tasks.

Mauksch (1974) identifies the linking process that occurs between family members as a process of interaction that results in modification of the properties of the other individual. The linking process also occurs through social interactions outside the family. Processes of interaction within the family may be positive, leading to pleasure and a sense of well-being, or negative, leading to stress and a sense of disorganization. Threats to a family's health may be the result of a weakening in the family linking system, with potential consequences for the health of individual members. Any dysfunction that affects an individual member also affects the family unit, creating a cyclical relationship. Consequently, as couples establish family roles and define attitudes and behaviors, they also initiate a family health estate that will influence the family unit and individual behavior in relation to health promotion, disease prevention, and illness susceptibility, management, and consequences.

Parenthood

The arrival of the first child changes a spouse into a parent and a marriage into a family with children. There are few other events that have more impact on a family than the birth of a child, whether one focuses on the general consequences of adding members to a group or views more specifically the changes that occur in the role and power structure of a marriage. The transition to parenthood usually describes movement from the early married stage to the stage in which the oldest child is under 2 years—a period that has received considerable attention in the literature. Several major themes predominate, including parenthood as crisis, the effect of parenthood on marital satisfaction, and patterns of interaction of families with infants.

Whether the addition of a child to a family constitutes a crisis and to what extent has been the focus of some studies. LeMasters (1957) and Dyer (1963) found that most couples identified the recent birth of a child as an extensive or severe crisis, whereas Hobbs (1965) and Hobbs and Cole (1976) found that the majority of couples experienced moderate or low levels of crisis. Significantly fewer couples in the later study viewed having a child as being important to their marital happiness, a substantial shift in attitudes toward marital and parental roles. The view of parenthood as a crisis event was also altered with the perception of parenthood as a transitional change (Hobbs & Cole, 1976).

A compromise position evolved when Entwisle and Doering (1981) conducted a study over a six-month period with white couples in stable relationships and found that the birth of a first child could be both crisis and transition. New parents may experience a period of stress, especially the mother, in part perhaps because women assume almost all of the responsibility for the infant. Another study suggests that the father's level of stress reflects the infant's characteristics and the father's involvement with the infant. Fathers tended to be more involved with the care of a son and also experienced decline in self-esteem, possibly due to struggling with unfamiliar parenting roles (Hawkins & Belsky, 1989). Thus, parenthood can be a stressful transition for both mother and father.

PARENTHOOD AS A CRITICAL TRANSITION

Support for the view of parenthood as a critical transition is generated by the impact of simultaneous stressors and changes in the family role complex (Merderer & Hill, 1983).

Among the stressors identified as contributing to the critical transition of first parenthood is the accession of an infant member and the plurality pattern change to a triad. Parental roles of mother and father are also activated, resulting in a major status change. For some families, another major status change may be the temporary or permanent withdrawal of the wife from the workforce to accommodate childrearing. Residential and location changes may also need to occur to accommodate the needs of a family with an infant. Usually, with the advent of the first child, kinship networks are also reactivated, including interaction with grandparents, aunts and uncles, and other members of the extended family. These structural events or changes in the family role complex occurring simultaneously generate major family reorganization, or a critical transition.

Marital Satisfaction

Marital satisfaction is also a major focus of the literature that explores the effect of children on the marital relationship, usually based on the attitudes of husbands and wives. Whitbourne (1986) states that there is substantial documentation of a curvilinear pattern across the stages of the family life cycle in couple marital satisfaction, with the period of lowest satisfaction coinciding with the presence of children in the home. One explanation of the negative effects of parenthood is based on the stress of everyday living, including fatigue, noise, and confusion in the home; additional household work; added financial burdens; and lack of control over routines. Rollins (1989) found that parental involvement in childrearing may result in less companionship, but when children leave home, parents have more time together. There may also be disagreement over childrearing practices, concerns about competence as a parent, and concerns for the welfare of the child. For the dual-worker household, a return to full-time work for both spouses is an impossibility without providing for their child's needs. Each parent must adjust emotionally to a plan that leaves children with someone other than themselves. Greater role stress is also experienced by parents who are attempting to coordinate two jobs with childraising responsibilities (Carter & McGoldrick, 1988). Direct negative effects on the expression of intimacy of the couple occur due to decreased communication, role strain, interference with a sexual relationship, and a segregation of husbands and wives based on traditional spheres of activity. For example, MacDermid, Huston, and McHale (1990)

found that spouses' activities became more child centered and less couple centered, and they tended to divide household tasks along traditional lines. Couples in this study also reported decreased marital satisfaction. Such decline is not universal. Belsky and Rovine (1990) found that some couples did experience diminished marital quality, but others reported no change or more satisfaction with their marriage.

There are significant data related to the positive effects of children on the marital relationship. Beginning with the sharing of the birth experience, which may be viewed by some couples as the high point of their lives, parenthood can be a source of mutual sharing and sense of pride for what they have created. Children can create a bond that solidifies the marriage. Marriages in which male children are present are less prone to dissolution, presumably because of fathers' institutionalized role in rearing sons (Morgan, Lye & Condran, 1988).

The couple shares many pleasant experiences with each other as they interact with the child throughout the various developmental phases. Other positive factors include the potential for moving away from traditional sex-role behavior to assist children in what were once considered typically masculine or feminine activities. Additional factors that contribute to marital satisfaction include the potential for fulfillment of personal needs as individuals and the possibility that satisfaction in the parental role may energize performance in other areas, benefiting the marital relationship. Finally, the personal and mutual growth that can result from open communication and resolution of problems focusing on the children, the equalization of power imbalances that may occur, and the reinforcement of commitment to one another may all serve to strengthen the bonds of intimacy (Whitbourne, 1986).

Single-Parent Families

The growth of single-parent families has been dramatic, is continuing, and can be largely attributed to an increasing divorce rate and an increase in never-married mothers (Norton & Glick, 1986). However, single-parent families are diverse forms, sometimes resulting from divorce or separation and sometimes from the choice to have children as a single person. Some single parents have custody of their children, others share custody, and some never see their children at all. Some single parents live heterosexual lifestyles and some homosexual lifestyles. The diversity of family forms, issues, and potential stressors is immediately apparent. Thus, becoming a single parent can also be perceived as a crisis, a life transition, or a critical transition, depending on changes in the family role complex.

Most single parents continue to be women, and consequently much of the research focuses on single mothers' experiences. Most single mothers face financial hardship, with over half living below the poverty level. The situation is even more dramatic for single-parent households headed by minority women and for those with preschool children (Dornbusch & Gray, 1988). Most single mothers are employed, however, and virtually all single fathers, leading to considerable stress as these parents attempt to manage both roles (Burden, 1986).

In a recent study of low-income single mothers, Hall, Gurley, Sachs, and Kruyscio (1991) found that high depressive symptoms occurred with more than half of the women interviewed. Higher depressive symptoms were associated with everyday stressors, fewer social resources, and greater use of avoidance coping. Neither social resources nor coping strategies buffered the relationship between everyday stressors and depressive symptoms. Depressive symptoms predicted parenting attitudes, which in turn predicted child behavior. These findings suggest that considerable attention needs to be directed to low-income single mothers to determine more effective ways to assist them and their children to develop effective coping strategies.

Thomas (1992) notes that noncustodial fathers may encounter difficulties when attempting to implement court-ordered visitation arrangements and may face prolonged, costly legal battles to have court-ordered visitation orders enforced. However, there is an increasing tendency to award custody of children to single fathers. Risman and Park (1988) found that the gender of the custodial parents was unrelated to intimacy in the parent-child bond, the child's development, or division of household duties in single-parent homes. For the most part, single fathers are likely to have better incomes than single mothers. They are older, better educated, and less likely to be living with a relative (Dornbusch & Gray, 1988). The increasing number of single fathers indicates the need for more research in this area to explore the unique facets of this role. Clearly, single parenthood presents considerable challenges. The variant forms of single parenthood preclude a comprehensive overview of the considerable research in this area, but such efforts are essential to encourage the development of effective support services and to influence policy development at the micro and macro level.

Single-Parent Families and Health

There is little information available concerning single-parent families and health. However, based on their analysis of governmental policies, statistics, and related research. Dornbusch and Gray (1988) conclude that the link of single parenthood to poverty, particularly in households headed by women, implies increased health problems, both mental and physical. Single-parent households may be forced to cut back on health-related expenditures more than other groups in our society. It is difficult to find data on the direct impact of single parenthood on the health of family members. Those studies that are available indicate that this may not be the case for many single-parent families. Loveland-Cherry (1986) found no difference between the personal health practices of single-parent families headed by women and the personal health practices of two-parent families. In investigating the characteristics of health in single-parent families, Hanson (1986) found that in general both the physical and the mental health of the male and female single parents and of their children appeared to be good. She found that children living with female parents reported higher overall health than children living with male parents. Boys living with their mothers had the best overall health, whereas girls living with their fathers had the least. Single mothers had poorer overall health than did single fathers. Risman (1986) found that custodial fathers were very concerned about the health of their children, noting that nine out of ten have a family physician and that the majority visit the dentist at least once a year. The majority of these children did not have serious health problems.

Although mothers may assume the role of nurturer and caregiver in conventional families and assume many health-related functions, Risman (1986) states that when males assume full responsibility for child care, they usually develop intimate and affectionate relationships with their children. Therefore, it appears that the situational demands of role requirements influence adult behavior and that both men and women are able to carry out health-related functions as couples or in single-parent families.

Adoption

Parenting, whether mothering or fathering, is often thought of as a role for biologic parents, but adults can become parents through adoption. Just as couples have different reasons for having children, they give a variety of reasons for adopting children. Many adoptions involve stepparents and other relatives, but infertility of one or both partners is another major factor.

In the past, the traditional adoptive family was usually middle or upper class, with the husband working and the wife assuming the homemaker and child care roles. Now, adoptive parents can be of all income levels, be unmarried, have birth children, or be disabled in some way themselves yet meet the standards set by adoptive agencies (Schaffer & Kral, 1988).

Choosing to adopt when infertility has been a problem may involve ambivalent feelings. Only recently have the crisis dimensions of involuntary childlessness begun to be explored. Choosing to become an adoptive parent may necessitate coming to terms with the reality of infertility, which can lead to lower self-esteem.

Advances in technology and the increasing availability of in vitro fertilization programs provide infertile couples with an alternative to adoption. Couples may wish to explore this option prior to considering adoption to determine the feasibility in their situation. Assistance in exploring alternatives and making decisions is available from health professionals, adoption agencies, and mutual self-help or support groups.

Stress and Adoption

Additional stressors faced by adoptive parents include the grim reality of the shortage of available infants and the unknown timetable involved. The unpredictable nature of the adoption process may create its own distress. Bachrach (1986) notes an increase in the number of babies available for adoption since the mid-1970s, a finding that needs to be interpreted with caution, as well as an increase in the number of adoptions. However, adopting couples may find that their experience is unique and that their circle of family and friends have not experienced the stressors involved, nor are they necessarily supportive or encouraging. In some cases, family members may be openly negative, addressing concerns of incompatibility and biologic deficits. These factors add to the anxieties of the adoptive parents, who may need to seek support and assistance outside their circle of family and friends.

In general, societal beliefs about adoption tend to create informal social sanctions that make it difficult to obtain support from other sources as well. In her study of involuntarily childless women's perceptions of societal beliefs about adoption, Miall (1987) found that the majority of women in her sample identified these beliefs as (1) biologic ties are important for love and bonding, and consequently, love and bonding in adoption are second best; (2) adopted children are second rate because of their unknown genetic past; and (3) adoptive parents are not "real" parents. The willingness to select adoption as an alternative or to be successful in the process may be influenced by social values that ultimately affect the self-image of potential adoptive parents. Although some couples may find that their support systems are quite adequate, others may be very stressed by perceived social sanctions and may benefit from involvement with positively oriented professionals and successful adoptive families. Berry (1990) indicates that family, friends, and helping professionals can facilitate adaptive coping by allowing adoptive families to develop their own coping strategies in creative and unconventional ways.

In some situations, adoption may be an expensive process that may create an additional financial strain besides that normally involved in the addition of a child to a household. Financial burdens coupled with anxieties concerning adjustment may place a considerable strain on the couple. However, when the adoption occurs, the need of the couple to parent may be fulfilled, giving them an opportunity to grow as individuals and as a couple (Sell, 1985).

In addition to the many changes incurred in the transition to parenthood, Hultsch and Deutsch (1981) describe the unique situation facing adoptive parents concerning the child's biologic parents. A consistently recurring problem involves the reconciliation of the conflict between the biologic and the social parentage of the child. Concerns about what to tell the child and when, as well as the possible involvement of the child with the biologic parents, may be sources of stress to adopting families. Adoptive parents' concern with successful parenting and the older child's concern about biologic parents may lead to feelings of failure on the part of parents as well as inner conflict for the child. A more recent trend toward reuniting children with biologic parents and more open discussion of the risks and benefits may facilitate future research and decision making in this area. Campbell, Silverman, and Patti (1991) found that adoptees who were reunited with their biological parents experienced greater self-esteem. Their relationship with their adoptive parents was either strengthened or did not change. However, Berry (1991) notes that sharing information or contact between biological and adoptive families is emotional and controversial and concerns balancing rights among three parties.

Social trends and technologic advances, including management of infertility problems, surrogate motherhood, and adoption of children by single adults, add many new dimensions to the concept of adoptive families that are not addressed here but merit consideration in future research. Some attention has also been given to the adoption of children with special needs (Groze & Gruenewald, 1991), and this area is of increasing concern in developing supportive programs for families who undertake this challenge. However, these trends in themselves may be a further indication that regardless of the stress involved in decision making or the transition to the parental role, the joint venture of the parent-child relationship is a rewarding undertaking.

Remarriage

When the previous family life cycle is interrupted by death or divorce, a remarried family must undergo a complex process to stabilize and redefine relationships and roles. Terminology associated with families attempting to negotiate these roles is indicative of the problems and stressors these families encounter. They are referred to as stepfamilies, blended families, or restructured and reconstituted families. Carter and McGoldrick (1988) state that the term *blended* suggests a degree of integration that is rarely possible, while *stepfamily* has a negative connotation. *Reconstituted* or *restructured* gives the connotation that a rearranging of parts is all that is necessary to form the new family. The term *remarried* is suggested because it emphasizes that the marital bond forms the basis for the complex arrangement of several families in a new constellation.

Carter and McGoldrick (1988) identify a family model that would help remarried families to be more successful in dealing with this complex situation. First, they suggest that permeable boundaries should be established around members of different households to permit children to come and go easily according to custody agreements. A second factor is the acceptance of the parental responsibilities of the other spouse without carrying out his or her responsibilities, competing with the parent-child attachment or interaction with the ex-spouse. Finally, they recommend the revision of traditional family gender roles. Rigidly applied traditional roles may be very disruptive in remarried families if sources of income and expenditure are not always within the husband's control (due to alimony and child support) and women are called upon to rear children who may be strangers. This complex family form creates an unusual set of demands on its members, who must relinquish some roles and relationships and take on others, a process requiring considerable time, patience, and recognition of the emotional demands generated.

Stressors Affecting Remarriage

Among the problems specific to remarriages is the complexity of the kinship network and the lack of institutionalized social regulations concerning relationships and social roles. Previously divorced parents acquire additional children while maintaining a parental role with their biologic children, and children acquire an additional parent. Various ties may exist between sets of grandparents and stepfamilies. The situation is complicated by lack of social guidelines, frequently creating a sense of uncertainty and confusion in persons who remarry, especially concerning parenting roles and relationships with grandparents or other blood relatives (Giles-Sims & Crosbie-Burnett, 1989).

Another issue concerns unresolved emotional issues from a prior marriage or divorce. Feelings from the past, such as a sense of abandonment or unresolved grief, may adversely affect the remarriage (Carter & McGoldrick, 1988). In other cases, persons have adjusted well to being single and may have difficulty giving up their independence or may be reluctant to involve a new stepparent in co-parenting issues.

The economic aspect of remarriage may be complicated by obligations for the noncustodial parent or dependency on a former spouse for child support. The economic situation is frequently marked by unpredictability, adding another stressor. Remarriage after a divorce means that a person takes on an additional family, setting up competing rights and responsibilities. Although the legal ties of parent and child continue following divorce, there is no legal definition of the stepparent-stepchild subsystem. These issues are usually left to the discretion of the individuals involved, adding another dimension to role obscurity (Giles-Sims & Crosby-Burnett, 1989)

The joining of households with primary biological ties linking them together suggests that boundary ambiguity and role ambiguity may be another source of stress. A nonresident father may still have decision-making power that influences the functioning of the remarried family. Stepchildren who do not live within the household may still be very much within the boundary due to visitation agreements and the necessary decisions of everyday living. Role ambiguity exists for stepparents and for stepchildren in remarried families. Issues of discipline, loyalty, visitation, and distribution of household tasks are sources of stress related to role ambiguity.

Conflicting life cycle stages are another potential source of stress for remarried families. The newly joined couple may need to have time for themselves, but the presence of children may preclude time alone. On the other hand, the couple may wish to create a cohesive family but adolescent children may be desiring more freedom and time spent with peers. A stepfather who has raised one family may find himself involved with the task of parenting a new baby or very young children. Financial decisions regarding home purchase, vacations, and other economic concerns may conflict with the demands for college tuition or medical care of members from the previous family. The differing life cycle stages present another issue: sexual tension when children, adolescents, and adults of the opposite sex are brought together without benefit of the sexual taboo. This area is very delicate and can be threatening to parents and children alike, creating considerable stress in the family (Crosbie-Burnett, 1989).

Although there is the potential for considerable stress in remarried families, couples committed to a new relationship bring considerable experience to it—and perhaps the hope that the new marriage will be better than the previous one. Researchers have compared satisfaction with initial marriages and remarriages, with conflicting results. A meta-analysis of previous studies concerning marital satisfaction with remarriage indicates greater satisfaction among couples in their first marriage than for remarried couples. However, the difference in levels of satisfaction is small and lacks practical significance. For example, the results do not justify recommending to couples considering remarriage that they give the matter a second thought based on the data (Vemer et al., 1989).

Although findings suggest that remarriage may be problematic, the further question of why remains unresolved. Several reasons have been identified, including family relationships, economic considerations, and the lack of social norms guiding relationships. As further research in this area is undertaken and clinicians deal with the problems affecting remarried families, more definitive answers may emerge.

Remarriage and Family Health

Clearly the potential stressors affecting remarried families and the increasing evidence of decreased marital satisfaction suggest that remarriage may have some effect on the health of both men and women. Research exploring the health of remarried couples has been very sparse. Some research has compared remarried families to first-time married people and found a slightly greater number of physical health deficits and more frequent use of alcohol and drugs (Weingarten, 1980). A later study found no difference between these two groups in mental well-being, however, indicating that further exploration of this area is needed (Fine, Donnelly & Voydanoff, 1986).

Recognizing the sparseness of research concerning remarried families and the lack of information concerning the effect of remarriage on the health of husband and wife, Ganong and Coleman (1991) conducted a study to explore the health of remarried men and remarried women and examine the correlates of health complaints of remarried adults. They found no major health differences between men and women, although women experienced more changes in health complaints overall following remarriage than men did. In general, these researchers found that the health of both men and women was affected most by their feelings toward one another and by having decision-making power within the family. For women, positive feelings toward their spouse and less decision-making power were associated with health, while for men high marital satisfaction and more decision-making power in the family were associated with health. Women also had better health if there were fewer children in the family and if the children were theirs. Ganong and Coleman (1991) concluded that participants in their study did not perceive a decline in their health following remarriage, in spite of the complex stressors involved. However, a relationship did appear to exist between family dynamics and health for the remarried individuals in their study. Further research is indicated to explore the concept of social support in relation to remarriage and health and to integrate objective health measures as opposed to subjective measures. The importance of continued research in this area is indicated given the number of remarriages following divorce and the increasing evidence that more remarriages end in divorce than do first-time marriages (Martin & Bumpass, 1989).

LOSS OF FAMILY MEMBERS

The interpersonal relationships that develop across the periods of a family life cycle have the potential of playing an important role in an individual's identity. Often family relationships exist within the context of an intimate partnership. The intimate relationship joins the separate identities of two persons with intense, durable, and close bonds that are found in very few other social interactions. Because it represents the union of the two identities, the intimate relationship influences the process of identity assimilation and identity accommodation through which each person develops (Whitbourne, 1986). Therefore, the loss of an intimate relationship may have painful and far-reaching effects.

Each marital relationship falls somewhere on the continuum of emotional autonomy and emotional fusion. The greater the fusion between two people, the more one person's attitudes, beliefs, and behavior are influenced by the other, and consequently the degree of self-direction. If emotional fusion is extreme, the loss of one spouse may be followed by total dysfunction in the remaining spouse. A person with more emotional autonomy is likely to be able to negotiate sudden and serious losses of important family members with less stress and a set of self-defined goals after a period of some dysfunction (Beal, 1985).

Divorce and death both disrupt marital relationships, but the consequences may be very different. Widowhood has an institutionalized status. Therefore, when a spouse is lost through death, a different social perspective is given to the definition of becoming single, one frequently accompanied by sympathy and support. Divorce, in contrast, may result in social sanctions and blame laying. With death, the spouse is only psychologically present to affect self-concept, and widowed persons often romanticize the lost spouse. However, with divorce, the spouse can be both psychologically and physically present, and the divorced person can continue to feel guilt, frustration, and anger. There may also be differences based on whether the divorce was desired, the circumstances surrounding it, and whether it leads to a sense of failure. Both may engender a deep, intense feeling of loss. The following discussion concerns both of these transitions in family lives, the sources of stress that accompany them, and successful mechanisms for families to use to cope with these events.

Divorce

Marital separation is a particularly disruptive transition because it is usually accompanied by multiple, drastic changes in the individual's life. It involves the loss of significant others, loss of the role of wife or husband, a change in the routines of living in one's own home, and probable economic loss. In addition, there is sometimes the loss of close friends and the loss of status in the community, resulting in the undermining of an entire family lifestyle (Thomas, 1992).

Given the stressful nature of the divorce transition, considerable attention has been focused on those factors that incline couples to continue or terminate their relationships. Kingsbury and Minda (1988) identified intimacy and love as the best indicators of whether couples will remain together or separate. These affective-type variables were more important than factors such as exchange of resources, conflict tactics, or self-disclosure. Since emotional bonds seem to play a central role in marital relationships, it is important to consider what factors contribute to their deterioration. Kersten (1990) examined the process of marital disaffection to determine if there is a pattern that evolves, to explore how love declines in marriage that may or may not lead to dissolution, and to suggest more effective interventions for spouses experiencing this process.

Marital disaffection is the gradual loss of an emotional attachment, a decline in caring about the partner, an emotional estrangement, and an increasing tendency toward indifference. A positive affect is replaced by a neutral affect in the process of disaffection. Kersten (1990) defines the beginning phase as characterized by feelings of anger, hurt, and disillusionment. The process begins with initial disappointment in the partner, combined with hope that the marriage will improve as attempts are made to solve problems.

The middle phase is characterized by an escalation of hurt and anger as problem-solving attempts yield little change in the partner or the relationship. Increasing apathy occurs during this phase, indicating an eroding of attachment and love of the partner. During the middle phase, thoughts continue to center on the negative evaluation of the partner and the assessment of costs and rewards in the marriage. At this time, there appears to be a more in-depth and complex analysis of the choice of staying or leaving. Barriers to leaving include children, finances, and religious beliefs. Problem-solving attempts continue during the middle phase but are direct and more assertive than initially. Unsuccessful attempts to solve problems lead to emotional, and in some cases physical, withdrawal.

The final phase of the process of disaffection is characterized by anger, a significant decline in feelings of hurt, and a significant increase in apathy. Thoughts of ending the marriage become more real as actions are taken to dissolve the relationship. Hope for the marriage significantly declines as the individual continues to focus on the negative traits of the partner and evaluates the rewards and costs of the marriage and staying versus leaving. During the ending phase, an individual may pursue professional counseling as a last effort to save the marriage. The disaffected spouse may have decided that the marriage is at an end but may need assistance in terminating the relationship. In general, Kersten (1990) found that the disaffected spouses in this study followed a sequence of phases of marital disaffection. Certain thoughts, feelings, and behaviors occurred in each phase in fairly predictable ways.

During the actual phase of separation, Carter and McGoldrick (1988) note that the more reactive the family is, the greater is the crisis. Each spouse may be in a state of emotional vulnerability that can interfere with normal functioning and affect health adversely. Ambivalence is a frequent occurrence, as is lingering attachment, despite anger and resentment. During the stage of separation, each spouse is subject to considerable emotional turmoil, a situation that continues to exist and may take as long as several years to resolve. For those who functioned marginally before the divorce occurred, the separation may increase the difficulties they face. Others may find that the divorce stimulates their growth in a way that was not possible during their marriage.

Sources of Stress

Divorce is viewed as a transitional crisis, forcing an interruption of the developmental tasks usually associated with a family's particular life cycle phase. A series of adjustments related to the separation and divorce occur that may place all family members in a state of disequilibrium for up to three years. The lack of societal support or guidelines for families going through this process adds to the problem. Carter and McGoldrick (1988) suggest that major individual adjustments must be made at two levels: the emotional and the practical. Individuals must deal with the emotional upheavals accompanying various phases of the separation process, as well as adjust to the practicalities of a new life. Many interrelated factors influence the response: the circumstances leading to the marital disaffection and separation, the nature and quality of postseparation life, sex, length of marriage, education, socioeconomic level, ethnic context, prior experience with stress, other stressors that occur simultaneously, and the availability of appropriate support.

Many stressors revolve around changes in intimate family relationships, as well as friendship patterns. The emotional bonding that takes place between mates seems to continue after divorce, creating unsettled, ambivalent feelings. Despite the negative emotions leading up to divorce, many people find that they still have feelings of attachment to their former spouse. These feelings of attachment may hinder adjustment, since reducing such attachment is essential to establishing another relationship or some sort of equilibrium as a single person (Tschann, Johnston & Wallerstein, 1989). In addition, virtually every subsystem within the family is affected, and membership, roles, boundaries, and hierarchical structures are altered. Relationships with all systems outside the nuclear family change as well: extended family, work, school and community. Initially, married friends may be supportive, but there is usually a sharp decline in support, especially for women. The social network of separated people usually shifts from friends who are married to new, single, more casual acquaintances. All of these changes in the absence of social supports and cultural ambiguity may create considerable conflict and added stress (Carter & McGoldrick, 1988).

An additional source of stress concerns the changes in lifestyle that accompany divorce, including a change in socioeconomic status and changes in responsibilities. Frequently, a divorce results in a change of housing, possible relocation, and assumption of different household responsibilities, depending on former role patterns. For both men and women, a shift in work responsibilities may occur as both attempt to make up for the loss of income related to the divorce. For some women, it may mean entering the workforce, and for some men, it may mean increasing their workload in order to meet support payments.

The economic impact of divorce is particularly difficult for women, with many divorced women experiencing significant declines in income and increased rates of poverty. Economic recovery brought about by fiscal reorganization of the household, job seeking, or enhanced careers is not the experience of most women, but it does occur in some cases. Women who are most at risk are those with little education or work experience with large families or young children (Morgan, 1991).

For both mothers and fathers, the assumption of new roles and changes in existing roles is not without a certain degree of stress. The long period of adjustment following divorce is often marked by emotional and behavioral problems in children, adding to parental stress and leading to feelings of anxiety, depression, and decreased self-esteem. The dysfunctional cycle of parent-child relationships during transition may be the result of depressed parents using poor parenting skills, which leads to dysfunctional family relationships both within and outside the system. In spite of the degree of stress involved in the loss of a family through divorce, constructive adjustment over time is possible for both parents and children.

Divorce and Health

The impact of divorce can be considerable for all family members. The increased amount of stress and heightened emotional vulnerability can interfere with normal functioning. In describing the actual period of separation, Carter and McGoldrick (1988) examine some of the commonly experienced symptoms that have been re-

ported, including inability to work effectively, weight changes, insomnia and other sleep disturbances, sexual dysfunction, poor health, and use of alcohol, tobacco, and other substances. Divorce is becoming a significant issue as research links stress and ineffective coping to physical and emotional aspects of health (Monat & Lazarus, 1985).

The effect of divorce on the emotional aspects of health has been explored by Wheaton (1990), who found a significant symptom reduction in distress when marital stress was high before the divorce, indicating that transition out of a stressful role has a beneficial effect on mental health. He suggests that this transition may act as a catharsis that resolves earlier problems but notes that this effect occurs not immediately but after two years have passed. Further, Wheaton states that divorces are not described in the stress literature as having positive benefits to mental health under any circumstances. Baron (1989) explored the relationship between women's causal explanations for divorce and their present emotional health. She found that causal dimensions did predict self-esteem and emotional distress, but only for women who perceived the divorce as personally uncontrollable. Women with greater emotional distress had significantly greater concerns about their overall wellness and energy. Overall, she found that the divorcing women in her study perceived themselves as being only moderately anxious, angry, overwhelmed, and depressed and demonstrated levels of self-esteem comparable to general societal norms. However, she notes that these women had been in the process of divorce for a time and had been coping with various stressors. These studies indicate the need for continued exploration from a longitudinal perspective of the effects of prior role stress, the stress of life transitions, and their relationship to physical and emotional health.

Adjusting to divorce is a long, often difficult process, characterized by functional and dysfunctional responses. Recovery from divorce is characterized by periods of progress and regression, with a general trend of progress viewed as very positive. Although anger, rage, repression, and denial may be appropriate responses initially, as well as sadness and grief, it is destructive to establish a long-term pattern of self-blame, guilt, or anger. Eventually the divorced person must come to accept that the relationship is over. Part of this acceptance rests with the ability to achieve a balanced view of the marriage and to recognize one's contribution to its deterioration. Divorces are most constructive if the process of dissolution leaves neither partner embittered, and punitive measures are avoided.

Reworking the parenting role is often very stressful but contributes significantly to the well-being of children and both partners. Lowery and Settle (1985) suggest that joint custody can help to eliminate the stress experienced by families by decreasing the incidence of other changes associated with divorce. A major focus for both parents should rest with assuring children that both parents still love them, avoiding the use of children as weapons, and discouraging behaviors that foster competition of the children's affection. Johnson (1986) identified certain factors as important to the child's adjustment when used as measures of parental well-being, concluding that the child's adjustment is closely related to parental adjustment. These factors include the emotional unavailability of the parent, the level of family conflict, the ability of the parent to be warm and affectionate, the parent's personal support system, the home organization, and the parental perception of financial well-being and of the presence of other stressors. Therefore, coping mechanisms that increase parental well-being and facilitate effective parent-child interactions can help to promote healthier family interactions following marital separation.

Ultimately, adjustment will be most constructive when the individual uses the opportunity for new growth. This involves making formal and informal contacts with individuals or groups who will provide emotional and material resources and finding sources of meaning in one's life other than one's former partner. Part of this growth process will involve the establishment of a new identity, the development of new roles, and the setting of new goals. The above coping patterns obviously represent the ideal rather than the typical process of adjustment, but they may be helpful in facilitating a positive adaptation under highly stressful circumstances.

Death

Loss of a family member has been identified as a primary area of stress in the lives of most individuals, resulting in disruption of family relationships and blurring of previously established roles. From the perspective of family members left to cope with the loss, death is a major familial concern and an area of primary responsibility. Efforts to determine the degree of stressfulness of life events have been the focus of research over the last decade and have consistently placed death of a family member very high, ranking death of a spouse as the most stressful life event.

Loss of a spouse is often viewed as a problem of older persons, especially of women. This may be attributed to the fact that three out of four women will become widows in this country, with the median age for onset at about 56 years. Women can be expected to live at least another 20 years, and the prospect of remarriage is unlikely since there is only one widower for every five widows, in addition to other detriments. Widows rank financial problems, loneliness, and unfamiliar duties such as home repairs among their greatest problems (Connidis, 1989). Some elderly widows

suffer not only from insufficient income but also lack of familiarity with family finances and financial management (O'Bryant & Morgan, 1989).

Widowers ordinarily have greater financial resources than widows, but they are more likely to have greater difficulty with loneliness and depression. This may be due to the fact that widowers tend to be older, with a majority in their 80s, and they are less likely to be able to cultivate new friendships. This may be due in part to the relative scarcity of same-sex widowed peers (Connidis, 1989). Although earlier studies found a higher incidence of natural death among the recently widowed, particularly in men, McCrae and Costa (1988) found no difference in mortality in a sample of widowed persons aged 25 to 74 when age and education were considered.

Loss of other family relationships can also be very stress producing. For parents, there may be no other stress greater than the loss of a child. Most parents view children as extensions of their dreams and hopes, and the death of a child is excruciating. A child's death is out of place in the family life cycle and may have serious negative effects on the spousal relationship (Carter & McGoldrick, 1988). The loss of a parent can also be a powerful event in shaping the life of a child. Kearl (1989) suggests that such a loss may increase vulnerability and distrust and lead to emotional problems. Anger for abandonment as well as feelings of guilt may occur. In some instances, the death of a parent can be a catalyst leading to the release of creative energy and subsequent accomplishments. Elderly parents' deaths are less disruptive and emotionally debilitating because they may be more predictable events, and adult children may rehearse the event as their parents grow frail (Norris & Murrell, 1990). The effects of dying on the family are personal, practical, legal, economic, psychologic, and social. They can be growth producing or destructive, positive or negative; they are usually profound.

Numerous variables affect familial response to death, including relationships, roles, support structures, and approach to management of family crisis. Many family adjustment difficulties and emotional reactions occur due to the lack of openness in the system. Openness implies that each family member is able to stay nonreactive to the emotional intensity in the system and to communicate feelings to others without expecting the others to act on them. The longer and more intense the degree of stress is, however, the less likely it is that a family will be able to remain well differentiated and communicate openly. The nature of death may isolate family members from external support networks such as work and social activities, further closing the system. Families that can communicate openly with one another, share information and options, and use support from other sources seem to stabilize better after the death of a member (Carter & McGoldrick, 1988).

Sources of Stress

Once the initial activities following the death of a family member have subsided, the attention of the family is turned to coping with the reality of the present and everyday living. A major stressor is the need to reapportion roles and establish boundaries. Some of the role tasks are instrumental and include financial management, transportation, and household tasks. Others are more expressive and include providing emotional support, a sense of security, and feelings of acceptance and belonging. Role reorganization is dependent on those vacated by the death of a family member and the ability of the remaining members to reapportion those roles successfully. At times it may be necessary to solicit the assistance of people outside the family or extended family members to fill roles, even temporarily, until the family is able to adjust satisfactorily.

Another basic stressor is that of loneliness and the lack of companionship that may result from the loss of a family member, depending on the intensity of the relationship and the daily involvement with the deceased (Connidis, 1989). Well-meaning friends may be available less frequently as they become impatient or uncomfortable with conversation about the deceased or bored with repeated anecdotes of the past. Parents who have experienced the death of a child may be lost without the daily involvement of child care, the parenting activities, or the social involvement with other parents. Widows and widowers may feel uncomfortable in joint activities with couples and out of place in a singles group. Family relationships may also be strained, adding to a sense of isolation as problems occur over interactions with children or a surviving parent or over property, legacies, and lifestyles.

Another stressor relates to working out practical living arrangements and managing the financial situation. For some, living with memories in the same home may be reassuring and healing, whereas for others it may be an intolerable burden. The changed reality of this situation may encourage families to make radical changes in lifestyle with insufficient preplanning or evaluation of consequences.

In addition, there may be an altered financial status due to the loss of a wage earner, health care costs, a poorly managed business, or numerous other factors. In some situations, lack of assets may not be the difficulty, but successful management in times of severe grief may be very difficult, whether it relates to settling an estate or simply going to work every day (O'Bryant & Morgan, 1989). Realignment of family roles, adjusting to loneliness and loss of companionship, and working out satisfactory living arrangements are some of the major stressors that confront families as they attempt to deal with loss of a family member. Families are able to mobilize their resources and successfully adjust over time, but readjustment is characterized by advances and retreats as family members encounter turning points and deal with the other situational and developmental stressors.

Coping, Adaptation, and Health

An open, functional family system is growth producing, integrative in blending the past and future realistically, and positive, because its members are able to work through the content of grief. Family reorganization and mobilization of resources are characterized as flexible, dynamic, and adaptable. The system must be flexible enough to adapt to the many changes family members will encounter and dynamic enough to flourish and grow as a result of their experience with loss.

Specific coping strategies for persons experiencing bereavement include keeping busy but not acting too hastily; accepting strong feelings and expressing them; participating in social groups and learning new skills; praying; reviewing the death; and maintaining ties to the deceased family member by recalling happy memories or sensing the presence of the deceased (Gass, 1987). Keeping a journal is an effective coping strategy for some because it serves as a mechanism for reviewing the death, expressing sorrow or other feelings, recalling happy times, and maintaining ties to the deceased. Thielman and Melges (1986) analyzed a widow's diary from the nineteenth century and found that coping strategies are associated with the culture and period in which one lives. They identified three strategies for coping: ritualized language that structures and redefines painful and distressing thoughts, associating the experience of loss to the larger Christian meaning of death; time marking, which includes annual commemoration and provides time for expressing feelings; and cognitive reframing, which transforms the loss into a new realization of personal meaning. Other effective coping mechanisms have been identified by Heinemann and Evans (1990), including attendance at support groups and the use of family, friends, and others who have experienced a similar loss. Pet ownership may be a source of companionship, a stimulus for activity, and a source of interaction. Gass (1987) identified some coping strategies that were not perceived as helpful in the course of normal grieving: taking medications (e.g., antidepressants, tranquilizers, sedatives), using alcohol, excessive sleep, avoiding others or getting angry with them, using fantasy, and bargaining with God or with oneself.

Coping and adaptation to the death of a spouse, identified as the life event associated with the greatest degree of stress, takes place over a longer period of time than previously identified and may have a significant effect on health and well-being. With regard to psychological well-being, Heinemann and Evans (1990) found that it takes from 2 to 11 or more years before the average scores of married women and widows are no longer significantly different. They also found that regardless of age, psychological health outcomes improve as length of time widowed increases, but relatively young widows are vulnerable to poor psychological health outcomes over time in comparison to their married counterparts. Many of the differences between married and widowed women with regard to health outcomes are related to inadequate financial resources. Women in their 70s who have lost their spouse within the past two years are another vulnerable group; the death of the spouse has an impact on their psychological health, with considerable intensity in the grief and mourning phase of coping and adaptation. Thus, age of occurrence and economic resources may have an effect on successful coping and adaptation.

Another view of psychosocial health dysfunction among spouses experiencing bereavement is described by Gass and Chang (1989). They explored problem-focused and emotion-focused coping strategies and found that they coexist and are used to manage stressful situations. Problem-focused strategies deal with problem-solving efforts that alter or manage problems associated with bereavement. Emotion-focused coping strategies are designed to reduce or manage emotional distress. Problem-focused strategies are more adaptive and reality oriented; emotion-focused coping strategies often prevent the person from confronting the reality of the situation by denying or avoiding it or wishing things were different. Gass and Chang (1989) found that lower threat appraisal, more problem-focused and less emotion-focused coping, greater resource strength, and younger age had direct effects on reducing psychosocial health dysfunction. Higher threat appraisal influenced the use of more problem- and emotion-focused coping strategies, while greater resource strength influenced lower threat appraisal. The results of these studies suggest that further research is indicated to assist health professionals in predicting the psychosocial health dysfunction of the bereaved and to help them to adjust. For the most part, health professionals should be able to empathize with bereaved persons, to understand that the grieving process can affect their health and recuperative process, and to facilitate the person's own potential for coping and adapting.

ILLNESS IN THE FAMILY

The onset of serious illness is a particularly dramatic crisis for the family because it adds a set of strains and hardships that interact with the normative changes most families experience. High levels of stress are generated, and constant adaptation is required by family members. Although a family may have standard ways of coping with any illness, there may be critical differences in their adaptation style and degree of success in coping with different disease processes (Rolland, 1988a). Illness may manifest in acute or chronic forms, necessitating temporary or long-term adjustments on the part of families as they redefine roles and attempt to accommodate necessary changes. Although chronic illness may be more difficult to adapt to than acute illness, the family's response to chronic illness may depend on the nature of the illness itself, as well as on the demands perceived by family members (Woods, Yates & Primomo, 1989; Hymovich & Hagopian, 1992).

Chronic illness, which has emerged as a major health problem in the United States, is defined as "the irreversible presence, accumulation, or latency of disease states or impairments that involve the total human environment for supportive care and self care, maintenance of function and prevention of further disability" (Lubkin, 1986, p. 6). At the same time, health care costs are soaring, resulting in greater levels of acuity, both on admission and on discharge, and shorter hospital stays. This means that the burden of care of people who are unable to function independently rests with family members, except in times of crisis or major complications. Over 6 million people have varying degrees of mobility problems, ranging from being confined to their homes to having difficulty in moving about freely. In addition, nearly half of the noninstitutionalized persons aged 65 years and older are limited by at least one chronic condition. All of these factors have a direct impact on the demands placed on family caregivers who provide assistance with activities of daily living, vigilance, monitoring of medication, and social support (Biegel, Sales & Schulz, 1991).

The number of dependent people of all ages is increasing, ranging from infants with birth defects to the frail elderly, now living into their 90s. As the degree of their impairment grows, the demands on families increase in terms of time, energy, emotional commitment, and financial resources. In most cases, families cannot assume the burden of long-term care without some assistance in negotiating the health care system and in maintaining the family structure. Many factors affect the ability of families to care for dependent members and merit consideration from a social and individual family perspective.

Social Factors Influencing Family Care of Dependent Members

Families have always cared for their dependent members, but recent demographic, economic, and social changes may affect the ability of families to provide such care, particularly in the home setting (Figure 20–2). Life expectancy and the aging of the population have increased dramatically during this century, leading to a large increase in the

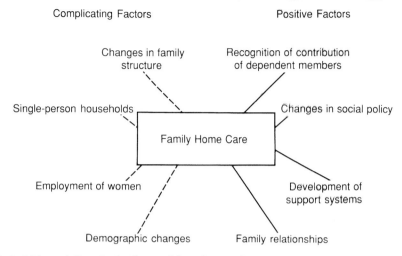

FIGURE 20–2. Social factors influencing family care of dependent members.

elderly population. The oldest cohort, those 85 years and older, is growing the fastest. This group is more likely to be at high risk for chronic illness, is characterized by greater functional dependency, and has the greatest need for health and social services (Beigel, Sales & Schulz, 1991). These changing demographics have led to the development of multigenerational families, with persons over age 60 sometimes responsible for their own aging parents, and some middle-aged persons responsible for two older generations. A recent survey conducted by the American Association of Retired Persons (1989) found that 20% of the respondents who identified themselves as primary caregivers were over 65 years of age.

Other changes that may influence family care of dependent members include the change in family structures due to declining fertility rates and increasing divorce rates. The total number of births is expected to decrease by 9.2% during the 1990s while the elderly population is expected to increase by 10%, indicating that there will be fewer children and siblings to share the burden of caring for dependent members (Older Women's League, 1989). Divorce rates have also increased over the past 20 years, as have remarriages, leading to a growing number of blended families. Thus, adult children may have multiple responsibilities for caregiving for former and present in-laws as well as their own parents. On the other hand, divorced children faced with multiple responsibilities, including single-parent obligations, may have less time and emotional energy for additional caregiving responsibilities (Biegel, Sales & Schulz 1991). The possibility of fewer people in the network raises concerns about social support for and isolation of dependent members. However, Chappell and Badger (1989) found that marital status and living arrangements are not related to subjective well-being, nor is having children. What does

seem to be important is companionship and the presence of confidants, which can be provided in other types of relationships such as friendships.

Another factor that threatens the capacity of the family to care for ill members is the rising employment of women, traditionally the caregivers of the disabled and the ill and with the chief responsibility for home care (Biegel, Sales & Schulz 1991). Over 55% of women were part of the civilian workforce by the mid-1980s (U.S. Bureau of the Census, 1987). Doty (1986) reviewed the literature in an attempt to determine the actual impact of women's employment on caregiving roles. Conflicting findings indicate that some women report diminished capacity for home care of relatives due to employment, while the results of other studies indicate no difference in the likelihood of providing care by working and nonworking caregivers. There is some concern regarding the multiple role responsibilities of women as wife, mother, and caregiver. Employment is another responsibility to be added and managed, probably at considerable cost to women who are expected to assume caregiving functions. Issues of how women manage work and caregiving and the impact of work on the purchase of caregiving services are issues that need further exploration.

Economic pressures and changes in the reimbursement structures in the health care system have put additional pressure on family caregivers. Shorter hospital stays and lack of coverage for long-term care in institutional or home settings have created considerable challenges for family members. Administration of medications, management of assistive devices, monitoring of the medical regime, and support of the activities of daily living may all be within the scope of family caregivers' responsibilities. Traditionally, there has been little government support for family caregiving functions or efforts unless family members were unable to provide care or when family resources were nonexistent. However, with the rising costs of institutional care, some states have instituted policies that support home care through tax supports and direct payment program. Although there has been considerable activity at the state level to support home care, few evaluations have been conducted (Linsk, Keigher & Osterbusch, 1988). Clearly, family caregivers provide significant amounts of assistance to dependent family members while managing competing demands. The multiple responsibilities coupled with lower incomes and lower self-reports of health indicate the need for supportive services, but availability of and access to such services continues to pose a social challenge (Biegel, Sales & Schulz 1991).

Although these demographic, social, and economic forces can impede the ability of families to care for dependent members, positive forces also exist that sustain the willingness and ability of family members to care for disabled members over protracted periods of time: increased recognition of the demands of the caregiver role and its impact on caregiver health status, trends in social policy that provide some support for family caregivers, and the development of support systems for families experiencing the stress of acute or chronic health problems in one of their members.

Stressors Influencing Family Care of Dependent Members

The typical family in our culture is a self-contained system that tends to be somewhat isolated and frequently depends on its own resources; it has few remedies for inadequate role performance and few resources to meet financial and medical emergencies. Although the stress of an acute illness can be significant, particularly if hospitalization is required, families who must manage a prolonged situation or deal with chronic illness throughout a significant period of time must be able to exert continuous effort. Rolland (1988b; 1988b) notes that while both gradual and acute onset illnesses may require major adjustments, acute situations require families to make both instrumental and affective changes relatively quickly. Illnesses with a more gradual onset allow for a greater period of adjustment, although considerable anxiety may occur due to a delay in diagnosis.

Among the stressors these families face are those related to role diffusion and discontinuity. Certain roles may be left unfilled or assumed by others on a shifting, inadequately defined basis. If the need for change is temporary, role allocation may return to its previously defined status. In the case of prolonged illness or death, families may experience chronic disorganization characterized by a lack of distinction between roles. Maladaptation may occur when family members sacrifice

personal development and growth, and the family's overall sense of order, coherence, and well-being drops (McCubbin & McCubbin, 1993).

Modifications of family activities and goals may need to occur. There may be reduced options in terms of career development and reduced flexibility in the use of leisure time. Vacations and short trips away from home may be unavailable options for families with dependent members. Worry and uncertainty may impede the ability of the family to plan for the future, both immediate and over the long term. Advanced planning is frequently relegated to the last minute, pending the condition of the ill or disabled family member.

Role strain may occur when individuals have difficulty meeting others' expectations and fulfilling obligations included in the various roles they accept (Fife, 1985). Providing direct care or being in a supportive role requires additional time commitments as extra tasks are undertaken. Hospitalizations result in family separation and the additional burden of travel time, visiting time, and time required for interacting with health care professionals. Home care may result in the additional tasks of personal care, daily treatments and therapies, appointments related to health care, and the preparation of special diets.

Social isolation may occur for a variety of reasons, decreasing the support available to families. At times, the reaction of relatives and friends or their expectations may be a limiting factor, or there may be embarrassment if visible abnormalities or mental dysfunction are present. Limited mobility or the unavailability of respite care may further impede socialization, making it impossible for family members to socialize together, if at all. Fear of accidents or exposure to infections or conditions that might exacerbate the illness may also place limitations on social life (Biegel, Sales & Schulz, 1991).

Increasing financial burdens frequently occur due to hospitalizations, medications, and equipment and therapy needs with variability of insurance coverage. Housing adaptation may also be required to accommodate needs for personal space, privacy, and special physical needs. As the situation is prolonged or stretches into a permanent situation, financial resources can be maximally strained, adding to family distress.

Health concerns may become a major focus for families as they attempt to obtain competent care and understanding and to clarify and verify medical information. Additional stress is involved in attempting to follow through with the prescribed medical regime and support the ill person. Families are also concerned about helping the ill or disabled person adjust to pain, a degree of dependency, and an altered lifestyle. They are also concerned about the prognosis, the present and future expectations of the family, and their own ability to cope successfully with the crisis of illness on a long-term basis. Grief is a common response as family members realize that a loved person will not maximize his or her potential (in the case of a young person) or will be unable to fulfill former roles (in the case of an older person).

Overall responses to caregiving have been negatively conceptualized as burdens, strains or stressors that produce negative psychological responses. Given, Stommel, Collins, King, and Given (1990) organize caregiver responses into four general categories. First, there are overall negative emotional reactions to the caregiving situation, which include future view, quality of life, and negative comparisons with other persons of age and gender. Second, caregivers experience role responsibilities and associate importance and meaning with these activities. Spouses may perform these roles out of personal commitment and a sense of moral obligation. Third, the demands of caregiving may lead other family members to withdraw from the process, leading caregivers to feel abandoned. Finally, caregiving intrudes on the daily lives of caregivers, including social activities and time for self and family relationships. The prolonged demands of caregiving may also affect the health and well-being of the primary caregiver, diminishing life satisfaction and potentially contributing to the development of stress-related illnesses.

Family Adaptation to Illness

Families who experience the illness of a member engage in a variety of coping and problem-solving approaches to reduce stress, obtain additional resources, and manage the ongoing tension within the family system. McCubbin and McCubbin (1993) have developed the Resiliency Model of Family Stress, Adjustment, and Adaptation, which characterizes the family system as a resource-exchange network in which problem solving and coping occur. They define family coping as involving coordinated problem-solving behavior of the whole system, as well as the complementary efforts of individual family members that fit together in a synergistic whole. In situations of illness and the accompanying stress, the function of coping is to maintain and restore the balance between demands and resources and reduce or eliminate the intensity of the illness. Coping facilitates adaptation to illness in a variety of ways.

According to McCubbin and McCubbin (1993), coping may involve direct action to decrease the intensity of the demands generated by the illness. For example, the family may seek the assistance of a respite care program, such as adult day care, to facilitate family functioning and reduce the pressure of constant care. In addition, family coping may be directed toward acquiring additional resources to improve their ability to function effectively. These resources may be directed to enhancing the skills and abilities of individual

members or providing social support. On the other hand, such resources may be directed toward meeting the specific needs of the ill member. Coping also facilitates family adaptation to illness through strategies directed toward managing the tension that occurs due to the ongoing demands placed on the family system. Frequently used approaches to managing the tension include talking and sharing experiences, using humor, openly expressing emotion in a constructive manner, and engaging in physical exercise. Finally, coping may involve family-level appraisal to interpret, create, and explore meanings related to the situation to make it more acceptable (Hymovich & Hagopian, 1992). Coping strategies may include changing individual family members or the total family schema of the situation, and using reframing techniques to relabel situations to reflect different, more acceptable meanings. A key appraisal-oriented coping strategy is maintaining an optimistic outlook and reaffirming the perspective that family members are doing the best they can under the circumstances.

Effective coping strategies facilitate synergizing, interfacing, and compromising, which are vital components necessary to achieve family adaptation. Successful family adaptation is achieved when the family's schema and patterns of functioning are congruent and when the growth and development of individual members are supported and family integrity is achieved. McCubbin and McCubbin (1993) maintain that it is not sufficient for families to restructure internally; they must also have a mutually supportive interface with the community. Finally, families successfully adapt to illness of a member through developing a shared sense of cohesion.

Crises of acute illness in the family or the prolonged strain engendered by chronic illness affords nurses and other health care professionals the opportunity to assess the degree to which the family has adapted and to facilitate the development of successful coping strategies. Health care providers can help families to improve problem-solving skills and mobilize resources for social support. Of prime importance is the role of the health care provider in helping family members to improve interpersonal relationships and enhance family well-being.

CHANGES IN FAMILY ROLES

Retirement

For most people, their place of employment and the activities involved in their work interact significantly with their identities. Occupation affects leisure time, friendships, hobbies, values, choice of residential location, financial well-being, social class, and social status. Although retirement does not represent a major life crisis for many men and women, it undoubtedly changes the individual's financial status, social relationships, and lifestyle. Retirement is frequently seen as a transition point since it marks the end of full-time work and the beginning of a period of relative leisure. Although many persons are content to retire in their 60s or 70s, a substantial number of persons continue to work part time by choice or economic necessity (Thomas, 1992). In any event, the decision to retire has many important ramifications and requires substantial adjustment in individual roles and family relationships. Retirees need to develop new approaches to active involvement and consider ways to fill a sizable time void. Achievements and commitments must be reevaluated, and one's outlook on life needs to be reconsidered in the light of role and lifestyle changes. Since health is an important consideration, a sense of health maintenance is essential for retirement planning and subsequent enactment (Antonovsky & Sagy, 1990).

Family relationships also merit some consideration, especially in dual-career families if one spouse chooses to retire and the other does not. When viewed as a transitional process, retirement encompasses the preparation phase, the event itself, and the adjustment phase.

Retirement may be one of the most crucial adjustments older persons face. A series of work-connected role changes must occur, and a sizable time void must now be filled with other activities. These adjustments must be made both by men and by women as they leave active work positions in which they have invested significant energy over time. If a spouse has been employed and now retires, or if both spouses retire, or if one remains employed and the other retires, significant adjustments must also be made in family roles and role relationships (Golan, 1986).

The Preparation Phase

The decision to retire may occur in a variety of different contexts. It may be a planned, systematic, voluntary decision; the result of ill health or illness of another family member; or the realization that one is no longer able to deal effectively with work requirements. For some, it may result from an involuntary process based on policy definitions or from the elimination of a position due to corporate restructuring. Ruhm (1989) reviewed the research on the labor force patterns of older adults and found that worsening health explained only a small fraction of the decline in labor force activity and that most persons choose when to retire, responding to economic incentives. The process of decision making has a great deal of variability depending on the context, and in some cases complications may result. When the decision to retire must be made before the individual is ready, before the family is able to reorient itself, or in the face of serious economic consequences,

the stress of the transition may take different forms from an anticipated desired event.

The responses to the prospect of retirement range from the view that retirement is a kind of social death, to ambivalence, to the view of a retirement as a wholly positive event. Karp (1989) explored the decade of the 50s as a point of transition in the development of professionals' consciousness about retirement. He assumed that the retirement process included a preretirement period and that one's feelings about retirement are formulated over many years. In examining the work contingencies influencing whether respondents anticipated retirement positively, Karp found that those who have unfinished agendas at work, have high job satisfaction, perceive retirement as financially unfeasible, and retain their health are least likely to anticipate retirement favorably. The results of this study have implications for further research in that many studies of adjustment to retirement have failed to consider previous attitudes people hold concerning the meaning of retirement in their lives and to explore the connection. Karp maintains that if retirement's the continuous process postulated, then researchers must adopt strategies that permit the documentation of the elements of that process.

Considerable anecdotal evidence encompasses fears about retirement, including concern about premature death. Such fears can be attributed to a cultural ideology that celebrates work as a source of self-worth and personal fulfillment, the tendency to see a prominent life event as the cause of change in health and overgeneralization from selective observations regarding retirement and negative occurrences. Fretz, Kluge, Ossana, Jones, and Merikangas (1989) examined the predictors of anxiety and depression about retirement and found that the best predictors of preretirement worry were a low sense of self-efficacy and a low degree of planfulness. Both were significant factors in addition to concerns about money or health. The low sense of self-efficacy includes a lower degree of planfulness, less accurate information on aging and retirement, less positive attitudes about retirement, less social support from others, and more commitment to one's job. They also noted no significant differences between those currently eligible for retirement and those two to three years from retirement. The results suggest a need for reconceptualizing the overall goal of preretirement programs beyond information providing to helping retirees to increase their own degree of planfulness and their own sense of ability to cope with impending transition.

Preretirement programs can be a very helpful approach to preparing for retirement, particularly when they encompass psychosocial and health issues as well as information concerning financial and legal issues. Ferraro (1990) notes that fewer than 10% of workers participate in these programs, however. Effective informal types of preparation exist outside formal programs and may include discussing retirement with friends and family; increasing one's knowledge about retirement, health, aging, and leisure-oriented lifestyle; and developing hobbies and interests outside the work environment. Additional aspects of preparation may include financial planning, decision making about relocation, preparing a will, and making arrangements for long-term care and health care decisions in the event of incapacity. Informal retirement planning may be affected by ethnicity and degree of education, with members of minority groups and those with less education participating less frequently (Ferraro, 1990). As with formal preretirement programs, those who might particularly benefit from informal planning are less likely to be involved. Retirement preparation involves significant differences in readiness, attitudes, and planfulness as well as differences in receptiveness to and availability of preretirement programs.

Adjustment to Retirement

Successful adjustment to retirement involves many aspects, including the factors leading to retirement, family relationships, cohort differences, and attitudinal factors. Antonosvky and Sagy (1990) identify four developmental tasks that confront increasing numbers of persons in Western society who are going through the retirement transition: active involvement, reevaluation of life satisfaction, reevaluation of a worldview, and a sense of health maintenance.

Active involvement concerns a reorganization of one's hierarchy of personal goals, including different ways of spending time. The dominant cultural values of Western societies place a premium on overt and evident active involvement in life. Work activity is viewed as a source of social legitimacy. If work activity has been a legitimating activity, then retirement poses distinct challenges. The second task involves reevaluation of life satisfaction. Retirement involves a formidable restructuring of life for most people in terms of family, social relations, spiritual life, and economic situation. The time structure of interaction changes radically, and one is confronted with what one wants to do as opposed to what worklife has required one to do. Retirement is a developmental transition that is likely to bring to the surface consideration of the degree to which one feels satisfied in the central areas of life. The third developmental challenge of retirement concerns the reevaluation of a worldview—the linkages between a person and his or her world. The familiar stimuli of one's work-life, including time structure, persons, tasks, and social role definition are replaced by multiple new stimuli. The resources used to cope with life demands previously may not be appropriate to the new ones. Persons who are retiring are faced with the issue of how to go

about constructing a new social world if they can or wish to. The fourth developmental task, the sense of health maintenance, has no formal link to retirement, but the issue of health becomes more personally significant as rates of morbidity and mortality increase among peers. Such an increase comes to the fore during the same period as "on-time" retirement. The challenge that confronts the individual concerns defining oneself as a person who will suffer a decline in health within a short period or one who will live and be well. Thus, retirement forces consideration of the issue of health vulnerability. Antovonsky and Sagy (1990) suggest that these tasks are issues before and after retirement, but they have a high degree of salience and poignancy and of centrality and criticalness at this time. Although this approach provides a firm basis for empirical research, it raises questions about whether coping with these tasks makes a significant contribution to wholeness in one's life, what factors influence coping, and whether gender, profession, or other variables influence successful coping.

Successful adjustment to retirement seems to be most consistently related to health, a comfortable retirement income, and social involvement. In addition, the individual's feelings about work are important factors. Men for whom work is not as important as other roles have a higher morale in retirement, while the saliency of work role is not related to women's morale (Matthews & Brown, 1987). Women may differ in their retirement experience from men due to an interrupted or delayed entry into the workforce and the occurrence of retirement at a different career phase. Single women are as likely as men to retire early, whereas married women—the larger portion of the female workforce—are unlikely to do so (Belgrave, 1988). In general, the retirement of a married woman is closely tied to the time of her husband's retirement (Hayward, Grady & McLaughlin, 1988). Predictors of retirement satisfaction among married women include financial adequacy and the frequency of support from friends; maintenance of preretirement friendships and frequency of contact with friends are important predictors of retirement satisfaction for widows (Dorfman & Moffett, 1987). Women are often called on to retire because of the illness of a spouse or parents who need help rather than at the preferred time. Belgrave (1988) noted that women are more often engaged in volunteer work than men, and more work part time. Considerable research is needed to explore the critical variables that may reveal gender differences, including the lower retirement benefits of women based on lower income.

Considerable retirement research reflects the white male experience, but more recent attention has focused on the retirement experience of African-Americans. Belgrave (1988) found that African-American women are less likely than white women to retire early and are more likely to have worked throughout adulthood. An ambiguous retirement status was identified by Gibson (1988), who found that a group of African-Americans are aged 55 and older and do not work but do not identify themselves as retired. Many have never had a full-time job, having experienced discontinuous patterns of labor force involvement. They continue to work sporadically as they grow older and are usually poor and poorly educated. The experiences of Mexican-Americans may parallel the labor market experiences of African-Americans, and the pattern of the "unretired retired" may emerge in these communities as well (Zsembik & Singer, 1990). Cultural, ethnic, gender, and economic variables merit further exploration concerning their effect on the process of adjustment to retirement.

Retirement adjustment can also be significantly affected by family relationships, and it can bring to the surface issues that have been obscured by occupational pursuits and childrearing. Although there has been some evidence that wives felt that their husband's retirement interfered with their personal activities, Vinick and Ekerdt (1989) found no studies that identified retirement as having a strong negative impact on the quality of a marriage. Adjustment issues are usually short-lived and may center on time impingement or unrealistic expectations of the spouse. Factors that may have negative consequences are illnesses or disabilities that impair the ability of one spouse and limit his or her participation in preplanned retirement activities. In a study of middle-income families, Vinick and Ekerdt (1989) found that almost half of them had an adult child living in the home, while others assumed the responsibility of caring for an aging parent. Retired couples found their plans and dreams altered by continuing responsibilities to generations both above and below. Thus, family relationships can be a major factor in contributing to a successful transition or can be major stressors that necessitate additional adjustment, support, and resources.

Retirement and Health

Issues concerning health and retirement have been explored from a variety of perspectives, including health limitations as a cause for retirement, health as a contributing factor to successful retirement, and the effect of retirement on health. Ruhm (1989) reviewed the literature concerning the decision to stop working and found that virtually all studies reviewed during the decade of the 80s reveal that retirement probabilities increase as self-assessed health status declines. However, self-classifications of health may be systematically self-biased in ways that overestimate its impact on labor force participation for two reasons. Poor health may be a more socially acceptable reason for retirement than preference for leisure, and poor health may be prerequisite for obtaining some benefit (disability insurance, early retirement, etc.). In spite of the limitations of self-assessed measures of health, declining health does contribute to small reductions in labor force participation, although economic and demographic variables are much more important.

Studies conducted over the past three decades indicate that retirement increases neither health deterioration nor risk of death. However, the notion that retirement harms health has persisted in the popular and health care literature and can influence professionals' approaches to persons of retirement age. Ekerdt (1987) attributes the persistence of this myth of aging to anecdotal reports from persons who may not be familiar with factors leading to retirement decisions or from health care professionals who overgeneralize from their experience with clients, and the tendency of people to overlook cumulative and interactive events in favor of a big event as a causative factor. In addition, negative views of retirement are consistent with a social view that identifies work as the source of personal fulfillment and identity, while retirement is portrayed as the inverse, eventually leading to health deterioration. Two theoretical perspectives also have encouraged the expectation that retirement negatively affects health: the early "activity theory" of aging, which equated successful aging with full social integration and participation, and the "stressful life events" paradigm, which focused additional attention on life stress as a factor increasing susceptibility to illness. Although retirement has been found to be stressful, it has not been shown to be stressful to the point of causing illness. While investigators have consistently concluded that retirement has no adverse impact on health, existing studies are regarded with some reservation due to limitations in design, sample, instrumentation, or other methodological flaws. This leads to continued speculation that retirement may influence health and that findings lack credibility, continuing the persistent notion that retirement may adversely affect health.

In a recent study of the retirement attitudes and health status of preretired and retired men and women, Daly and Futrell (1989) found that men and women did not differ on the three health components of symptoms, emotion, and social health. However, differences were found on physical health scores: men perceived their capacity to function physically at a higher level than did women. Several health dimensions varied by respondents' retirement status in that retirees experienced more symptoms and less optimal physical and social health than those preretired. Neither participants' age nor their retirement age were significantly related to the health dimension scores. Retirement attitude exerted significant effects in four dimensions of retired women's and men's health and in two dimensions of preretired women's and men's health—symptoms and emotional health—but it had virtually no effect on preretired women's physical and social health. The authors conclude that retirement attitudes play an important role in health and well-being.

Although resources concerning health status and retirement are somewhat ambiguous concerning the effect of health on the adjustment to retirement and the effect of retirement on health, the importance of both cannot be negated as families in later life adjust role requirements in relationships to life transitions. Perhaps the best approach to ensuring the health and adaptation of families to retirement in the future is the encouragement of effective health promotion activities in the preretirement years and realistic planning for the transition from active employment.

Unemployment

Sudden, unpredictable loss of employment has devastating effects on individuals and families because it adds a dimension of stress without opportunity for psychologic or financial preparation. Thomas (1992) states that unemployment may have effects on the mental and physical health of individuals and on family relationships and stability. Unemployment can lead to stress-related health problems such as elevated blood pressure, pulse rate, and cholesterol levels. Psychologically, unemployment is associated with feelings of anger, guilt, grief, loss, anxiety, reduced self-esteem, and depression. Middlebrook and Clark (1991) compared the emotional state of laid-off employees to the stages of grief experienced when a loved one dies. The experience of losing one's job may have multiple consequences since the work role may be a source of social integration and a structuring mechanism for daily living.

Hamilton, Broman, and Hoffman (1990) conducted a study of autoworkers from closing and nonclosing plants approximately three months before scheduled plant closings. Results revealed a pattern of interaction between unemployment and demographic variables, showing differential vulnerability to job loss. Less-educated blacks were particularly affected, and their more distressed mental health could not be attributed entirely to other prior stressors.

Reaction to unemployment varies with age, just as degree of job satisfaction is associated with age differences. Men in their 30s and 40s expressed greater distress than men in their teens and early 20s. They also expressed more employment commitment than did younger men (Rowley & Feather, 1987). Contrary to gender stereotypes that portray women as less traumatized by job loss than men, Leana and Feldman (1991) found no significant difference between women and men in psychological and behavior stress symptoms.

Patterns of Response

Various aspects of family life are seriously threatened with problems developing in relation to spending behavior, division of labor, parental authority, marital power, and, at times, family violence. The results of unemployment usually create financial hardship, ranging from insufficient income to serious economic deprivation. It also means the loss of a major role that has social value and is deemed essential by traditionalists and those whose profession is part of the identity.

Families differ in their ability to cope with sudden unemployment, depending on their perception of the event and their ability to mobilize resources. If unemployment is seasonal, is predictable, has a specified duration, or has occurred before, families may define the event somewhat differently and may encounter less stress. Anticipation of a layoff or termination can also be very detrimental to workers and their families but may lead to decreased stress after the job loss actually occurs. Wheaton (1990) found that in every marital status/sex combination except unmarried women, a high level of prior work problems has an ameliorative effect on the impact of job loss in most age groups. His findings indicate that life transitions are not always inherently stressful and there is a need to consider prior social circumstances.

In general, families of unemployed workers are characterized by more interpersonal problems than families of employed individuals (Shelton, 1985). The unemployed individual suffers as do other family members. Spouses may be particularly vulnerable since they may act as a source of social support and be particularly vulnerable to shifts in family roles. Penkower, Bromet, and Dew (1988) found that women whose spouses were continually or intermittently unemployed over a two-year period suffered considerably more stress than women whose husbands were continually employed. Although spouses share the trauma of unemployment, the marital relationship is an important stress buffer for unemployed persons (Liem & Liem, 1988).

Children may also be vulnerable if a parent becomes unemployed. Jones (1990) reviewed the research linking child abuse with unemployment and found various explanations for the linkage. They included economic stress, deterioration of the psychological state of the unemployed person, a loss of the breadwinner's status, and an increase in alcohol and substance abuse as outcomes of job loss. Other factors included the provision of child care by unemployed fathers, increased family isolation, and higher reporting of spouse and child abuse in times of unemployment in the community. Clearly the experience of unemployment has serious implications for family relationships, and the development of effective coping strategies is necessary to maintain stability.

Coping Strategies

Individuals vary in their response to the experience of job loss depending on the situation and the meaning of that particular work role in the individual's life. Some evidence of gender difference in coping style has been reported. Leana and Feldman (1991) found that both men and women experience psychological distress in response to job loss but use different coping strategies. Men relied more on problem-focused activities such as job search, while women relied on more symptom-focused activities such as seeking social support. Strategies that individuals may have found helpful in the other situations to deal with stress may also be of assistance, such as exercise, relaxation techniques, development of social outlets, and restructuring time commitments.

Effective coping mechanisms for families facing the stress of unemployment include maintaining the quality of family relationships and using social supports effectively. Strategies that enhance family flexibility and permit members to redefine roles and restructure their daily patterns can be helpful in maintaining morale. Family cohesiveness or attachment can be enhanced through open communication, avoidance of laying blame, and family activities that foster unity. Continued contacts with friends, relatives, and former coworkers may provide emotional and concrete support, assisting family members to avoid isolation and cope more effectively with restructured daily activities.

Additional coping methods relate to management of financial resources and exploring other sources of income. The employed person may seek part-time, temporary employment in other areas, and other family members may augment the family income by seeking jobs outside the home. This combined effort may reduce anxiety about loss of family assets in the future. Management of financial resources becomes a major source of family disagreement as the length of time extends and resources dwindle. A concerted effort is necessary to maintain family cohesion and develop strategies for budgeting and paying bills. At times the assistance of professionals may be necessary to help families plan and prevent the loss of home or means of transportation.

The ability to mobilize resources and to view the situation as an opportunity for life change is helpful to some families and leads to further education or a more desirable job situation. For others, the use of coping strategies may be an additional source of stress as family members may encounter difficulty with role shifts. For example, a woman may enjoy the newfound freedom of employment and develop personally and professionally, whereas her unemployed husband may be threatened and distressed by the situation. Strong support systems may delay the mobilization of a family's own resources or impede their progress in exploring other alternatives. For example, a helpful parent may offer financial support but at the same time create a dependency that undermines family cohesion. The process of coping with the multifaceted stressor of unemployment is complex, with certain strategies being successful in some situations and detrimental in others (Voydanoff, 1983).

FAMILIES AND RELOCATION

In an increasingly technologic society, attention has focused on understanding the interaction of work and workers, the safety of the work environment, and the effect of work on the families of the worker. Among the growing number of investigations concerning families and work, the effect of relocation on family life has emerged as a topic for serious concern. Geographic relocation may be considered a transition since it involves adaptation to a new environment, social structure, and, possibly, new roles. Although frequently associated with job transfers, the issue of relocation potentially affects individuals of all ages. It may be a factor for adolescents as parents move or as they decide to attend college out of state. It may figure importantly in retirement planning or may result from the loss of a spouse or the illness of an aging parent. In later years it may also be significant as individuals and families seek supportive care environments.

The decision to relocate may be inspired by many factors, including career advancement, higher income, prestige, personal gratification, or the desire to be closer to or more distant from relatives. In some situations, chronic illness or increasing frailty may lead to a decision to relocate to a life-care retirement facility that accommodates differing needs for activity and support. Every decision involves a balancing of gains and losses in relation to the individual and the family's existence. Family relationships, children's education and well-being, proximity to aging relatives, lifestyle, economic aspects, and concerns for security all enter the analysis if the decision is voluntary. In some situations, relocation is not voluntary, and additional stressors may be involved as families relocate due to political unrest, unemployment, or loss of significant, supportive relationships. Relocation may be an option that evolves from a family decision-making process; in other cases, individuals may be the prime decision maker, depending on sociocultural variables or family structure. The degree of stress involved in relocation can be substantial or less significant. For some, it may lead to the fulfillment of a long-desired goal and may not be perceived as stressful. The process of relocation may be perceived as growth producing and may even signal the end of a very stressful period in life. Given the variety of issues, situations, and developmental periods that could be involved, there are multiple opportunities to research the process of relocation and the effectiveness of interventions to support families through this transition.

Patterns of Response

The process of relocation affects approximately 20% of people annually each in the United States (Fisher, 1988). Such figures may be conservative in that they may not reflect relocation within the same city, migratory patterns between approximating countries or relocation that involves moves from or to institutional types of settings. Nevertheless, the impact is significant and is reflected in the various types of issues explored in the literature. Much of the research concerns the impact of relocation on women and children who may be part of traditional family structures, indicating that family relocation to further a woman's career goals or in families headed by a woman head of household are areas yet to be significantly explored. There is some attention to recent immigrant experiences as well as to adaptation to international temporary moves. Residential mobility has been a significant area of interest in relation to the aging family.

The effect of relocation on children is an area of continued exploration, and it is estimated that in many urban and suburban communities, 15% to 20% of children enrolled in public schools each year are transfers (Puskar & Dvorsak, 1991). For adolescents in particular, relocation can be a very stressful experience (Nernberg, 1990), ranking seventh among some 37 stressful life events as measured by Hutton, Roberts, Walker, and Zuniga (1987). The stressors related to moving expressed by adolescents included moving to a new school, leaving a former school, and separating from a former social circle. They also identified losing a best friend and seeking a new one as sources of stress (Raviv, Keinan, Abazon & Raviv, 1990). For the most part, adolescents experience the most stress in relation to social peer relationships, and adjustment may involve grieving over the loss. Vernberg (1990) found that mobile adolescents had less positive social experiences with their peers, had fewer contacts with friends, and experienced less intimate relationships with their best friends. The socialization process during adolescence is very important, and relocation can have an effect on the ability and confidence to develop relationships.

The effect of relocation on adults can be challenging or detrimental, and the impact of the move can be mediated by such factors as personality, psychological and situational variables, coping strategies, and social support (Starker, 1990). In a study of the accompanying spouse in dual-career couples, Niems (1986) found that higher levels of adaptation to a geographic move were associated with particular coping strategies, including a positive outlook toward change. In a study of males and females who had moved to a large metropolitan city, Starker (1990) found that over a three-month period the size of the new social network changed little and that it was unstable and in flux. In the first six months following a move, the support network was in a transitional phase, making it difficult to turn to superficial contacts for social support. Subjects relied heavily on their spouses, with the majority receiving moderate to considerable amounts of support from their husbands or wives. From a retrospective analysis, Starker concluded that it took between two and a half and four and a half years in a community to attain stable levels of intimacy. In this same study, approximately half of the participants identified moderate to considerable amounts of stress associated with their health during the first five to seven months following their move. Given the significant degree of importance attributed to social support as a buffer of stress, the limited support available following relocation has many implications, particularly for health care providers who may encounter family members in a variety of community settings.

Although any type of relocation can be stressful, Puskar (1990a) suggests that international relocation can be particularly challenging due to differences in forms of communication, lack of job opportunities for women, and cultural differences involved with activities of daily living. There can be considerable lack of social support, feelings of isolation, and dependency on nuclear family members for support. In a study of the wives of military and corporate men Puskar (1990a) found that women who coped poorly had been married longer and experienced more moves in their lifetimes. They were not involved in volunteer activities and did not work outside the home. A larger percentage of their children were unhappy about the move as well. These women viewed life events in a more negative manner, while women who coped well had a more positive and intense response to life events.

The issue of relocation has also been explored in terms of groups recently migrating to the United States. In a recent study of Vietnamese refugees Fox (1991) conducted interviews with women married to their husbands in Vietnam. They found that an increase in affectivity occurred without a decrease in spousal power differential. The women explained this change by describing increased mutual dependency and greater emotional involvement with their husbands after resettlement associated with being separated from family and friends. When wives were employed, husbands participated more in household tasks and child care, a situation related to functional need. There was also a tendency for spousal power differentials to decrease. This was associated with language competency and a residency of three or more years. These factors tended to increase women's exposure to more liberal attitudes concerning gender relations. However, employment itself did not guarantee more egalitarian exchange. This study is particularly interesting because it focuses primarily on communication processes and negotiating strategies rather than the outcomes of family process. This and other studies concerning immigrant groups have implications for health care providers who are attempting to promote healthier lifestyles within the context of changing cultural norms.

The issues of relocation are not limited to youth or persons of middle age; they affect aging persons as well. Although some moves may be associated with more relaxing lifestyles, better climate, or closer associations with family, the move from independent to dependent living often presents considerable stress for an older person as well as family members. This type of relocation can result in mental and physical illness, particularly if it is perceived to be a "last move." Gass, Gaustad, Oberst, and Hughes (1992) explored the meaning assigned to or appraisal of relocation to a nursing home and the relationship to a number of situational and demographic variables, including psychological and physical health. Positive, benign, and challenge appraisals were related to higher morale and functional independence, while threat appraisal was related to poorer psychological health and lower morale. Harm-loss appraisal was associated with lower morale and lower functional independence. The authors concluded that the assessment of people's appraisal of relocation is important to their positive adaptation. Nurses and other health care providers may be able to assess appraisal in advance of relocation and develop effective strategies to aid the transition. It is evident from this brief review that responses to relocation can be positive or negative and that it may result in varying degrees of stress for individuals and families. Therefore successful coping strategies are particularly important given the impact of relocation of all types on social and family relationships.

Coping Strategies

Due to the diversity of experiences involved in relocation, a variety of strategies have been recommended to strengthen the coping resources of individuals. For the most part, these strategies and programs are clinical approaches rather than well-documented intervention strategies. In describing the successful coping behaviors of women, Puskar (1990a) found that women who coped well identified various active behaviors, such as problem solving, seeking support from family and friends, using humor, getting involved in creative and community outlets, and not worrying. The women in her study who coped poorly with the relocation

experience used passive behaviors, such as eating, sleeping, crying, watching TV, getting angry at self and others, and expecting the worst. Based on the findings of this study, nurses and other health care providers might recommend that relocated women build relationships through community involvement and use hobbies as a way of contacting people with similar interests. An open attitude and a workable plan to maintain contact with family and friends remaining behind can also be very beneficial. Niems (1986) found similar results in a study of the accompanying spouse in dual-career couples. Coping strategies such as viewing change in general as providing more options, considering the relocation as a challenge, and assuming an active stance were all associated with higher levels of adaptation to a geographic move.

Several programmatic approaches to facilitating relocation for families and individual members have been suggested. Puskar (1989) recommends that a family health promotion model be used in dealing with this transition. One approach is to develop a school-based model designed to facilitate the transition of children and adolescents by integrating elements to help them successfully cope with relocation. She recommends that a multidisciplinary team be used that brings together both professionals and nonprofessionals to deal with the issues and especially emphasizes the importance of networking among families, students, teachers, school nurses, and other health care professionals. Multiple methods can be used within the context of health promotion, including individual counseling, supportive and educative groups, and outreach home visits. In some situations, the existence of a student assistance program is helpful in developing a systematic process by which students with problems can be identified and referred for help.

A similar approach is recommended to assist adults with relocation through the use of employee assistance programs. Starker (1990) recommends that these programs be expanded to address the stresses of relocation. Activities could include individual counseling, workshops, premove and postmove interviews, and referrals to community resources. Support groups have also been helpful in reducing feelings of loss and isolation and as a way of helping individuals express and deal with negative reactions (Puskar, 1990b). Such programs could be part of the wellness component of organizations and be integrated as a stress-reduction, illness-prevention strategy.

The issue of relocation can be very difficult for older persons, particularly when it involves giving up a home or moving from a fairly independent lifestyle to one that is more dependent and perhaps more controlled. Gass et al. (1992) found that preparation for a move was related to higher positive appraisal, higher morale, functional independence, and lower conceptions of harm and loss. The results of this study suggest a need to assess the meaning of the move to the individual in order to plan strategies that prevent relocation stress. In general, there is a need for individuals to have some control over the environment, have prior preparation, and be able to maintain familiar situations as much as possible. Since personal possessions help to affirm one's sense of self and one's personal history, maintaining familiar furnishings and objects may facilitate adaptation to a new environment. Variations in approaches may be necessary depending on the situation and whether relocation involves a home-to-institution move, an institution-to-institution move, or a residential move.

Regardless of the situation or where the family falls on the stress continuum, health care providers can give vital information and support and facilitate effective coping strategies. They might function in a variety of roles, including acting as a buffer in providing support, educating the family about relocation processes and coping strategies, and providing appropriate referrals or suggestions for networking. Successful adaptation is marked by tolerance to separation from old friends, formation of new friendships and social networks and acceptance by the community. Starker (1990) cautions against unrealistic expectations of their clients by health care providers, however, noting that delayed social distress and the inability to establish social networks in a brief period of time may be normative for persons experiencing relocation.

It is often difficult to predict how successful families will be in adjusting to the new environment because personality factors and coping mechanisms vary considerably in response to stressors inherent in the process of relocation. In addition, the research on mobility and its impact on families has been tentative and exploratory, frequently limited by methodologic difficulties. Most studies consider the viewpoint of individuals rather than the family perspective, creating another limitation concerning the subtler differences that may exist among families. Because the field is relatively unexplored, numerous opportunities exist for researchers to explore the family dimensions of relocation decision making, the process itself, and the period of adjustment that follows.

IMPLICATIONS FOR FAMILY HEALTH NURSING

Assessment of Life Transition and Health Effects

Family life events appear to be intimately related to health, and the family life cycle encompasses numerous transitions and events that may produce stress (Wheaton, 1990). Although most families are able to cope with normative events, loss of a significant other or unexpected major life changes increase stress by imposing demands that may seem insurmountable. When families encounter multiple stressors, health problems may arise, adding to the complexity of the situation. Therefore, health care professionals must be sensitive to the life cycle phase of the individual and the family, as well as family coping strategies.

Characteristically, nursing assessments of families include individual and family characteristics, the environment, and areas of client concern. In assessing families who may be experiencing the cumulative stress of transition, attention is focused on the psychosocial characteristics of each family member, incorporating data concerning life stage, value orientation, and previous experience with transition. Schlossberg (1981) defines the attributes of environment as inclusive of interpersonal support systems, institutional supports, and the characteristics of the setting, such as neighborhood, living arrangements, and workplace. All of these factors may have specific implications for families in transition. Areas of client concern may not be specifically related to transition but could be explored for relevance to the family. Specific topics include whether individuals are engaged in the addition or loss of roles, whether the change is external or internal, and whether the transition is viewed as a positive or negative occurrence. Additional variables are the life cycle timing of the event, the suddenness of onset, and the permanent or transitory nature of the change. Because adaptation to transition is dependent on individual and family resources or deficits, environmental differences, and involvement of various support systems, nursing assessments are inclusive of these areas as a means of identifying the degree of stress and potential family strengths.

Golan (1986) provides input on the nature of transitional problems that may be helpful assessment data to family health nurses in structuring interventions. Families may be unable to separate themselves from the past or to distance themselves from relationships with persons, places, or things over which they have little control. Second, they may be unable to make a decision about which direction to take or the consequences inherent in their decision. In addition, some individuals or families have difficulty in implementing a decision, such as locating and mobilizing resources, obtaining information, or coping with the new conditions inherent in their choices. Finally, some families experience problems of adjustment and have difficulty adapting to new roles and changed conditions until the situation stabilizes (Fig. 20–3). Although Golan (1986) identifies these as "stuck points" in the process of transition and adaptation, other problems may be present that are less directly connected with transitions, such as substance abuse, nutritional deficiencies,

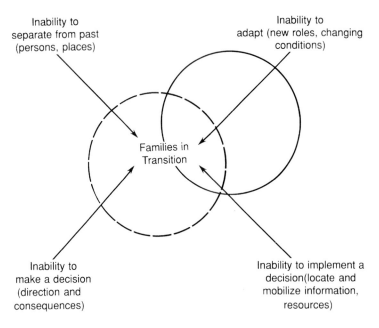

Inability to separate from past (persons, places)

Inability to adapt (new roles, changing conditions)

Families in Transition

Inability to make a decision (direction and consequences)

Inability to implement a decision (locate and mobilize information, resources)

FIGURE 20–3. Nursing assessment of potential problems in families experiencing transitions. (Data from N. Golan (1986). *The Perilous Bridge*. New York: Free Press.)

insomnia, or other physical symptoms that may not be resolved until the underlying issue is explored. As part of a family nursing history, nurses need to be cognizant of these transitional elements and their effect on health and incorporate them into the assessment process.

Facilitating Family Coping

Specific nursing interventions for families in transition are tailored to the individual family needs, which can vary considerably depending on the setting, the goals of the client and family system, and the availability of resources that can be mobilized to facilitate family adaptation. Following assessment, a mutual exploration of concerns may assist family nurses and their clients to narrow the focus and establish specific problems or needs. There may be an initial concern with a current issue that reaches back to the disruption or event that triggered the current response, followed by a return to the present and the development of specific goals. Emphasis is placed on assisting families to resume a forward momentum if they are unable to separate themselves from the past or to determine a more appropriate direction if difficulties have occurred.

Using a problem-solving approach, Golan (1986) has identified a series of behavior-oriented coping tasks for families, both instrumental and affective. Instrumental tasks involve the recognition of a lack or insufficiency and the need to change; the exploration of possible alternatives, resources, and roles; the implementation of a decision and use of new solutions and resources to function in a new role; and adaptation to the new situation with the development of increasing competence.

Affective coping tasks incorporate both cognitive and emotional components and involve coping with insecurity and dealing with feelings of loss; dealing with the anxiety involved in making decisions and the feelings of pressure and ambivalence; handling the pressure initiated during implementation; and adjusting to the new solution with its attendant shifts in role position and potential initial lack of satisfaction. Finally, the family may need to develop different standards of daily living until the level of functioning rises to acceptable norms and the family comes to terms with the new reality. Some of these coping tasks may be easily undertaken by family members, whereas others may require considerable support, education, and mustering of individual and family strengths. In some situations, family health nurses may be in the unique position of establishing a helping relationship that is sufficient to provide the necessary information, support, and mobilization of resources. Due to the stressful nature of transitions and the implications for changes in health status, family health nurses may be the first professional contact families have as they attempt to resolve their current concerns. Therefore, they become important sources for assessment, intervention, and appropriate referral. However, the expertise of another type of health care professional may be needed to facilitate family adaptation, or a different type of institutional support may be more useful.

Nursing Roles and Family Transitions

Family health nurses are probably more effective in handling situations in which families have histories of adequate, positive coping and there is no entrenched pathology or intractable social problems that would limit nursing intervention. In addition to providing a supportive relationship directed toward helping families to use their own resources to achieve a desired goal and serving as a resource for referral, family health nurses are well qualified to develop and implement educational programs directed toward families in transition. The ability to combine health promotion with specific information regarding the complexities of life transitions is a unique function of family health nurses that is sorely needed by families as they experience parenthood for the first time, attempt to blend families with children of other family groups, or move to a new location lacking extended family or supports. These types of programs can be adapted to hospital, home, school, or office settings as family health nurses expand their scope of practice to meet community needs and become more involved in the public sector. Consultation in developing educational materials and media consultation are other facets of this educational role.

Finally, it is apparent from this brief review of the literature concerning families in transition that it is a fairly recent field of exploration for a variety of disciplines. A lack of theoretical framework, inherent methodologic problems, a heavy reliance on cross-sectional data, lack of appropriate instrumentation, and conflicting findings are criticisms of existing data. Therefore, family health nurses are able to contribute significantly to this growing body of knowledge, particularly in relation to the effects of life transitions on the health of the families and the processes involved as families negotiate these transitions. Because family health nurses function in many settings and have access to families experiencing transitions, they can work collaboratively with other disciplines to establish longitudinal approaches to data collection in order to delineate family strengths and needs more effectively as families move through life transitions.

REFERENCES

AARP. (1989). *Working Caregivers Report, March 1989.* Washington, DC: American Association of Retired Persons.

Antonovsky, A., & Sagy, S. (1990). Confronting developmental tasks in the retirement transition. *Gerontologist,* 30(3), 362–368.

Bachrach, C.A. (1986). Adoption plans, adopted children and adoptive mothers. *Journal of Marriage and the Family,* 48(2), 243–253.

Baron, C.R. (1989). Causal explanations and emotional health of women during divorce. *Archives of Psychiatric Nursing,* 3(5), 266–271.

Beal, E.W. (1985). A systems view of divorce intervention strategies. In J.C. Hansen & S.C. Grebe (Eds.), *Divorce and Family Mediation* (pp. 17–32). Rockville, MD: Aspen.

Belgrave, L. (1988). The effects of race differences in work history, work attitudes, economic resources and health on women's retirement. *Research on Aging,* 10(3), 383–401.

Belsky, J., & Rovine, M. (1990). Patterns of marital change across the transition to parenthood: Pregnancy to three years postpartum. *Journal of Marriage and the Family,* 52, 5–19.

Berry, M. (1990). Stress and coping among older child adoptive families. *Social Work and Social Sciences Review: 1989–1990,* 1(2), 71–93.

Berry, M. (1991). The effects of open adoption on biological and adoptive parents and their children. *Child Welfare,* 70(6), 637–651.

Biegel, D.E., Sales, E., & Schulz, R. (1991). *Family Caregiving in Chronic Illness.* Newbury Park, CA: Sage.

Burden, D.S. (1986). Single parents and the work setting: The impact of multiple job and homelife responsibilities. *Family Relations,* 35, 37–44.

Burr, W.R. (1990). Beyond I—Statements in family communication. *Family Relations,* 39, 266–273.

Campbell, L.H., Silverman, P.R., & Patti, P.B. (1991). Reunions between adoptees and birth parents: The adoptees' experience, *Social Work,* 36(4), 329–335.

Carter, B., & McGoldrick, M. (1988). *The Changing Family Life Cycle: A Framework for Family Therapy.* New York: Gardner Press.

Caycedo, J.C., Wange, G., & Bahr, S.F. (1991). Gender roles in the family. In S.J. Bahr (Ed.), *Family Research: A Sixty-Year Review, 1930–1990* (pp. 435–491). New York: Lexington Books.

Chappell, N.L., & Badger, M. (1989). Social isolation and well-being. *Journal of Gerontology: Social Sciences,* 44(5), 169–176.

Connidis, I.A. (1989). *Family Ties and Aging.* Toronto: Butterworths.

CHAPTER HIGHLIGHTS

Maintenance of family health promotion is crucial to reduce family stress during critical family transitions and demarcation of new family stages.

Major family transitions and demarcations include addition and loss of family members, parenthood, illness of family members (particularly chronic illness), changes in family roles, and family relocation.

Critical family transitions have the potential to be perceived as a crisis by families because any change in one member of the unit may influence the quality of health of the family and/or individual family members.

Family stress is a common phenomenon during critical family transitions and demarcations in family life stages.

The role of the family nurse is to assess family transitions, determine the impact on the family system, and participate with the family in planning interventions to reduce stressful effects of the transition on family health.

Crosbie-Burnett, M. (1989). Application of family stress theory to remarriage: A model for assessing and helping stepfamilies. *Family Relations,* 38, 323–331.

Daly, E.A., & Futrell, M. (1989). Retirement attitudes and health status of preretired and retired men and women. *Journal of Gerontological Nursing,* 15(1), 29–32.

Dorfman, L.T., & Moffett, M.M. (1987). Retirement satisfaction in married and widowed rural women. *Gerontologist,* 27, 251–221.

Dornbusch, S.M., & Gray, K.D. (1988). Single-parent families. In S. Dornbusch & M. Strober (Eds.), *Feminism, Children and the New Families* (pp. 274–296). New York: Guilford Press.

Doty, P. (1986). Family care of the elderly: The role of public policy. *Milbank Quarterly,* 64(1), 34–75.

Duvall, E.M., & Miller, B.C. (1985). *Marriage and Family Development.* New York: Harper & Row.

Dyer, E. (1963). Parenthood as crisis: A restudy. *Marriage and Family Living,* 25(2), 196–201.

Ekerdt, D.J. (1987). Why the notion persists that retirement harms health. *Gerontologist* 27(4), 454–457.

Entwisle, D.R., & Doering, S.G. (1981). *The First Birth: A Family Turning Point.* Baltimore: John Hopkins University Press.

Erickson, E.H. (1963). *Childhood and Society.* New York: W.W. Norton.

Ferraro, K.F. (1990). Cohort analysis of retirement preparation, 1974–1981. *Journal of Gerontology: Social Sciences,* 45, S220–227.

Fife, B.L. (1985). A model for predicting the adaptation of families to medical crisis: An analysis of role integration. *Image: The Journal of Nursing Scholarship,* 17(4), 108–112.

Fine, M., Donnelly, B.N., & Voydanoff, P. (1986). Adjustment and satisfaction among parents from intact, single-parent and stepparent families. *Journal of Family Issues,* 7, 391–404.

Fisher, S. (1988). Leaving home: Homesickness and the psychological effects of change and transition. In P. Fisher & J. Reason (Eds.), *Handbook of Life Stress, Cognition and Health* (pp. 41–59). New York: Wiley.

Fox, P.G. (1991). Stress related to family change among Vietnamese refugees. *Journal of Community Health Nursing,* 8(1), 45–56.

Fretz, B.R., Kluge, N.A., Ossana, S.M., Jones, S.M., & Merikangas, M.W. (1989). Intervention targets for reducing preretirement anxiety and depression. *Journal of Counseling Psychology,* 36(3), 301–307.

Ganong, L.H., & Coleman, M. (1991). Remarriage and health. *Research in Nursing and Health,* 14, 105–211.

Gass, K.A. (1987). The health of conjugally bereaved older widows: The role of appraisal, coping and resources. *Research in Nursing and Health,* 10(1), 39–47.

Gass, K.A., & Chang, A.S. (1989). Appraisals of bereavement, coping, resources and psychosocial health dysfunction in widows and widowers. *Nursing Research,* 38(1), 31–36.

Gass, K.A., Gaustad, G., Oberst, M.T., & Hughes, S. (1992). Relocation appraisal, functional independence, morale and health of nursing home residents. *Issues in Mental Health Nursing,* 13(3), 239–253.

Gibson, R.C. (1988). The work, retirement, and disability of older black Americans. In J.S. Jackson (Ed.), *The Black American Elderly: Research on Physical and Psychosocial Health* (pp. 304–324). New York: Springer.

Giles-Sims, J., & Crosbie-Burnett, M. (1989). Step-family research: Implications for policy, clinical interventions and further research. *Family Relations,* 38, 19–23.

Given, B., Stommel, M.S., Collins, C., King, S., & Given, C.W. (1990). Responses of elderly caregivers. *Research in Nursing and Health,* 13, 77–85.

Glenn, N.D., & Shelton, B.A. (1985). Regional differences in divorce in the United States. *Journal of Marriage and the Family,* 47(3), 641–652.

Golan, N. (1986). *The Perilous Bridge.* New York: Free Press.

Gottman, J.M., & Krokoff, L.J. (1989). Marital interaction and satisfaction: A longitudinal view. *Journal of Consulting and Clinical Psychology,* 57(1), 47–52.

Groze, V., & Gruenewald, A. (1991). PARTNERS: A model program for special-needs adoptive families in stress. *Child Welfare,* 70(5), 581–589.

Hall, L.A., Gurley, D.N., Sachs, B., & Kruyscio, R.J. (1991). Psychosocial predictors of maternal depressive symptoms, parenting attitudes and child behavior in single-parent families. *Nursing Research,* 40(4), 214–220.

Hamilton, V.L., Broman, C.L., & Hoffman, W.S. (1990). Hard times and vulnerable people: Initial effects of plan closing on autoworkers' mental health. *Journal of Health and Social Behavior,* 31(2), 123–140.

Hanson, S.M.H. (1986). Healthy single-parent families. *Family Relations,* 35(91), 125–132.

Hawkins, A.J., & Belsky, J. (1989). The role of father involvement in personality change in men across the transition to parenthood. *Family Relations,* 38, 378–384.

Hayward, M.D., Grady, W.R., & McLaughlin, S.D. (1988). The retirement process among older women in the United States: Changes in the 1970's. *Research on Aging,* 10(3), 358–382.

Heinemann, G.D., & Evans, P.L. (1990). Widowhood: Loss, change and adaptation. In T.H. Brubaker (Ed.), *Family Relationships in Later Life* (pp. 142–168). Newbury Park, CA: Sage.

Hill, R. (1973). *Family Life Cycle: Critical Role Transitions.* Paper presented at the Thirteenth International Family Research Seminar, Paris.

Hobbs, D.F., Jr. (1965). Parenthood as crisis: A third study. *Journal of Marriage and the Family,* 27(3), 367–372.

Hobbs, D.R., Jr., & Cole, S.P. (1976). Transition to parenthood, a decade replication. *Journal of Marriage and the Family,* 38(4), 723–731.

Hultsch, D.F., & Deutsch, F. (1981). *Adult Development and Aging.* New York: McGraw-Hill.

Hutton, J.B., Roberts, G.B., Walker, J., & Zuniga, J. (1987). Ratings of severity of life events by ninth-grade students. *Psychology in Schools,* 24, 63–68.

Hymovich, D.P., & Hagopian, G.A. (1992). *Chronic Illness in Children and Adults: A Psychosocial Approach.* Philadelphia: Saunders.

Johnson, B.H. (1986). Single mothers following separation and divorce: Making it on your own. *Family Relations,* 35(1), 189–197.

Jones, L. (1990). Unemployment and child abuse. *Families in Society,* 71(10), 579–588.

Kamo, Y. (1988). Determinants of household division of labor. *Journal of Family Issues,* 9, 177–200.

Karp, D.A. (1989). The social construction of retirement among professionals 50–60 years old. *Gerontologist,* 29(6), 750–760.

Kearl, M.C. (1989). *Endings: A Sociology of Death and Dying.* New York: Oxford University Press.

Kersten, K.K. (1990). The process of marital disaffection: Interventions at various stages. *Family Relations, 39,* 257–265.

Kimmel, D.C. (1990). *Adulthood and Aging: An Interdisciplinary, Developmental View.* New York: Wiley.

Kingsbury, N.M., & Minda, R.B. (1988). An analysis of three expected intimate relationship states: Commitment, maintenance and termination. *Journal of Social and Personal Relationships, 5,* 405–422.

Leana, C.R., & Feldman, D.C. (1991). Gender differences in response to unemployment. *Journal of Vocational Behavior, 38*(1), 65–77.

LeMasters, E.E. (1957). Parenthood as crisis. *Marriage and Family Living, 19*(4), 352–355.

Liem, R., & Liem, J.H. (1988). The psychological effects of unemployment on workers and their families. *Journal of Social Issues, 44,* 87–105.

Linsk, N.L., Keigher, S.M., & Osterbusch, S.E. (1988). State policies regarding paid family caregiving. *Gerontologist, 28*(2), 204–212.

Loveland-Cherry, C.J. (1986). Personal health practices in single-parent and two-parent families. *Family Relations, 35*(1), 133–139.

Lowery, C.R., & Settlel, S.A. (1985). Effects of divorce on children: Differential impact of custody and visitation patterns. *Family Relations, 34,* 455–463.

Lubkin, I.M. (1986). *Chronic Illness: Impact and Interventions.* Boston: Jones and Bartlett Publishers.

MacDermid, S.M., Huston, T.L., & McHale, S.M. (1990). Changes in marriage associated with the transition to parenthood: Individual differences as a function of sex-role attitudes and changes in the division of household labor. *Journal of Marriage and the Family, 52,* 475–486.

Martin, T.C., & Bumpass, L.L. (1989). Recent trends in martial disruption. *Demography, 26*(10), 37–51.

Matthews, A.M., & Brown, K.H. (1987). Retirement as a critical life event: The differential experiences of men and women. *Research on Aging, 9,* 548–571.

Mauksch, H.O. (1974). A social science basis for conceptualizing family health. *Social Science and Medicine, 8,* 521–528.

McCrae, R.R., & Costa, P.T. Jr. (1988). Psychological resilience among widowed men and women: A 10 year follow-up of a national sample. *Journal of Social Issues, 44*(3), 129–142.

McCubbin, M.A., & McCubbin, H.I. (1993). Families coping with illness: The resiliency model of family stress, adjustment and adaptation. In C.B. Danielson, B. Hamel-Bissel & P. Winstead-Fry (Eds.), *Families, Health and Illness: Perspectives on Coping and Intervention.* St. Louis: Mosby.

Merderer, H., & Hill, R. (1983). Critical transitions over the family life span: Theory and research. In H.I. McCubbin, M.B. Sussman & J.N. Patterson (Eds.), *Social Stress and the Family: Advances in Family Stress Theory and Research,* (pp. 39–60). New York: Haworth Press.

Miall, C.E. (1987). The stigma of adoptive parent status: Perceptions of community attitudes toward adoption and the experience of informal social sanctioning. *Family Relations, 36*(1), 34–39.

Middlebrook, S., & Clark, E. (1991). Emotional trauma of job loss. *Employee Assistance Quarterly, 7*(2), 63–65.

Monat, A., & Lazarus, R.S. (1985). Introduction: Stress and coping—some current issues and controversies. In A. Monat & R.S. Lazarus (Eds.), *Stress and Coping: An Anthology* (pp. 1–12). New York: Columbia University Press.

Morgan, L.A. (1991). *After Marriage Ends: Economic Consequences for Midlife Women.* Newbury Park, CA: Sage.

Morgan, S.P., Lye, D.N., & Condran, G.A. (1988). Sons, daughters and divorce: Does the sex of children affect the risk of marital disruption? *American Journal of Sociology, 94,* 110–129.

Niems, M. (1986). The effects of relocation on the accompanying spouse in dual career couples. Unpublished doctoral dissertation, University of Florida.

Norris, F.H., & Murrell, S.A. (1990). Social support, life events and stress as modifiers of adjustment to bereavement by older adults. *Psychology and Aging, 5,* 429–436.

Norton, A.J., & Glick, P.C. (1986). One parent families: A social and economic profile. In *The Single Parent Family: Special Issue of Family Relations.* Minneapolis, MN: National Council on Family Relations.

O'Bryant, S.L., & Morgan, L.A. (1989). Financial experience and well-being among mature widowed women. *Gerontologist, 29,* 245–251.

Older Women's League. (1989). *Failing America's Caregivers: A Status Report on Women Who Care.* Washington, DC: Author.

Penkower, L., Bromet, E., & Dew, M.A. (1988). Husbands' layoff and wives' mental health: A prospective analysis. *Archives of General Psychiatry, 45,* 994–1000.

Puskar, K.R. (1989). Promoting health through family relocation adaptation. *Family and Community Health, 11*(4), 52–62.

Puskar, K.R. (1990a). International relocation: Womens' coping methods. *Health Care for Women International, 11,* 263–276.

Puskar, K.R. (1990b). Relocation support groups for corporate wives. *American Association of Occupational Health Nursing Journal, 38*(1), 25–31.

Puskar, K.R., & Dvorsak, K.G. (1991). Relocation stress in adolescents: Helping teenagers cope with a moving dilemma. *Pediatric Nursing, 17*(3), 295–298.

Rapoport, R. (1963). Normal crises, family structure and mental health. *Family Process, 2*(1), 68—80.

Rapoport, R., Rapoport, R.N., & Streilitz, A. (1977). *Fathers, Mothers, and Society.* New York: Basic Books.

Raviv, A., Keinan, G., Abazon, Y., & Raviv, A. (1990). Moving as a stressful life event for adolescents. *Journal of Community Psychology, 18,* 130–140.

Risman, B.J. (1986). Can men "mother"? Life as a single father. *Family Relations, 35*(1), 95–102.

Risman, B.J., & Park, K. (1988). Just the two of us: Parent-child relationships in single-parent homes. *Journal of Marriage and the Family. 50,* 1049–1062.

Rolland, J.S. (1988a). Chronic illness and the family life cycle. In B. Carter & M. McGoldrick (Eds.), *The Changing Family Life Cycle: A Framework for Family Therapy* (pp. 433–456). New York: Gardner Press.

Rolland, J.S. (1988b). A conceptual model of chronic and life threatening illness and its impact on families. In C.S. Chilman, E.W. Nunnally & F.W. Cox (Eds.), *Chronic Illness and Disability.* Newbury Park, CA: Sage.

Rollins, B.C. (1989). Marital quality at midlife. In S. Hunter & M. Sundel (Eds.), *Midlife Myths: Issues, Findings and Practice Implications* (pp. 184–194). Newbury Park, CA: Sage.

Rowley, K.M., & Feather, N.T. (1987). The impact of unemployment in relation to age and length of unemployment. *Journal of Occupational Psychology,* 60, 323–332.

Ruhm, C.J. (1989). Why older Americans stop working. *Gerontologist,* 29(3), 294–298.

Schaffer, J., & Kral, R. (1988). Adoptive families. In C.S. Chilman, E.W. Nunnally & F.M. Cox (Eds.), *Variant Family Forms* (pp. 165–184). Newbury Park, CA: Sage.

Sell, C.M. (1985). *Transition.* Chicago: Moody Press.

Schlossberg, N.K. (1981). A model for analyzing human adaptation to transition. *Counseling Psychologist,* 9(2), 1–18.

Shelton, B.K. (1985). The social and psychological impact of unemployment. *Journal of Employment Counseling,* 22, 18–22.

Starker, J.E. (1990). Psychosocial aspects of geographic relocation: The development of a new social network. *American Journal of Health Promotion,* 5(1), 52–57.

Steggell, G.L., & Harper, J.M. (1991). Family interaction patterns and communications processes. In S.J. Bahr (Ed.), *Family Research: A Sixty-Year Review, 1930–1990* (pp. 97–170). New York: Lexington Books.

Thielman, S.B., & Melges, F.T. (1986). Julia Rush's diary: Coping with loss in the early nineteenth century. *American Journal of Psychiatry,* 143, 1144–1148.

Thomas, J. (1992). *Adulthood and Aging.* Boston: Allyn and Bacon.

Tschann, J.M., Johnston, J.R., & Wallerstein, J.S. (1989). Resources, stressors, and attachment as predictors of adult adjustment after divorce: A longitudinal study. *Journal of Marriage and the Family,* 51, 1033–1046.

U.S. Bureau of the Census. (1987). *Statistical Abstract of the United States* (108th ed.). Washington, DC: U.S. Government Printing Office.

Vemer, E., Coleman, M., Ganong, L.H., & Cooper, H. (1989). Marital satisfaction in remarriage: A meta-analysis. *Journal of Marriage and the Family,* 51, 713–725.

Vernberg, E.M. (1990). Experiences with peers following relocation during early adolescence. *American Journal of Orthopsychiatry,* 60(3), 466–472.

Vinick, B.H., & Ekerdt, D.J. (1989). Retirement and the family. *Generations,* 13(2), 53–57.

Voydanoff, R. (1983). Unemployment: Family strategies for adaptation. In C.R. Figley & H.K. McCubbin (Eds.), *Stress and the Family, Vol. 2: Coping with Catastrophe* (pp. 90–102). New York: Brunner/Mazel.

Weingarten, H. (1980). Remarriage and well-being: National survey evidence of social and psychological effects. *Journal of Family Issues,* 1, 533–559.

Wheaton, B. (1990). Life transitions, role histories and mental health. *American Sociological Review,* 55, 209–223.

Whitbourne, S.K. (1986). *Adult Development.* New York: Praeger.

Woods, N.F., Yates, B.C., & Primomo, J. (1989). Supporting families during chronic illness. *Image: Journal of Nursing Scholarship,* 21(1), 46–50.

Zsembik, B.A., & Singer, A. (1990). The problem of defining retirement among minorities: The Mexican Americans. *Gerontologist,* 30, 749.

SOCIAL POLITICAL ENVIRONMENT AND FAMILY HEALTH PROMOTION

21

ROSEMARY GOODYEAR

> Politics is too serious a matter to be left to politicians.
>
> CHARLES DE GAULLE

OBJECTIVES

On completion of this chapter the reader will be able to:

1. Explain the purpose of the policy formation and its effect on the family
2. Understand the steps of the policy-making process
3. Examine a historical review of twentieth century family and health care policies
4. Identify the health care issues that are currently affecting the family
5. Analyze the nurse's role as a shaper of policy for family health
6. Examine future health care issues that could affect the family
7. Examine future family policy issues

INTRODUCTION

Recently the family has become a focus for policy decisions in political campaigns. The family, regardless of the membership, ethnicity, or geographic location, is a force that currently dominates the thinking of policy makers in this country. One critical issue for our legislators is the need for health care reform. The resurgence of interest in the family unit and the development of policy that affects the family signal a change in the agenda of many elected officials of government, as well as nongovernment institutions such as big business. Because of this attention to the family by both private and public policy makers, nurses must become knowledgeable about the policy-making process so that they can be advocates for the family, particularly in the area of health care. Nurses need to gain insight into the issues and policies that affect this unit of society so that they may guide the formation of policy that supports it. In addition to the issues, nurses interested in becoming involved as advocates must comprehend the process by which policies are formed.

Policies are the guidelines or rules by which a society operates. *Family policies* are the government laws, legislation, and programs that directly or indirectly affect family (a group of people related by blood, marriage, or adoption, or two or more persons in a committed relationship). *Health* relates to one's state of being sound in body and mind; often the term *family well-being* is used, which is based on the notion that whatever affects one member affects the larger family unit as well. *Health policies* can include specific policies that involve family health, such as improving access to health, resources for the handicapped, prevention of child abuse, funding for prenatal care, and school screening for vision and hearing deficits, and also can be indirectly involved with a family's health through such services as housing, education, unemployment income, or care for children whose parents are both working outside the home (Zimmerman, 1992).

This chapter will focus on the purpose of policy formation, provide a background of prior health care policy and its relationship to family, review the process of moving policy through the decision-making channels for future health and family policy issues, and finally, identify ways for nurses to be involved as advocates for family policy.

PURPOSE OF POLICY FORMATION IN SOCIETY

Policies are described as the guidelines or rules by which a society operates. All functioning societies have established methods for maintaining order to which the people conform; this provides a sense of survival, maintenance, and progress. Furthermore, the values and norms form the foundation for the rules/policies by which people will live; these do not arise easily or without conflict among the members of a society (Anderson, 1984; Diers, 1985). When different needs surface from different voices in a given society, one method of addressing them is to establish a policy, guideline, or rule that will provide direction toward resolving the conflict. Different forms of government have devised a variety of approaches to the process of addressing conflict, and in the United States it is the democratic process. Specifically, this process of policy making is the duty of the elected public officials through a representative form of government with a responsibility to the sovereign people of the country. Policies guide societies toward order, maintenance, resolution of conflict, and advancement of the people (Lindblom, 1968).

Conflict, Resolution, and Policy Making

Conflict is present when the competing needs and desires of people, families, or groups of families arise and there are limited available resources. When the conflict becomes a public matter, resolution is needed if the people are to move forward in a peaceful manner. A policy can be formed by drawing on the espoused value system of the people and following the established formation process. However, conflict must be recognized as a real and vital part of the policy-making process and not set aside as simply the "politics" of policy making. It could be said that policies are guides for orderly decision-making and that policy formation facilitates conflict resolution (Anderson, 1984; Kalisch & Kalisch, 1982).

Divergent perspectives is another concept of policy making that must be addressed by elected officials. Perhaps the most succinct point is that makers of public policy are representatives of society and they are elected to the position by their constituents. In the United States there is a recognized system for selection, service, duties, and responsibilities of these officials. Lindblom (1968) expands on the role of the elected officials as policy makers with respect to their different roles when they are making decisions on a policy issue.

Just as conflict is necessary for policy making, politics is also inherent in the policy-making process of elected officials. We can say that politics is a form of public decision making and policy is the outcome of the people's decision. Therefore, the study of issues and policies and their effect on families cannot be introduced unless the political arena and the dynamics of action that evolve are fundamentally understood. It therefore can be said that (1) policy making will only be set in motion when there is a conflict that requires resolution, and (2) the elected officials must take into consideration the divergent perspectives of the people they represent.

Policy Formation and Politics

Policy formation essentially has the purpose of shaping the behavior of our society or members of our society. In this chapter, it is discussed in relation to health policy and goals for health. Inherent in policy formation is the art of politics, or the process of negotiating for the best outcome for all involved.

Politics can be defined as the way we interact with one another, or the specific relations or conduct between individuals in a society, using authority, scarce resources, and the allocation of these to bring about change (Anderson, 1984; Kalisch & Kalisch, 1982). We may also include in this definition the parameters of this interaction, such as where it takes place, the topic that is being addressed, what is at risk, and what will change as a result of this action. When we change the behavior of members in society through policy formation, we mean political change through legislation, through policies that will give direction to those individuals in society. Therefore, policy formation is the enactment of political actions to bring about change in a formalized way.

Another way to view policy formation is as the legitimation of political action and the interacting of members of one group, several small groups, or a group as large as the Congress of the United States. The legislators in this type of policy formation listen to their constituents, bring their ideas to the table, and assess the salience of these ideas for future change. Therefore, in order to better understand this process the issues need to be identified and tracked from inception to policy implementation. This will provide insight into the political action of policy formation.

Change is difficult for any individual or group regardless of when it occurs. Major change in society is impossible unless a crisis, such as war, is confronting the people; therefore public policy takes the form of incremental change (Lindblom, 1980), that is making small changes to policy over time. Due to this process it can be said that policy making is ongoing and never ending.

Policy formation is also seen as a method of developing an acceptable course of action or problem solving. When this action takes place in the public arena it is public policy; in private organizations it is referred to as organizational policy. Both these processes have their roots in the same framework of change and serve the same purpose as that of resolving conflict. Forming public policy is a representation of the constituent's values on a specific issue, so the purpose of public policy formation is to try to bring together in a unifying way the resolution of a problem brought into the public arena by members of society (Anderson, 1984; Kalisch & Kalisch, 1982; Lindblom, 1980.

As Wisensale pointed out (1993), the development of family policy in the United States has been slow and disjointed because of four main factors: (1) the importance of individualism, (2) the use of state decisions for family law because of decentralization from central government, (3) the lack of long-range planning and use of "band-aid" solutions, and (4) the existence of a pluralistic society which precludes a good definition of family or policy. As a result, family policy in the 1980s suffered from incrementalism and increased responsibility under the Republican regime to state governments, and responded to a conservative Supreme Court as guardians of the "traditional family."

HISTORICAL REVIEW OF POLICIES FROM 1900 TO THE PRESENT

1900 to the 1950s

There are marker events that have had a driving impact on policy making in the United States since the early 1900s: (1) technological advances, (2) a decrease in philanthropy with a concomitant increase of the federal government's involvement, and (3) wars. The focus of the following discussion will be on national rather than state or local policy because of its all-encompassing nature.

For the first half of this century, as can be seen in Table 21–1, the environment was greatly affected by technological advances as well as war and economic hardship. The health of the people reflected a lack of sanitation (dysentery), an increase in communicable disease (tuberculosis), and the traumatic results of combat (amputees and respiratory insults). Industrialization produced a positive change in the economic environment, but it also brought with it an increase of child labor in the factories as well as work-related injuries. Eventually this resulted in the child labor laws, which were the grandparents of our current child abuse laws. Worker's compensation was also a result of industrialization. The depression com-

TABLE 21–1. HISTORICAL REVIEW OF FACTORS INFLUENCING POLICIES

	1900–1935	1936–1965	1966–PRESENT
Environment	World War I Depression	Post-war boom Vietnam Civil rights/poverty Women's movement	International peace Big business Recession Homelessness
Major health problems	War trauma Sanitation Communicable disease	War trauma Lifestyle illness Accidents Infectious disease	↓ Access to health care Communicable disease Lifestyle illness CVD, CA
Technological advancements	Anesthesia Surgery Penicillin Public health	Artificial organs Drugs and devices Research	Transplants Research Media/information
Social/organization Involvement	Philanthropy Begin state and federal intervention Private	Voluntary organization (+/−) Federal Government ↓ Philanthropy	↓ Federal Government ↑ State/local ↑ Voluntary organization
Legislative makers	Child abuse laws 1900s Worker's Compensation 1910 Social Security 1935	Hill Burton 1946 Community Mental Health Centers Act 1963 Medicare & Medicaid 1965 Health Planning & Resource Development Act 1974	Omnibus Budget and Reconciliation Act 1981 Tax Equity & Fiscal Responsibility Act Child Abuse Prevention and Treatment Act amended 1984 Family Leave 1994

pounded the plight of the poor and their multiple problems with disease; it spurred the initiation of the Social Security Act, which addressed some of their needs, such as assistance to the disabled, blind, and widowed (Litman, 1984; Starr, 1982). The Social Security Act of 1935 is perhaps the most significant piece of health care legislation of this century because it formed the basis for ideologic change as well as the roots for future health policy.

An example of the technological and scientific advances of this period is the introduction of anesthesia and the ability of surgeons to perform life-saving operations in our hospitals. The growth of public health departments resulted in limiting the spread of communicable disease during this era, and signaled a greater cooperative involvement between the state and federal governments. This was the beginning of an ideological shift from health care as a private concern to that of a public concern, and is important in the development of health policy. Another significant advancement in the health field was the discovery of penicillin for the fight against infectious diseases (Anderson, 1984; Starr, 1982).

Between 1946 and 1965, the era began with a post-war boom and ended with Civil Rights legislation forbidding discrimination because of race, color, or national origin. The health problems of World War II veterans resulted in increased long-term and rehabilitative care at VA centers. Despite the post-war years of jobs, prosperity, a move to suburbia for a segment of the United States (the white middle class), there remained an income inequality between the classes, and the relative distribution of national income was relatively unchanged, with one-fourth of the population still living in poverty in the 1960s (Miller, 1990).

Ongoing wars and "police actions" helped proliferate scientific and technologic advancement. During this period, orthopedic devices for the purpose of rehabilitation were promoted, as well as the development of many pharmaceutical products such as the birth control pill. There was a post-war resurgence of psychological/psychiatric services and chemical management, and this triggered a change in the management of patients in hospital to community-based centers. The Community Mental Health Centers Act (1963) is an example of an identified need receiving Federal Government attention, and legislation being enacted to meet that need (Starr, 1982). It was also during this time that the Federal Government intervened through expanding legislation in the Veteran's Administration and Hill Burton Acts. The voluntary organizations that had been at an all-time high during World War II began to diminish their support and involvement in health care programs.

The legislation that evolved was incremental and generally improved or expanded on an exist-

ing health policy. Examples include the Indian Health Assistance Act, which provided money for construction of health facilities for the Indians, the Social Security Amendment that authorized grants to states for medical assistance for the aged, and the Vaccination Assistance Act of 1962 that sought to prevent whooping cough, poliomyelitis, diphtheria, and tetanus. Until the Economic Opportunity Act of 1964 was passed, and the social Security Amendments of Medicare (Title XVIII) and Medicaid (Title XIX) became law in 1965, there was a notable absence of new major health legislation between 1950s and the 1960s (Kalisch & Kalisch, 1982). Medicaid introduced a comprehensive medical care assistance program by allocating funds to the states so that they could provide health care for the poor. This is an amendment that requires meeting a specific level of financial eligibility; whereas Medicare, Part A, is an example of an entitlement amendment that provides full payment for all persons over 65 for in-hospital care.

1960s to the Present

The Vietnam War, ongoing discrimination issues, and the women's movement all had an impact on policy formation during the years between 1960 and 1980. In contrast to the prior period of limited legislation, this era produced over eighty policies that addressed the health needs of the people; this reflects an increase in the federal government's involvement as a policy maker (Litman, 1991; Starr, 1982). Lifestyle changes of the counterculture, with its drugs and sexual freedom, produced a new series of health problems. In addition, diseases of the cardiovascular system, cancer, and accidents became the focus of research as the incidence continued to rise. The international competition between the superpowers resulted in major federal government funding shifts to research-seeking scientific advancements, but the rivalry also produced an increase of stress in the workplace. The space program is an example of competition between the superpowers. Advancement in health field technology included the use of artificial organs, transplantation, and research into the management of diseases with many new drugs. Another major influence during this period was the overwhelming increase in information exchange; the development of computer technology, communication links, and media coverage has had a great influence on both politics and policy formation. In addition, both the women's movement and civil rights' groups demanded policy attention and resolution; they attempted to secure equal opportunity in the work, education, and health fields (Bullough & Bullough, 1984; Kovner, 1990; Litman & Robins, 1991).

This era of turmoil was also a period of prolific policy formation with an intent to reduce inequity and restructure the health system to improve access to care. Some of the eighty health and safety bills enacted include the National Traffic and Motor Vehicle Safety Act, the National Health Planning Act, the Child Nutrition Act, the Occupational Safety and Health Act (OSHA), and the Social Security Amendment that was concerned with end-stage renal disease.

A change in political party leadership during the 1980s signaled a major change in government control. Factors such as international peace, an increase in big business, a recession that resulted in loss of work and propagation of homelessness, and the skyrocketing cost of health care all produced major health problems from societal distress. Communicable diseases such as AIDS, hepatitis B, and a return of tuberculosis are a product of the multiple factors of IV drug use, immigration, lifestyle variations, and crowded housing, reminiscent of the health problems of the people living in America in the early 20th century (Brown, 1987).

Family policies are affected by many trends that can be seen as part of contemporary American life. The changing family is a product of an increasing divorce rate, a larger number of female-headed households, a greater percentage of women in the labor force, an increase in teen pregnancy out of wedlock, and so on. The aging of America demonstrates a large increase of people over 65 and over 85. With the migration of ethnic groups, particularly Hispanics, the United States has become a larger multiracial, multicultural society. Economically there is a decreasing middle class and increasing poverty among women and children; this has helped to create higher levels of domestic violence, family abuse, drug use, suicide, and homelessness (Marshall, 1991; Wisensale, 1993).

Scientific advances include diagnosis by noninvasive imagery, micro surgeries, and transplantation. The media has broadcast military invasions as a common informational event from the nation's capitol into the living room, and has made it appear that problem solving can be accomplished in 30 minutes. Deregulation by the federal government of business, as well as financial containment of health care and cutbacks of past programs, has also been covered by news commentators. Federal government support for some health programs has been lateralized to state and local governments, and has changed the focus of health policy formation; this has encouraged the increase of voluntary organization involvement in family health programs, especially for the underserved (e.g., Habitat for Humanity, which creates homes for the poor) (Etzioni, 1991; Kovner, 1990).

Signing into law the family and medical leave legislation and lifting the "gag rule" that limited information during family planning visits were examples of policies that were enacted under President Clinton and have had an impact on family health. The legislation authorizing seat belts and the Americans with Disabilities Act signed under the prior administration also affected the family and their quality of life. The defeat of health reform legislation in 1994, in its simplest explanation, demonstrated a lack of readiness on the part of the public and policymakers to approve a massive change in the funding and provision of health care. As a result 37 to 40 million people remain uninsured and this issue continues to confront today's policymakers, regardless of partisan alignment (Lee, Soffel, & Luft, 1994).

The transition from private to public responsibility for health care services and scientific research on health and disease were the foundation of policy formation for the past 90 years of this century. The environmental milieu must be recognized as a powerful shaper of the policy as well as the political preferences of our elected representatives (Navarro, 1987).

POLICY-MAKING PROCESS

The formation of policy occurs through a process which is viewed by some as an orderly, logical method of establishing rules for large organizations as well as for government. However, for the latter, the process seems neither orderly nor logical; "messy" has been used to describe policy making in the government arena!

Through the policy process, both the wants and the needs of a population are considered, and converted into policies, rules, and regulations. The process includes all the steps for a proposal to be considered, amended, enacted, set aside, or vetoed. Although the process is complex, the steps that can be identified sound familiar to those of us who have worked with the nursing process; they are a guide to follow in planning patient care. However, the process has limitations when describing the actual decisions and activities the nurse undertakes in order to implement a plan of care. In the same way, the policy formation process, particularly as it applies to public policy, has limitations due to the concepts of conflict, politics, and scarce resources. It is the unwritten steps and the moving interaction of political origin that are more difficult to identify and quantify.

The four steps of the policy-formation process include problem formation, issue adoption, implementation, and evaluation (Table 21–2). When a need of an individual or a group of people is articulated and brought to the attention of an elected official, the first step of problem formation is introduced. An example is the lack of ability to care for an aging parent or pre-school child because everyone in the family setting is working

TABLE 21–2. THE POLICY FORMATION PROCESS

PROBLEM FORMATION
Awareness of need
Recognition of significance
Gains broad public support

ISSUE ADOPTION
Meets test of saliency
Prioritized by public's readiness

IMPLEMENTATION
Refining and interpreting language
Establish rules and regulations

EVALUATIONS
Revisiting the policy outcomes
Gathering feed back from constituents
Re-identification of need

full time. Within the first step, in order for any issue to gain sufficient status to be placed on a policy-making agenda, it must meet certain criteria; for example, the issue's relevance and feasibility must be determined by the policy makers (Anderson, 1984). The issue must be considered with respect to its degree of shared public concern so that it can be prioritized according to the urgency of the need as well as the degree of support it can be expected to receive. If the problem is relevant to the larger population and less of a focus for special groups of the polity, this will provide a greater assurance that the issue will gain a place on the policy-making agenda. An issue is relevant if it has an impact on one's life or work or family and can possibly ease a stressful situation. This criteria also can be applied to the family leave issue.

The feasibility of a problem is the potential for this issue to become a policy; the elected officials use their expertise for considering the availability of resources, colleague support, and a thorough understanding of the problem to move the issue to agenda status. Knowledgable constituents can provide a strong support by serving as expert informants to the legislators framing potential policy during this phase of problem development (Anderson, 1984; Kalisch & Kalisch, 1982). One can see that (1) the availability of resources and having a large population concerned with turning the issue into a law could be key factors in assuring that a particular issue would be placed on the agenda. If all these criteria are favorably disposed, the first step of the process is completed.

The second step, issue adoption, includes the formal and the informal list of issues that come forward from the people, organizations, and elected officials (Lindblom, 1980). In the public policy arena, this process is well delineated as a formal process in the Congress of the United States. The informal list of issues (grassroots issues) that evolve from the expressed needs of the people travel a less clear-cut adoption process. Each issue, regardless of its origin, undergoes a test of salience with regard to widespread interest, the shared public concern or commonly perceived need by the general population; that is, the issue is not a focused or parochial need of one segment of a geographic region. For example, the policy of family leave does share broad public concern in that childbearing families, families with members suffering from chronic or terminal illness, and families with aging parents can all identify with this need. Opposition may be raised by employers who must continue to operate without a valued employee, insurance carriers who may have to reimburse an organization for lost time, and others who may perceive this policy as limiting their business rights. The commonly perceived need is then measured on a scale of public readiness that consensus can be reached when negotiation ensues. The issue is given prioritization, or ranking on the agenda, and this will reflect the urgency of the need for the policy to be enacted as well as the sum of support and shared value by the polity. The adoption of an issue is affected by the art of the elected officials to negotiate and collaborate, while recognizing their own goals, values, stakes, and stands (Goodyear & Hautman, 1989). Once the issue has been adopted, the formalized steps of enactment lie ahead.

The third step in the policy-making process, implementation, is when the formulated policy is turned over to an administrative agency with the purpose of refining and interpreting policy language and turning it into rules and regulations. This phase is perhaps the most misunderstood and underutilized part of the formal policy-making process in terms of influencing outcome. Each individual, as a citizen of this country, has the right to provide input into the language of every policy during its regulatory process. The people within the agencies doing the interpretation, articulation, and listing of rules in their order of importance are not the elected officials, but life-long bureaucrats, with an expertise in government and the authoring of policy (Nichols, 1989). Nonetheless, the potential for individual input into this part of the policy-making process exist, and we can influence the regulators as they turn the policy into fair and workable rules.

The last step of the process, evaluation, is also called oversight or review. This retrospective step assesses the success of the implementation of a policy. Policy making, as Lindblom (1980) has noted, is an incremental process. The milieu needed for change for a specific issue depends on environmental factors, including the state of the economy, specific health problems, the type of leadership, and world conditions of peace or turmoil for the people who will be affected by the change. Collaboration between the elected officials and the regulatory personnel must be present, and feedback from constituents and agencies will help provide the data for altering or leaving a policy as originally formulated. Questions that guide the personnel evaluating the policy include (1) What was the relevancy of the policy to a given population? (2) Did it address the intended need? (3) Did the intended change come about? With these answers in hand, the decision for change is addressed and the process of issue identification can begin again. This is a vivid demonstration that policy formation is a dynamic process. It must be recognized, however, that people are generally unwilling to make major changes all at one time; historically change evolves slowly and new rules must be tested over time before acceptance is achieved (Anderson, 1984; Kalisch & Kalisch 1982; Litman & Robins, 1991).

NURSES' ROLE IN POLICY MAKING

The breadth of policy making at the national level may seem remote for nurses but political campaigns have demonstrated that it is as close as a 1-800 number. Being a family advocate by fostering the advancement of those health policies which could improve family conditions is a challenge that can be undertaken by nurses (Abdellah, 1991). Nurses hold qualities and characteristics of policy makers that few other professionals possess: a knowledge of family theory, the value of preventive care, inclusion of patient education for the individual and family, and the understanding of the needs of the terminally ill and their significant others. The continuous exposure of nurses to patients and their families in inpatient, outpatient, and home environments allows them to gain insight into the strengths, problems, and special needs of the family.

If nurses are to be family advocates in the health care arena they must be *involved*; that is, they must make a commitment to become knowledgeable about the needs and wants of the families that they encounter every day in their work, such as a group with special needs or families with general problems requiring an improved health status. Therefore, this commitment will include knowing the issues and how to access and use the policy-making process. Other characteristics are commitment to an ideal of quality health care; having access to a colleague network; and having expert, referent, and informational power. Referent power is the strength that emanates from being identified with a person or role that commands respect. Nursing draws respect from both families and policy makers and therefore is a holder of referent power. This power, coupled with the nurse's ability to communicate with families as well as legislators who are official policy makers, provide the nurse with an armada of resources necessary to implement the role of a family policy advocate (Del Bueno, 1987; Kalisch & Kalisch, 1982).

Any nurse who is both professionally committed and involved in nursing organizations that address the ideals of practice and advancement has taken the first step to becoming an advocate. As a member of an organization, the nurse is assured of support from colleagues who speak with a shared voice, and who have a good chance of being recognized by official policy makers. This approach is often referred to as "interest group politics" and has been commonly used in the field of nursing (Lindblom, 1980; Mason & Talbott, 1985). The professional organization often has formalized its commitment to quality health care through its position statements, which can become the basis for shaping family policy needs (ANA, 1991).

Nurses often overlook, and some even deny, that they have expert and informational power. Nursing education currently teaches theories of family growth and development (Abdellah, 1991; Kalisch & Kalisch, 1982; Lindeman, 1980). The nurse can be the communicator, caregiver, and advocate for the family within the health care system, social system, and often within the community. The expansion of this role into the policy arena is a logical next step. Who can better represent or convey the needs of the family than the nurse who already considers all members of the family when providing care? This intimacy provides the nurse with the expert and informational power that a policy maker must have prior to initiating policy, and referent power is already a strong characteristic of nurses. There are some very practical ways for any nurse interested in effecting change to accomplish the role of family advocate (Bagwell & Clements, 1985).

The strategies for activating the dimensions of advocacy include the following

- Use public relations with nonnursing groups
- Collaborate with interdisciplinary groups
- Educate colleagues about the political process
- Educate nonnurses about family issues
- Learn the negotiation process
- Work in the campaign of elected officials
- Work in the political party of your choice
- Be a delegate and attend conventions

If a nurse is involved and committed, he or she has set the stage to be a family advocate for issues arising in today's policy arena, such as long-term care, family leave, access to health care, and family planning. These problems have been recognized, adopted, and prioritized and are currently being written or amended so that acceptable legislation can come forward. The point at which the nurse enters the policy-making arena as an advocate can vary, from the local level working with families to organize a support group, to meeting with policy makers as an expert in a specific area of health care delivery, to functioning at a higher level as an official policy maker and elected official. Regardless of the level, there are several important points to understand about the advocate role. The nurse must recognize (1) the presence of conflict in every issue; (2) the true issue that is being addressed; (3) the multiple players interested in the issue, both supporters and detractors; (4) the presence of one's own interests and goals for the issue as well as the areas of compromise and concession when negotiating the process; and (5) the resources that will be needed to implement the process with a constructive method for appropriation. The advocate for family change policy must realize that the redistribution of scarce resources often is synonymous with money. To have an articulate and succinct policy with the regulatory language already developed but no available resources to enact this policy is to have no policy at all. This raises the question as to whether the official policy maker did all of the necessary homework and negotiation during the adoption and implementation phases of the process. Crises will always occur when there is a monetary shortfall, and an incomplete information base will impede the process and deter the formation of policy. Knowing the action channels that are necessary to move the policy through to its fruition will enable the nurse to transform an issue into policy with minimal frustration (Goodyear & Hautman, 1989).

FUTURE HEALTH CARE ISSUES

Family trends and issues can be health related whether or not they have the term "health" in their title. For example, the issues of unemployment, access to health care, and ability to pay for health care were major topics in the 1992 United States presidential campaign. President Clinton addressed these problems and has achieved both success and failure on these issues. Unemployment dropped in all segments of the country and was at the lowest rate for many years. However, after a protracted struggle over reforming the American health care system, the legislation was defeated in the fall of 1994. During periods in American history (1935, 1945, 1965, and 1994), national health insurance has been considered by lawmakers. The ideology of the American people was not at the point of acceptance for this form of government control over the health care system, and policy promoting national health insurance

was defeated. The legislation introduced in 1993 moved away from a single control and single payer to "managed competition" through coalitions of insurance companies, but this was also defeated. The issue of coverage for the millions of uninsured has now moved to the agendas of each state instead of the national agenda (Knickman & Thorpe, 1990; Reinhardt, 1992; Inglehart, 1993).

FUTURE FAMILY POLICY ISSUES

Other issues that directly impact the American family have most recently been identified as long-term care, family planning, immunizations, and budget-cutting measures in assistance programs such as AFDC (Aid to Families with Dependent Children), nutrition programs of WIC (Women, Infants, and Children), and school lunch programs. Today adequate bills have not been drafted to satisfy the concerns of the people. It is suggested that family policies should support families in the discharge of their functions when possible, not simply to provide as their substitutes for families (UN, 1991). Easing the tensions of families created by the employment of women will require family support policies that include the maintenance of maternity leave, dependent child care at work, sick child care, nursing care for the infirm, family leave, child allowances, and flexible work schedules. The availability of birth control and abortion are unresolved issues. The reform of the welfare system, which provides few incentives for Aid to Families with Dependent Children (AFDC) recipients to work suggests the need for work programs for low-income people, quality preschool services, and the restructuring of schools to improve the education of adolescents (Marshall, 1991; Himall, 1995; Zimmerman, 1992).

Polluted air, water, and soil, pesticides, acid rain, and oil leaks are all current problems that have a health care impact. In addition, teenage pregnancy and child and elder abuse are issues with which nurses are confronted in their speciality area each day of their working life. The increased incidence of communicable diseases such as HIV, tuberculosis, hepatitis, and chlamydia all require additional funding to combat and control; nurses need to be involved in the policies related to these illnesses. Nurses also need to be involved with the transaction between family and community, and attuned to the impact of changes in members and on the family. As agents of the family, nurses need to understand that family well-being is affected by both social policies and clinicians who affect access to care and its outcomes (Meister, 1993). Whether a nurse supports the right-to-life or right-to-choose issues; the values and ideology of the individual client are inherent in that decision. As a change agent and family advocate, it is critical for each nurse to take

CHAPTER HIGHLIGHTS

Families currently are the focus of policy makers in the United States.

Implementation of public policy is a process that requires ongoing, never-ending small changes over time.

Family policy development in the United States has been slow and disjointed because of an emphasis on individualism, decentralization of government, lack of long-range planning, and a pluralistic society that precludes a clear definition of family policy.

Family policies are influenced by such trends as an increasing death rate, an increasing number of female-headed households and working women, an increase in teen pregnancy, a larger proportion of people over 65 and 85, increasing migration, a decreasing middle class while poverty increases, family domestic violence, drug abuse, homelessness, and suicide.

The policy-making process includes problem formation, issue adoption, implementation, and evaluation.

Nurses must be knowledgeable about the policy-making process and should be family advocates for policies that will significantly influence family health.

a stand and become involved in the policy-making arena to assure the quality of health in individuals, families, and communities.

REFERENCES

Abdellah, F.G. (1991). Nursings' role in the future: A case for health policy decision making. *Sigma Theta Tau International. Monograph Series 1991*: Indianapolis, IN: Sigma Theta Tau International.

American Nurses' Association (1991). *Nursings Agenda for Health Care Reform*. Kansas City, MO: Author.

Anderson, James, E. (1984). *Public-Policy Making* (3rd ed.). New York: Hall, Rinehart & Winston.

Bagwell, M., & Clements, S. (1985). *A Political Handbook for Health Professionals*. Boston: Little, Brown.

Brown, L. (Ed.) (1987). *Health Policy in Transition*. Durham, NC: Duke University Press.

Bullough, V., & Bullough, B. (1984). *History, Trends and Politics of Nursing*. Norwalk, CT: Appleton Crafts.

Del Bueno, D. (1987). How well do you use power.? *American Journal of Nursing*, 87, 1495–1498.

Diers, D. (1985). Policy and politics. In D. Mason & S. Talbott (Eds.), *Political Action Handbook for Nurses*. Reading MA: Addison-Wesley.

Etzioni, A. (1991). Healthcare rationing: A critical evaluation. Commentary. *Health Affairs* (Summer), 88–95.

Fox, D. (1986). *Health Policies, Health Politics*. Princeton, NJ: Princeton University Press.

Goodyear, R., & Hautman, M.A. (1989). Conflict resolution: Applying the political model to the RCT proposal. *Nurse Practitioner*, 14(9), 50–56.

Himali, U. (1995). The 104th Congress: A whole new ball game. *The American Nurse, 27*(2), 18.

Inglehart, J. (1993). From the editor. *Health Affairs, 12*(2), 5.

Kalisch, P., & Kalisch, B. (1982). *Politics of Nursing,* (2nd ed.) Philadelphia: J.B. Lippincott.

Kovner, A. (1990). *Health Care Delivery in the United States* (4th ed.). New York: Springer.

Lee, P., Soffell, D. & Luft, H. (1994). Cost and coverage: Pressures toward health care reform. In P.R. Lee & C.L. Estes (eds.). *The Nation's Health* (pp. 204–213). Boston: Jones & Bartlett.

Lindblom, C.E. (1968). *The Policy-Making Process*. Englewood Cliffs, NJ: Prentice-Hall.

Lindblom, C.E. (1980). *The Policy-Making Process*. Englewood Cliffs, NJ: Prentice-Hall.

Lindeman, C. (1980). Implications of social, political and economic changes for nursing and nursing organizations. *Washington State Journal of Nursing*, 52, 40–46.

Litman, T. (1991). Government and health: A sociopolitical overview. In T. Litman & L. Robins (Eds). *Health Politics and Policy* (2nd ed.). Albany, NY: Delmar.

Litman, T., & Robins, L. (Eds.). (1991). *Health Politics and Policy* (2nd ed.). Albany, NY: Delmar.

Marshall, R. (1991). *The State of Families: Losing Diection*. Milwaukee: Family Service America.

Mason, D., Talbott, S. (1985). *Political Action Handbook for Nurses*. Reading, MA: Addison-Wesley.

Meister, S.B. (1993). The family's agent. In S.L. Feetham, S.B. Meister, J.M. Bell, & C.L. Gillis (Eds.), *The Nursing of Families: Theory, Research, Education, Practice*. Newbury Park, CA: Sage.

Miller, S.M. (1990). Race in health of America, In P. Lee & C. Estes (Eds.), *The Nation's Health* (3rd ed.). Boston: Jones & Bartlett.

Navarro, B. (1987). Federal health policies in the United States: An alternative explanation. *The Millbank Quarterly*, 65(1), 81–107.

Nichols, B. (1989). Regulatory initiatives: Instruments for leadership. *Nursing Outlook*, 37(2), 62–100.

Starr, P. (1982). *The Social Transformation of American Medicine*. New York: Basic Books.

Wisensale, S.K. (1993). State and federal initiatives in family policy: Lessons from the eighties, proposal for the nineties. In T.H. Brubaker (Ed.), *Family Relations: Challenge for the Future*. Newbury Park, CA: Sage.

United Nations (1991). *1994 International Year of the Family*. Vienna, Austria: United Nations.

Zimmerman, S.L. (1992). *Family Policies and Family Well-Being: The Role of Political Culture*. Newbury Park, CA: Sage.

ADDITIONAL READINGS

Hogan, J.M. (ed.). (1995). *Initiatives for Families: Research, Policy, Practice, Education*. Minneapolis, MN: National Council on Family Relations.

Journal of Health Politics, Policy, & Law. Durham, NC: Duke University Press.

Knickman, J.R., & Thorpe, K.E. (1990). Financing for health care. In A.R. Kovner (ed.), *Health Care Delivery in the United States*. (4th ed.). New York: Springer.

Monroe, P. (1995). Family policy: A special collection. *Family Relations, 44*(1), 3–68.

Price, S., & Elliott, B. (eds.). (1993). *Vision 2010: Families and Health Care.* Minneapolis, MN: National Council on Family Relations.

Red, I., Harrington, C., & Estes, C. (1994). *Health Policy and Nursing: Crisis and Reform in the U.S. Health Care Delivery System.* Boston: Jones & Bartlett.

Reinhardt, U.E. (1991). Breaking American health policy gridlock. *Health Affairs,* 10,(2), 96.

Sidel, R. (1992). Women and children first: Toward a U.S. family policy. *American Journal of Public Health, 85*(5), 664–665.

Smith, M.D., et al. (1992). Taking the public's pulse on health system reform. *Health Affairs,* 2(11), 125.

INDEX

Note: Page numbers followed by the letter t refer to tables those in *italics* refer to figures.